BEHAVIORAL MEDICINE
The Biopsychosocial Approach

ENVIRONMENT AND HEALTH

Andrew Baum and Jerome E. Singer,
Series Editors

BEHAVIORAL MEDICINE
The Biopsychosocial Approach

Edited by

NEIL SCHNEIDERMAN, Ph.D.
Professor of Psychology,
Director of Behavioral Medicine Program
University of Miami

JACK T. TAPP, Ph.D.
Adjunct Professor of Psychology
University of Miami
Associate Professor
NOVA University Professional School of
Psychology and President,
Psychological Health Services

LAWRENCE ERLBAUM ASSOCIATES, PUBLISHERS
1985   Hillsdale, New Jersey   London

Lawrence Erlbaum Associates, Inc., Publishers
365 Broadway
Hillsdale, New Jersey 07642

Library of Congress Cataloging in Publication Data

Main entry under title:

Behavioral medicine.

    Includes index.
    1. Medicine and psychology.   2. Medicine, Psychosomatic.   I. Schneiderman,
Neil.   II. Tapp, Jack T., 1934-   . [DNLM: 1. Behavioral medicine. WE 100 B4188]
R726.5.B4258   1985   616.08   83-14105
ISBN 0-89859-292-5

Typography by Dimensional Graphics, Roselle, N.J.

Printed in the United States of America
10   9   8   7   6   5   4   3   2   1

TO Ellie, Jon, Laura, Eric,
Nathan, and Dorothy

—Neil Schneiderman

TO Judith Garnier Tapp

—Jack T. Tapp

Table of Contents

III. ASSESSMENT AND TREATMENT
IN BEHAVIORAL MEDICINE

IV. LIFE-STYLES AND HEALTH

V. BEHAVIORAL ASPECTS OF HEALTH DISORDERS

LIST OF CONTRIBUTORS

John B. Anderson, *Predoctoral Maytag Fellow, Department of Psychology, University of Miami, P.O. Box 248185, Coral Gables, Florida*

Nancy Blaney, Ph.D., *Associate Professor of Psychology, Department of Psychology, Florida International University, Miami, Florida*

Paul Blaney, Ph.D., *Department of Psychology, University of Miami, P.O. Box 248185, Coral Gables, Florida*

Bernard Brucker, Ph.D., *Assistant Professor of Orthopedics and Rehabilitation, and Psychology, Director of Biofeedback Research Laboratory and Chief of Psychology in Orthopedics and Rehabilitation, Department of Orthopedics and Rehabilitation, University of Miami School of Medicine, Miami, Florida*

C.S. Carter, Ph.D., *Associate Professor, Department of Ecology, Ethology and Evolution, Department of Psychology, University of Illinois at Urbana–Champaign, Champaign, Illinois*

Charles S. Carver, Ph.D., *Professor of Psychology, Department of Psychology, University of Miami, P.O. Box 248185, Coral Gables, Florida*

Robert S. Davidson, Ph.D., *Director, Behavioral Medicine and Automated Assessment Laboratories, Veterans Administration Medical Center, and Professor, Department of Psychology, Florida International University, Miami, Florida*

Eric L. Diamond, Ph.D., *Assistant Professor of Clinical Psychology, Department of Clinical Psychology, University of Florida Health Science Center, Gainesville, Florida*

Terence A. Gerace, Ph.D., *Assistant Professor of Epidemiology and Psychology, Division of Nutrition, Department of Epidemiology and Public Health, University of Miami School of Medicine, Miami, Florida*

Catherine J. Green, Ph.D., *Assistant Professor of Psychology and Clinical Coordinator, Department of Psychology , University of Miami, P.O. Box 248185, Coral Gables, Florida*

Daryl Greenfield, Ph.D., *Associate Professor of Psychology and Pediatrics, Department of Psychology, University of Miami, P.O. Box 248185, Coral Gables, Florida*

David Hammer, Ph.D., *Assistant Professor of Psychology, Department of Psychology, University of Miami, P.O. Box 248185, Coral Gables, Florida*

Susan Hendrick, Ph.D., *Adjunct Assistant Professor, Department of Psychology, University of Miami, P.O. Box 248185, Coral Gables, Florida*

Charlene Humphries, Ph.D., *Research Associate, Department of Psychology, University of Miami, P.O. Box 248185, Coral Gables, Florida*

Annette M. La Greca, Ph.D., *Associate Professor of Psychology and Pediatrics and Coordinator of Clinical-Child/Pediatric Training, Department of Psychology, University of Miami, P.O. Box 248185, Coral Gables, Florida*

Philip McCabe, Ph.D., *Assistant Professor of Psychology, Department of Psychology, University of Miami, P.O. Box 248185, Coral Gables, Florida*

Elbert Russell, Ph.D., *Director of Neuropsychology Laboratory, Veterans Administration Medical Center, Miami, Florida*

Neil Schneiderman, Ph.D., *Professor of Psychology and Director of Behavioral Medicine Program, Department of Psychology, University of Miami, P.O. Box 248185, Coral Gables, Florida*

David Schwartz, *Research Assistant and Department of Psychology, Biofeedback Research Program, Department of Orthopedics and Rehabilitation, University of Miami School of Medicine, Miami, Florida*

Wendy Stone, Ph.D., *Pediatric Psychologist, Private Practice, Chapel Hill, North Carolina*

Jack T. Tapp, Ph.D., *Adjunct Professor, Department of Psychology, University of Miami; Associate Professor, NOVA University Professional School of Psychology; and President, Psychological Health Services, Miami, Florida*

Ronald Vorp, Ph.D., *Predoctoral Fellow in Behavioral Medicine, Department of Psychology, University of Miami, P.O. Box 248185, Coral Gables, Florida*

Rebecca Warner, Ph.D., *Associate Professor of Psychology, Department of Psychology, University of New Hampshire, Durham, New Hampshire*

Ray Winters, Ph.D., *Professor of Psychology, Department of Psychology, University of Miami, P.O. Box 248185, Coral Gables, Florida*

FOREWORD

The application of behavioral principles to health and disease has undergone explosive growth during the past few years. This growth is reflected in the emergence of Health Psychology as a distinct specialty area within the discipline of Psychology, and in the interdisciplinary field of Behavioral Medicine, which has integrated behavioral and biomedical science knowledge with regard to health and disease.

Behavioral Medicine: The Biopsychosocial Approach represents the efforts of the two editors, Neil Schneiderman and Jack Tapp, to provide a concise overview of the field of Behavioral Medicine and the multi-system biopsychosocial foundations that represent its underpinnings. Professor Schneiderman brings to this volume the perspective of a basic research scientist who has worked extensively in the biomedical sciences; Professor Tapp brings the perspective of a clinician involved in behavioral applications to prevention, diagnosis, treatment and rehabilitation. Both are experienced in the field of Behavioral Medicine, and share a profound appreciation of the cooperative efforts necessary for interdisciplinary research and practice to succeed. The content of the chapters that make up this volume indicates that the contributing authors share convictions, passions and ideals similar to those of the editors. The result is an ecumenical document that presents a balanced overview of Behavioral Medicine from a biopsychosocial perspective.

The present volume is rooted in the development of Health Psychology and Behavioral Medicine at the University of Miami over a period of several years. Although interdisciplinary research involving faculty of the Department of Psychology and various Medical School departments has existed for more than a decade, the Department of Psychology first adopted health-related behavior as a guiding theme for all psychology doctoral programs in 1977. This theme has been highly productive. Relevant health-related coursework in several specialties including Clinical Psychology and Applied Developmental Psychology was developed, and a basic science program in Behavioral Medicine was started under the able leadership of Dr. Schneiderman. Impetus was added to the program by a training grant from the National Heart, Lung and Blood Institute awarded to him. Ongoing research grants, several in collaboration with the School of Medicine, have appreciably bolstered the health theme and provided a distinct interdisciplinary Behavioral Medicine emphasis to the department's milieu. Most recently, a Behavioral Medicine Research Building was constructed by the University to house the multiple research and training functions performed by the Behavioral Medicine program. I consider myself privileged to have served as the Chair of Psychology during this exciting period of innovation.

This volume is in a sense the most recent outcome of the Behavioral Medicine program. The book presents Behavioral Medicine successfully at different disciplinary levels—biological, psychological and social. The title *Behavioral Medicine: The Biopsychosocial Approach* is exactly on target in its intention and delivery. The mix of contributors also reflects the intention to select authors having interests in behavioral aspects of health and disease who for the most part have ties to the University of Miami's Department of Psychology and/or Behavioral Medicine program. It was felt that this approach provided a commonality of purpose sufficient to craft a fine, cohesive book. The high quality and compatibility of the chapter offerings indicate that the assumptions were accurate. I am delighted to be associated with this book and the fine scholars who have written it.

Clyde Hendrick

PREFACE

Until this century most people in the western industrialized nations died of infectious diseases. Medical research focused upon identifying the single microorganism that caused the disease and upon finding agents that could kill the microorganism without harming the diseased individual. Today most deaths in our society can be traced to disorders which in part are related to life-style and hence behavior. Cigarette smoking, an imprudent diet, psychosocial stress, and accidents associated with the excessive consumption of alcohol have all been implicated in premature mortality. Although modern medicine is still concerned with identifying and treating infectious diseases, advances in disease prevention and treatment have increasingly become dependent upon understanding how (a) multiple features of life-style interact with genetic and constitutional factors to contribute to the development of illness, and (b) changes in life-style can help prevent illness.

The great strides that have been made in medicine and public health during this century have increased our life-span, but have also brought an increase in chronic diseases. This is due both to more people surviving to an advanced age and to more people surviving illnesses that subsequently leave them impaired. In any event, the increase in chronic diseases has left many of our citizens with disorders that require behavioral management.

The gradual changes that have taken place in our perspectives of health care have led to the emergence of a field, which has come to be known as *Behavioral Medicine*. In 1978, a meeting of senior behavioral and biomedical scientists at the National Academy of Sciences defined behavioral medicine as ... "the interdisciplinary field concerned with the integration of behavioral and biomedical science knowledge and techniques relevant to health and illness and the application of this knowledge and these techniques to prevention, diagnosis, treatment and rehabilitation" (Schwartz & Weiss, 1978).

The purpose of the present volume is to provide a broad overview of this emerging field. Let us begin by examining the definition. At the outset it should be recognized that behavioral medicine is not a single discipline but an interdisciplinary enterprise. As such it requires teamwork and effective communication among such disparate disciplines as cardiology, oncology, pediatrics, epidemiology, neurology, nursing, psychology and sociology. Moreover, its multi-systems' view of health and disease requires imaginative integration of biological, behavioral and social perspectives. For this reason we have called the book *Behavioral Medicine: The Biopsychosocial Approach.*

An important aspect of the definition of behavioral medicine is that it not only encompasses prevention, diagnosis, treatment and rehabilitation, but also an integration of behavioral and biomedical science knowledge to provide new information about etiology and pathogenesis. This is extremely important, because advances in the treatment of the sick have in the long run always benefitted from a rational understanding of disease. It is our belief that advances in the field of behavioral medicine will continue to be contingent upon maintaining (a) an intimate relationship with the fundamental aspects of the scientific enterprise, and (b) two way channels of information flow between scientific research and clinical practice.

One of the major impetuses for the growth of the field of behavioral medicine has been the successful application of the learning principles governing the treatment of behavioral disorders to the treatment of organic dysfunctions. Occasionally this has fostered the naive assumption that training in behavioral medicine merely requires the transfer of behavioral principles and technology to the treatment of physical disorders. This assumption is incorrect, because the behavioral treatments of organic disorders require working within the boundary conditions set by the pathology. Often, when dealing with organic problems, a great deal is known about antecedent pathophysiological events, and this must be carefully considered in designing appropriate behavioral treatments.

At present the training of practitioners in behavioral medicine leaves room for both cautious optimism and concern. The optimism is based upon (a) development of *health psychology* as an important subarea in the discipline of psychology, (b) introduction of behavioral science instruction into medical school curricula, (c) incorporation of behavioral medicine training into some medical residency programs, (d) creation of clinical psychology internships emphasizing behavioral medicine and postdoctoral training opportunities in behavioral medicine for behavioral and biomedical scientists, and (e) increases in the number of qualified behavioral scientists available for teaching, research and service in health care settings. Concern is expressed because the training of clinicians has not emphasized as strongly as it should the importance of instruction in (a) behavioral contributions to the mechanisms of disease (i.e., pathophysiology), and (b) the biobehavioral and psychosocial foundations of behavioral medicine.

The major objectives of the present volume are to provide the reader with an overview of the field of behavioral medicine and an appreciation of the multisystems biopsychosocial approach that provides its underpinning. As such, it is intended neither as a "how-to-do-it" type volume nor as an encyclopedia. The volume begins with an introductory orientation chapter, followed by sections on (a) basic perspectives, (b) general approaches to assessment and treatment, (c) life-styles and health, and (d) health disorders.

In general, the earlier chapters in this book are designed to provide the tools for better understanding later ones. Thus, for example, the chapter on the neurologic bases of behavior sets the stage for subsequent chapters on the psychophysiology of stress and on neuropsychological assessment, and the chapters on behavioral epidemiology and the psychophysiology of stress are intended to lay the groundwork for later chapters such as the one on biobehavioral aspects of cardiovascular disorders. Similarly, issues such as compliance/adherence and psychosocial interactions run as continuous threads throughout the volume. Thus, while this is an edited book, the intent has been to provide a view of behavioral medicine as an integrated biopsychosocial approach from a variety of perspectives.

REFERENCES

Schwartz, G. E., & Weiss, S. M. Behavioral medicine revisited: An amended definition. *Journal of Behavioral Medicine*, 1978, *1*, 249 – 251.

ACKNOWLEDGMENTS

The editors and authors would like to acknowledge and thank the many students who read drafts of our manuscripts and suggested improvements. We would also like to thank the administrative and secretarial staff of the Department of Psychology who helped with this project. These included Alice Knight, Beryl Murray, Sally Miller, Veronica Murphy, Rebecca White, Linda Cahan, and Dr. Shelley Slapion. Our thanks are due also to Dr. A. Rod Wellens, Associate Chairperson, who helped coordinate these efforts. Most especially, however, we would like to gratefully acknowledge the contribution of Sandra Racoobian. Mrs. Racoobian's dedication to the quality of the work, attention to detail, and personal commitment to perfection were accompanied by the grace, charm, and goodness of spirit that made the project pleasurable.

The editors would like also to acknowledge the National Heart, Lung, and Blood Institute, whose award of training grant HL07426, "Behavioral Medicine Research in Cardiovascular Disease," served as the catalyst for this volume.

INTRODUCTION

1 The Multisystems View of Health and Disease

Jack T. Tapp
University of Miami and Nova University

Rebecca Warner
University of New Hampshire

INTRODUCTION

The health care system is in the midst of a change in perspective. The past 60 years have produced extensive scientific research on understanding the biological basis of disease, yet with increasing prevalence there is recognition that the traditional biomedical model is limited in its scope. As a result, a search for a new model has begun, which emphasizes the health of the total individual as the appropriate subject of research and health care delivery. This shifting viewpoint reflects an alteration of the perspective in health and disease similar to the scientific revolutions outlined by Kuhn (1970). The accompanying paradigm shift has put individual behavior as one focus of health care both as antecedent to the attainment of health and as a consequent to the effects of disease. As a result, social scientists have become involved in research on the pathogenesis, etiology, diagnosis, treatment, rehabilitation and prevention of disease.

The scientific study of psychosocial factors in disease is in relative infancy. It does not yet offer the amount of quantitative or objective information that has accumulated with the biomedical sciences. Yet it is evolving as a research discipline of considerable importance, as becomes apparent from the chapters in this book. Behavioral medicine has an important role to play in this evolving zeitgeist. Furthermore the biopsychosocial model provides a means for conceptually integrating the diverse perspectives of this field into a comprehensive viewpoint.

CHANGING PERSPECTIVES ON DISEASE

A variety of historical factors have contributed to the evolving holistic perspective on health and disease. As with all historical changes, no single factor seems

1

primary; rather, diverse historical forces seem to be at work to effect the demand for change.

Disease Incidence

Examination of data from the United States Statistical Abstracts on incidence of selected reportable diseases and causes of death shows that major changes have occurred during the past 50 years. Coe (1978) suggests a useful distinction between acute/communicable disorders (diphtheria, malaria, measles, mumps, poliomyelitis, smallpox, typhoid, etc.) and chronic/degenerative disorders (diabetes, hypertension, arthritis, etc.). The communicable diseases have shown great declines in the number of cases. Communicable diseases no longer rank high among causes of death in the United States. In fact, as of 1976, about 70% of all deaths were due to cardiovascular diseases and malignancies (Statistical Abstracts, 1978, Table No. 108). The control of the communicable diseases was due in part to the successes of the biomedical model. Discoveries of disease-causing microorganisms by Koch, Pasteur, and others paved the way for development of vaccines and antibiotics. Improved sanitation also helps to control communicable diseases (Coe, 1978).

While the incidence for many communicable disorders has been falling, the number of persons with chronic activity limitations due to heart conditions, arthritis, hypertension, and other chronic disorders has been increasing (from 23.2 million in 1969 to 30.2 million in 1976; Statistical Abstracts, 1978, Table No. 187). Chronic disorders have replaced communicable disorders as the leading causes of death. For chronic/degenerative disorders, the biomedical model has been less successful in finding causes and cures. Thus, although it is still true that the vast majority of illnesses seen by general practitioners are minor, self-limiting gastro-intestinal or respiratory disorders (Rogers, 1977), there has been a change in the types of serious disorders that physicians are called upon to deal with—away from acute communicable diseases toward chronic degenerative disorders.

This shift in disease pattern toward chronic disorders has raised several problems. First, efforts to isolate a single biological pathogen as a cause for each chronic disorder (in line with the assumptions of the traditional biomedical model) have so far been largely unsuccessful. As a consequence, basic assumptions of the biomedical model are being challenged and reexamined.

Second, different treatment and prevention strategies are called for in dealing with chronic disorders. Infectious diseases and physical injuries can be dealt with by means of drugs or surgery that require little active cooperation from the patient. However, the measures that are typically prescribed for prevention or treatment of chronic diseases include changes in life-style. Compliance with such recommendations is typically poor (Sackett & Haynes, 1976).

As a result of these changes, Engel (1977) has proposed that we need a new multifactorial view of etiology that includes social and psychological factors as precursors of physical disorders. The factors included in the biopsychosocial model would supplement our understanding of specific biological agents in the etiology of disease. Such a model would recognize that social stress and personality styles of coping may either directly produce wear and tear on the organism, or they may affect the host's susceptibility to disease-causing biological pathogens, or both.

Drews (1980) has pointed to the importance of biobehavioral factors in the scientific study of the disease process. He points out the need for the behavioral factors to be "studied objectively and quantitatively so that the information will be compatible with traditional pathophysiology [p. 6]."

Specialization

Another frequently noted trend in medicine is that the proportion of physicians in specialties has been increasing, with a corresponding drop in the proportion of general practitioners. Roughly 64% of physicians were general practitioners in 1949; by 1973 this had dropped to 24% (Rogers, 1977). Sophisticated biomedical technology is partly responsible for the pressures toward specialization; physicians can more easily stay abreast of new technical developments if they specialize, and expensive, specialized equipment requires highly trained specialized personnel to operate and utilize. Undoubtedly biomedical technology has led to great improvements in the technical aspects of medicine, but as Field (1971) has noted, the disappearance of the general practitioner and lack of continuity of primary care contribute an overemphasis on curing or technical aspects of medicine, to the detriment of the personal or caring aspect.

Some authors have suggested that this change has resulted in an alienation between physicians and patients, creating further problems in the quality of health care services (Illich, 1975). The need for generalists has resulted in a reexamination of medical specialties (Millis, 1966) and the creation of efforts to train primary care physicians. But this has created new sets of problems in defining the limits and scope of training in the areas of biopsychosocial interventions.

Expenditures

A third notable trend is the rapid rise in expenditures, and the increasing involvement of the government in financing health care for individuals. According to several sources (e.g., Thomas, 1977) health care expenditures now comprise approximately 10% of the gross national product, and health care costs are rising at a faster rate than the general rate of inflation. The reasons for this increase are complicated, but certainly the availability of expensive new technologies, the cost of correcting past inequities in the availability of medical services through programs designed to benefit the poor and elderly, and a high priority on health-related research by public policy makers are all critical factors.

Mechanic (1978) has described the impact of major federal funding programs such as Medicare and Medicaid and has noted that rational allocation of resources and reorganization of the medical care system could be accomplished in part by placing restrictions on the use of these funds. Political scientists and economists specializing in the health care sector provide valuable input into government policy decisions both by providing descriptions of the existing system and by predicting probable outcomes of various alternative courses of action. The contributions of these two disciplines are briefly discussed by Adler and Stone (1979).

Medicalization

Fox (1977) has noted a tendency toward reclassification of problems such as drug addiction, alcoholism, schizophrenia, hyperactivity, and criminal behavior as illnesses. Historically these conditions were generally regarded as indications of weakness or immorality. Mechanic (1978) discussed the general sociological concept of deviance and pointed out that most deviant behaviors are labeled as either "sick" or "bad," depending on whether the sufferer is held personally responsible for his or her condition. By redefining many "bad" behaviors as sickness, many social control problems are turned over to the medical care system for solution. This reclassification has resulted in attempts to use the biomedical model to search for a biological basis for other forms of deviant behavior: for example, the claim that an XYY chromosome abnormality leads to criminal propensities.

Though the appropriateness of the biomedical model for mental illness and other forms of deviance has been challenged (Szasz, 1961), the fact remains that this reclassification brings new disorders within the domain of the medical care system. Hyperactivity, once viewed as a classroom discipline problem, is frequently treated with medication. Like the chronic degenerative disorders, many of the recently reclassified problems such as alcoholism and drug abuse have not yielded successfully to a purely biomedical approach. Behavior management, attitude change and social system interventions are needed, placing additional demands for these types of services on the medical care system. Consequently new roles for behavioral management personnel have arisen, both as direct patient care providers, and as researchers examining the etiology and treatment/prevention techniques that are appropriate for "medical" problems.

Prevention and Health Focus

Popular cultural changes have their impact on health care delivery. The period of the recent past witnessed an increased focus on the health value of preventive activities such as diet changes, exercise, decreased smoking, food and alcohol consumption. This has had an impact on health care in Western culture that is yet to be fully evaluated. It reflects a shift in attitude toward self-care and health, with a focus on individual behaviors as a means to the achievement of health.

This cultural change has been strongly influenced by biomedical research on health and the factors that contribute to chronic disease. Much of the material in this text reviews data that have produced this view and has pointed to the relationships between health practices and chronic diseases.

Summary

For a variety of historical reasons there has been a demand for change in the traditional health care delivery model, including a change in perspective on disease. The increasing involvement of biomedicine with the social sciences has produced a melding of the viewpoints of these disciplines with a concomitant search for alternative models to replace the traditional biomedical view.

THE HOLISTIC PHILOSOPHY

The mechanistic-reductionistic view of man has dominated inquiry into the nature of disease and its impact on the human condition. The search for an "ultimate cause" has reflected a search for the explanation of disease at the lowest and simplest possible level. The biochemical hypothesis of affective disorders is a classic example of this process and its basis in historical thinking.

Greek physicians believed that the liver purged food of its toxic humors including black bile. If the liver malfunctioned and black bile built up in the body, melancholia resulted. In contemporary theory, black bile has been replaced by neural transmitters such as the catecholamines and serotonin. The brain, rather than the liver, is the organ within which these humors exert their action.

The contemporary view is more sophisticated and considers a broader range of evidence in the explanation; nonetheless it focuses on a chemical imbalance within the body's functioning nervous system and implies that this malfunction is the "cause" of the disease. Biomedical treatment strategies designed to cure depression focus on alterations of the chemical imbalance via psychopharmacological interventions. As a result, antidepressant medications are among the most widely used drugs in contemporary medicine.

This "single-cause" view is obviously limited. Depression is not solely a biochemical disorder. The behavior of depressed people has notable characteristics that impact on other physiological symptoms and the social environment within which they function. Depression is a complex disease with broad ramifications for intervention strategies that extend beyond taking a pill.

Contemporary theories of disease are thus shifting from the reductionistic, single-cause point of view to a holistic perspective. Stress is now viewed as a major source of distress that contributes significantly to the manifestations of those diseases that lead the list in modern Western society.

This alteration in the perception of disease has dictated a change in the basic assumptions that underlie the examination and treatment of disease. This change in viewpoint reflects a paradigmatic shift. In this section we outline some of the philosophical tenets of this paradigm and discuss their implications for theory development in behavioral medicine.

Philosophical Fundamentals

All theories and research rest on a set of basic assumptions that define a view of the universe. Science, in other words, is built on a philosophy that defines: (1) the nature of reality (metaphysics); (2) how we know about that reality (epistemology); and (3) what accounts for change and stability in that reality (the means of explanation).

All sciences, including the medical sciences, have made advances over the last 100 years because they have adopted a mechanistic view of reality. The world, according to this view, is made up of objectifiable matter-energy and space-time phenomena. Truth resides in the world of this reality and can be known by empirical methods. The experimental method in which the world is altered and the consequent results are measured is the means for understanding this reality. The mechanical forces of the universe play themselves out in a totally determined manner moved by energy that is temporal, linear, and dimensional.

Behavioral medicine and the multisystems perspective reflect a partial shift in these basic assumptions to a paradigm that has been labeled "holistic." According to this view, the world is seen from a hierarchial perspective within which matter, energy, space, time, life, and nonlife are transformations within the same ordered unity. The metaphysics of the holistic paradigm is thus monistic, stressing the unity of the phenomena of the universe.

For the holistic paradigm, truth is to be found in the interaction between the knower and the external world and involves both inner experience and external verification. To obtain verification one creates a model of the phenomenon to be explained and attempts to determine if the properties of the model match the properties of the phenomenon. The model serves as the isomorphic analogy for the phenomenon to be explained and reflects the same order of complexity as the phenomenon rather than making reference to a lower-order mechanistic force.

Understanding stability and change within the holistic paradigm necessitates an understanding of general systems theory. In brief, stability reflects the mainte-nance of the *form* of a system; change is the transformation of a system resulting in the reorganization of a set of mutually dependent probabilistic variables. The particulars of the holistic paradigm are summarized in more detail in an excellent paper by Battista (1977). Many of the ideas presented here are derived from that work.

General Systems Theory in Brief

General systems theory is a set of knowledge about the nature and dynamics of systems. It conceives of the universe as a system comprised of hierarchial subsystems, each composed of its particular set of interdependent variables. A system is an abstract concept made up of the concrete elements that are capable of taking on different characteristics over time. These elements are the system variables. The form of the system at any point in time is reflected in the particular characteristics of the system variables. The state of the variable and the state of their interaction reflects a stop-action view that defines the form of the system at a particular point in time.

The formal aspects of a system are reflected in the rules that functionally define the relationship between system variables. These rules define the organization of the system and are known as its structure. Understanding a system necessitates a knowledge of both its properties and its structures.

System Properties. There are six identifiable properties that are characteristic to any system. These are: wholeness, hierarchical organization, interdependence, activity, self-maintenance, and self-transformation. For any system these properties exist and make up the unity of the total system.

Wholeness reflects the inherent organization of a system and is made up of the definition of the boundaries of the system (what it is not) and the state of its component variables. A system exists as an entity in its own state and is greater than the sum of its parts.

Hierarchical organization asserts that any system is both a part of a more encompassing and comprehensive system and the synthesis of component subsystems. Thus any system can be identified in terms of its particular level of complexity. The human body, for example, consists of the synthesis of seven levels: elementary particles, atoms, compounds, molecules, cells, organs, and the physical body. Each subsumes the preceding and all are implicit in the body's hierarchy of organization.

Structural analysis combines wholeness with hierarchical organization. Because systems exist in their own right as the synthesis of their parts, any given system can be understood structurally by analyzing the way its parts are coordinated. Reductionistic analysis is not necessary, as each part of any system in the hierarchy is the synthesis of its parts.

Interdependence exists within any system in such a manner that altering the state of any variable within the system alters the state of all the variables within a given hierarchical level. Interdependence is essential for the definition of a system because it identifies the functional organization properties of the system. Without this relationship among elements an organization is not a system. By implication the state of each variable is partially determined by the state of every other variable within the system via feedback loops.

Activity is a property of systems that emphasizes the process of transformations that constitute the continual interaction among system elements. Systems are neither static nor reactive. The feedback loops that interrelate system elements insure activity as a constant condition of the system within and between hierarchies.

Self-maintenance refers to the ability of systems to maintain their form and properties over prolonged periods of time and through a great number of influences from the environment surrounding the system.

Self-transformation refers to the capacity of systems to transform their properties, including their form and structure, over time. Such changes can occur at the same or at higher or lower hierarchical levels. Alterations in the structure of systems thus become an essential component to system survival.

Self-transformation leading to hierarchical reorganization has two characteristics that require further mention. Hierarchical reorganization requires the differentiation of elements into distinct entities along with their reintegration at a higher level. In addition, hierarchical transformation is a discrete phenomenon occurring in quantal jumps and not through a gradual linear process of change.

Given the perspective of hierarchical interrelated systems that are mutually influential and that seek to maintain wholeness, change within any given level will alter systemic balance and potentially produce disequilibrium throughout the systems.

In the classical view of systems developed by von Bertalanffy (1968), open systems are in continual interaction with the environment, bringing in elements from outside the system and transporting others out of the system. In this process the system maintains a constant ratio among the elements within the system—a steady state. Energy is brought into the system to allow the system to do the work necessary to maintain disequilibrium against the forces of entropy. The ratio of elements within the system is self-regulating such that alterations in one element of the system will be compensated for by alterations in another. The maintenance of the steady state is dependent on the ratio of constants between input and output reactions.

By this view, systems are regulated by the necessity to maintain a steady state reflecting system constancy. Alterations in constancy produce compensatory reactions of system elements to return the system to equilibrium. These transformations are effected by feedback loops within the system that test the state of particular system variables against defined, prescribed limits. If the system is outside these limits, correcting operations are initiated in which alternative feedback loops may be called into play to control the variable that is out of bounds. The new feedback system is strengthened by its capacity to restore the equilibrium within the system and terminate the motivating properties associated with disequilibrium.

The importance of these self-maintenance activities lies in the explanatory power they offer to changing the structure of the system. Overlapping and alternative feedback loops allow the system to transform itself (i.e., to learn, within any given level of the hierarchy).

It is particularly important to be able to account for change across levels of the hierarchy. Because all systems are part of the whole, the imbalance within any level will reflect itself in the imbalance across the hierarchy. Thus change that alters the functional and/or structural properties of a system at any given level will produce consequent changes throughout the hierarchy to accommodate to the demand for self-regulation.

Though this perspective is implicitly valid to general systems theory and follows as a logical consequence of the theory organization, it lacks sufficient detail to provide one with a satisfactory understanding of how such cross-hierarchical transformations might occur. This reflects a contemporary limitation of the development of the metatheory.

Battista (1977) has suggested that structuralism such as that outlined by Piaget (1970) might provide the method of systems analysis that would be responsive to the need for cross-hierarchy transformations. Structures are conceived as open and evolving processes reflecting an integrated system of transformations that is self-regulating. They are hierarchically ordered such that each level encompasses all the levels below it. They are interrelated by form and content. The form of one level constitutes the content of the next level in the hierarchy. Alterations in the structural form of one level of the hierarchy that occurs as the result of the self-regulatory accommodation to the demands of the environment would produce changes in the content of the next level and produce demand for changes in structure. Changes in one level of the hierarchy will emerge as changes in the elements of the next level of the hierarchy. This process has been elaborated in an excellent article by Carver & Scheier (1982).

Control Systems.   The concept of homeostasis is used to express the maintenance of a constant internal environment. To maintain this steady state, the human organism has thousands of interrelated control mechanisms. Imbalance in one control system can produce imbalance in others and cause wide-spread disequilibrium. Some of these systems are discussed throughout the remainder of this book.

Most control systems operate on the basis of negative feedback. It is to be assumed that within every system there is an internal sensing device whose function is to monitor the state of the internal environment. When deviations occur outside the range of "normal" the control mechanism is initiated. The detector system continues to test the state of the environment and when balance is restored the control mechanism is shut off.

This simplified model has been elaborated by Miller, Galanter and Pribram (1960) as the TOTE system, an acronym for Test, Operate, Test, Exit. O'Kelly (1963) put the model into a biological perspective by elaborating the motivational properties that are associated with such a system. Carver and Scheier (1982) have elaborated a hierarchical view of control systems that has direct relevance to human behavior in a variety of applications. Leventhal and his colleagues have applied a control systems model to symptom appraisal (Leventhal, Nerenz, & Straus, 1980).

The control of a system can be presented schematically as shown in Fig. 1.1. This is a simple control mechanism, but even in this simplicity there are several

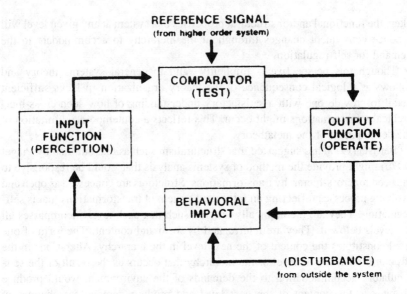

FIG. 1.1. Feedback Control System

potential alterations that could occur within the system to produce a malfunction in the maintenance of the steady state. Within this simple system there are many error sources: an inability to sense the existence of an abnormal value by the detector; failure or inaccuracy in transmitting information about abnormal values; comparator reading malfunctions; incorrect stored values of normal; failure in the initiation or operation of the correcting response; to name a few. When systems become more complex, they compound the errors and the difficulties in detecting their source.

Control systems are not always stable in their performance. Corrections can often produce oscillation in response as the system attempts to correct itself. In an unstable system there is little inertia in the systems response—a property called *damping*. Mild disruptions in system function can increase to severe disruptions. If there is a great deal of damping, oscillation tends to decrease quickly. Some systems with moderate damping properties will continue to oscillate.

Some systems reflect chronic oscillation by the nature of their organization. These are said to *reverberate*. The signal for cessation in one part of the system becomes a signal for initiating a response in another part of the system. These cybernetic-information models provide the means for measuring and analyzing the characteristics by which the system performs.

From the multisystem perspective, the models provide a means for analyzing and understanding the controls that operate within any level of a hierarchy. The elements of a system are definable in terms of the units of the control mechanism. The properties of the system are defined in terms of the interaction among elements.

Scientific investigation of phenomena from the biopsychosocial perspective ultimately necessitates the integration of the interactions among systems and their elements at different levels of the hierarchy. The methods of observation and the establishment of scientific "proof" via probabilistic models applies in the operations of the system at any given level of discourse. Quantitative measurements, and the objective gathering of data with appropriate controls form the basis of the study of the phenomena and allow assertions to be made about the elements of the system and their interactions. These models of investigation apply for any source of data whether they be chemical, physiological, behavioral, or familial.

The capacity to study interactions scientifically across systems is lacking. These interactions may require different mathematical-statistical models such as those embodied in multivariate correlational techniques. Causal inference may demand extending these models (e.g., pattern analysis), the use of quasi-experimental designs at several levels, or the development of new models that account for systemic transformations (e.g., catastrophe theory; Thom, 1975).

ILLNESS AND HEALTH FROM A MULTISYSTEMS PERSPECTIVE

It follows from the foregoing discussion that the state of health represents a relative balance within which all systems are simultaneously in harmony. There is some consensus in the literature that such a state of affairs does reflect the abstract meaning of health. The World Health Organization has defined health as a "state of complete physical, mental and social well-being."

In a more concrete sense, the state of health is difficult to define. Davies (1975) has suggested that there are five features of health that need to be assessed separately: (1) physical health defined by objective means that may or may not be associated with symptoms; (2) presence or absence of reportable symptoms; (3) the functional capacity of the individual; (4) emotional and mental status; (5) the subjective state of well-being. In effect each of these categories provides a test of systemic integrity, though from different vantage points or different hierarchical levels. In what follows, we examine the meaning of health from these multiple perspectives with the idea of developing a multisystems view of health. It is our assumption that behavioral medicine must address the issues of defining health from this perspective and must work towards a meaningful definition of health as the endpoint of treatment.

Biological Basis of Health and Disease

The physiological sciences have addressed the definition of health from the perspective of physiological systems. For almost every physical parameter of bodily function, constants have been identified that define the range of health—or "normal" functioning. These are *signs* of dysfunction and they can be measured by objective, quantifiable means. Some of the values that are frequently used in physical diagnosis are summarized in Table 1.1. These are physical constants of the operations of chemical and cellular systems within the human body. They reflect the simultaneous operation of different systems. Deviations from normal are signs of potential disorders in the functions of the body. However, deviations are not conclusive indicators of which system(s) is dysfunctional nor do normal values reflect the absence of disease. They are partial indicators of abnormality. When taken together, the pattern of values is used to reflect deviations from health and to pinpoint systemic involvement. No single parameter is indicative of a single system dysfunction.

Blood pressure, for example, is an easily obtainable and familiar measure of bodily function. Systolic pressure in a "normal" young adult is about 120 mm of mercury; diastolic pressure is about 70 mm Hg. These are easily obtainable measures and for 50 cents they can be read on machines placed in the supermarket or the drug store. Arterial blood pressure is a measure of cardiac output times the total peripheral resistance as distributed throughout the body. This measure is therefore a reflection of both short-term and long-term reactions of the body to a variety of influences. In the short-term (1 second to 2 days) there are at least eight control mechanisms that respond to changes in blood pressure. Some of these are neural-reflexive responses designed to maintain immediate constancy of blood pressure. Others are hormonal or volume controls, designed to stabilize pressure over a longer time period. These systems influence both changes in cardiac output and total peripheral resistance. On this basis, deviations from normal ranges in blood pressure may indicate only a transitory state wherein there is no abnormality other than that related to systemic oscillation.

Health is also defined in terms of an absence of *symptoms*. According to Stedman (1972), symptoms are: the "morbid phenomena or departures from the normal in function, appearance or sensation, experienced by the patient and indicative of the disease [p. 1231]." They reflect the subjective experience of the patient in his or her assessment of deviations from normal. The absence of symptoms, however, is not exclusively indicative of health. Symptoms are not always present for many diseases. Hypertension has no reportable symptoms in most instances and the diagnosis is based primarily on a reading of arterial blood pressure. Furthermore, the individual is often an inaccurate observer of the state of symptoms. Denial, lack of awareness of body changes, acceptance of wide deviations from normal, all will render the patient's judgments about disease inaccurate.

Historically the conjoint criteria of absence of signs and symptoms has been used as the operational definition of health (World Health Organization, 1958). The annual physical has been based on this definition and allowed the examiner to pronounce good health as "the absence of any identifiable disease." This has been the basis of the movement toward prevention and programs of lifetime health monitoring (Breslow & Sommers, 1977).

TABLE 1.1
Normal Values for Common Clinical Tests
(Assumes 12-hour Fasting)

Blood, Plasma, or Serum	Normal Value	
Glucose	65 – 115	mg/dl
Urea nitrogen (BUN)	5 – 25	mg/dl
Creatinine	.7 – 1.4	mg/dl
Uric acid	2.3 – 8.1	mg/dl
Electrolytes		
Potassium	3.8 – 5.0	meg/l
Sodium	135 – 145	meg/l
Chloride	79 – 108	meg/l
CO	25 – 32	meg/l
Calcium	8.5 – 10.5	meg/l
Proteins—Total	6 – 8	g/dl
Iron	50 – 200	g/dl
Albumin	3.5 – 5.5	g/l
Globulin	2.0 – 3.5	g/dl
Lipids		
Cholesterol	150 – 300	mg/dl
Triglycerides	30 – 150	g/dl
Enzymes (Proteins)		
Lactic dehydrogenase (LDH)	100 – 225	/l
Serum glutamic oxaloacetic		
transaminase (SGOT)	0 – 40	/l
Bilitrulin	0.1 – 1.2	mg/dl
Blood Cells		
White blood cell count (WBC) X 10	4.8 – 10.8	
Red blood cell count (RBC) X 10	4.2 – 6.1	
Hemoglobin (HGB)	12 – 18	g/dl
Mean corpuscular volume (MCV)	80 – 99	
Mean corpuscular hemoglobin (MCH)	27 – 31	
Mean corpuscular hemoglobin concentration		
(MCHC)	32 – 36%	
Urine		
Calcium	150	mg/day
Catecholamines		
Epinephrine	20	g/day
Norepinephrine	100	g/day
Protein	150	mg/day
Steroids		
17-Ketosteroids	4 – 26	mg/day
17-Hydroxysteroids	3 – 8	mg/day

Functional Illness and Health

The perspective on health just described is limited in one major respect; it fails to
consider the functional capacity of the individual. The assertion that an individual

has a disease based on the presence or absence of signs and symptoms makes no allowance for the capacity to perform. This criterion becomes an important consideration in defining the health of an individual who has a chronic disease or a physical or mental disability.

The introduction of functional criteria into the assessment of health expands the operational criteria for defining health status to include optimal health for a particular individual and risk for disease at some future point in time. More importantly, the introduction of functional criteria into the definition of health expands the concept of health (and disease) into a psychosocial sphere that extends well beyond bodily limitations. It therefore gives endorsement to behavioral criteria of health based on the individual's capacity to perform relative to a standard. It shifts the conceptual definition of illness from a conjoint presentation of signs and symptoms to an inability to perform at the functional level that defines health. The disability that accompanies disease (as the antithesis of health) becomes operationally defined in terms of limitations in performance.

These considerations are exemplified in definitions of impairment. According to the American Medical Association (1971): "Impairment is a medical condition defined as an anatomic or functional loss occurring after medical rehabilitation which is stable or non-progressive over time." A disability occurs as the result of an impairment when the "actual or presumed activity is reduced or absent [p. 47]."

An evaluation of an impairment reflects an appraisal of the nature and extent of illness or injury as it affects personal efficiency in the activities of daily living (i.e., self-care, communication, normal living postures, ambulation, elevation, traveling, and nonspecific hand activities). An impairment is evaluated in terms of the function of specific organ systems but its impact is assessed in terms of its effect on the "whole person."

In the evaluation of an impairment, it is recognized that the physiological systems of the body have an identifiable set of functions that can be measured quantitatively or evaluated by some combination of measurements and impressions. For example, a dysfunction in the knee is measured against a criteria of 150 degrees of flexion-extension in the joint in a lying and sitting position. Amputation of the limbs at the knee is a 90% impairment of the lower extremity. It is a 36% impairment of the whole person. A 50-degree active flexion as the maximal range of flexion of the knee is a 35% impairment of the lower extremity; a 5% impairment of the whole person.

Evaluating a permanent impairment of a cardiovascular disease is considerably more subject to impression and judgment than assessing the percentage of impairment of a lower extremity. A permanent impairment is described as that "condition which persists after medical and surgical therapies and rehabilitation and after a period has elapsed to permit collateral circulation and other adjustments of nature after an acute insult" (AMA, 1971). Impairment due to heart disease is rated on a 1 to 4 scale of classification that incorporates multiple criteria of functioning. Level 2 is defined as resulting in 20% to 45% impairment. For this level, there is "organic heart disease but without symptoms at rest; walking freely on level ground or climbing at least one flight of stairs and the performance of usual activities doesn't produce symptoms; prolonged exertion, emotional stress, hurrying, hill climbing, recreation, or similar activities produce symptoms; signs of congestive heart failure are not present."

It is clear from these considerations that functional impairments and their assessment are tied to a set of criteria that reflect organ system functioning against a variety of diverse behavioral events. The inclusion of rehabilitation, efficiency in living, and the concept of the "whole person" expands the evaluation of disability into areas of behavioral capacity. "The evaluation of a permanent disability is an appraisal of the patient's present and future ability to engage in gainful activity as it is affected by such diverse factors as age, sex, education, economic and social environment, in addition to the definite medical factor-permanent impairment [AMA, 1971]."

It is recognized that the evaluation of a disability is an administrative decision reflecting the patient's entitlement. For the purposes of this discussion the criteria are definitely the result of social-psychological considerations that transcend the presence of signs and symptoms. In this context, disability reflects a social judgment based on an idiosyncratic criteria of performance. The evaluation of disability extends the criteria for illness and health in three critical dimensions: (1) relative health is defined in functional terms; (2) health is reflected in the behavior of the individual; and (3) health is defined in terms of social functioning against standards set by society.

Illness Behavior.   From the foregoing considerations, illness can be viewed as a complex set of biological, psychological, and social events that put the individual outside the boundaries of "normal." There is often a fine line between labeling an individual as "sick" versus "bad." Goffman's (1963) notion of stigma is a valuable concept in relation to illness. He described how visible physical deformity can inspire reactions of pity, revulsion, and curiosity in observers. This often means that a person with a medical problem such as blindness or paralysis is frequently faced with a social problem in that other persons react to him or her in an unnatural way. Being labeled as "sick" can thus decrease an individual's feelings of attractiveness and social worth. Furthermore, there is a tendency to blame victims for their misfortunes, as Lerner and Simmons (1966) have shown. To retain a belief in a just and orderly world where people have control over their outcomes, there is a tendency to assume that people who are sick or injured have done something to bring about misfortune (Janis & Rodin, 1979). The sick person often blames himself or herself for the disease. Sontag (1978) has argued that cancer carries strong social stigma. Thus, illness labels can have dramatic effects on the emotions, behaviors, and social experiences of individuals.

The social context of illness and its associated behaviors has some potential benefits for the ill person. Parsons (1951) has outlined these in his analysis of the sick role. According to his view, when an individual becomes ill, he or she adopts a social role that carries with it an altered set of norms that are advantageous. Specifically, the sick person is exempt from normal social responsibilities, has the obligation to want to get well, and the obligation to seek technically competent medical care and to cooperate in the process of getting well. Clearly there are situations where exemption from normal responsibilities is attractive; a soldier facing combat or a child facing a day in school may seek to adopt the sick role as a way out of a threatening situation. Furthermore, the physician may be viewed as a source of attention, comfort, and help when a person is overcome by problems with living; many of the "worried well" who consult a physician with concern about their health may be trying to adopt the sick role as a means of obtaining emotional reassurance.

The sick role concept has been criticized on the grounds that it does not apply to many disorders—particularly chronic disorders for which there is no hope of recovery, and illnesses that are unpleasant or painful but that do not interfere with the ability to carry out normal responsibilities. Much research has been done on the impact of illness on the individual's ability to carry out responsibilities to the family (Croog & Levine, 1977), the willingness of health care professionals or social workers to extend the sick role to other groups such as alcoholics (Chalfant & Kurtz, 1971), and other aspects of the sick role.

More recent work has turned to an analysis of the behavior patterns associated with illness (Kasl & Cobb, 1966). This work acknowledges that illness carries with it expectations that define the parameters of behavior of the ill person. This behavior is culturally learned and reflects norms that define the "approved" ways of manifesting illness (Kleinman, Eisenberg, & Good, 1978). The particular expressions of these behaviors will depend on a variety of factors.

The Fabrega (1974) 9-step model outlines the expectations that make up an illness behavior pattern. (1) Recognition and labeling defines the existence of disease based on internal or external information (symptoms or signs). This initiates illness behavior depending on (2) the perceived disvalue of the illness (e.g., how much it disrupts "normal" functioning for the patient). (3) Treatment plans are developed and (4) assessed to determine the probability that they will alter the disvalue of the illness. (5) Treatment costs are assessed relative to (6) their benefits, and (7) a utility estimate is made of the net benefit of the cost relative to the gains from treatment. A selection of the treatment plan is made in Stage 8 and preevaluates the condition in Stage 9 before returning to Stage 1. Thus illness behavior patterns reflect the variety of behaviors involved in the expression of symptoms and the seeking of help to remove the distress from the illness.

Suchman (1965) has outlined stages that occur in response to illness that potentially lead to a patient career wherein the illness behavior pattern is sustained over an extended period of time. These stages include: (1) the initial symptom experience; (2) the assumption of the sick role; (3) medical care contact; (4) the dependent patient role; and (5) recovery or rehabilitation. At any point in the process, the person may either deny (and retreat to an earlier stage), accept and go on to the next stage, or exit from the model. Fixation at any stage can occur as the result of the expectations of the individual and the social-psychological reinforcement patterns accompanying behaviors exhibited at that stage (see Carver & Scheier, 1982, for a discussion of the influence of expectations on behavior controls).

In effect these theories address the psychosocial consequences of perceived biological diseases. They reflect the fact that disease is not defined merely in terms of its consequences on biological or physiological systems, but that the disease manifestation is a multisystem phenomenon with consequences on the behavior of individuals who engage in corrective actions and the behavior of familial and social systems within which the actions take place.

Health Behavior. In contrast, there has been less work on the analysis of health behaviors (i.e., those behaviors designed to preserve or promote good health where there are no observable signs of disease). This differential emphasis no doubt reflects the focus on disease that is implicit in the American Health Care system (Kass, 1975; Kristein, Arnold, & Wynder, 1977).

The Health Belief Model has promoted some research in this area. Becker and Maiman (1975) have outlined the details of this model. There are two critical factors that seem to focus the individual on actions to promote health: (1) readiness to take action; and (2) belief that the action will be beneficial. Readiness is based on the perceived vulnerability of an individual's health based on a potential serious threat to health. Perceived benefit reflects a subjective cost-benefit analysis based on the beliefs that the individual holds about the probable consequences of the actions to be taken.

Studies on preventative behavior have supported the general theory implicit in the model (Kirscht & Rosenstock, 1977; Rosenstock, 1974), though many of the variables influencing beliefs and readiness need further definition, refinement, and analysis. There are studies of health behaviors that directly link physical health to health behavior. Studies by Palmore (1970) and Pratt (1971) demonstrated that people over 60 and mothers who visited a health clinic had fewer health problems and a higher level of health when they avoided smoking, kept moderate weight, exercised, and pursued other health practices.

In a more comprehensive study of 6928 adults, Belloc & Breslow (1972) studied the relationship between health practices and rated health. Low alcohol consumption, not smoking, not eating between meals, usually eating breakfast, maintaining a desirable weight, and being physically active each correlated with good health to some degree. More notably, the study showed that the more of these practices pursued, the higher the overall health rating regardless of which particular practices were involved. In a study conducted 5 1/2 years later, Belloc (1973) reported that individuals who followed six or seven good health practices had the lowest mortality rates when adjustments were made for the relationship between age and mortality. The proportion of men and women over 55 who died from the initial sample who followed six or seven health practices was less than half that of those who followed three or fewer health practices. The expected remaining life-time of 55 to 64-year-old men who followed six or seven of the health practices was 25 years. For those who followed three or fewer practices, there was an expected 14 remaining years. For women, the differences in these values were slightly less (20 to 28 years for this age group).

The origin of health behaviors has received limited investigation, though there is the general belief that health practices such as daily dental care develop early in a person's life. Pratt (1977) studied family health behavior, finding that those families who practiced the best health care showed an "energized family structure." They made discriminating choices about health, sought information, and assertively negotiated their needs with the health care system. Though they represented a minority of the families studied, the results support the implication that the origins of good health habits are early patterns of health practices in the home.

Other lines of research point to the importance of family and social involvements in health. Kobrin and Hendershot (1977) analyzed a sample of 20,000 deaths occurring from 1966 to 1968. Mortality was lower for married persons than for nonmarried persons, and lower for married persons with children than for those without. A follow-up study by Berkman and Syme (1979) of the Alameda County subjects indicated that married people had lower mortality than nonmarried people. People who belonged to religious groups or one or more other groups also had lower mortality rates. Over all age groups, the risk was roughly twice as great for the isolated individuals, regardless of sex.

The mechanisms by which such results might be produced is obscure. They could reflect a selection process wherein healthier people get married and have children. On the other hand, involvement with others may exert influences that are protective from disease either in terms of neurochemical-hormonal effects or social influences.

A study by Langlie (1977) stresses the importance of social variables as a correlate of health behavior patterns. She found that behaviors that promote health by indirectly reducing risk (e.g., good nutrition, using seat belts, medical and dental checkups) were significantly related to family socioeconomic status and frequent interactions with friends. This relationship was not observed for health behaviors she described as direct risk-preventative health behaviors (e.g., safe driving and pedestrian practices, not smoking, and personal hygiene).

Tapp and Goldenthal (1982) have observed three primary dimensions related to self-reported health practices. They found three factors that describe health behaviors in a sample of patients visiting a family physician's office. The first of these reflected positive health practices requiring active pursuit of health (e.g., good nutrition habits, exercise, rest and relaxation, and regular checkups). The second factor was characterized by avoiding health risk (e.g., not smoking, using good road and water safety practices). A third factor reflected a low frequency of negative emotions (depression, anxiety, and anger) and good personal health habits in contrast to drug and alcohol abuse. There is clearly a need for further investigation of interrelationships among those variables that influence and describe habits used in pursuit of health.

Stress and Disease

The interaction between stress and disease has been studied from a number of vantage points. Selye's (1976) research reflects a biological perspective in which a noxious and therefore stressful stimulus activates a physiological response he called the General Adaptation Syndrome. This syndrome is characterized by activation of the pituitary-adrenocortical hormonal system, which defends the body against stress by mobilizing body reserves of glucose, decreasing peripheral blood flow, activating thymus glandular secretions, etc. (see Chapter 5 by McCabe & Schneiderman). Continued exposure to the noxious stimulus prolongs this response but ultimately weakens the organism by lowering the body's resistance. After an extended time period the organism weakens to the point of exhaustion.

During this process, the body is vulnerable to various diseases of adaptation. Constitutional or acquired organ weaknesses tend to make some systems more vulnerable to the effects of prolonged stress than others, thus accounting for individual differences in the origins of illness.

Much research has focused on the consequences of life changes as a precipitant of stress. Significant relationships have been reported between life changes (e.g., moving, job loss, loss of spouse) and the onset of various illnesses (e.g., myocardial infarctions, multiple sclerosis, accidents, injuries, and other medical complaints [Bramwell, Masuda, Wagner, & Holmes, 1975]). Undesirable changes were better predictors of behavioral impairment in children (Gersten, Langner, Eisenbert, & Orzek, 1974), self-reported tension and distress in adults (Vinokur & Selzer, 1975), anxiety, depression, neuroticism and hypochondriasis (Sarason & Sarason, 1979), and self-reports of the total number of illness symptoms (Antoni, 1981).

Sarason and Sarason (1979) have suggested that moderation variables influence the impact of life change on stress. Personality characteristics, coping style, social supports, and internal physiological states influence stress reactions. For example, individuals who show high "internal" scores on a measure reflecting the extent to which individuals believe they have control over their own fate also report higher levels of stress than low internals (Gilbert & Mangelsdorf, 1979). Similarly low internals (high externals) report better "adjustments" to the effects of cancer and to myocardial infarctions. Individuals who score high in social conformity have less illness following life changes than people who score low on this measure (Garrity, Somes, & Marx, 1977). These personality factors seem to mitigate the effects of stress.

Stress is a constant of life. The manner in which the individual reacts to those events that induce stress is a determinant of their effects. Denial, for example, seems to promote recovery from myocardial infarction in that those individuals who deny the severity of their illness return to work sooner and have fewer complications than those who do not deny their disease (Croog & Levine, 1982). Lazarus (1966) has addressed a diversity of coping styles and found that denial was an effective mechanism for minimizing stress reactions. Indeed, this work has direct implication on the treatment of stress via cognitive stress innoculation procedures.

It is generally acknowledged that social isolation is a demographic variable contributing to illness. Cobb (1976) and others have made the assertion that belonging to a social network of communication and mutual support facilitates coping with crisis and adaptation to life change. The level of social support defined by the frequency of social contacts moderates the reported intensity of stressful life events (Goplerud, 1980). Women with many social supports have significantly fewer birth complications than those with fewer supports (Nuckolls, Cassell, & Kaplan, 1972). Individuals who possess good social supports do not have as severe asthma attacks as those who have fewer supports (de Araujo, Van Arsdel, Holmes, & Dudley, 1973). In a study of 163 naval enlisted men, Antoni (1981) found that only those with low social supports showed significant correlations between adverse life events and self-reported illness.

Though these studies do not specify the mechanisms by which stress might be moderated by personality variables and social supports, they are suggestive of the fact that stress is affected differentially depending on characteristics of the individual and his or her social environment. The specification of these interactions and the delineation of how these mechanisms might be mediated in regulating the organism's physiological response to stress is the key question of future research.

Summary and Conclusions

The purpose of this chapter has been to introduce the factors that have influenced the need for expanding the scope of medicine to include behavioral antecedents and consequences of disease. The establishment of empirical and theoretical relationships among social, behavioral, and physiological process in disease demands scientific standards of investigation and proof within models of inquiry that will allow the simultaneous examination of these processes and the elucidation of their interactions. The study of the social psychology of illness and health has begun the elaboration of such models and has indicated ways for integrating social-psychological-behavioral thought into medicine. The nature of stress and the psychosocial contributors to biological responses have identified the sources of variation to be examined.

In what follows in this book we examine the biological bases of these phenomena, the processes they serve, the manner of their investigation and treatment, and how this multisystems way of viewing diseases can integrate the multiple viewpoints and sources of scientific study that impact on disease.

REFERENCES

Adler, N. E., & Stone, G. C. Social science perspectives on the health system. In G. C. Stone, F. Cohen, & N. E. Adler (Eds.), *Health psychology*. San Francisco: Jossey-Bass, 1979.

American Medical Association *Guides to the evaluation of permanent impairment*. American Medical Association, Chicago, 1971.

Antoni, M. *Life events, social supports and physical illness in Navy personnel*, MA thesis. New London, Conn.: Connecticut College, 1981.

Battista, J. R. The holistic paradigm and general system theory. *General Systems*, 1977, Vol. 22, 65–71.

Becker, M., & Maiman, L. Social behavioral determinants of compliance with medical care recommendations. *Medical Care*, 1975, *13*, 10–23.

Belloc, N. B. Relationship of health practices and mortality. *Preventive Medicine*, 1973, *2*, 67–81.

Belloc, N. B., & Breslow, L. Relationship of physical health status and health practices. *Preventive Medicine*, 1972, *1*, 409–421.

Berkman, L., & Syme, S. L. Social networks, host resistance and mortality: A nine-year follow-up of Alameda County residents. *American Journal of Epidemiology*, 1979, *109*, 186–204.

Bertalanffy, L von. *General systems theory*. New York: Braziller, 1968.

Bramwell, S., Masuda, M., Wagner, N., & Holmes, T. Psychosocial factors in athletic injuries: Development and application of the social and athletic readjustment rating scale (SARRS). *Journal of Human Stress*, 1975, *1*, 6–20.

Breslow, L., & Sommers, A. A life-time program of health monitoring. *New England Journal of Medicine*, 1978, *172*, 1234–1237.

Carver, C. S., & Scheier, M. Control theory: A useful framework in conceptualizing human behavior. *Psychological Bulletin*, 1982, *92*, 111–135.

Cobb, S. Social support as a moderator of life stress. *Psychosomatic Medicine*, 1976, *38*, 300–314.

Coe, R. *Sociology of medicine* (2nd ed.). New York: McGraw-Hill, 1978.

Chalfant, H. P., & Kurtz, R. A. Alcoholics and the sick role: Assessment by social workers. *Journal of Health and Social Behavior*, 1971, *12*, 66–72.

Croog, S. H., & Levine, S. *The heart patient recovers: Social and psychological factors*. Port Washington, N.Y.: Human Sciences Press, 1977.

Croog, S. H., & Levine, S. *Life after a heart attack: Social and psychological factors eight years later*. Port Washington, N.Y.: Human Sciences Press, 1982.

Davies, D. F. Progress toward the assessment of health status. *Preventive Medicine*, 1975, *4*, 282–295.

de Araujo, G., Van Arsdel, P. O., Holmes, T. H., & Dudley, D. L. Life change, coping ability and chronic intrinsic asthma. *Journal of Psychosomatic Research*, 1972, *17*, 359–363.

Drews, P. Introduction and overview in F. Solomon, P. B. Dews., & D. L. Parron (Eds.), *Biobehavioral factors in sudden cardiac death*. Conference summary, National Academy of Sciences, 1980, Washington, D.C.

Engel, G. L. The need for a new medical model: A challenge for biomedicine. *Science*, 1977, *196*, 129–136.

Fabrega, H., Jr. *Disease and social behavior*. Cambridge: MIT Press, 1974.

Field, M. G. The health care system of industrial society: The disappearance of the general practitioners and some implications. In E. Mendelsohn, J. P. Suazey, & I. Taviss (Eds.). *Human aspects of biomedical innovation*. Cambridge, Mass.: Harvard University Press, 1971.

Fox, R. C. The medicalization and demedicalization of American society. In J. H. Knowles (Ed.), *Doing better and feeling worse: Health in the United States*. New York: Norton, 1977.

Garrity, T. F., Somes, G. W., & Marx, M. B. Personality factors in resistance to illness after recent life changes. *Journal of Psychosomatic Research*, 1977, *21*, 23 – 32.

Gersten, J., Langner, T., Eisenbert, J., & Orzek, I. In B. S. Dohrenwend & B. P. Dohrenwend (Eds.), *Stressful life events – their nature and effects*. New York: John Wiley & Sons, 1974.

Gilbert, L. A., & Mangelsdorf, D. Influence of perceptions of personal control on reaction to stressful events. *Journal of Counseling Psychology*, 1979, *26*(6), 473 – 480.

Goffman, E. *Stigma: Notes on the management of spoiled identity*. Englewood Cliffs, N.J.: Prentice-Hall, 1963.

Goplerud, E. N. Social support and stress during the first year of graduate school. *Professional Psychology*, 1980, 283 – 290.

Illich, I. *Medical nemesis: The expropriation of health*. London: Calder and Boyars, 1975.

Janis, I. L., & Rodin, J. Attribution, control and decision making: Social psychology and health care. In G. C. Stone, F. Cohen, & N. E. Adler (Eds.), *Health psychology*. San Francisco: Jossey-Bass, 1979.

Kasl, S. V., & Cobb, S. Health behavior, illness behavior and sick role behavior. *Archives of Environmental Health*, 1966, *12*, 246 – 266.

Kirscht, J. P., & Rosenstock, I. M. Patient adherence to antihypertension medical regimes. *Journal of Community Health*, 1977, *3*, 115 – 124.

Kleinman, A., Eisenberg, L., & Good, B. Culture, illness and care. *Annals of Internal Medicine*, 1978, *88*, 251 – 258.

Kobrin, F. E., & Hendershot, G. E. Do family ties reduce mortality? Evidence from the United States, 1966 – 1968. *Journal of Marriage and the Family*, 1977, 737 – 745.

Kass, L. R. Regarding the end of medicine and the pursuit of health. *The Public Interest*, 1975, *40*, 11 – 42.

Kristein, M. M., Arnold, C. B., & Wynder, E. L. Health economics and preventive care. *Science*, 1977, *195*, 457 – 462.

Kuhn, T. S. *The structure of scientific revolutions*. Chicago: University of Chicago Press, 1970.

Langlie, J. K. Social networks, health beliefs, and preventive health behavior. *Journal of Health and Social Behavior*, 1977, *18*, 244 – 260.

Lazarus, R. S. *Psychological stress and the coping process*. New York: McGraw-Hill, 1966.

Lerner, M. J., & Simmons, C. Observer's reaction to the innocent victim: Compassion or rejection? *Journal of Personality and Social Psychology*, 1966, *4*, 203 – 210.

Leventhal, H., Nerenz, D., & Straus, A. Self-regulation and the mechanism for symptom appraisal. In D. Mechanic (Ed.), *Psychosocial epidemiology*. New York: Neale Watson, 1980.

Mechanic, D. *Medical sociology* (2nd ed). New York: Free Press, 1978.

Miller, G. A., Galanter, E., & Pribram, K. H. *Plans and the structure of behavior*. New York: Holt, Rinehart, & Winston, 1960.

Millis, J. S. *Graduate education of physicians*. Report of Citizen's Commission. Chicago: American Medical Association, 1966.

Nuckolls, K. B., Cassell, J., & Kaplan, B. H. Psychosocial aspects, life crisis and the prognosis of pregnancy. *American Journal of Epidemiology*, 1972, *95*, 431 – 441.

O'Kelly, L. I. The psychophysiology of motivation. *Annual Review of Psychology*, 1963, *14*, 57 – 92.

Palmore, E. Health practices and illness among the aged. *The Gerontologist*, 1970, *4*, 313 – 316.

Parsons, T. *The social system*. New York: Free Press, 1951.

Piaget, J. *Structuralism*. New York: Harper & Row, 1970.

Pratt, L. Changes in health care ideology in relation to self-care by families. *Health Education Monographs*, 1977, *5*, 121 – 135.

Rogers, D. E. The challenge of primary care. In J. H. Knowles (Ed.), *Doing better and feeling worse: Health in the United States*. New York: Norton, 1977.

Rosenstock, I. M. The healthy belief model and preventive health behavior. *Health Education Monographs*, 1974, *2*, 354 – 386.

Sackett, D. L., & Haynes, R. B. *Compliance with therapeutic regimens*. Baltimore: Johns Hopkins University Press, 1976.

Sarason, I. G., & Sarason, B. R. *The importance of cognition and moderator variables in stress*. Office of Naval Research Technical Report, No. N00014-75-C-0905, NR 170 – 804. Arlington, Virginia, 1979.

Selye, H. *The stress of life* (revised edition). New York: McGraw-Hill, 1976.

Sontag, S. *Illness as metaphor*. New York: Random House, 1978.

Statistical Abstracts of the United States: 1978 (99th edition). Washington, D.C.: United States Bureau of the Census, 1978.

Stedman's Medical Dictionary. Baltimore: Williams & Wilkins, 1972.

Suchman, E. A. Stages of illness and medical care. *Journal of Health and Human Behavior*, 1965, *6*, 114 – 128.

Szasz, T. The myth of mental illness. *Foundations of a theory of personal conduct*. New York: 1961.

Tapp, J. T., & Goldenthal, P. A factor analytic study of health habits. *Preventive Medicine*, 1982, *11*, 724 – 728.

Thom, R. Structural stability and morphogenesis. Reading, Mass.: Benjamin, 1975.

Thomas, L. On the science and technology of medicine. In J. H. Knowles (Ed.), *Doing better and feeling worse: Health in the United States*. New York: Norton, 1977.

Vinokur, A., & Selzer, M. L. Desirable versus undesirable life events: Their relationship to stress and mental distress. *Journal of Personality and Social Psychology*, 1975, *32*, 329 – 337.

World Health Organization. *Constitution of the World Health Organization, Annex I*. Geneva, WHO, 1958.

II PERSPECTIVES ON BEHAVIOR AND HEALTH

2 Epidemiology and Behavior

Terence A. Gerace
University of Miami, School of Medicine

Ronald Vorp
University of Miami

INTRODUCTION

Epidemiology is the scientific study of disease and injury, with a special emphasis on their differential distribution by place, population, and time. Through descriptive, analytic, and experimental studies of groups of people, epidemiologists seek clues to the etiology of disease and injury. Their ultimate goal is applying this knowledge to the prevention of illness.

Behavioral components can be seen in two aspects of disease development. First, behaviors influence risk factors for certain diseases. *Risk factors* are characteristics of groups of individuals that designate them as being at above average risk for a specified disease. For instance, groups of people eating foods high in saturated fatty acids usually have elevated serum cholesterol levels, a risk factor for coronary heart disease (Keys, 1980).

Second, behaviors themselves can be risk factors. The smoking of cigarettes is considered a major risk factor for both coronary heart disease and lung cancer, because the probability of getting either of these is greater in smokers than in nonsmokers (*Smoking and Health*, 1979).

Chronic diseases such as diseases of the heart, cancer, and cerebrovascular diseases account for more than two-thirds of all deaths in the United States (US Bureau of the Census, 1980). The analysis of causes of death shows that risk factors for these diseases have significant behavioral components that can be studied by epidemiological methods. Behavioral factors have been suggested for each of the characteristics listed in Table 2.1 which emerged as predictors of death from coronary heart disease in a study of over 40,000 former male college students (Paffenbarger, Wolf, Notkin, & Thorne, 1966). Because cancer rates vary dramat-

25

TABLE 2.1
Characteristics of College Students and Mortality Ratio
for Coronary Heart Disease

Characteristic	Mortality Ratio*
Smoking greater than or equal to 10 cigarettes per day	2.34
Systolic blood pressure more than or equal to 130 mm Hg	1.64
Ponderal index less than 12.8	1.72
One or both parents dead	1.67
Only child	1.56
Height less than 68 inches	1.72
Sense of exhaustion	2.25
Varsity athletics	0.47

*Mortality ratio is the death rate with the characteristic divided by the death rate without the characteristic.
Adapted from Paffenbarger et al. (1966).

ically across countries and within countries, epidemiologists can examine differences in diet, smoking, exposure to industrial carcinogens, and personality characteristics that might account for the disparity in rates. Differences in the incidence of stomach cancer in Japan as shown in Table 2.2 are presumed to be due, in part, to dietary differences.

Accidents rank first as the cause of death in people 15 to 34 years of age in the United States and fourth as the cause of death overall (*Vital Statistics,* 1980). Vehicular accidents, falls, fires, drownings, industrial accidents, and poisonings rank as the leading categories of accidents, accounting for 81% of all cases in 1977. Poisoning accidents involve one in 500 preschool children with one of every four children being a repeater, a rate 125 times that expected by chance (Wehrle,

TABLE 2.2
Stomach Cancer Rates for Males by Geographical Area

Geographical Area	Age Adjusted Rate/100,000	Rank
Japan	56.6	1
Singapore	30.2	10
Yugoslavia	24.0	19
Switzerland	18.1	28
Greece	14.0	37
United States	7.2	42
Thailand	2.2	46

Adapted from Silverberg (1980).

DeFreest, Penhollow & Harris, 1961). Behavioral factors are operative in accidents of all types.

Suicides and homicides rank ninth and eleventh, respectively, as causes of death in the United States (*Vital Statistics*, 1980). The suicide and homicide rates by country presented in Table 2.3 suggest psychosocial factors that might be related to the rate of death. For instance, the five countries lowest in suicide rate are strongly influenced by the Roman Catholic or Greek Orthodox Churches. In contrast, none of the top five countries is predominantly Roman Catholic or Greek Orthodox.

Epidemiological analysis can be applied to nonfatal diseases that are related to behavior. Sexually transmitted diseases present a major health problem throughout the world (World Health Organization, 1977). In the United States, reported cases of gonorrhea increased from 324,925 in 1965 to 999,937 in 1975 (MMWR, 1979). The increase in sexually transmitted diseases may be related to the increasing number of sexually active teenagers (MMWR, 1979; World Health Organization, 1977). Furthermore, changes in the number of young men adopting an "alternative life-style" may be responsible for the four to tenfold increase in cases of shigellosis, amoebiasis, and hepatitis A and B over a 3-year period in San Francisco (Dritz, Ainsworth, Black, Boucher, Garrard, Palmer, & River, 1977).

Nosocomial (hospital acquired) infections affect approximately 5% of patients (Cluff & Johnson, 1972). This translates into nearly 2,000,000 cases each year in nonfederal hospitals alone. Infections could be reduced if hospital personnel consistently practiced hygienic behaviors. A recent study revealed that only 41% and 28% of contacts with patients in intensive care units were followed by handwashing in a university hospital and a private hospital, respectively (Albert & Condie, 1981).

TABLE 2.3
Suicide and Homicide Rates Per 100,000 Persons
(Age greater or equal to 15 years) for the Top Five and
Bottom Five Locations in a Study of 25 Geographical Areas, 1975

	Suicides		*Homicides*	
	Location	*Rate*	*Location*	*Rate*
Top Five:	Finland	31.9	Puerto Rico	16.1
	Austria	31.3	N. Ireland	11.4
	Denmark	31.1	United States	10.0
	Switzerland	28.8	Finland	3.6
	Germany, F.R.	26.4	Canada	2.7
Bottom Five:	Ireland	6.9	Greece	.8
	Spain	5.3	Netherlands	.7
	N. Ireland	5.1	Norway	.7
	Greece	3.6	Denmark	.6
	Philippines	1.5	Spain	.6

Adapted from World Health Organization data (cited by US Bureau of the Census, 1979).

In addition to the analysis of behavioral influences on death and disease, there are new areas that may contribute to our understanding of the etiology and prevention of disease. For example, Gerace and Vorp (1983) examined the relationship between the interpersonal distance of pairs of people from different countries, and the incidence of mortality and morbidity from various causes in those countries. Specifically, they hypothesized there would be a higher incidence of infectious diseases spread by direct airborne transmission in countries where people position themselves closer to each other than in countries where they position themselves further apart. No significant relationships were found between interpersonal distance and the incidence of disease (e.g., tuberculosis and meningococcal meningitis).

These studies show how epidemiological investigations relate to a variety of behavioral phenomena. In the sections that follow we review some of the specific language and methods of epidemiology and show how these can be used to examine behavioral influences on disease.

The Language of Epidemiology

Mortality refers to death and is useful to the epidemiologist when causes can be ascribed. *Morbidity* refers to disease. Generally, diseases are labeled either in terms of the "consequences" of causal factors, or in terms of the "causal agents." For example, carcinoma of the lung is a "consequence," whereas tuberculosis results in part from the presence of a specific pathogen, the tubercle bacillus, which is a "causal agent."

Endpoints in epidemiological studies are dependent variables. "Hard" endpoints are those with little chance for diagnostic error (e.g., mortality from all causes). "Soft" endpoints are those with greater probability of diagnostic error such as adult onset diabetes mellitus.

For a given population, one may be obliged to provide the *prevalence* and *incidence* rates of a disease or a risk factor. The prevalence rate is equivalent to the number of people with a disease or risk factor per number of people in the population at a given point in time or in a given period of time. In 1978 for example, the prevalence rate per 100,000 for smoking in females 20 years of age and older was 30,000 (US Bureau of the Census, 1980). Incidence refers to the occurrence of new events, such as new cases of diabetes mellitus. The incidence rate is the number of new cases per population base per time period.

Incidence data can be used to estimate the risk of disease for individuals with certain characteristics. For instance, male smokers 35 years of age with systolic blood pressures of 165 mm Hg and serum cholesterol levels of 260 mg/dl have a 3 in 100 chance of developing coronary heart disease in 6 years (*Coronary Risk Handbook,* 1973). In contrast, 35-year-old male nonsmokers with systolic blood pressures of 120 mm Hg and serum cholesterols of 185 mg/dl have an 8 in 1000 chance. The first group is 3.75 times (.03/008) more likely to develop coronary heart disease in 6 years than the second group.

Attributable risk is the difference between the risk with the risk factor and the risk without the risk factor. For instance, the risk of neonatal death is .014 with smoking mothers and .012 with nonsmoking mothers (Meyer & Tonascia, 1977). The attributable risk is therefore .002. Although this difference is not numerically large, the impact is substantial in terms of public health. With a prevalence rate of 30,000 smokers per 100,000 females of maternal age, approximately 2000 excess neonatal deaths would occur each year. This example assumes that the birthrate is the same for smokers and nonsmokers.

Incidence and prevalence rates are generally expressed in number of cases per 1000, 10,000, or 100,000 people. To obtain the incidence rate per 100,000 people for cancer mortality in the United States in 1977 the following calculations were made:

(1) $\dfrac{X(\text{rate per } 100,000)}{100,000} = \dfrac{386,686 \text{ Cancer deaths}}{216,400,000 \text{ U.S. population in 1977}}$

(2) $\underline{X} = \dfrac{386,686}{216,400,000} \text{ times } \dfrac{100,000}{1}$

(3) $\underline{X} = 178.7$ Deaths from cancer per 100,000

In some epidemiological studies, certain people may be observed for longer periods of time than others. To compute the incidence rate in these studies, the denominator must be "person-years" instead of number of people. If 500 people in a study were observed for 2 years (500 times 2 = 1000 person-years) and another 500 for 3 years (500 times 3 = 1500 person-years), the incidence rate would be based on the number of new cases per 2500 person-years.

Generally, epidemiologists classify changes in disease rates over time as being either *secular, cyclic,* or *epidemic.* Secular chages refer to those that occur over relatively long periods of time. A recent example is the decreasing mortality rate from ischemic heart disease observed since 1968 (Fig. 2.1). Behaviorally related events such as the decreasing rate of smoking in adult males, the decreasing intake of saturated fats, and the improved management of hypertension may be contributing to this decline (Havlik & Feinleib, 1979; Levy, 1978).

Cyclic changes are those that vary with some periodicity. Cyclic changes in death rates have been examined in relationship to holidays, birthdays, elections, and other important personal events (Phillips & Feldman, 1973; Schulz & Bazerman, 1980). The question being asked is: "Do people postpone dying until after an important event, resulting in a lower than chance mortality rate prior to the event and an excess of deaths following the event?" Recently, Rabkin, Matthewson, and Tate (1980) reported that sudden cardiac death in men with no previous clinical evidence of ischemic heart disease occurs disproportionately on Mondays compared with other days of the week. Suicides in the United States also show cyclic changes with peaks occurring in the fall and spring (Frederick, 1978).

Epidemics occur when there is an increase in the occurrence of a disease in a relatively short period of time. Epidemics are commonly associated with infec-

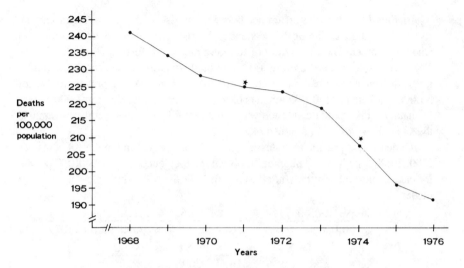

FIG. 2.1.   Age-adjusted death rates for ischemic heart disease during influenza-epidemic and non-epidemic years: United States 1968–1976. Source: Division of Vital Statistics, National Center for Health Statistics; and Center for Disease Control, Report No. 91, 1975–1976, issued July 1977 cited in Havlik and Feinleib, 1979.

tious diseases. Presently, an infectious disease with a large behavioral component, gonorrhea, is considered to have reached epidemic proportions in the United States (Fig. 2.2) (MMWR, 1979).

Host characteristics are those attributes of the individual (intrinsic) that may affect health status by interacting with environmental (extrinsic) factors. For example, host characteristics associated with increased prevalence of cancer of the cervix in women are being married, having early experience in sexual activity, and having multiple partners (Martin, 1967).

Epidemiological studies often require large cohorts, groups defined by one or more demographic characteristics (e.g., age), so that sufficient endpoints from chronic diseases will occur in a reasonable amount of time. To obtain large groups with certain known characteristics often requires the use of rapid screening techniques administered to even larger numbers of people.

For a screening test to be useful, it should be *sensitive*. A 100% sensitive test detects all those with the characteristic of interest. For example, a rapid paper and pencil test for the Type A behavior pattern when compared against a standard (Rosenman-Friedman Structured Interview; Rosenman, Friedman, Straus, Wurm, Kositchek, Hahn, & Werthessen, 1964) should identify all those designated as Type A by the standard.

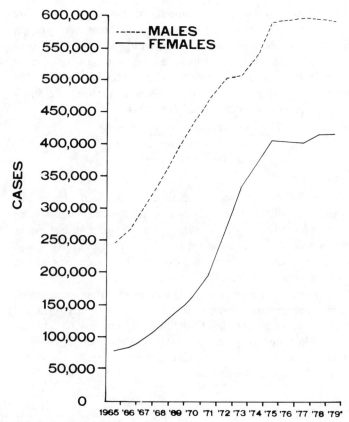

*Data for 1979 are estimates.

FIG. 2.2.   Reported gonorrhea cases by sex, United States, 1965 – 1979.

The actual calculation for *sensitivity* presented for a paper and pencil test of Type A behavior, the Jenkins Activity Survey (Jenkins, Rosenman, & Friedman, 1967) is as follows:

(4) Sensitivity = $\dfrac{113 \text{ True Positives*}}{\substack{113 \text{ True Positives plus} \\ 60 \text{ False Negatives**}}}$ times 100

(5) Sensitivity = 65%

---

*True Positives: Number determined positive for Type A by paper and pencil test and by the standard.

**False Negatives: Number determined negative for Type A by the paper and pencil test and positive by the standard, the Structured Interview.

For research and treatment purposes it is also important that the screening test not designate individuals as having a behavioral characteristic or disease if they do not in fact possess it. The test should be *specific* or correct in its labeling of those without the characteristic. The test should have few "false positives," that is, individuals said to have the characteristic (positive) but not having it (false). The *specificity* for the Jenkins Activity Survey for Type A behavior using the Structured Interview as the standard was determined as follows:

(6) Specificity = $\dfrac{\text{126 True Negatives*}}{\substack{\text{126 True Negatives plus} \\ \text{31 False Positives**}}}$ times 100

(7) Specificity = 80%

In epidemiological studies, data must sometimes be adjusted to take into account differences in the distribution of ages or other variables across study groups. The following hypothetical data illustrate how adjusting for age can be important. The prevalence of Type A behavior in children from a country of high coronary heart disease incidence (United States) and from a country of low coronary heart disease incidence (Greece) are given in Table 2.4.

To compare the percentage of Type A in the United States group to the Greek group, one can simply multiply the columns (1) and (3) for the United States and (2) and (4) for Greece for each age category. Then, the total number of Type A's can be obtained for each culture and the percentage of Type A's can be calculated by dividing by the total number of children in each country.

United States

		(1)		(3)		
8 – 9 year old Type A's	=	30	times	.30	=	9
10 – 11 year old Type A's	=	30	times	.40	=	12
12 – 13 year old Type A's	=	40	times	.50	=	20
Total Type A's	=				=	41

$\dfrac{41 \ \ (\text{Type A's})}{100 \ (\text{Total USA children})}$ times 100 = 41% Type A

Greece

		(2)		(4)		
8 – 9 year old Type A's	=	80	times	.20	=	16
10 – 11 year old Type A's	=	10	times	.30	=	3
12 – 13 year old Type A's	=	10	times	.40	=	4
Total Type A's	=				=	23

$\dfrac{23 \ \ (\text{Type A's})}{100 \ (\text{Total Greek children})}$ times 100 = 23% Type A

*True Negatives: Number of negatives as determined by the paper and pencil test and by the standard.

**False Positives: Number of negatives as determined by standard, but labeled positive by the paper and pencil test.

TABLE 2.4
The Percentage of Type A Children in the United States and Greece
by Age in a Hypothetical Study

	Number of Children		Proportion Type A	
	(1)	(2)	(3)	(4)
Age (Years)	USA	Greece	USA	Greece
8–9	30	80	.30	.20
10–11	30	10	.40	.30
12–13	40	10	.50	.40

The foregoing calculations give the impression that there are many more Type A children in the United States (41%) than in Greece (23%). In reality, the difference between countries is inflated because the age distributions are not similar in the two samples.

When the characteristic of interest (e.g., Type A behavior) may be related to chronological age, differences in the distribution of ages among study populations must be taken into account in analyzing and interpreting the data. To control for unequal distributions in age, epidemiologists adjust the data by applying the proportions of the characteristic of interest at each age category for the study groups to some known distribution of ages, for example, the distribution of ages in the United States in 1940. This "standard distribution" or any other will do, provided it is not extremely different from that in the populations being studied. The combined populations of the groups being compared can also be used as the standard. The Type A data previously presented are adjusted for age as follows, using the combined populations as the standard.

Combining the populations from each group gives the following "standard population" in column (1).

		Proportion Type A		Type A's	
	(1)	(2)	(3)	(4)	(5)
Age (Yrs.)	Standard population	USA	Greece	USA	Greece
8–9	110	.30	.20	33	22
10–11	40	.40	.30	16	12
12–13	50	.50	.40	25	20
Total:	200			74	54

Multiplying columns (1) and (2) for the USA and (1) and (3) for Greece at each age category provides the total number of Type A's adjusted for age within each country—columns (4) and (5), respectively. Next, the totals from columns (4) and (5) are divided by the total number in the "standard population," 200, giving the percentage of Type A's for the USA and Greece, 37% and 27%, respectively.

The summary that follows shows that the adjustment reduced the differences in percentage of Type A's between the two countries by more than 44%.

	Percentage of Type A's		
	USA	*Greece*	*Difference*
Unadjusted rate	41%	23%	18%
Adjusted rate	37%	27%	10%

Methods of Epidemiology

Naturalistic Observation.   Often the earliest suggestions relating behavior to a specific disease come from naturalistic observation. These observations are made in natural settings with minimal intrusion by the investigators. Populations can be examined for differences in incidence of disease and customary behaviors. For example, observations in East and West Finland revealed remarkably different 10-year coronary heart disease mortality rates (992 per 10,000 versus 351 per 10,000, respectively) and differences in smoking behavior (31% versus 15% smoking greater than or equal to 20 cigarettes per day, respectively) (Keys, 1980).

The most common uses of naturalistic observation are to answer the traditional epidemiological questions: (1) Where does the disease occur? (2) Who gets the disease? and (3) When does the disease occur? Where the disease occurs refers specifically to geographical location. As a matter of convenience, place is frequently studied as a function of political boundaries because: (1) the boundaries often coincide with cultural divisions; and (2) governments are often the source of health-related data. When national boundaries are used to define population groups, care must be taken to assure that diagnostic and reporting procedures are comparable across countries.

An example of naturalistic observation within political boundaries is the World Health Organization's study of dental problems in the villages of Papua, New Guinea (Schmschula, Adkins, Barnes, Charlton, & Davey, 1978). Dental examinations revealed a significant difference in the incidence of dental caries, up to fourfold, between certain villages that are geographically separated. After examining characteristics of the villagers that might explain the difference in the incidence of the caries, the investigators concluded that inhabitants of villages that had the fewest caries had a "betel-chewing habit." The villagers chew the fruit of the areca palm, mixed with slaked lime and betel leaves. A significant negative correlation was found between the number of areca nuts chewed per day and caries per person.

Naturalistic observations provide descriptive data and generate hypotheses related to the etiology of disease. Frequently, these observations depend on the alertness and intuition of the investigator. Causal inferences made from naturalistic observations always require further verification.

Cohort Study.   A cohort study identifies a group of people (e.g., military unit or residents of a community) and follows it for a period of time to see whether certain characteristics are associated with different rates of morbidity and/or mortality. Because potentially useful information is collected prior to the occurrence of new cases of death, disease, or injury, the design is a *prospective study*. An example of this approach is the classic Framingham Study (Dawber, Meadors, & Moore, 1951). A cohort from the town of Framingham, Massachusetts was observed for over 30 years to determine which variables measured at entry into the study were associated with various incidence rates for coronary heart disease and other diseases. The Framingham Study is primarily responsible for identifying the major traditional risk factors for coronary heart disease in the United States—sex, age, serum cholesterol, blood pressure, smoking, and diabetes mellitus.

A major advantage of cohort studies is that they allow calculation of the incidence of the disease. If the cohort is representative of the general population, it can provide projected incidence rates associated with different risk factor levels for the population. Because cohorts are usually not representative of the entire population, incidence data must be applied cautiously. For example, in the Paffenbarger et al. (1966) study of variables associated with coronary heart disease, the cohort was a group of male former students from the University of Pennsylvania and Harvard University. The incidence data from this study might not apply to other population groups that differ in socioeconomic class, sex, or other characteristics.

A major disadvantage of cohort studies arises in studying a disease with a low incidence. To gather enough cases to profit from the study, one must begin with an extremely large cohort and/or continue the study for a long time. This disadvantage can be reduced by looking at a cohort higher in risk than the general population. Then, a greater number of cases could be seen per number studied.

Case-Control Study.   A case-control study compares people having a disease, the cases, with people without the disease, the controls. The two groups can be examined for differences in their behavior that may account for their difference in health status. A recent case-control study assessed whether those with bladder cancer, the cases, differed from a control group in their use of artificial sweeteners and exposure to other carcinogens (Hoover, Strasser, Child, Austin, Cantor, Thomas, Sullivan, Swanson, Mason, Myers, Silverman, Altman, Stemhagen, Narayana, Culp, Key, Kutvirt, West, & Lyon, 1979). Interviewers obtained information from cases and controls on their past use of artificial sweeteners and exposure to known carcinogens. Because the past histories were recorded after identifying persons with and without the disease, this is a *retrospective study*.

One common practice in conducting a case-control study is to match the cases and controls on variables known to be associated with the disease. Matching allows some factors to be controlled so that the effects of other factors can be assessed. In the bladder cancer and artificial sweetener study (Hoover et al., 1979), cases and controls were matched for gender because males have a much higher prevalence of bladder cancer than females. Care must be taken not to match on variables that are suspected to be "intermediate stages" between a behaviorally related cause, and the disease entity. Matching on such variables might interfere with determining whether the hypothesized causal factors are present in differential amounts between cases and controls (Mausner & Bahn, 1974). For instance, in one of the early case-control studies of lung cancer, cases and controls were matched for other respiratory ailments, such as bronchitis. Because cigarette smoking is strongly associated with bronchitis, the cases did not show a large difference in smoking behavior compared to the controls.

Characteristics on which groups are commonly matched are age, race, socioeconomic status, and "presence of a disease." "Presence of a disease" can be controlled for by selecting controls from the same hospital records from which the cases were chosen. This procedure also provides for control of such factors as utilization of the health care system and certain psychological factors that may be related to using a particular hospital.

An important advantage of the case-control design is that it allows study of a disease that has a relatively low prevalence in the population, such as bladder cancer. A prospective cohort study would be very inefficient for studying these diseases, as it would require a long time to accumulate enough cases to assess suspected precursors of the disease.

Community-Based Study.   Most experimental studies that test treatments or hypotheses concerning health-related behaviors are clinic based. In clinic-based trials, treatment is provided either individually or in small groups. In contrast, community-based intervention projects evaluate the impact of programs on whole communities. One community may receive the intervention program, while another may serve as the control or contrast community. Intervention in these studies may take place through the use of public speakers, brochures, television, newspapers, or some combination of these.

In the Stanford Heart Disease Prevention Program, for instance, the mass media were used to increase knowledge about risk factors and to reduce cardiovascular risk factors (Meyer, Nash, McAlister, Maccoby, & Farquhar, 1980). Two communities received mass communication; one received nothing as the control community. In addition, the protocol provided for face-to-face intervention for a high risk group in one of the intervention communities.

Community-based studies may provide important public health models for intervention. A large number of people can receive intervention at less cost per person than would be necessary for screening and clinic-based intervention. However, it is more difficult to evaluate community studies than randomized clinical trials because of the lack of randomization, possibility of contamination due to unmeasured factors influencing behavior, and the difficulty of assessing compliance with suggestions for behavioral changes.

To evaluate the intervention component of the Stanford Heart Disease Prevention Program, the investigators randomly selected members of each community between the ages of 35 and 59 and measured their reduction in coronary heart disease risk factors and knowledge of risk factors for coronary heart disease (Meyer et al., 1980). (See Chapter 3 by Warner for a further discussion of this study.)

Quasi-Experimental Design.   A quasi-experimental design is one in which the investigator chooses two or more groups that differ on the independent variable, but does not manipulate this variable.

For example, the degree of "Westernization" was used as the independent variable in a quasi-experiment that examined the development of coronary heart disease risk factors in males 8 to 17 years of age (Christakis, Kafatos, Fordyce, Kurtz, Gerace, Smith, Duncan, Cassady, & Doxiadis, 1981). The study included 1500 youngsters from two rural and two urban sites in Greece, a country of low coronary heart disease incidence; and one urban site in the United States (New York City), a country of high coronary heart disease incidence. The children from the urban site in the United States were divided into three cohorts: children born in Greece who migrated to the United States, children of Greek origin born in the United States and non-Greek American children.

A specific type of quasi-experiment in epidemiology is the "migratory study," which attempts to unravel the role of cultural, environmental, and genetic factors in the etiology of specific diseases. The migratory study compares the morbidity and mortality rates of migrants to: (1) the rates of those who remain at home, and (2) the rates of the original inhabitants of their new homeland. Migratory studies have been used primarily to: (1) determine if disease rates in certain countries are intrinsic to the inhabitants of the countries; (2) demonstrate that certain places possess characteristics that influence the development of disease regardless of who lives there; and (3) assess the effects of having spent specific amounts of time in the host area relative to the homeland (MacMahon & Pugh, 1970).

One example of a migratory study is Haenszel and Kurihara's (1968) examination of site-specific cancer mortality rates for Japanese who immigrated to the United States. They found the mortality rate from stomach cancer in the migrant population was similar to that observed in Japan, but different from that observed in the United States for whites. This finding suggests that stomach cancer may be causally related to genetic factors, traditional customs that the migrants retain, or some interaction of both. The same pattern obtained for the incidence of breast cancer in females. In contrast, cancer of the colon showed the opposite pattern. Mortality from cancer at this site had risen to a point comparable to the rate in the United States, suggesting that the increased rate may have been due to environmental factors, or customs acquired in the United States.

Although migratory studies can provide unique opportunities for investigating diseases and their determinants, they have limitations (MacMahon & Pugh, 1970). First, it is difficult to assess accurately the degree to which migrants have retained cultural patterns similar to those of their homeland, or adopted those of the host area. Second, a migrant population may not be representative of the population of its former homeland, and therefore may possess unique characteristics that have an effect on disease frequency.

Clinical Trials.   A clinical trial is a human experiment in which the independent variable (e.g., purported health-related behavior) is purposefully manipulated by the investigators, and the dependent variable (morbidity or mortality) is measured following this manipulation. A clinical trial is designed so that two or more groups of participants differ only in the independent variable.

Specific criteria determine who may participate in a clinical trial. For instance, the participants recruited for the Multiple Risk Factor Intervention Trial (MRFIT) were required to be in the upper 10 or 15% risk category for having a fatal myocardial infarction within 6 years of entry into the trial. This designation resulted from entering the serum cholesterol level, diastolic blood pressure reading, and number of cigarettes smoked per day of males who went through a mass screening into a multiple logistic function equation based on the Framingham Study (Multiple Risk Factor Intervention Trial Group, 1977).

After participants have been selected for a trial, they must be assigned to groups for differential treatment. Assignment to groups should be done randomly so each participant has an equal chance of being placed into one of the groups. Then any differences among groups prior to intervention can be attributed to chance variation. Table 2.5 shows the effectiveness of randomization in producing equal groups in the MRFIT.

The treatment group (Special Intervention Group) in the MRFIT received an

TABLE 2.5
Comparison of Usual and Special Intervention Groups in the
Multiple Risk Factor Intervention Trial on a Number of
Variables Measured Prior to Randomization

Variable	Usual Care Group $n = 6438$	Special Intervention Group $n = 6428$
Age	46.3 yrs.	46.3 yrs
Weight	189.1 lbs.	189.3 lbs.
Body mass index	27.7 kg/m^2	27.7 kg/m^2
Serum cholesterol	253.5 mg/dl	253.8 mg/dl
Fasting serum glucose	99.3 mg/dl	99.5 mg/dl
Alcoholic beverages	12.7 drinks/wk	12.5 drinks/wk
Diastolic blood pressure	99.2 mm Hg	99.2 mm Hg
Cigarettes	21.7/day	21.5/day
Smokers	63.5%	63.8%
Forced vital capacity	3700 cc	3691 cc

Adapted from Sherwin, Kaelber, Kezdi, Kjelsberg, and Thomas, Jr., 1981.

extensive intervention program aimed at reducing coronary heart disease risk factors, while the contrast group (Usual Care Group) was referred to its usual source of medical care (Multiple Risk Factor Intervention Trial, 1976). (See Chapter 17 by Schneiderman and Hammer.)

Clinical trials may be defined as explanatory or management (Sackett & Gent, 1979). Explanatory trials attempt to find out whether a treatment is efficacious (i.e., they examine cause-effect relationships). In the case of the MRFIT, does lowering serum cholesterol, diastolic blood pressure, and cigarette consumption reduce mortality and morbidity from coronary heart disease?

Management trials are used to determine if an intervention program is successful in producing the desired consequences. For instance, in the MRFIT, can risk factors and subsequent mortality be reduced more effectively by including participants in a special intervention program than by referring them to their usual source of medical care? Three issues are addressed in a management trial: (1) facilitating compliance with the behavioral regimens, (2) the efficacy of the behavioral regimens in changing risk factors, and (3) the cost–benefit ratio of the behavioral strategies relative to other procedures (e.g., drugs). Because the endpoints for compliers and noncompliers in the Special Intervention Group are being summed and compared to those in the Usual Care Group, the MRFIT is being treated as a management trial.

One difficulty with not being able to distinguish a trial clearly as either explanatory or management is that the results of the trial may be interpreted as if the trial were entirely explanatory, when in reality it is also a management trial. For instance, Rose and Hamilton (1978) concluded that although their intervention and control groups differed in smoking behavior, the difference did not affect chronic lung disease. Unfortunately, self-reports were used to verify the presence of the independent variable. Because participants often say they have quit smoking cigarettes when in fact they have not (Vogt, Selvin, Widdowson, & Hulley, 1977), it is questionable whether the hypothesis that smoking cessation reduces chronic lung disease was in fact tested by the aforementioned study. There is no assurance that the treatment group did, in fact, reduce their smoking behavior relative to the control group. Supporting this argument, absentee records showed that the intervention and control groups were equal in days missed from work for all causes, whereas self-reports from the intervention group indicated a 30% reduction in days missed (Rose & Hamilton, 1978).

Care must be taken in interpreting clinical trials so that one does not automatically conclude that favorable results are simply a function of the treatment. To illustrate, in the Hypertension Detection and Follow-Up Program (1979) the Stepped-Care Intervention Group had a 17% lower 5-year mortality rate than the Referred Care Group. The Stepped-Care Group did better in five of seven categories generally related to blood pressure (e.g., cardiovascular and renal disorders). Close examination of the data, however, reveals the Stepped-Care Group also did better in six of nine categories not generally related to blood pressure. The apparent lack of "specificity" of the treatment suggests that further analyses are needed before concluding that better control of hypertension reduced the mortality from all causes. For example, an examination should be made of the level of blood pressure control in those who survived and those who died in both groups.

Bias can also be introduced into a clinical trial by the investigator or participants' knowledge of the hypothesis (Rosenthal, 1976). Attempts to control this type of bias are made by "blinding" study diagnosticians and/or participants. This is accomplished by preventing the diagnosticians and participants from knowing into which group participants were assigned. Studies in which diagnosticians and participants are not informed of the group assignment are called "double blind" studies.

Although double blind procedures usually are not possible in behavioral trials, evaluation of the endpoints can still be made without bias. For example, electrocardiographic evaluations in the MRFIT are made without knowledge of group membership.

Although clinical trials can provide more rigorous tests of hypotheses than other epidemiological research designs, they are not without their problems. Clearly, to test the relative efficacy of one treatment compared to another, differences must be produced between the groups. In clinical trials where behavioral changes are being tested for their effect on subsequent health, the control group may also change, thus reducing the difference between the intervention and control groups. Simply being included in a health study may enhance the health-related motivation of some control participants. In addition, members of the control group may respond to the same factors that cause secular trends, and to "intervention" procedures that may have been unknowingly and/or unavoidably introduced by the clinical trial. In the MRFIT it was not uncommon for a Usual Care man to have ten or more contacts with the staff and/or materials in a single year.

There are certain difficulties in implementing and interpreting the results of long-term clinical trials where the behavioral component is large. For one, secular trends in the contrast group (e.g., MRFIT Usual Care Group) cannot be controlled. Consequently, the risk factor status of this group over time may approach that of the intervention group. For example, during the course of the MRFIT and the Hypertension Detection and Follow-Up Program, substantial efforts were made by the National High Blood Pressure Education Program and major pharmaceutical houses to "increase the number of hypertensives under adequate blood pressure control" (NHBPEP, 1980). In both clinical trials, the results of this effort most likely decreased the difference between the group treated in the clinic versus the contrast group. To illustrate, at the sixth annual examination in MRFIT, 47% of the Usual Care Group were on antihypertensive drugs compared with 58% of the Special Intervention Group (Multiple Risk Factor Intervention Trial Research Group, 1982).

Evaluating the behavorial intervention techniques in clinical trials is hampered by a number of factors. Because reducing risk factors is the *sine qua non* of the trial, a large number of techniques, many of them quite individualized and hard to document, may be used. Consequently, it is extremely difficult to specify what brought about the changes in risk factors.

Although trials concentrate on particular changes (e.g., smoking cessation), the question must be asked, "Do those in either group change in other ways that could affect the outcome of the trial?" For example, did those men in the Special Intervention Group of MRFIT exercise more, lose weight to a greater extent, or cope with stressors better than those in the Usual Care Group? These potentially confounding variables can be examined statistically if the appropriate data are collected. To accomplish this in the MRFIT, information was collected on leisure time physical activity, weight, life events, and self-esteem, among other variables.

In evaluating the effect of the MRFIT intervention program on risk factors, yearly comparisons were made between the Usual Care and Special Intervention Groups' percentage change from baseline. One assumption that was made was that the difference between the two groups represents that which intervention has added to the changes that have occurred in the Usual Care and Special Intervention Groups following regression to the mean, secular trends, and other outside influences on change.

A second assumption is that community events such as antihypertension programs and advertisements for low fat food items will affect both groups equally. This assumption may be false for a number of reasons, thus making the estimate of the intervention program's effect less accurate—either by overstating or understating its impact. For example, the intervention program may: (1) prime participants to be extra sensitive to community efforts, or (2) inadvertently desensitize them through "overkill" so they hardly react at all. In the first case, the apparent effect of intervention may be inflated due to the interaction of community events and previous intervention being included in the results for what appears to be an intervention effect alone. Likewise, if the intervention program has produced "overkill" the Special Intervention participants may be insensitive to community efforts. In this case, a new community program may differentially affect the Usual Care Group due to desensitization engendered by the intervention program on the Special Intervention Group. When this happens the apparent effect of the intervention program may look less impressive.

Just as medications sometimes have untoward side-effects, behavioral changes can have undesirable consequences in addition to their positive ones. The epidemiologist must be vigilant in evaluating the consequences of a behaviorally controlled disorder. The disorder may lessen in prevalence, but at what expense? During the MRFIT, it was hypothesized that informing Usual Care men they were at above average risk for coronary heart disease, but not providing specific treatment, may increase anxiety and depression (Benfari, McIntyre, Eaker, Blumberg, & Paul, 1979). After 2 years of the Trial the Usual Care Group did not differ from the Special Intervention Group on a questionnaire assessing anxiety-depression.

In conclusion, for the clinical trial to be a powerful tool for examining cause and effect relationships between behavior and disease, scientific vigor must be applied in the design, implementation, and interpretation of results.

Summary

This chapter has demonstrated the inseparable link between epidemiology and human behavior by noting behavioral factors that have contributed to the uneven distribution of death, disease, and injury across population groups. In addition, epidemiological terms and methods have been defined and described using studies that illustrate the relationship between epidemiology and behavior.

REFERENCES

Albert, R. K., & Condie, F. Hand washing patterns in medical intensive care units. *New England Journal of Medicine*, 1981, *304*(24), 1465 – 1466.

Benfari, R. C., McIntyre, K., Eaker, E., Blumberg, S., & Paul, O. The psychological effects of differential treatment of a high risk sample in a randomized clinical trial. *American Journal of Public Health*, 1979, *69*(10), 996 – 1000.

Christakis, G., Kafatos, A., Fordyce, M., Kurtz, C., Gerace, T., Smith, J., Duncan, R., Cassady, J., & Doxiadis, S. Cultural and nutritional determinants of coronary heart disease risk factors in adolescents: A USA-Greece cross-cultural study, preliminary results. In A. E. Harper & G. K. Davis (Eds.), *Nutrition in health and disease and international development: Symposia from the XII International Congress of Nutrition*. New York: Alan R. Liss Incorporated, 1981.

Cluff, L., & Johnson, J. *Clinical concepts of infectious diseases*. Baltimore: The Williams and Wilkins Company, 1972.

Coronary Risk Handbook. New York: American Heart Association, 1973.

Dawber, T. R., Meadors, G. F., & Moore, F. E., Jr. Epidemiological approaches to heart disease: The Framingham study. *American Journal of Public Health*, 1951, *41*, 279 – 286.

Dritz, S. K., Ainsworth, T. E., Black, A., Boucher, L. A., Garrard, W. F., Palmer, R. D., & River, E. Patterns of sexually transmitted enteric diseases in a city. *Lancet*, 1977, *2*(1), 3 – 4.

Frederick, C. J. Current trends in suicidal behavior in the United States. *American Journal of Psychotherapy*, 1978, *32*(2), 172 – 200.

Gerace, T. A., & Vorp, R. *Social distance, morbidity and mortality*. Unpublished manuscript, University of Miami, 1983.

Haenszel, W., & Kurihara, M. Studies of Japanese migrants: I. Mortality from cancer and other diseases among Japanese in the United States. *Journal of the National Cancer Institute*, 1968, *40*, 43 – 68.

Havlik, R. J., & Feinleib, M. (Eds.). *Proceedings of the conference on the decline in coronary heart disease mortality*. (NIH Publication No. 79 – 1610). Bethesda, Md.: U. S. Department of Health, Education, and Welfare, 1979.

Hoover, R., Strasser, P. H., Child, M., Austin, D., Cantor, K., Thomas, D., Sullivan, J. W., Swanson, M. W., Mason, T. J., Myers, M., Silverman, D., Altman, R., Stemhagen, A., Narayana, A., Culp, D., Key, C., Kutvirt, D., West, D., & Lyon, J. *Progress report to the Food and Drug Administration from The National Cancer Institute concerning The National Bladder Cancer Study*, 1979.

Hypertension Detection and Follow-Up Program Cooperative Group. Five-year findings of the hypertension detection and follow-up program: I. Reduction in mortality of persons with high blood pressure, including mild hypertension. *Journal of the American Medical Association*, 1979, *242*, 2562 – 2571.

Jenkins, C. D., Rosenman, R. H., & Friedman, M. Development of an objective psychological test for the determination of the coronary prone behavior pattern in employed men. *Journal of Chronic Diseases*, 1967, *20*, 371 – 379.

Keys, A. *Seven countries: A multivariate analysis of death and coronary heart disease.* Cambridge, Mass. and London: Harvard University Press and Commonwealth Fund, 1980.

Levy, R. I. Progress in prevention of cardiovascular disease. *Preventive Medicine*, 1978, *7*, 464 – 475.

MacMahon, B., & Pugh, T. F. *Epidemiology: Principles and methods.* Boston: Little, Brown & Co., 1970.

Martin, C. E. Marital and coital factors in cervical cancer. *American Journal of Public Health*, 1967, *57*, 803 – 814.

Mausner, J. S., & Bahn, A. K. *Epidemiology: An introductory text.* Philadelphia: W. B. Saunders Company, 1974.

Meyer, A. J., Nash, J. D., McAlister, A. L., Maccoby, N., & Farquhar, J. W. Skills training in a cardiovascular health education campaign. *Journal of Consulting and Clinical Psychology*, 1980, *48*(2), 129 – 141.

Meyer, M. B., & Tonascia, J. A. Maternal smoking, pregnancy complications, and perinatal mortality. *American Journal of Obstetrics and Gynecology*, 1977, *128*, 494 – 502.

MMWR. Gonorrhea: United States. *Morbidity and Mortality Weekly Report*, 1979, *28*, 533 – 534.

Multiple Risk Factor Intervention Trial (MRFIT). A national study of primary prevention of coronary heart disease. *Journal of the American Medical Association*, 1976, *235*(8), 825 – 827.

Multiple Risk Factor Intervention Trial Group. Statistical design considerations in the NHLI Multiple Risk Factor Intervention Trial (MRFIT). *Journal of Chronic Diseases*, 1977, *30*, 261 – 275.

Multiple Risk Factor Intervention Trial Research Group. Multiple risk factor intervention trial: Risk factor changes and mortality results. *Journal of the American Medical Association*, 1982, *248*(12), 1465 – 1477.

NHBPEP, National High Blood Pressure Education Program. *Long-range objectives of NHBPEP.* Enclosure from Conference Headquarters, National Conference on High Blood Pressure Control, 1501 Wilson Boulevard, Suite 600, Arlington, Va., 22209, October, 1980.

Paffenbarger, R. S., Jr., Wolf, P. A., Notkin, J., & Thorne, M. C. Chronic disease in former college students: I. Early precursors of fatal coronary heart disease. *American Journal of Epidemiology*, 1966, *83*(2), 314 – 328.

Phillips, D. P., & Feldman, K. A. A dip in deaths before ceremonial occasions: Some new relationships between social integration and mortality. *American Sociological Review*, 1973, *38*, 678 – 696.

Rabkin, S. W., Matthewson, F. A. L., & Tate, R. B. Chronobiology of cardiac sudden death in men. *Journal of the American Medical Association*, 1980, *244*, 1357 – 1358.

Rose, G., & Hamilton, P. J. S. A randomized controlled trial of the effect on middle-aged men of advice to stop smoking. *Journal of Epidemiology and Community Health*, 1978, *32*, 275 – 281.

Rosenman, R. H., Friedman, M., Straus, R., Wurm, M., Kositchek, R., Hahn, W., & Werthessen, N. T. A predictive study of coronary heart disease. *Journal of the American Medical Association*, 1964, *189*(1), 103 – 110.

Rosenthal, R. *Experimenter effects in behavioral research* (Enlarged ed.). New York: Irvington Publishers, Halstead Press Division of Wiley, 1976.

Sackett, D. L., & Gent, M. Controversy in counting attributing events in clinical trials. *New England Journal of Medicine*, 1979, *301*(26), 1410 – 1412.

Schmschula, R. G., Adkins, B. L., Barnes, D. E., Charlton, G., & Davey, B. G. *WHO study of dental caries etiology in Papua, New Guinea.* Geneva: World Health Organization, 1978.

Schulz, R., & Bazerman, M. Ceremonial occasions and mortality: A second look. *American Psychologist*, 1980, *35*(3), 353 – 361.

Sherwin, R., Kaelber, C. T., Kezdi, P., Kjelsberg, M., & Thomas, H. E., Jr. The Multiple Risk Factor Intervention Trial (MRFIT):II. The development of the protocol. *Preventive Medicine*, 1981, *10*, 402 – 425.

Silverberg, E. Cancer statistics, 1980. *Ca—A Cancer Journal for Clinicians*, 1980, *30*(1), 23 – 38.

Smoking and health: A report of the surgeon general. (DHEW Publication No. (PHS) 79 – 50055). Washington, D.C.: US Government Printing Office, 1979.

US Bureau of the Census. *Statistical abstract of the United States: 1979 (100th ed).* Washington, D.C.: United States Government Printing Office, 1979.

US Bureau of the Census. *Statistical abstract of the United States: 1980 (101st ed).* Washington, D.C.: United States Government Printing Office, 1980.

Vital Statistics of the United States: 1977 Volume II—Mortality part B. Hyattsville, Md.: US Department of Health and Human Services, 1980.

Vogt, T. M., Selvin, S., Widdowson, G., & Hulley, S. B. Expired air carbon monoxide and serum thiocyanate as objective measures of cigarette exposure. *American Journal of Public Health, 1977, 67,* 545 – 549.

Wehrle, P. F., DeFreest, L., Penhollow, J., & Harris, V. G. The epidemiology of accidental poisoning in an urban population: The repeater problem in accidental poisoning. *Pediatrics, 1961, 27,* 614 – 619.

World Health Organization. *Social and health aspects of sexually transmitted diseases (Public Health Papers No. 65).* Belgium: World Health Organization, 1977.

3   Communication in Health Care

Rebecca Warner
University of New Hampshire

INTRODUCTION

Applied social psychology of health care has focused principally on the study of interpersonal relations (Friedman & DiMatteo, 1979). There are numerous facets to this theme that impact on a broad range of more traditional social – psychological phenomena. For example, the function of attribution in symptom recognition, self-blame, and placebo effects has been discussed in recent reviews (Janis & Rodin, 1979; Ross & Olson, 1981). Personal beliefs and their influence on health behaviors (Becker, Maiman, Kirscht, Haefner, Drachman, & Taylor, 1979; Wallston, Wallston, Kaplan, & Maides, 1976), social power of the physician (Janis & Rodin, 1979), reactance and noncooperative behaviors (Taylor, 1979), social isolation as a risk factor (Lynch, 1977), and the effects of illness on social relationships (Wortman & Dunkel-Schetter, 1979) are areas of investigation that reflect the traditions of applied social psychology in the medical arena. It is a growing field of study with a great deal of potential for future research.

To exemplify the breadth of applied social psychology in health care, this chapter focuses on communication. This is one problem area that has been investigated in depth from an interdisciplinary perspective. Medical anthropology, sociology, counseling psychology, communications and medicine have been concerned with communication and its impact on the delivery of health services. Studies have ranged from those examining face-to-face communication between practitioners and their patients to those utilizing communication technology to effect changes in risk behaviors. The problem of communication is central to the application of social – psychological research to health care.

Major Research Strategies

Four major types of research on communications in medicine have been done: (1) There are correlational studies in which the behaviors of patient and physician are systematically observed during a clinical interview; patient outcomes such as satisfaction, adherence to treatment regimen, and medical condition are assessed; and correlations between communication process and patient variables are examined (Korsch & Negrete, 1972). (2) There are experimental studies in which a treatment group receives a communication intervention that provides information and/or psychological support, and the outcomes of this treatment group are compared to the outcomes of a control group that received no special attention (Mumford, Schlesinger, & Glass, 1982). Such studies usually focus on a medical crisis event such as surgery or recovery from myocardial infarction; communication interventions are most frequently administered by nurses, although physicians, psychologists, anesthetists, and other personnel have also been used. (3) There are pretest – posttest studies in which medical students are exposed to an interview skills training program; assessments of attitudes or specific interview behaviors are made to evaluate the impact of training (Carroll & Monroe, 1979). (4) Moving away from this focus on face-to-face interaction, other investigators have been interested in evaluating the effectiveness of mass media health education programs in modifying risk factor behaviors such as smoking, diet, and exercise (Meyer, Nash, McAlister, Maccoby, & Farquhar, 1980). If mass media can be shown to be effective, then it may be possible to reach a larger number of persons at lower cost than is feasible through individual practitioner – patient contacts. The motivating rationale in these four research areas is similar in spirit if not in detail. In all instances, the concern is to design communication interventions with effective content and style, and to provide the most beneficial mixture of information, psychological support, and specific skills training. Each of these four research areas is reviewed in subsequent sections.

Patient Outcome Assessment

The problem of identifying and assessing patient outcomes is a methodological problem common to three of these four research domains. Several major classes of patient outcomes have been studied. These are: patient satisfaction with medical care (Hulka, 1979); adherence to therapeutic regimens (Haynes, Taylor, & Sackett, 1979); and medical outcomes such as postsurgical complications, speed of recovery, amount of medication requested, etc. (Mumford, Schlesinger, & Glass, 1982). In addition, psychological adjustment to chronic or terminal illness may be viewed as an important outcome of medical intervention (Kastenbaum, 1979). Other important nonmedical outcomes that have been considered by some investigators are termination of the doctor – patient relationship (Hayes-Bautista, 1976) and malpractice suits (Vaccarino, 1977). More generally, these outcomes can be described as beliefs or attitudes of the patient toward the physician and the treatment regimen; the health actions that the patient takes; the degree to which the disorder is managed or successfully cured; the emotional response of the patient; and the legal or contractual status of the practitioner – patient relationship. It is important to note that the priorities that the physician and patient have toward these goals may be different. The patient may place a higher value on emotional outcomes such as reduction of anxiety and distress, whereas the practitioner may be more concerned with successful management of a disorder (such as hypertension) that the patient is not particularly aware of as a problem.

The three major outcomes that have been most extensively studied (satisfaction, compliance, and medical outcomes) are obviously not independent (e.g., dissatisfaction may lead to noncompliance; noncompliance may lead to poor medical outcomes; poor medical outcomes may lead to dissatisfaction). Unraveling the direction of "causation" among these three outcome variables is difficult because they tend to be confounded. Each of these outcome variables poses special assessment problems.

Assessment of patient satisfaction with medical care is often used because paper and pencil questionnaires are easily administered. However, patients are often reluctant to express criticism, so ceiling effects and limited response variability are common. Furthermore, satisfaction may not be unidimensional; Hulka (1979) has devised one of the better known assessment procedures, in which three separate components are tapped: satisfaction with professional competence, with personal qualities of the physician, and with the convenience and cost of care. Respondents may provide more accurate information when they are asked about specific grievances (e.g., "Did the doctor use words that you could understand?") than when they are asked to give global satisfaction ratings (Korsch & Negrete, 1972).

Assessment of compliance with medical regimens is difficult, as self-reports tend to overestimate actual behavioral compliance, and objective measures such as pill counts and analysis of blood or urine are expensive. Furthermore, such assessments are probably reactive, because patients may be much more likely to comply when they know that their compliance can be accurately monitored (Gordis, 1979).

Medical outcome variables are often easy to observe but difficult to evaluate. Data on the length of hospital stay after surgery, frequency of requests for analgesics or tranquilizers, postsurgical complications, and so forth are relatively easy to obtain. However, it is debatable whether some of these outcome measures actually represent benefits (e.g., a speedy release from the hospital might not be optimal for all patients; failure to request analgesic medication does not necessarily imply that the patient is comfortable). Furthermore, the inconvenience and expense of long-term follow-ups leads to an overemphasis on short-term consequences, for which information is more easily obtained.

Studies reviewed in subsequent sections demonstrate that practitioner – patient communication can have an effect on all three types of outcomes. However, there are many other factors (severity of illness, complexity of treatment regimen, the emotional stability of the patient prior to illness, etc.) that are known to affect these outcomes. It is not clear how important doctor – patient communication processes are compared to other factors. However, unlike these other factors, the face-to-face communication process can be modified to improve outcomes (Taylor, 1978) and, therefore, knowledge about the relationship between communication process and patient outcomes is important, suggesting effective interventions.

CORRELATIONAL STUDIES OF COMMUNICATION PROCESS AND PATIENT OUTCOMES

Interview Structure

Stiles, Putnam, Wolf, and James (1979) outline three phases of the typical initial clinical interview: medical history, physical examination, and conclusion. These three phases are distinguished by different content, different interaction modes, and different goals. In the medical history phase the physician asks for a presenting complaint, explores some fairly standard content areas (see Enelow & Swisher, 1979, pp. 187 – 222), formulates hypotheses about the nature of the disorder, and decides what evidence is needed to confirm or disconfirm these hypotheses (Elstein & Bordage, 1979). In terms of style, this portion of the interview may be characterized as either directive or nondirective. A directive style occurs when the physician formulates hypotheses quickly and begins asking closed-ended yes-or-no questions to obtain evidence. This may be efficient if the initial guess was correct, but this closed-ended approach may make it difficult for patients to mention their greatest concerns or to introduce information that might lead to the formulation of different diagnostic hypotheses. By contrast, a less directive style occurs when the physician asks open-ended questions and encourages the patient to talk and ask questions. Evidence reviewed here suggests that this less directive style encourages active patient participation and leads to greater satisfaction and compliance. Furthermore, this form of interview need not result in a much longer interview than more direct questioning. Most of the research on interview style and most of the training in interview skills has focused primarily on the phase of the interview in which the physician is obtaining information from the patient.

The second phase found in most typical clinical interviews is the physical examination phase. During this phase, the physician collects further data to evaluate the diagnostic hypotheses. Relatively little work has been done on the interpersonal aspects of this phase of the interview. Physical examination techniques are generally taught separately from interviewing skills and interpersonal skills training (Kahn, Cohen, & Jason, 1979). There are suggestions in the literature that the way in which the practitioner touches the patient during examination may affect the patient's perceptions of the practitioner's concerns and feelings toward the patient (Blondis & Jackson, 1977).

In the conclusion phase, the physician gives information about the diagnosis and the treatment regimen; the patient gives acknowledgements and perhaps asks questions. The primary direction of information transmission thus shifts: from patient to physician early in the interview; from physician to patient later in the interview. Studies of physician – patient interaction suggest that a major source of dissatisfaction with the interview is inadequate information in the conclusion phase. The skills involved in transmitting information to the patient—particularly emotion-laden information—have not been included in the majority of the interview training programs in medical schools (Kahn et al., 1979). This appears to be an area where better knowledge and new intervention strategies are particularly needed.

Interview Style

Throughout the interview, information exchange is affected by interview style characteristics. Several features of information style have been identified as common sources of problems in practitioner – patient communication. The use of medical terminology or slang often creates communication gaps. Employing a questioning style that is excessively directive may prevent patients from being able to raise concerns, present information, or ask questions; it may force them into a passive role. Lack of ability to recognize and respond appropriately to patient anxiety, depression, or distress may be detrimental to patient outcomes in several ways: (a) it can lead to dissatisfaction; (b) the lack of rapport may prevent the practitioner from being able to obtain emotionally colored or potentially embarrassing information about symptoms or problems; and (c) lack of positive expectations and hope by the patient may lead to less positive response to treatment.

One way in which emotions may be communicated is through nonverbal channels such as facial expression, body position, gaze, touch, tone of voice, and interpersonal distance; the ability of the physician to encode and decode nonverbal emotional messages may be an important component of this ability to establish rapport. Subsequent sections of this chapter review the research that elaborates on each of these aspects of style.

Two major types of research have been done examining the relationship between communication process and patient outcome. The first approach involves systematic observation of the doctor – patient interaction, coding the actions of the doctor and the patient as instances of particular response modes (e.g., "seeks information" or "releases tension"), and looks for correlations between the frequency of use of various response types and patient outcomes. This coding process relies primarily on the verbal content of the communication actions, although some coding systems also make use of nonverbal behaviors (Bales, 1970). The second strategy is based on the premise that the ability to establish emotional rapport depends on physician skill in encoding and decoding nonverbal emotional messages; thus correlations between physician skill and patient satisfaction are examined (DiMatteo & Taranta, 1979).

Systematic Observational Studies

The landmark work in this area was done by Korsch and her associates (Francis, Korsch, & Morris, 1969; Freemon, Negrete, Davis, & Korsch, 1971; Korsch & Negrete, 1972) using a modified version of social interaction coding categories developed by social psychologist Freed Bales (1970). Bales listed twelve categories of behavior such as "seems friendly," "gives information," etc. Each action in the interview is coded as an instance of one of these 12 categories of actions. Nonverbal cues such as facial expression are used along with verbal content to make these coding decisions. Korsch and her associates coded 800 interviews between physicians and mothers who brought their infants to a pediatric clinic. Each mother was interviewed immediately after her interaction with the physician to assess her reaction to the physician and was followed up within 2 weeks to determine the extent to which she had complied with the physician's instructions. They also took additional information from the transcripts of the doctor – patient interactions. Their work documents some common communication problems and also demonstrates a positive relationship between effective communication and patient satisfaction and compliance.

Korsch and Negrete (1972) reported that overall, the majority of mothers (76%) reported that they were moderately or highly satisfied with the conference with the physician when they were asked for global satisfaction ratings. However, the mothers did voice many specific complaints in response to more specific questions. Nineteen percent of the mothers felt that they had not received a clear statement of what was wrong with the baby, and almost half were still unsure what had caused their child's illness. Examination of the transcripts showed that in many cases the physician had indeed failed to provide a clear diagnostic statement. In other cases, a diagnostic statement was given, but the mother was evidently too upset to listen. Twenty-six percent of the mothers told interviewers that they had not had an opportunity to mention their greatest concern to the physician, or were not encouraged to do so.

Detailed analysis of the Bales category system indicated that on the average, the physicians talked more than the mothers. Physicians displayed friendly behavior toward the mother less than 5% of the time. About 10% of the mothers' behaviors indicated nervousness or tension, but in a large number of cases the physician did not offer any reassurance in response to this display of anxiety.

Korsch and Negrete (1972) reported that sessions in which the mother asked questions and participated actively in the interview tended to have more successful outcomes (high satisfaction with the interview, and better compliance with instructions) than interviews in which the mother was a less active participant. Expression of friendly interest by the physician and attention to the mother's worries and concerns also led to better satisfaction and compliance. The overall length of the interviews did not correlate with the goodness of outcomes; but the interviewing style of the physician did.

Their research also documented the frequent use of confusing medical slang or technical terminology. Korsch and Negrete (1972) reported that in more than half of the interviews, physicians used technical terms (e.g., "Coombs titres," "antigen – antibody reactions") that were not understood by the mothers, or employed euphemistic phrases that were misinterpreted (e.g., the use of the term "explore" to refer to surgery). Other authors have provided additional documentation of difficulties that most patients have in comprehending medical terminology (Boyle, 1970; Samora, Saunders, & Larson, 1961). However, most patients have greater capability to comprehend explanations of their medical conditions than physicians believe they have, at least when these explanations are phrased in ordinary language (DiMatteo & Friedman, 1982, chap. 5).

The work of Korsch and her associates led to increased interest in systematically studying doctor – patient interaction, and training medical students in interpersonal skills.

Another research program that utilized a different coding system has found convergent evidence. Stiles et al. (1979) analyzed the verbal interaction between physicians and patients using Stiles' (1978) method of discourse analysis. He identified eight types of communication, based on a 2 times 2 times 2 typology (focus on speaker versus other; use of speaker or other's frame of reference; reference to experience of speaker or other). This coding system was applied separately to the three phases of the medical interview: medical history, physical examination, and conclusion. Factor analysis was used to identify various communication styles, each consisting of a cluster of specific communication behaviors (e.g., "exposition" or "feedback" styles). The affective satisfaction of patients was positively correlated to an "exposition" style during the medical history phase; this corresponds to an open-ended, nondirective interviewing style in which the patient is allowed to tell his or her story. Patient cognitive satisfaction was positively associated with a "feedback" mode during the conclusion of the interview (this mode consisted of provision of information by the physician, and acknowledgement and questioning by the patient). The single behavior by the physician that correlated most strongly with patient satisfaction was "edification," or providing information in the conclusion segment. These results are consistent with those of Korsch et al., because they point to the importance of the following aspects of the interview: opportunity for the patient to express concerns and ask questions, taking an active role in the interview; and provision of adequate information about the medical condition and treatment regimen. Stiles et al. (1979) also concluded that interview length per se was not a crucial determinant of satisfaction; rather, a style that maximized patient participation was most conducive to satisfaction.

Not all studies have collected direct observational data on the physician – patient interaction. Some have examined indirect evidence as a means of describing communication effectiveness. For instance, Hulka (1979) and her associates have used the accuracy of the medical practitioner's predictions of patient response to each item on a questionnaire about concerns as an indication of how effective the communication process was. Along different lines, Schulman (1979) asked patients to evaluate their medical treatment in terms of the degree to which the patient felt like an active participant: she found that patients who perceived themselves as highly actively involved showed much better management of hypertension and reported higher adoption of many health-enhancing behaviors. Although these studies provide less direct information about the actual communication process, they illustrate complementary methods of looking at the relationship between communication and outcome.

Sensitivity to Nonverbal Cues

DiMatteo and Taranta (1979) have suggested that it may be possible to define "empathy" more specifically by looking for specific skills that contribute to accurate perception of patient's emotions, effective communication of concern for the patiénts, and positive expectations about treatment outcome. Because nonverbal behaviors (such as facial expression, body movement, gaze, touch, tone of voice, and interpersonal distance) are often self-consciously less controlled than verbal content, it is thought that people often "leak" their feelings of distress or uneasiness over deception through nonverbal behaviors. Through attention to these nonverbal cues, particularly when they are discrepant with the verbal messages, a medical practitioner may acquire valuable information about the patient's emotional state (Blondis & Jackson, 1977; Enelow & Swisher, 1979, pp. 55 – 61). Nonverbal communication channels may be particularly important when the patient is unable to communicate verbally (due to speech disorder, surgical interventions such as tracheotomy, etc.).

The confusing and frustrating aspect of the nonverbal communication literature, when it is consulted as a guide for action, is that it does not provide comprehensive "dictionaries" telling what each facial expression or gesture means. (Ekman & Friesen, 1975, have attempted to provide a dictionary for the emotional meanings of facial expressions, but the validity of some of their suggested meanings has been challenged.) The meaning of a given nonverbal action (such as touching someone on the hand, or raising the pitch of the voice, or positioning oneself within 3 feet of the conversation partner) differs depending on the cultural context, the social relationship between the interactors, and so forth (Weitz, 1979). There are, of course, some gestures that are fairly easily decoded (e.g., frequently touching a body part may indicate pain; grooming gestures such as pulling up the socks, adjusting necktie, and smoothing the hair may indicate flirtation between therapist and client; etc.). However, there are other gestures whose meaning is more variable, such as a touch on the hand. This kind of touch is interpreted very differently depending on whether it is perceived as socially appropriate, and whether it conveys comfort, social dominance, sexual intimacy, impersonal examination (as in taking the pulse), or administration of a potentially painful treatment. Lynch (1977) reports that patients in a CCU who are touched by a nurse show dramatic changes in heart rate; some show increased heart rate and more arrhythmia (as they evidently interpret the touch as threatening in some way); others show decreased heart rate and less arrhythmia. Similar disparities in response were found by Whitcher and Fisher (1979), a study that is discussed later in this chapter.

In spite of the fact that there are many nonverbal gestures whose meaning cannot be determined outside of the interaction context in which they occur, it is possible to study the impact of nonverbal communications on physician – patient rapport. The most fruitful approach has been assessment of nonverbal sensitivity of the physician (DiMatteo & Taranta, 1979). The Profile of Nonverbal Sensitivity (PONS) test (Rosenthal, Hall, DiMatteo, Rogers, & Archer, 1979) provides an assessment of skills in decoding nonverbal communication. To create the PONS, an actress was videotaped acting out various scenarios involving positive or negative emotions; test stimuli were produced by isolating several nonverbal communication channels (face alone, no voice; body from neck to knees, no voice; face and body down to thighs, no voice; electronically content-filtered voice, no picture; and randomized spliced voice, no picture). Each stimulus presented included one or two of these five channels. After presentation of each stimulus, the test respondent is asked to choose between two descriptions of the scenario, and points are given for correct choices. Separate scores are given for accuracy in each of the five channels, as well as overall accuracy. Extensive work has been done to establish the reliability and validity of this test (Rosenthal et al., 1979).

DiMatteo and Taranta (1979) reported that physicians who score high on the body channels of the PONS (i.e., those who are adept at judging emotion from body movement and posture) were rated as more caring and sensitive by their patients, $r = + .35$. Ability to judge emotions from facial expressions and tone of voice was not significantly correlated to patient satisfaction. Thus, one specific decoding skill appears to be a predictor of patient satisfaction.

DiMatteo and Taranta (1979) also considered skill of physicians in encoding emotions. Each physician was asked to communicate three neutral sentences in four different affective states (happiness, sadness, anger, surprise); videotapes of their portrayals were shown to student judges, and the proportion of judges who were able to correctly identify the intended emotion served as an index of each physician's encoding skill. Physicians' ability to encode positive emotions (happiness and surprise) correlated positively with patient satisfaction (DiMatteo & Taranta, 1979). Along similar lines, Milmoe, Rosenthal, Blane, Chafetz, & Wolf (1967) found that physicians whose tone of voice suggested concern for the patient were more successful in getting patients to follow through on referrals to an alcoholism treatment program than physicians whose voice tone suggested a businesslike, impersonal attitude toward the patient.

A somewhat less productive approach to analysis of nonverbal communication between physicians and patients involves observer ratings of the frequency of certain nonverbal behaviors (eye contact, bodily positioning, touch) during medical interviews. Comstock, Hooper, Goodwin, and Goodwin (1982) found no correlation between these nonverbal communication variables and patient satisfaction. They did find that satisfaction was related to other interview style features such as physician courtesy (formally greeting and discharging the patient), and with information-giving and listening behavior. It appears that simply looking at the frequency of certain nonverbal behaviors (such as touch) is not sufficient; however, assessment of the skilled and appropriate use of such behaviors may be useful, along lines suggested by the work of DiMatteo and Taranta (1979).

COMMUNICATION INTERVENTION STUDIES

The correlation studies reviewed in the previous section looked at existing communication patterns and attempted to identify those components of interaction style that are good predictors of patient outcome. In this section, evaluation of communication interventions, mostly in the context of field experiments, is discussed.

Mumford et al. (1982) noted two major kinds of communication intervention frequently employed with surgical and myocardial infarction patients: information provision and psychological support. The 34 studies included in their review each compared a treatment group that received special attention from a health care practitioner, to a control group that received ordinary care. The interventions were most commonly delivered by nurses, although physicians and psychologists were the care providers in other studies. A typical communication intervention package includes many components. Kendall and Watson (1981) outlined these components as follows: (1) psychological support, often in the form of brief individual psychotherapy (Gruen, 1975); (2) provision of information about medical procedures or sensory experience such as pain (Egbert, Battit, Welch, & Bartlett, 1964); (3) training in specific skills such as diaphragmatic breathing, leg and foot exercises, etc. (Lindeman & Van Aernam, 1971); (4) hypnosis and relaxation training (Miller, 1977); (5) observation of filmed models undergoing medical procedures (Shipley, Butt, Horwitz, & Farbry, 1978); and (6) cognitive – behavioral interventions to affect attention to pain and sense of personal control (Langer, Janis, & Wolfer, 1975). Any particular intervention package often includes more than one of these components. This confounding of variables makes it difficult to evaluate which component was necessary for the observed improvement in patient outcome.

Mumford et al. (1982) reviewed selected studies that employed reasonably good experimental controls and found evidence that both information provision and psychological support interventions had beneficial impact. Effect size (ES) is the difference between the treatment and control group means, divided by the standard deviation of the control group. They used average ES as a means of summarizing results across these studies that employed so many different patient populations, intervention strategies, and outcome variables. Intervention packages that included both information provision and psychological support were more effective on the average than interventions that used only information or only psychological support. For these combined interventions, ES was plus .65 (i.e., the treatment group scored more than half a standard deviation above the control group, averaged across outcome variables and across studies). In terms of specific benefits, they reported that communication intervention groups tended to have durations of hospitalization approximately 2 days shorter than control groups. None of these studies provided any detailed information about the practitioner–patient interaction. The emphasis was more on program content than practitioner skill.

A specific example of an intervention derived from social psychological background is the widely cited study by Langer et al. (1975). Two types of intervention with surgical patients were included: a preparatory information package (information about skin preparation, elimination, preoperative medication, anesthesia, and expectations about the postoperative experience); and a cognitive coping device (involving selective attention, self-distraction from pain, and stressing a sense of patient control over the experience of pain). Four groups were included in a factorial design: no treatment, information only, coping device only, and both information and coping device. They found that patient outcomes such as staff ratings of anxiety and ability to cope, requests for pain relievers or sedatives, and length of hospitalization were favorably affected by the coping device, but that the preparatory information produced no significant effects. Langer et al. noted that it was not possible to infer from this study whether the apparently beneficial effects of the coping device were due to increased perception of control over pain, or distraction, or some combination of these factors.

Another field experiment that derived its rationale from social psychology compared surgical patients who were touched on the hand by the nurse during an educational session to patients who were not touched (Whitcher & Fisher, 1979). Based on the social — psychological literature about touch as a means of conveying intimacy and dominance, they expected to find that the effect of touch would depend on whether the touch was perceived as socially appropriate. They reasoned that women are accustomed to being touched and tend to interpret touch as a supportive or comforting gesture; whereas men are touched less often and may interpret touch as an attempt to dominate, or as a sexual advance, and therefore find touch threatening and upsetting. Their results were consistent with this rationale; they found that female patients who were touched by the nurse had more favorable outcomes (lower blood pressure, read more of an instruction booklet, etc.) than female patients who were not touched. Male patients who were touched showed less favorable reactions than male patients who were not touched. This study is unusual among intervention studies, in that it isolated one specific variable (touch) rather than using a multicomponent intervention.

A few of the methodological problems in the assessment of communication interventions have been mentioned. Most of these studies employ interventions with multiple components, making it impossible to sort out the contributions of the various components. Often the intervention program is provided by a single practitioner, so that practitioner interpersonal style and skill are confounded with other aspects of the intervention. Not all studies provide adequate controls (control groups should receive some form of attention) to control for the possibility that the apparent benefit of the intervention is not due merely to the extra attention. It is often impossible to randomly assign subjects to groups, and evaluation of nonequivalent control group designs is difficult (Cook & Campbell, 1979). There may be ethical objections to withholding a potentially valuable intervention from some patients in order to assess its effects. If treatment and control patients are on the same wards, they may be aware of the differences in treatment received, and the control group may actually be a "resentment" group, as Campbell suggested. Finally, an intervention may not affect all patients in the same way (as illustrated by Whitcher & Fisher, 1979). For instance, Auerbach, Kendall, Cuttler, and Levitt (1976) found that persons who score in the external direction on the Rotter Locus of Control scale adjust better if they are given general information about treatment, whereas internals adjust better if they are given specific information.

Mumford et al. (1982) cited five additional studies that suggest that the benefits of intervention vary according to the individual coping style of the patient. They suggested that the reason that interventions combining information provision and psychological support appeared to be more effective overall than interventions that provided information only or psychological support only was that this combination increased the chance of meeting the individual needs of more patients.

The studies reviewed here, and the more extensive reviews by Mumford et al. (1982) and Kendall and Watson (1981), demonstrate the efficacy of providing patients with additional opportunities to interact with medical practitioners, information, and psychological support.

INTERVIEW SKILLS TRAINING PROGRAMS

The research reviewed so far indicates that interpersonal skills can contribute to better patient outcomes. The next question considered is whether these interpersonal skills are teachable. In a recent survey of 4-year medical schools in the United States, Kahn, et al. (1979) found that about 68% of the medical schools had training in interpersonal skills and that the majority of these programs had been established since 1974. Most teachers are psychologists or psychiatrists, and the courses are taught mostly during preclinical years with rather little follow-up during the clinical years. Almost all the programs used videotaping of real or simulated patient interviews as demonstrations of desirable interview behaviors, or as a means of providing students with feedback about their own interview behaviors. Detailed questions about the specific skills being taught show that the majority of programs emphasized skills such as listening, observing, responding, information gathering, demonstrating empathy, providing psychological support, and responding to patient feelings. (Kahn et al. remarked that there may have been a bias toward overinclusion when program administrators were asked to report on the skills being taught, however.) By contrast, less than one-third of the programs included any training on information giving, counseling, sharing diagnostic findings, giving advice, or educating patients; and less than one-quarter dealt specifically with such issues as suicide prevention, sexual counseling, death and dying, etc.

Carroll and Monroe (1979) surveyed 73 studies on teaching medical interviewing and arrived at the following conclusions. Overall, instruction in medical interviewing had promoted significant gains in interviewing skills (as assessed by a variety of self-report and behavioral measures). Although most programs were intended to facilitate nondirective interviewing, many different conceptualizations were evident. The majority of studies evaluating the impact of training were one-group pretest − posttest studies. This design does not adequately control for the effects of history, maturation, testing, instrumentation, and other threats to internal validity (Cook & Campbell, 1979).

Five studies that used true experimental designs were reviewed by Carroll and Monroe (1980), and most showed improvements in interview skills after training. Carroll and Monroe (1980) argued that the use of videotaped feedback to provide students with information about their own interview behaviors was an essential component of interview skills training. Standardized presentations were probably more useful than live, spontaneous demonstrations of patient interviews. They also concluded that programs that included specific statements of skills tended to be more effective than programs that were less structured. They pointed out the need for more research to identify specific interpersonal skills; to define the proper role of adjunct instructions; to evaluate the long-term retention of skills; and to assess the impact of instruction in interviewing on actual patient outcomes.

The majority of the training programs that report a specifically psychological rationale are based on counseling psychology, particularly work by Kagan (1979) and Truax and Carkhuff (1967). Kagan (1979) has developed a method called Interaction Process Recall (IPR), in which a student is videotaped while interviewing a patient; afterward, the student reviews the tape with the assistance of an instructor, who asks the student to recall feelings that were experienced at various points in the interview and teaches the student to recognize specific questioning strategies that are more and less effective. Kagan outlined four types of physician responses to patients: exploratory, listening, feeling, and honest labeling responses. Kagan has developed a rating scale to evaluate interview behaviors and assess the extent to which training program goals have been realized. Modified versions of his system have been widely adopted (Kagan, 1979; Robbins, Kauss, Heinrich, Abrass, Dreyer, & Clyman, 1979; Werner & Schneider, 1974; Kauss, Robbins, Heinrich, & Abrass, 1981).

Truax and Carkhuff (1967) have also been influential, although their original work dealt with communication effectiveness in psychotherapy rather than medicine. Their research on communication skills and psychotherapy outcome led them to argue that three aspects of communication style were associated with better patient outcomes: accurate empathy, genuineness, and nonpossessive warmth. They developed rating scales to assess these skills in the context of clinical interviews, and modified versions of their scales have been employed in the assessment of medical interviewing courses.

Yet another approach to the assessment of interview behavior is the Brockway rating scale (Brockway, 1978). The components of this rating system include relationship skills (e.g., eye contact, body posture, questioning style); and problem solving skills (statement of goals for session, checking on patient information, requesting information about health of other family members, etc.). Based on limited data ($N = 10$), Brockway suggested that the interpersonal and problem-solving components of physician skills are not significantly correlated. The assumption that these components of interview skill are independent seems like an important question both from a pragmatic and a theoretical perspective. This deserves further study.

Rather few programs have attempted to teach information giving or patient education skills. It has been suggested that role playing with simulated patients is an effective way to teach medical students how to convey emotion-laden information (Woolraich, Albanese, Reiter-Thayer, & Barratt, 1981; Woolraich & Reiter, 1979). This problem merits attention, particularly because studies cited in earlier sections indicated that information giving and psychological support influence patient satisfaction and compliance (Korsch & Negrete, 1972; Stiles, 1978). Typically, patients say that they prefer more detailed disclosures about medical conditions than physicians routinely offer (Faden, Becker, Lewis, Freeman, & Faden, 1981). Discussion of issues that arise when dealing with chronically or terminally ill patients is offered by Wortman and Dunkel-Schetter (1979) and Kastenbaum (1979). A key problem with disclosure of negative information (such as surgical risks or side effects of drugs) is that negative placebo effects may occur when negative expectancies are suggested to the patient (Loftus & Fries, 1979).

THE ROLE OF MASS MEDIA IN HEALTH EDUCATION

Up to this point in the discussion, only the face-to-face interpersonal aspects of medicine have been considered. The question has arisen whether it is possible to effectively improve the health beliefs, knowledge, and actions of a wider audience through mass media communication programs that are far less expensive on a per-person basis than face-to-face instructional programs. Social psychologists have been among the contributors in this research area.

The Health Belief Model

The Health Belief Model (HBM) is a theoretical formulation that was developed in the early 1950s by social psychologists (including Hochbaum, Kegeles, Leventhal, & Rosenstock) to address the problem of how people's beliefs affect their involvement in preventive health behaviors, medical help seeking, and compliance with medical regimens (Kirscht & Rosenstock, 1979; Rosenstock & Kirscht, 1979). Its essential elements were recently reviewed by Becker et al. (1979). The HBM is a value expectancy theory involving valence (perceived attractiveness of the goal) and subjective probability (personal estimate of likelihood of goal attainment). Whether or not an individual engages in a particular behavior (such as quitting smoking) is theoretically related to beliefs about: (1) level of personal susceptibility to illness; (2) perceived severity of illness; (3) the health action's potential benefits or perceived efficacy in reducing susceptibility; and (4) perceived barriers or costs associated with the health action. The theory also suggests that cues to action (either internal cues such as symptoms, or external cues such as mass media messages) are necessary to trigger the health action, by making the health threat salient. The original HBM formulation has undergone revisions to make it applicable to specific situations, such as pediatric compliance (Becker et al., 1979).

The implications of the HBM have been extensively researched. Positive correlations have been found between patient compliance and health beliefs in many, although not all, of these studies. Based on the HBM, there has been speculation that compliance and other health behaviors might be modifiable through provision of information that affects the health beliefs specified as the essential elements of the HBM. Most designers of health education campaigns share this fundamental assumption (that behavior can be modified through changes in health knowledge and attitudes), and many of them have used the HBM as a guide for selection of target beliefs.

During the 1950s and 1960s there was great interest in the efficacy of fear-arousing communications (which included information intended to heighten perceived susceptibility and/or perceived severity of the illness) (Dabbs & Leventhal, 1966; Leventhal & Niles, 1964). Some studies also included information about the efficacy of specifically recommended health actions, or specific skills training (such as methods for flossing teeth), or information intended to reduce perceived barriers to action. According to the original HBM formulation, high threat messages ought to increase the likelihood that the individual will engage in health action. The majority of the fears arousal studies reviewed by Leventhal (1970) did find that increased fear led to greater expressed intention to take health action. However, a substantial minority of these fear-arousal studies have found curvilinear or negative relationships between fear arousal and health action (Janis & Feshbach, 1953). It has been suggested that if fear is aroused and there is no effective course of action available to deal with fear, denial may occur, blocking rational and effective action to deal with the threat. This controversy about the effects of fear arousal on health action has never been entirely resolved. Furthermore, although fear arousal may be an acceptable means of trying to motivate healthy people to floss their teeth, it seems like an inappropriate strategy to adopt with high risk or seriously ill persons, who may already be distressed and fearful.

More recent interventions still reflect the influence of the Health Belief Model in many cases, but they frequently focus more on the efficacy of health actions and the specific behavioral and social skills that are helpful in carrying out the health actions (Evans, 1980).

There are some additional problems with HBM as a rationale for intervention. First of all, the majority of the existing studies focus on changes in attitudes or beliefs rather than actual changes in health behavior (Leventhal, 1970, p. 135). There is not always a close association between health beliefs, expressed intentions to engage in health actions, and actual health behaviors (Evans, 1980). One study suggests that health beliefs develop along with health behavior, and that health beliefs do not precede and determine health actions (Taylor, in Becker et al., 1979). If this is so, then efforts to modify health behavior solely through provision of information to change health beliefs may not be very successful.

To summarize, available data suggest that the health beliefs that correspond to elements of the HBM are correlated with health actions. However, behavior cannot always be changed simply by providing information; it is also necessary to motivate or persuade people to take action, and sometimes to train them in specific skills. Although fear arousal may be an appropriate method of increasing motivation for relatively innocuous problems (such as motivating healthy people to wear seat belts, floss their teeth, or take tetanus shots), it seems inappropriate for high risk persons, and it is incompatible with the goal of "providing psychological support" to patients that was articulated earlier. It may be possible to appeal to more positive motivations (the feelings of well-being that result from better diet and exercise, cosmetic or social motivations for health, etc.; Rosenstock & Kirscht, 1979). Information about illness, the efficacy of health actions, and the specific instructions about health diet and life-style appear to be a necessary, but not sufficient condition for behavior change. Recent mass media health education campaigns have done much more than merely provide information; they have supplemented information with other elements such as skills training and social support (e.g., the North Karelia Project, McAlister, Puska, Salonen, Tuomilehto, & Koskela, 1982).

Mass Media Health Education Campaigns

Two major ongoing projects examine multifaceted interventions designed to modify cardiovascular risk factor behaviors, particularly smoking, diet, and exercise: the North Karelia Project in Finland (McAlister et al., 1982) and the Stanford Heart Disease Prevention Project (SHDPP, Meyer et al., 1980).

The North Karelia Project was intended to affect cardiovascular risk factors in an entire province. The project has six major objectives: improved preventive services, health information, persuasion to motivate people to take health actions, skills training, community organization, and environmental change. The strategies developed for dissemination of information and persuasion are compatible with the HBM and other social-psychological approaches to persuasion. For instance, based on the "communications" approach to persuasion (that focuses on source credibility and message content), endorsements by prestigious individuals and organizations were sought, and messages were carefully designed to anticipate and suppress counterargument. Any fear-provoking messages (such as informing certain individuals that they belonged to a high risk category) were accompanied by clear and attainable recommendations for fear reduction, as suggested by the HBM. The "affective" approach to persuasion relied on emotional associations and appealed to provincial pride (e.g., "Do it for North Karelia"). The "behavioral" approach to persuasion involved asking everyone associated with the project to make at least minor behavioral commitments, such as displaying stickers and posters. Information, persuasion, and skills training were provided through many media including newspapers, radio, television, formal and informal group meetings. In addition to the messages directed at individuals, the project attempted to generate social support for the program by using family units and existing social networks; and major environmental changes were accomplished, such as promoting the development of entirely new low cholesterol meat and dairy products.

Difficulties arise in evaluating the impact of the North Karelia project because it was designed to be a demonstration, rather than a vehicle for testing social psychological theories. The confounding of the many components of the intervention makes it difficult to evaluate the specific contributions of mass media educational campaigns to the overall reduction in risk factors that was reported (Klos & Rosenstock, 1982; Wagner, 1982). Furthermore, it is difficult to disentangle the effects of their intervention from the general international trend toward reduction of cardiovascular risk factors.

The Stanford Heart Disease Prevention Project was somewhat smaller in scale and had more of the characteristics of a field experiment (Meyer et al., 1980). A comparison was made among risk factor reduction rates in towns that received a mass media health campaign only; a town that received mass media supplemented by face-to-face instruction for selected high risk individuals; and a town that received neither mass media nor face-to-face instruction. Their targets were cardiovascular risk factor behaviors such as smoking, diet, and exercise. In the mass media program, radio and television spots, newspapers, and other printed materials were used to disseminate information about the probable causes of cardiovascular disease and specific risk factor behaviors. The face-to-face instruction package varied from individual to individual including components such as smoking cessation counseling, dietary instruction, prescriptions of aerobic activity. Behavior modification and social learning principles were the basis for most of this instruction.

Meyer et al. reported that the mass media plus face-to-face instruction subjects showed the greatest risk factor reduction; however, mass media alone was reported to have a significant impact on risk factor reduction in the target communities.

Evaluated as a field experiment, this study has methodological shortcomings that limit the conclusions that can be drawn (Leventhal, Safer, Cleary, & Gutmann, 1980). However, it serves as a unique demonstration that mass media alone may be an effective tool for modification of risk factor behavior. This finding is important because it calls into question the pessimistic assertions that have been made about the effectiveness of mass media for behavior change (e.g., Etzioni, 1972; and the literature on selective attention and selective exposure reviewed by Milburn, 1979). This study suggests that mass media alone may be an effective method for reducing risk factor behaviors at relatively low cost per individual; but clearly, even greater effectiveness is possible when mass media are supplemented with additional skills training and other face-to-face interventions.

Smaller Scale Intervention

Evans (1980) has developed a program to deter the onset of smoking in adolescents that is derived from the same general theoretical background as the social psychology of persuasion, but that also incorporates some novel features. His program emphasizes social skills training for adolescents to help them to anticipate and cope with the social pressures to smoke from peers, adult models such as parents, and mass media advertisements. He also notes that most health threat messages usually used to discourage smoking focus on distant future outcomes (such as lung cancer) that are not meaningful to teenagers. Instead, his program focuses on the immediate effects of smoking, such as carbon monoxide in the breath. Evans and his associates have demonstrated that a videotaped program incorporating the social skills training appears to be an effective deterrent to the onset of smoking. His work suggests new directions for health education: away from information-centered, fear-arousing communications, and toward the development of skills for coping with social pressures for poor health habits.

SUMMARY

The research reviewed here leads to several conclusions. It is clear that the interpersonal skills of medical practitioners can affect patient satisfaction, compliance with medical regimens, and medical outcomes. Systematic observational studies have identified common problem areas in communication, such as the use of medical terminology; an excessively directive questioning style; failure to respond to emotional concerns of patients; and inadequate information provision during the conclusion phase of the interview. Intervention studies have shown that communication packages that provide additional information and psychological support can be beneficial to patients in a variety of situations. Assessment of medical curriculum indicates that the interpersonal skills that have been identified as targets for training can be improved through education; however, most training programs seem to underemphasize information-giving skills, and the survey by Kahn et al., (1979) suggests that more follow-up of interpersonal skills training during the clinical years is needed. Finally, although there is some evidence that mass media health education campaigns that primarily provide information may have an impact on health behaviors, it is clear that greater benefits are obtained when mass media campaigns are supplemented by face-to-face instruction and social support. Interventions that combine psychological support, skills training, and other features generally appear to be more effective than communication interventions that only provide information.

REFERENCES

Auerbach, S. M., Kendall, P. C., Cuttler, H. F., & Levitt, N. R. Anxiety, locus of control, type of preparatory information, and adjustment to dental surgery. *Journal of Consulting and Clinical Psychology*, 1976, *44*, 809 – 818.

Bales, R. F. *Personality and interpersonal behavior.* New York: Holt, 1970.

Becker, M. H., Maiman, L. A., Kirscht, J. P., Haefner, D. P., Drachman, R. H., & Taylor, D. W. Patient perceptions and compliance: Recent studies of the Health Belief Model. In R. B. Haynes, D. W. Taylor, & D. L. Sackett (Eds.), *Compliance in health care.* Baltimore: Johns Hopkins University Press, 1979.

Blondis, M. N., & Jackson, B. E. *Nonverbal communication with patients.* New York: John Wiley, 1977.

Boyle, C. M. Differences between patients' and doctors' interpretations of some common medical terms. *British Journal of Medicine,* 1970, *2*, 286 – 289.

Brockway, B. S. Evaluating physician competency: What difference does it make? *Evaluation and Program Planning,* 1978, *1*, 211 – 220.

Carroll, J. G., & Monroe, J. Teaching medical interviewing: A critique of educational research and practice. *Journal of Medical Education,* 1979, *54*, 498 – 500.

Carroll, J. G., & Monroe, J. Teaching clinical interviewing in the health professions: A review of empirical research. *Evaluation and the Health Professions,* 1980, *3*, 21 – 45.

Comstock, L. M., Hooper, E. M., Goodwin, J. M., & Goodwin, J. S. Physician behaviors that correlate with patient satisfaction. *Journal of Medical Education,* 1982, *57*, 105 – 112.

Cook, T. D., & Campbell, D. T. *Quasi-experimentation: Design and analysis issues for field settings.* Chicago: Rand McNally, 1979.

Dabbs, J. M., & Leventhal, H. Effects of varying the recommendations in a fear arousing communication. *Journal of Personality and Social Psychology,* 1966, *4*, 525 – 531.

DiMatteo, M. R., & Friedman, H. S. *Social psychology and medicine.* Cambridge, Mass.: Oelgeschlager, Gunn, & Hain, 1982.

DiMatteo, M. R., & Taranta, A. Nonverbal communication and physician – patient rapport: An empirical study. *Professional Psychology,* 1979, *10*, 540 – 547.

Egbert, L. D., Battit, G. E., Welch, C. E., & Bartlett, M. K. Reduction of post – operative pain by encouragement and instruction of patients: A study of doctor – patient rapport. *New England Journal of Medicine,* 1964, *270*, 825 – 827.

Ekman, P., & Friesen, W. V. *Unmasking the face.* Englewood Cliffs, N.J.: Prentice – Hall, 1975.

Elstein, A. S., & Bordage, G. Psychology of clinical reasoning. In G. Stone, F. Cohen, & N. Adler (Eds.), *Health psychology.* San Francisco: Jossey – Bass, 1979.

Enelow, A. J., & Swisher, S. N. *Interviewing and patient care* (2nd ed.). New York: Oxford University Press, 1979.

Etzioni, A. *Human beings are not very easy to change after all.* Saturday Review, June 3, 1972.

Evans, R. I. Behavioral medicine: A new applied challenge to social psychologists. In L. Bickman (Ed.), *Applied social psychology annual I.* Beverly Hills, Calif.: Sage, 1980.

Faden, R. R., Becker, C., Lewis, C., Freeman, J., & Faden, A. I. Disclosure of information to patients in medical care. *Medical Care,* 1981, *19,* 718 – 733.

Francis, V., Korsch, B. M., & Morris, M. J. Gaps in doctor – patient communication: Patients' response to medical advice. *New England Journal of Medicine,* 1969, *280,* 535 – 540.

Freemon, B., Negrete, V. F., Davis, M., & Korsch, B. M. Gaps in doctor – patient communication: Doctor – patient interaction analysis. *Pediatric Research,* 1971, *5,* 298 – 311.

Friedman, H. S., & DiMatteo, R. M. Health care as an interpersonal process. *Journal of Social Issues,* 1979, *35,* 1 – 11.

Gordis, L. Conceptual and methodological problems in measuring inpatient compliance. In R. B. Haynes, D. W. Taylor, & D. L. Sackett (Eds.), *Compliance in health care.* Baltimore: Johns Hopkins Press, 1979.

Gruen, W. Effects of brief psychotherapy during the hospitalization period on the recovery process in heart attacks. *Journal of Consulting and Clinical Psychology,* 1975, *43,* 223 – 232.

Hayes-Bautista, D. E. Termination of the patient – practitioner relationship: Divorce, patient style. *Journal of Health and Social Behavior,* 1976, *17,* 12 – 21.

Haynes, R. B., Taylor, D. W., & Sackett, D. L. (Eds.). *Compliance in health care.* Baltimore: Johns Hopkins University Press, 1979.

Hulka, B. S. Patient – clinician interactions and compliance. In R. B. Haynes, D. W. Taylor, & D. L. Sackett (Eds.), *Compliance in health care.* Baltimore: Johns Hopkins University Press, 1979.

Janis, I. L., & Feshbach, S. Effects of fear arousing communications. *Journal of Abnormal Psychology,* 1953, *48,* 78 – 92.

Janis, I. L., & Rodin, J. Attribution, control and decision making: Social psychology and health care. In G. Stone, F. Cohen, & N. Adler (Eds.), *Health psychology.* San Francisco: Jossey – Bass, 1979.

Kagan, N. Counseling psychology, interpersonal skills, and health care. In G. Stone, F. Cohen, & N. Adler (Eds.), *Health psychology.* San Francisco: Jossey – Bass, 1979.

Kahn, G., Cohen, B., & Jason, H. The teaching of interpersonal skills in US medical schools. *Journal of Medical Education,* 1979, *54,* 29 – 35.

Kastenbaum, R. "Health dying": A paradoxical quest continues. *Journal of Social Issues,* 1979, *35,* 185 – 206.

Kauss, D. R., Robbins, A. S., Heinrich, R., & Abrass, I. Interpersonal skills training: Comprehensive approach versus brief instruction. *Journal of Medical Education,* 1981, *56,* 663 – 665.

Kendall, D. C., & Watson, D. Psychological preparation for stressful medical procedures. In C. K. Prokop & L. A. Bradley (Eds.), *Medical psychology: Contributions to behavioral medicine.* New York: Academic Press, 1981.

Kirscht, J. P., & Rosenstock, I. M. Patients' problems in following recommendations of health experts. In G. Stone, F. Cohen, & N. Adler (Eds.), *Health psychology.* San Francisco: Jossey – Bass, 1979.

Klos, D. M., & Rosenstock, I. M. Some lessons from the North Karelia project. *American Journal of Public Health,* 1982, *72,* 53 – 54.

Korsch, B. M., & Negrete, V. F. Doctor – patient communication. *Scientific American,* 1972, *227,* 67 – 74.

Langer, E. J., Janis, I. L., & Wolfer, J. A. Reduction of psychological stress in surgical patients. *Journal of Experimental Social Psychology,* 1975, *11,* 155 – 165.

Leventhal, H. Findings and theory in the study of fear arousing communications. In L. Berkowitz (Ed.), *Advances in experimental social psychology* (Vol. 5). New York: Academic Press, 1970.

Leventhal, H., & Niles, P. A field experiment on fear arousal with data on the reliability of questionnaire measures. *Journal of Personality,* 1964, *32,* 459 – 479.

Leventhal, H., Safer, M. A., Cleary, P. D., & Gutmann, M. Cardiovascular risk modification by community-based programs for lifestyle change: Comments on the Stanford study. *Journal of Consulting and Clinical Psychology*, 1980, *48*, 150–158.

Lindeman, C. A., & Van Aernam, B. Nursing intervention with the presurgical patient—the effects of structured and unstructured preoperative teaching. *Nursing Research*, 1971, *20*, 319–331.

Loftus, E. F., & Fries, J. F. Informed consent may be hazardous to health. *Science*, 1979, *204*, 11.

Lynch, J. J. *The broken heart: The medical consequences of loneliness.* New York: Basic Books, 1977.

McAlister, A., Puska, P., Salonen, J. T., Tuomilehto, J., & Koskela, K. Theory and action for health promotion: Illustrations from the North Karelia project. *American Journal of Public Health*, 1982, *72*, 43–50.

Meyer, A. J., Nash, J. D., McAlister, A. L., Maccoby, N., & Farquhar, J. W. Skills training in a cardiovascular health education campaign. *Journal of Consulting and Clinical Psychology*, 1980, *48*, 129–142.

Milburn, M. A. A longitudinal test of the selective exposure hypothesis. *Public Opinion Quarterly*, 1979, *43*, 507–517.

Miller, M. P. The effects of electromyographic feedback and progressive relaxation training on stress reactions in dental patients. (Doctoral dissertation, University of Oklahoma, 1976.) *Dissertation Abstracts International*, 1977, *37*, 6340B.

Milmoe, E., Rosenthal, R., Blane, H. T., Chafetz, M. L., & Wolf, I. The doctor's voice: Postdictor of successful referral of alcoholic patients. *Journal of Abnormal Psychology*, 1967, *72*, 78–84.

Mumford, E., Schlesinger, H. J., & Glass, G. V. The effects of psychological intervention on recovery from surgery and heart attacks: An analysis of the literature. *American Journal of Public Health*, 1982, *72*, 141–151.

Robbins, A. S., Kauss, D. R., Heinrich, R., Abrass, I., Dreyer, J., & Clyman, B. Interpersonal skills training: Evaluation in an internal medicine residency. *Journal of Medical Education*, 1979, *54*, 885–894.

Rosenstock, I. M., & Kirscht, J. P. Why people seek health care. In G. Stone, F. Cohen, & N. Adler (Eds.), *Health psychology.* San Francisco: Jossey–Bass, 1979.

Rosenthal, R., Hall, J. H., DiMatteo, M. R., Rogers, R. L., & Archer, D. *Sensitivity to nonverbal communication: The PONS test.* Baltimore: Johns Hopkins University Press, 1979.

Ross, M., & Olson, J. M. An expectancy – attribution model of the effects of placebos. *Psychological Review*, 1981, *88*, 408–437.

Samora, J., Saunders, L., & Larson, R. F. Medical vocabulary knowledge among hospital patients. *Journal of Health and Human Behavior*, 1961, *2*, 83–89.

Schulman, B. A. Active patient orientation and outcomes in hypertensive treatment. *Medical Care*, 1979, *17*, 267–280.

Shipley, R. H., Butt, J. H., Horwitz, B., & Farbry, J. E. Preparation for a stressful medical procedure: Effect of amount of stimulus pre-exposure and coping style. *Journal of Consulting and Clinical Psychology*, 1978, *46*, 499–507.

Stiles, W. B. Verbal response modes and dimensions of interpersonal roles: A method of discourse analysis. *Journal of Personality and Social Psychology*, 1978, *36*, 693–703.

Stiles, W. B., Putnam, S. M., Wolf, M. H., & James, S. A. Interaction exchange structure and patient satisfaction with medical interviews. *Medical Care*, 1979, *17*, 667–669.

Taylor, S. E. A developing role for social psychology in medicine and medical practice. *Personality and Social Psychology Bulletin*, 1978, *4*, 515–523.

Taylor, S. E. Hospital patient behavior: Reactance, helplessness, or control? *Journal of Social Issues*, 1979, *35*, 156–184.

Truax, C. B., & Carkhuff, R. R. *Toward effective counseling and psychotherapy.* Chicago: Aldine, 1967.

Vaccarino, J. M. Malpractice: The problem in perspective. *Journal of the American Medical Association*, 1977, *238*, 861–863.

Wagner, E. H. The North Karelia project: What it tells us about the prevention of cardiovascular disease. *American Journal of Public Health*, 1982, *72*, 51 – 53.

Wallston, B. S., Wallston, K. A., Kaplan, G. D., & Maides, S. A. Development and validation of the health locus of control (HLC) scale. *Journal of Consulting and Clinical Psychology*, 1976, *44*, 580 – 585.

Weitz, S. (Ed.). *Nonverbal communication: Readings with commentary.* New York: Oxford University Press, 1979.

Werner, A., & Schneider, J. M. Teaching medical students interpersonal skills: A research-based course in the doctor – patient relationship. *New England Journal of Medicine*, 1974, *290*, 1232 – 1237.

Whitcher, S. J., & Fisher, J. D. Multidimensional reaction to therapeutic touch in a hospital setting. *Journal of Personality and Social Psychology*, 1979, *37*, 87 – 96.

Woolraich, M., Albanese, M., Reiter-Thayer, S., & Barratt, W. Teaching pediatric residents to provide emotion-laden information. *Journal of Medical Education*, 1981, *56*, 438 – 440.

Woolraich, M., & Reiter, S. Training physicians in communication skills. *Developmental Medicine and Child Neurology*, 1979, *21*, 773 – 778.

Wortman, C. B., & Dunkel-Schetter, C. Interpersonal relationships and cancer: A theoretical analysis. *Journal of Social Issues*, 1979, *35*, 120 – 155.

4 The Neurologic Bases of Behavior

Ray Winters

John B. Anderson
University of Miami

INTRODUCTION

Behavioral medicine is a psychobiological discipline that seeks to advance our understanding of the relationship between disease and behavior. The brain is an organ of behavior and as such can be treated as a health care system (Schwartz, 1980). This conceptual framework is based on cybernetic theory (Wiener, 1948) and general system analysis (Von Bertalanffy, 1968) and therefore utilizes the concepts of positive and negative feedback, regulation and disregulation (See Chapter 1). The human organism is viewed, therefore, as a composite of self-regulatory feedback systems that are designed to maintain a steady state condition of emotional and physical health by effectively processing feedback from the external and internal environments. Disregulation, and hence poor physical and/or emotional health, occurs when there is attenuation, distortion, disconnection, or dissattention to feedback from the external environment or the internal milieu. Consider the following example of disregulation. The cardiovascular system is designed to regulate blood flow so that nutritional needs of the various body tissues are met. Suppose that an individual has established a compulsive behavior pattern in which most of the individual's time is devoted to a stressful job (as in the Type A pattern discussed in Chapter 16). Also, suppose that the individual is overweight and does not exercise. The stress of the job leads to the mobilization of fatty acids from lipid stores in the body and because the individual does not exercise, the fatty acids are not utilized and cleared from the blood stream. Chronic hypertension and/or atherosclerosis could develop because the free fatty acids would be attached directly to the arterial walls or be converted to triglycerides by the liver and later deposited on the arterial walls as atheromas. The narrowing of the arterial walls of the coronary blood vessels could eventually lead to a heart attack because of inadequate oxygenation of the heart muscle.

The hypothetical case described in the previous paragraph is said to exemplify disregulation because there is dissattention to feedback to the brain. Undoubtedly this individual would receive verbal feedback regarding his or her work habits, weight problem, and lack of exercise. The visual feedback (the individual could look at his or her own body) must be attenuated, and at some point he would receive somatic sensory feedback regarding his or her physical condition: an attempt to walk up several flights of stairs would provide significant information. Moreover, in the advanced stages of the disease, an internal regulatory mechanism would be in a state of dysfunction because blood pressure would not be maintained at normal levels. Blood pressure is regulated, in part, by baroreceptors located in arterial walls. The signals generated by these receptors would become attenuated if sustained hypertension develops.

The nervous system, thus, provides the integrative force in physiological and behavioral control systems. As such it is essential to the understanding of behavioral medicine, and it is important that one have a working knowledge of the functions and the actions of its various regulatory subsystems.

ANATOMY AND PHYSIOLOGY OF NEURONS

The human nervous system is a complex network of billions of cells that regulate internal bodily functions and provides a means for an organism to adapt to the external environment. Information about the internal milieu and the external environment flow to the central core of the nervous system, the brain, and the spinal cord, via individual nerve cells, and hormonal circulation through the vascular system. The *central nervous system* then conveys the appropriate information to body organs so that internal and/or behavioral adjustments may be made.

The functional unit of the nervous system is the *neuron*. Each neuron serves as an individual communication channel in an extremely complex information-processing system. The typical neuron in the human nervous system consists of four structures: the *soma* or cell body, the *dendrites,* the *axon,* and the *terminal boutons.* The soma embodies the machinery for the metabolic processes that sustain the life of the cell. Protruding from the soma are small processes called dendrites, and a long process, the axon. The dendrites receive information from other cells and transmit this information to the cell body; information is carried away from the cell body by the axon, the longest process of the neuron. The message that is sent is electrochemical in nature and is called the *nerve impulse* or *action potential.* It results from the sequential movement of ions across the cell membrane. Action potentials are propagated along the axon to the terminal boutons. The communication between neurons is chemical in nature. Once action potentials reach the terminal boutons a *neurotransmitter* is released and passed to another cell or cells. The junction between two neurons is referred to as a *synapse*.

A chemical transmitter is stored in small packets called *synaptic vesicles*. When action potentials reach the terminal bouton the synaptic vesicles migrate to the *presynaptic cell membrane* and cause the release of a chemical transmitter into the *synaptic cleft*—the space between two cells. Chemical transmitters bring about changes in the electrical activity of the *postsynaptic* cell by transiently altering the distribution of ions across the neuron's cell membrane at specialized regions on the membrane called *receptors* or *receptor sites*. When a neurotransmitter (or hormone) stimulates a receptor, changes take place in the membrane, or within the cell, that ultimately lead to the movement of ions across the cell membrane.

The synapse serves as a means to process information in that the postsynaptic cell integrates spatially and/or temporally the chemical inputs that it receives from a number of neurons. These inputs have either an excitatory—*excitatory postsynaptic potential* (EPSP) or inhibitory—*inhibitory postsynaptic potential* (IPSP) effect. The EPSP is small (5 to 10 mV) and graded and if it is large enough will produce an action potential. The IPSP is also graded and small but opposite in polarity to the EPSP; thus it tends to prevent the formation of action potentials. Most neurons in the brain and spinal cord receive chemical inputs from a large number of neurons and whether or not any given cell produces an action potential is dependent on the relative amounts of excitatory and inhibitory neurotransmitters it receives.

Chemical Transmitters and Diseases of the Nervous System

The neurochemical nature of neuronal activity has broad implications for the biological basis of disease. As a case in point, several diseases of the nervous system can be treated by increasing the amount of transmitters available at synapses. One such disorder, *Parkinson's disease*, is a motor disorder characterized by a tremor at rest, and muscle rigidity. It is a disease of the brain involving neurons that control movement but the symptoms also may be shown as a side effect of several drugs used to treat schizophrenia. The disorder results from a deficiency of the neurotransmitter *dopamine* (Ehringer & Hornykiewicz, 1960). The cell bodies of the neurons involved in the disorder are located in a *nucleus* in the brain known as the *substantia nigra*. A nucleus is a group of cell bodies (and dendrites) that serve a similar function. Axons of the dopaminergic neurons connect to neurons in the *neostriatum* (two nuclei); hence the pathway (axons) between the brain structures is referred to as the *nigrostriatal dopaminergic system* (Fig. 4.1). In Parkinsonian patients as many as 90% of these dopaminergic neurons have degenerated or are in the process of doing so. Dopamine is an inhibitory

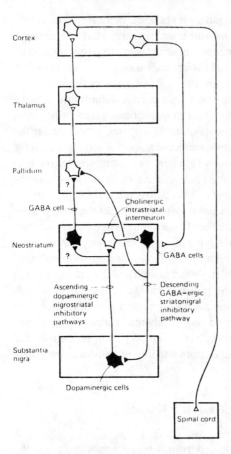

FIG. 4.1.   Interactions of the neurons in the nigrostriatal system that are involved
in Parkinson's disease. Shaded neurons are inhibitory; white neurons are excitatory.
From Cote, L., Basal ganglia and the extrapyramidal system. In E. R. Kandel &
J. H. Schwartz (Eds.), *Principles of neural science*. New York: Elsevier/North
Holland, 1981.

transmitter, so a deficiency would cause muscle rigidity—too many action potentials sent to the muscles from neurons in the spinal cord in Fig. 4.1. Note in Fig. 4.1
that a decrease in the transmitter acetylcholine would also reduce muscle rigidity.

   Thus it is an increase in the ratio of dopamine to acetylcholine that is important
in alleviating the symptoms of the disorder. Antischizophrenic drugs block
dopamine receptors and the Parkinsonian side effects are often treated with
anticholinergic drugs (i.e. ones that block acetycholine at receptors). Parkinson's
disease usually is treated with the drug *L-dopa*. Upon entering dopaminergic
neurons in the brain L-dopa is chemically transformed into dopamine by the
enzyme dopa decarboxylase.

Tardive dyskinesia is a movement disorder involving involuntary movements of the facial muscles, rolling of the tongue, lip smacking and puckering, and rapid eye blinks. The disorder also may be a side effect of the long-term use of drugs used to treat *schizophrenia,* hyperkinesis, or Parkinson's disease. The disease appears to occur when the ratio of dopamine to acetylcholine transmission is too high. In some cases the disease has been treated successfully with *choline,* which in the presence of the enzyme choline acetylase, combines with acetyl coenzyme A to form acetylcholine. The dietary source of choline is *lecithin,* which is found in soybeans, eggs, and liver.

FUNCTIONAL ORGANIZATION OF THE NERVOUS SYSTEM

In order that an organism adapt to the external environment and regulate the internal milieu, information (action potentials) must flow to and from the central nervous system. Neurons that transmit information to the CNS are referred to as *afferent neurons;* they are activated by receptors located in sense organs such as the eye or within the body itself (e.g., in blood vessels or the bladder). This provides the CNS with information regarding environmental changes and sends feedback to the CNS regarding the consequences of the organism's behavior or physiological responses. Sensory receptors perform the function of *transduction,* in that they convert one form of energy to another. For example, photoreceptors in the eye convert electromagnetic radiation into the electrochemical energy of the nervous system. Baroreceptors in the arteries convert mechanical energy to electrochemical energy, thereby providing information about changes in blood pressure.

Efferent neurons transmit nerve impulses from the CNS to muscles and glands. Afferent and efferent neurons are a part of the *peripheral nervous system.* A third type of neuron, the *interneuron,* is found in the CNS. Interneurons perform processing, integrative, and control functions as mediators between afferent and efferent neurons. Thus neurons concerned with cognition, attention, arousal, motivation, and emotions would be interneurons.

The nervous system is composed of various subsystems of neurons involved in the regulation of a number of behaviors and physiological functions. For example, there are subsystems—networks of interconnected neurons concerned with movement, emotions, motivation, and various sensory functions such as vision, hearing, and taste. The *autonomic nervous system,* which has neurons in both the central nervous system and peripheral nervous system, is involved in the regulation of internal body functions.

Superficially the brain looks very much like a mushroom. It has a stem, called the *brainstem,* and an overlying cap, the *cerebral hemispheres.* The spinal cord represents a caudal extension of the brainstem. Afferent and efferent neurons that connect to the CNS are contained within the *cranial nerves,* which connect to the brain, and the *spinal nerves,* which connect to the spinal cord. A nerve is an aggregate of axons.

The responses that the organism makes to internal changes, external changes, and feedback depend, of course, on many factors. If the situation demands movement on the part of the organism, motor neurons of the CNS are activated and nerve impulses are sent to *skeletal muscles* via efferent neurons. If the situation requires changes inside the body, either the autonomic nervous system is activated or hormones are released into the bloodstream, or both. The target organs of the autonomic nervous system are the *smooth muscle, cardiac* (heart) *muscle,* and *glands.* Smooth muscle is found in the various internal organs associated with digestion and excretion, the iris muscle that controls the size of the pupil of the eye, the bronchi, the piloerector muscle of the skin (that causes goose bumps and erection of hair on the skin), and blood vessels.

Hormones may be released by glands under the control of the autonomic nervous system (e.g., the medulla of the adrenal glands, lacrimal tear glands), and the salivary glands; or the hormonal secretions may result from hormones released into the blood stream by the *pituitary gland,* located at the base of the brain. Because it controls other glands like the thyroids, the reproductive glands, and the cortex of the adrenal glands, the pituitary gland is often referred to as the "master gland." The pituitary gland is divided into two parts, an anterior portion, called the adenohypophysis, and a posterior portion called the neurohypophysis. Both portions are controlled by the *hypothalamus,* a brain region located above the stalk of the pituitary. The adenohypophysis is controlled by hormones circulated through the local vascular bed around the hypothalamus; the neurohypophysis is controlled by nerve impulses sent along axons originating in the hypothalamus.

The Autonomic Nervous System

The autonomic nervous system (ANS) is the portion of the nervous system that is essential to the control of the internal environment. It is involved in the regulation of such vital processes as digestion, excretion, body temperature, blood pressure, and heart action. In addition to its internal homeostatic function, this division of the nervous system plays an important role in the organism's adaptation to the external environment. External events that threaten the physical or psychological well-being of the organism trigger responses from the ANS that prepare the individual for immediate action. The ANS has two major subdivisions, the *sympathetic* and *parasympathetic* divisions. The autonomic pathway from the CNS to the target organ usually contains two neurons: a preganglionic cell, whose cell body is located in the central nervous system, and a postganglionic cell, whose cell body is found in the peripheral nervous system. The preganglionic cell bodies of the sympathetic division are located in the spinal cord; the preganglionic cell bodies of the parasympathetic division are found in the brainstem and the spinal cord. The terminal boutons of the preganglionic axons synapse with the cell bodies of the postganglionic cell and the axons of the postganglionic neurons convey information to the target organs by secreting a neurotransmitter. This transmitter is usually, but not always, acetylcholine for the parasympathetic division and nor-epinephrine for the sympathetic division. Acetylcholine is the transmitter between the preganglionic and postganglionic cells of both systems.

Role of the ANS in Adaptation to the Environment.   The sympathetic division of the ANS is activated by a wide variety of physical and psychologically stressful stimuli including exercise, exposure to cold, and pain. In general, sympathetic activation is designed to mobilize energy to prepare the organism for immediate action. Energy transformations in the body require oxidation of foodstuffs and the production of heat, particularly in the skeletal muscle—the tissue that enables the organism to take action. Thus the sympathetic division increases cardiac output so that more oxygen is supplied to the muscle. Respiration is facilitated by dilation of the bronchi, gastrointestinal function is inhibited, and blood is shunted to the active muscles. Glucose levels in the bloodstream increase. Epinephrine and norepinephrine are released into the bloodstream by the adrenal glands to increase metabolism; these hormones also enhance the effects of the sympathetic division because their effects mimic sympathetic effects on autonomic target organs. The sympathetic division also increases sweating so that body temperature does not rise during the increased metabolic and muscular activity.

The parasympathetic division appears to work in a complementary way to the sympathetic division in that it serves to increase the body's supply of stored energy and to protect and conserve these supplies for times of stress. Thus the parasym-pathetic division controls various functions associated with digestion like sali-vation, gastric motility, secretion of gastric juices, and movements of the esophagus important in swallowing.

The Asymmetries of the Human Brain

One of the most striking features of the brain is that there are two distinct hemispheres. Even though, for the most part, the structures in the two hemispheres are anatomically identical, it is natural to speculate about possible functional differences between the two halves of the brain. There is now rather convincing evidence that substantiates this idea.[1] The evidence comes from three sources: brain damaged patients, studies using the Wada technique for anesthetizing one half of the brain, and from studies of the split-brain patient, in which the two hemispheres are surgically disconnected.

The findings of studies of patients suffering from cortical damage on one side of the brain were the first to suggest the lateralization of language function in the human brain. In right-handed patients, language ability, in general, is severely impaired with extensive damage to the left hemisphere but is only minimally affected by damage to the right hemisphere. Many left-handed patients show the

---

[1]A concise review of the literature on asymmetries of the brain is provided by Springer and Deutsch (1981). *Left brain, right brain.* San Francisco: Freeman.

same impairment, but for many left-handers, language dysfunction is often found to result from damage to the right hemisphere, or to either hemisphere. In general the loss in language ability was found not to be as severe, or as permanent, with left-handers as with right-handers.

The Wada (1947) technique can be used to assess cerebral lateralization by temporarily disrupting the neural activity in one hemisphere. This technique involves injecting the barbiturate sodium amytal into one of the carotid arteries, thereby anesthetizing one side of the brain. If the anesthetized hemisphere is dominant for speech, a temporary language dysfunction occurs. For example, subjects may misname objects, show reversals in the order of words in a sentence, stutter, or have difficulties comprehending language. The effect is temporary because the barbiturate is eventually metabolized. Milner, Branch, and Rasmussen (1966) used the Wada technique to study 169 patients. They found that 92% of the right-handed patients had speech representation in the left hemisphere, 7% in the right hemisphere, and 1% with bilateral representation. Among the 74 left-handed patients, 69% showed left hemisphere dominance for speech, 18% right hemisphere dominance, and 13% had bilateral representation.

Split-Brain Patients.   Motor epilepsy is typically treated by anticonvulsant drugs such as Dilantin. In some severe cases brain surgery is required. Neurosurgeons have found that many patients can be helped by surgically severing the axons that connect the two hemispheres, particularly the corpus callosum, the largest group of fibers that connect the two halves of the brain. Controlled experiments with the split-brain patients have advanced substantially our understanding of the specialized functions of the two cerebral hemispheres.

The typical experiment with a split-brain patient is designed to stimulate one hemisphere without stimulating the contralateral one. This is accomplished by presenting a stimulus to one side of the body or in one side of the visual environment. The nervous system is organized such that stimulation of one side of the visual environment or one side of the body activates neurons in the contralateral cerebral hemisphere. Thus, an object placed in the right hand activates neurons in the left hemisphere, and an object in the left part of the visual field increases the neural activity of neurons in the right visual cortex. Similarly, the right hemisphere controls movements of the left side of the body and the left hemisphere controls movements on the right side of the body. It should be pointed out that it is not possible to selectively stimulate one hemisphere with individuals in which the two hemispheres are connected because the information that initially arrives in one hemisphere would be conveyed to the contralateral hemisphere via interhemispheric structures like the corpus callosum.

The fundamental differences between the two hemispheres becomes readily apparent when they are stimulated separately. If an object, say a cup, is placed in the right hand of a blindfolded split-brain patient, he or she has no difficulty in naming the object. When the cup is placed in the left hand, however, the patient is unable to identify the object verbally. The question that arises is whether the inability to verbally identify the object in the left hand is due to a deficit in sensory processing or in the ability of the right hemisphere to produce language. If it is simply a speech production problem we need only to find an appropriate means of communicating with the right hemisphere. Sperry and colleagues (Meyers & Sperry, 1958; Sperry, 1968; Sperry, 1974) have accomplished this in a number of ways. One method is to ask the patient to choose, with his or her left hand, from among a group of objects, the one that had been placed in his or her left hand. Another way is to have the patient pick out the object, with his or her left hand from among a series of slides. It is essential that the object be chosen with the left hand because this hand is directed by the right hemisphere, the only hemisphere that has received the information. Indeed, studies of this type have demonstrated conclusively that the right hemisphere is capable of identifying stimuli. Moreover, the right hemisphere is superior to the left hemisphere in a number of skills including visual/spatial tasks and some aspects of music ability. For example, the left hand of a split brain patient is much more adept at drawing a scene in perspective than the right hand, even though the patients are typically right-handed. The notion that the right hemisphere predominates in visual/spatial tasks is supported by clinical observations that patients with damage to the right hemisphere (but not the left hemisphere) often show a *facial agnosia*—an inability to recognize familiar faces. Also, these patients often neglect the left side of space and the left side of their bodies. For example, they may eat food on the right side of a plate but not the left side. A paralyzed limb on the left side of the body may be denied by these individuals.

Several studies provide evidence that the right hemisphere is specialized for the processing of emotional information. When a cerebral hemisphere is specialized for a particular function and it is processing information, the eyes move laterally in the contralateral direction. For example, when language information is being processed in the left hemisphere, the eyes move laterally to the right. Similarly, when a question is asked requiring visual/spatial processing (e.g., Is Hawaii north or south of Mexico?) left lateral eye movements occur. Schwartz, Davidson, and Maer (1975) found that in response to emotional questions most people move their eyes to the left, thereby indicating processing in the right hemisphere. In addition, patients with brain damage to the right hemisphere often have a difficult time comprehending the affective component of speech. Also, Sackheim, Gur, and Saucy (1978) demonstrated that emotions are expressed more intensely on the left side of the face (which is controlled by the right hemisphere) than on the right side of the face.

These findings are particularly interesting in regard to disregulation resulting from CNS processing of information. Repression of negative emotions, particularly anger, has been thought to be linked to various psychosomatic disorders such as hypertension (G. Schwartz, 1977). One might postulate, therefore, that these individuals are able to suppress affective information from the right hemisphere. In support of this view, Gur and Gur (1975) report that people who show left lateral eye movement regardless of the type of question have higher scores on tests of denial and also report a higher incidence of psychosomatic complaints. Thus it may be possible that the brain can learn to cope with anger by functionally severing the connections between the two hemispheres.

Brain Mechanisms Mediating Language.   Our knowledge about the manner in which the brain processes and produces language is based on studies of brain damaged patients. Two of the most important brain areas concerned with language are *Broca's Area,* located in the frontal lobe, and *Wernicke's Area,* in the temporal lobe. A lesion in Broca's area results in an *expressive aphasia.* With this type of language disorder there is an impairment in the ability to express language in either written or oral form. If a brain lesion is restricted to this region, language comprehension is usually normal. Most of the patients with an expressive aphasia exhibit very little speech and the speech that is emitted is usually abnormal. Syntactical errors are quite common. For example, one patient describing his state of health said "I haven't been headache troubled not for a long time [Brain, 1961]." Penfield and Roberts (1959) give an example of a patient attempting to describe an operation:

> Well, I thought thing I am going to the tell is about my operation and it is not about all I can tell is about the preparation the had was always the time was when they had me to get ready that is they shaved off all my hair was and a few odd parts of pencil they gave me in the fanny. (p. 382)

Naming problems are also common with the expressive asphasic. A pen might be called a shoe, a house may be called a car. In attempting to name a bunch of keys one patient made the statement: "Indication of measurement of piece of apparatus or intimating the cost of apparatus in various forms [Brain, 1961]."

The most devastating language dysfunction is the *receptive aphasia.* This disorder, which results from the destruction of Wernicke's area, is characterized by an inability to comprehend language in oral or written form. The patient hears and sees words but they have no meaning. The receptive aphasic is able to produce speech and is able to write, but the end product is devoid of meaning.

Wernicke's area is connected to Broca's area by a band of axons called the *arcuate fasciculus.* A lesion that severs these axons results in a *conduction aphasia.* The patient is able to understand words, both spoken and written, but cannot repeat words that he or she hears or reads. Even though speech may be fluent, it is unrelated to the language material that is heard or read. For example, if asked a question, the answer will be totally unrelated to the question. For obvious reasons, a conduction aphasia is often referred to as the "politician's syndrome."

Another cortical area important in language is the *angular gyrus* (Fig. 4.2). Geschwind (1972) suggests that this region serves to convert language from a visual form to an auditory and vice versa. According to Geschwind's view, language material that is being read must be converted to an auditory form in order

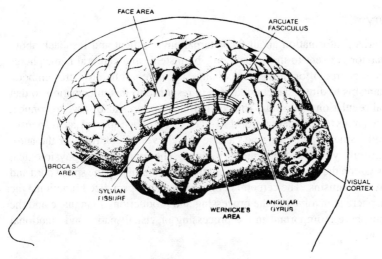

FIG. 4.2.   Primary language areas of the brain. From Geschwind, N. Language and the brain. *Scientific American*, 1972, 226, 76 – 83.

to be processed in Wernicke's area. Thus, since the visual projection area is in the occipital lobe it must be converted to an auditory form by the angular gyrus before reaching Wernicke's area in the temporal lobe. The angular gyrus is not involved in the comprehension of spoken language because the information is already in an auditory form. Thus this information would be passed directly from the auditory area in the temporal lobe to Wernicke's area.

   One symptom of a lesion in the angular gyrus is *alexia*—the inability to read. Alexia is believed to occur because the material is not converted to an auditory form by the angular gyrus. The patient with a lesion in the angular gyrus shows no deficit in the ability to respond to language presented in an auditory form because, as mentioned previously, it is already in an auditory form. Writing ability, however, is impaired, a condition called *agraphia*. There is an area in the parietal lobe involved in writing, and information from Wernicke's area must, according to Geschwind's view, be converted to a visual form by the angular gyrus before reaching this area.

   A question that naturally arises from studies of language areas in the left hemisphere is: What is the function of the anatomically corresponding language areas in the right hemisphere? Studies of patients with brain damage in the right hemisphere strongly suggest that the affective aspects of language are represented in these areas in the right hemisphere and that the anatomical organization mirrors the organization in the left hemisphere (Heilman, Scholes, and Watson, 1975; Ross, 1981). Thus the comprehension of the emotional aspects of language takes place in the region in the right hemisphere that corresponds to Wernicke's area, and the expression of the emotional aspects of language occurs in the region that corresponds to Broca's area.

Summary

To summarize, information about the external environment and feedback about one's behavior are sent to the spinal cord, brainstem, and cerebral hemispheres (via afferent neurons) for further processing. The cerebral hemispheres embody the mechanisms to direct skeletal muscles in response to this information so that behavioral regulation can occur. The cerebral hemispheres also serve to connect the hypothalamus to the external world so that it can produce appropriate responses from glands, smooth muscles, and cardiac muscle via its control over the autonomic nervous system and the pituitary gland. The regulation of physiological responses within the internal milieu are controlled primarily by the spinal cord and brainstem mechanisms. The cerebral hemispheres have specialized functions: the left hemisphere is involved in the processing and production of language and the right hemisphere is important in the processing of visual/spatial and emotional information.

NEURONAL SUBSTRATES OF HUMAN CONSCIOUSNESS

Human consciousness is not only important to the adjustment of the individual to the environment, but irregularities in the modulation of consciousness may lead to decrements in behavioral performance or may, in fact, be symptomatic of disregulation. Short-term irregularities in sleeping schedules, for example, may lead to performance decrements and long-term irregularities may lead to sleep disorders such as narcolepsy (Schrima, 1981). Moreover, one symptom of inadequate adjustment to the environment is variations in the sleep/waking cycle.

Awareness of the external world is an essential component of human consciousness. In fact it could be argued that human consciousness evolved to deal with the variability of the external world, allowing the organism to delay responses and plan future responses. Energy fluctuations in the external environment are transformed into electrical activity by sensory receptors located in sense organs, and information is sent to the brain for interpretation. One of the most important portions of the human brain involved in conscious perceptions is the cerebral cortex. It is the outermost layer of the cerebral hemispheres. This area is, on the average, about 2.5 mm thick and contains over 50% of the neurons in the nervous system.

Each sensory modality, except pain, has a projection area in the cerebral cortex. Destruction of that area causes a loss of conscious perceptual experiences associated with the sense.

If sensory experience is dependent on the activity of neurons in the cerebral cortex it should be possible to generate perceptual experiences by electrically stimulating the projection area. This in fact, has been demonstrated by neurosurgeons on countless occasions but more importantly, it is possible to utilize this fundamental fact to assist people with sensory dysfunctions. Dobelle, Meadjowsky, and Girvin (1974), for example, are in the process of developing a prosthetic eye that utilizes electrical stimulation of the visual cortex in the occipital lobe. The device, which has been partially developed, consists of a glass eye with a miniature camera. The camera transmits, electronically, variations in light patterns to a small computer, which converts information about light to an electrical current. The current is then sent to electrodes that produce artificial sensations (phosphenes) by activating visual neurons in the cerebral cortex. This system has now been developed to the point where blind patients can discriminate letters of the alphabet.

Alerting Mechanisms

The human brain does not passively process all information about the external world. Neural activity in the CNS is in a constant state of flux and the organism's reaction to a stimulus is, in part, determined by its state at the time the stimulus arrives. In this regard, the brain's state of arousal contributes significantly to the fate of a stimulus arriving at a sense organ.

A major advance in our understanding of the physiological mechanisms of arousal came in 1949 when Morruzzi and Magoun reported that electrical stimulation of the brainstem led to the arousal of sleeping animals. Similarly, destruction of neurons in this region caused somnolence. The *brainstem activating system* is actually a network of interconnecting neurons that make either direct or indirect connections with neurons throughout the central core of the brain, particularly the cerebral cortex. It is thought to prepare the rest of the brain for incoming information by increasing the background activity of neurons. The activation of specific nuclei, like the locus coeruleus and the *ventral tegmental nucleus* of the mesolimbic system, are probably responsible for the arousal resulting from the stimulation of the brainstem activating system (reticular formation).

Effects of Psychoactive Drugs on the Brainstem Activating System.   There are several drugs that are believed to alter consciousness by their effects on the alerting mechanisms of the brainstem. Among these are the sedative-hypnotic drugs and various stimulants.

Included within the category of sedative-hypnotic drugs are: alcohol, barbiturates, the antianxiety tranquilizers (e.g., Miltown, Librium, Valium, Equinil), and methaqualone. The effects of the drugs within this category are dependent on the dosage. The sedative-hypnotic drugs in general, depress synaptic activity throughout the nervous system. At low doses they are believed to depress inhibitory synapses without depressing excitatory synapses. Thus, at low doses they behave as stimulants, increasing activity, arousal, and releasing social inhibitions. At higher doses they depress excitatory synapses also, and their effects on the reticular formation are thought to underlie the effects that they have on general arousal level. These effects, at progressively greater doses include: antianxiety effects, sedation, sleep, general anesthesia, coma, and death. Death is a result of the depression of respiratory neurons in the brainstem.

Stimulants like the amphetamines and cocaine have the opposite effects on the reticular formation. Both these drugs increase the *catecholamines* (norepinephrine and dopamine) at synapses in the brainstem activating system.

Sleep and Dreaming

Sleep is a circadian alteration in state of consciousness that is characterized by several distinct physiological changes. There are two major stages of sleep and these stages may be distinguished by three physiological measuring devices: the EEG (electroencephalogram), the EOG (electrooculogram) and the EMG (electromyogram).

The EEG measures electrical brain potentials recorded from electrodes placed on the scalp. These potentials are believed to be generated by electrical activity at synapses, particularly in the cerebral cortex. If the individual is awake and attending to something in the environment or engaged in mental activities, the EEG is characterized by relatively fast (18-30 per second) waves of low amplitude (50 to 100 microvolts). The activity is also said to be desynchronized in that the wave pattern is irregular and arrhythmic. Desynchronized activity may be taken to represent a high level of synaptic activity. These waves, *beta waves,* are replaced by *alpha waves* if the individual is awake, relaxed, but not attending to anything. Alpha waves have a frequency of 8-13 waves/second and are relatively synchronized. Synchrony in the EEG is believed to mean that activity at synapses is in a resting or depressed state. The waves of the EEG are desynchronized during most of our waking hours and synchronized during most of our sleeping hours.

As an individual enters the first stage of sleep, *S-sleep* (synchronized sleep), the EEG shows an increasing amount of low frequency, high voltage, synchronized activity. Sleep becomes progressively deeper during the first 90 minutes with *delta waves* appearing in the EEG after 25 minutes. Delta waves are high amplitude, low frequency, synchronized waves associated with deep sleep. They also are seen when an individual is in a coma or is anesthetized. Sleep walking, talking, and snoring occur during S-sleep.

The EMG is used to measure muscle tone. During S-sleep muscle tone is reduced significantly from the waking level. Eye movements, as assessed by the EOG, are minimal during S-sleep.

After about 90 minutes of S-sleep the individual enters *D-sleep* (desynchronized sleep). Its onset is signaled by a number of abrupt physiological changes. The EEG changes to a desynchronized pattern. This pattern is difficult to distinguish from the beta waves observed when the subject is awake and alert. The EOG recordings often show rapid eye movements during D-sleep. The rapid eye movements (REMs), usually indicate that the sleeper is dreaming. Although we may see occasional twitches of the muscle, the EMG indicates a profound loss of muscle tone. In effect the brain paralyzes the muscles during D-sleep. This paralysis serves to prevent the sleeper from acting out his or her dreams and therefore is a protective mechanism.

The initial episode of D-sleep lasts about 10 minutes. For the rest of the night there is an alternation between S-sleep and D-sleep, with the cycle variation lasting about 90 minutes. The duration of D-sleep periods becomes progressively longer as the night wears on with later periods of D-sleep lasting as long as 1 hour. About 20-25% of sleep is spent in D-sleep.

Sleep Deprivation. In 1959, Peter Tripp, a New York disc jockey, stayed awake for 200 consecutive hours. He developed an acute paranoid psychosis in which he believed that people were attempting to put drugs into his food and beverages to make him sleep; he also had auditory hallucinations. This finding led many investigators to believe that sleep is essential to normal emotional functioning. However, several years later, Randy Gardner, a 17-year-old high school student, deprived himself of sleep for 264 hours without any ill effects.

Controlled laboratory studies of sleep deprivation show that subjects selectively deprived of D-sleep show more D-sleep on subsequent nights (Dement, 1960). This *D-sleep rebound* underlines the importance of this stage of sleep. D-sleep rebound is also a symptom of withdrawal from sedative-hypnotic drugs. During withdrawal, the addict may spend close to 100% of his sleeping hours in D-sleep.

The most significant effect of D-sleep deprivation appears to be on learning and memory. Several studies have shown that selective deprivation of D-sleep impairs the recall of material that has emotional content (Cartwright, Gore, & Weiner, 1974; Greiser, Greenberg, & Harrison, 1972; Tilley & Empson, 1978) or novel material (McGinty, 1969). If the material has no emotional content or is not unusual, D-sleep deprivation does not impair memory (McGrath & Cohen, 1978). Animals that have engaged in learning tasks during the day spend more time in D-sleep at night (Bloch, Hennevin & Leconte, 1977; Lucero, 1970). Also, human patients with Korsakoff's syndrome, where memory storage is impaired, show less D-sleep than normals (Greenberg, Mayer, Brook, Pearlman, & Hartmann, 1968). Memory consolidation almost certainly requires protein synthesis; protein synthesis occurs at a higher rate during D-sleep than S-sleep, or during waking hours, (Drucker-Colin & Spanis, 1976). Moreover, inhibiting protein synthesis by the administration of anisomycin reduces D-sleep (Drucker-Colin, Spanis, Cotman, & McGaugh, 1975). Starvation, which also decreases protein synthesis, reduces the amount of D-sleep (McFayden, Oswald, & Lewis, 1973).

Brainstem Mechanisms. There are several regions in the brainstem that are involved in sleep. The locus coeruleus is probably a part of a general arousal mechanism. Lesioning this nucleus causes hypersomnia (Jones, Bobillier, & Jouvet, 1969). Some of the projections of the locus coeruleus are essential to the inhibition of muscle activity during D-sleep (Jones, Harper, & Halaris, 1977).

The *raphe nuclei* of the brainstem appear to be essential to the inhibition of D-sleep events such as dreaming and rapid eye movements (Hendricksen, Dement, & Barchas, 1974). Jacobs and Trulson (1979) contend that dreams and hallucinations have some brain mechanisms in common. If this is true it is not surprising that cats whose brains have been depleted of serotonin, the major transmitter of raphe neurons, appear to hallucinate when they are awake (Hendricksen et al., 1974). Similarly, cancer patients treated with parachlorophenylalanine, which reduces the amount of serotonin levels in the brain, often experience hallucinations as a side effect of the treatment (Engelman, Lovenberg, & Sjoerdsma, 1967). Other drugs that are serotonin antagonists, like LSD and mescaline, also produce hallucinations. Drugs like MAO inhibitors, which are potent agonists of serotonin, decrease the amount of D-sleep (Wyatt, 1972).

The *nucleus of the solitary tract* appears to inhibit the arousal mechanisms within the brainstem activating system. This nucleus receives information from the tongue and digestive organs. Perhaps this is why we feel drowsy after a large meal.

The onset of S-sleep and D-sleep are controlled by neurons in the brainstem but the locations of the trigger zones are not known. It does appear, however, that acetylcholine agonists facilitate D-sleep (Sitaram, Nurnberger, Gershon, & Gillin, 1980; Sitaram, Wyatt, Dawson, & Gillin, 1976; Stoyva & Metcalf, 1968). Also, cells in the hypothalamus, which are sensitive to temperature, are capable of producing sleep. Thermoreceptors in the skin relay information to this area. Perhaps the drowsiness associated with a fever or being in the sun for an extended period of time results from activation of this region.

Sleep Disorders

Insomnia.   This is by far the most common sleep disorder, affecting at least 20% of the population at some time in their lives. It is characterized by difficulty in going to sleep, staying asleep, awakening prematurely, or some combination of these symptoms. In some cases this disorder is related to situational stress that the individual may experience, and the symptoms disappear when the stress has abated.

The physiological characteristics of the sleep pattern of the insomniac are usually different from the normal sleeper. There are more body movements, and elevated body temperature and heart rate, reflecting a higher level of arousal during sleep. This is consistent with the idea that most cases of insomnia are due to stress. Stress would be expected to lead to an increased level of activity in the brainstem activating system.

Insomnia is often treated by drugs. The nonprescription varieties such as Compoz, Nytol, and Sominex contain antihistamines, which cause drowsiness— probably by depressing neurons in the brainstem activating system. Because histamine is a transmitter secreted by many neurons in the brainstem, as a temporary measure they may be effective for some insomniacs.

Barbiturates like Seconal and Nembutal also have been prescribed for insomnia. As discussed earlier, barbiturates are CNS depressants and thus, if the dose is high enough, would decrease the activity within the brainstem activating system, thereby decreasing the background activity of the brain.

The long-term use of barbiturates as sleeping aids is ill-advised. As is true for all sedative − hypnotic drugs, barbiturates are addicting and the withdrawal symptoms are life-threatening. Moreover, they decrease the quality of sleep. Initially they depress D-sleep, and even though D-sleep reemerges after long term use of the drug, the qualitative characteristics of dreams change, not being as vivid as normal dreams (Carroll, Lewis, & Oswald, 1969). When the medication is discontinued, D-sleep rebound occurs and the patient usually experiences intense nightmares and sleepiness during this period and often demands more sleeping pills. A vicious cycle emerges from this pattern. Some investigators have gone so far as to say that the major cause of insomnia is sleep medication (Carlson, 1981).

Pseudoinsomnia and sleep apnea are special forms of insomnia. The pseudoinsomniac believes that he or she does not sleep, when in fact, he or she does. Stated another way, the patient dreams that he or she is awake. The causes of this condition are poorly understood.

Sleep apnea is a disorder in which the patient cannot breathe and sleep at the same time. Because the individual is, in effect, holding his or her breath, there is a change in blood gases: oxygen levels decrease and carbon dioxide levels rise. Eventually the changes in the blood gases are detected by specialized respiratory neurons in the brainstem. A regulatory mechanism is automatically set into motion and the sleeper awakens and begins to breathe again. He or she stays awake only long enough for the blood gases to normalize. The patient then falls asleep and the cycle is repeated. During an 8-hour period the sleeper may awaken as often as 500 times.

Treatment of sleep apnea varies. In some cases it may be as simple as removing the tonsils to open the breathing passage. A more drastic measure is to perform a tracheotomy and allow the patient to breath through a tube inserted into the trachea.

Jet Lag Syndrome.   The human body is a finely tuned physiological instrument. A large number of its functions are regulated by internal mechanisms that cause rhythmic changes over a 24-hour period. At least 100 body functions are known to show this circadian rhythm. Among these are blood pressure, body temperature, hormone levels, amino acid levels, activity levels in organs like the liver and kidney, motor efficiency, and of course, consciousness. As an example, body temperature for most people is lowest at 4:00 a.m. and highest during the middle of the day.

A disruption of one's natural body rhythms often leads to fatigue, irritability, loss of efficiency, nausea, or insomnia. These symptoms often are experienced by those who travel across time zones, hence the term "jet lag." As an example, someone flying from the west coast to the east coast may find it difficult to fall asleep at his or her normal sleeping time because the "body time" is out of phase with "clock time." Until a phase shift in body rhythms takes place there is usually a decrement in performance and in the quality of sleep. This applies to anyone whose sleep schedule varies; the doctor or nurse who works the day shift on Tuesday and the night shift on Thursday; the college student who goes to bed at midnight during the week and 6:00 a.m. on the weekends (Dement, 1974).

The performance loss is not due to a decrease in sleep; it results from an attempt of the body to become synchronized with the environment. The internal mechanism, which is probably controlled by the brain, will adjust to changes in sleep/waking schedules but it usually takes several days and, during the time at which the phase shift is occurring, the individual does not perform at an optimal level.

Narcolepsy. This illness, which affects at least 100,000 people in the United States, is characterized by several symptoms, including periodic occurrences of overwhelming sleepiness during the day. The narcoleptic may fall asleep at any time. Dement (1974) cites one case in which a narcoleptic woman fell asleep when scuba diving and another case of a fireman who had an attack while climbing a ladder in a burning building. It can be a very dangerous disorder because of the increased likelihood of sleepiness during monotonous activities like driving a car.

Another symptom of narcolepsy is *cataplexy.* Cataplexy refers to a complete or partial muscle paralysis triggered by a strong emotion. A narcoleptic may become paralyzed and fall to the ground when experiencing any emotion like anger, sadness, joy, or fear, or just general excitement. One narcoleptic reported that he had to discontinue duck hunting because the excitement of seeing the birds caused him to drop his gun and fall to the ground. The patient remains fully awake during these seizures.

Normally an individual spends the first 90 minutes of sleep in S-sleep but the narcoleptic enters D-sleep immediately. In addition, he often experiences *sleep paralysis* and *hypnogenic hallucinations.* Sleep paralysis refers to the condition where the patient is aware that he or she cannot move just before falling asleep. Hypnogenic hallucinations are vivid dreams that occur immediately before the onset of sleep.

All the symptoms of narcolepsy strongly suggest that it is a sleep disorder involving intrusions of D-sleep at inappropriate times. The cataplexy attacks probably represent the muscle paralysis that occurs during D-sleep. Because a prominent feature of dreams is their emotional content, it is not surprising that emotions trigger the seizures. The D-sleep mechanism is so strong that the narcoleptic immediately enters this stage when he or she goes to sleep and in many cases experiences the D-sleep paralysis just prior to the transition from wakefulness to sleep. The hypnogenic hallucinations are probably the vivid dreams associated with D-sleep.

The raphe cells are responsible for inhibiting many of the D-sleep mechanisms when an individual is awake. It is not unreasonable to speculate that these cells are involved in the symptoms of narcolepsy. The symptoms of narcolepsy are treated with stimulants such as amphetamines or methylphenidate, to reduce sleepiness, but these drugs do not prevent the other symptoms of the disorder. Typically tricyclic antidepressants such as imimpramine and protriptyline are used to allay the symptoms of cataplexy, hypnogogic hallucinations, and sleep paralysis.

NEURAL SUBSTRATES OF MOTIVATION AND EMOTION

In terms of viewing the brain as a health-care system, motivation and emotions are considered to be processing variables because they are major factors in determining which of a variety of stimuli receive the attention of the organism. In order to illuminate the neuronal mechanisms underlying motivation and emotions we focus here on processes associated with two sets of circumstances that motivate behavior: a caloric imbalance and reward. Then behavioral disorders involving motivation and emotions are discussed.

An appropriate balance of nutrients is necessary for cellular metabolism and hence the maintenance of life itself. Changes in behavior that act to preserve a constant internal milieu are homeostatic. Homeostatic mechanisms allow an animal to adapt to a wide range of environments and hence are essential to the survival of the species. Homeostasis is a feedback controlled process. The body must have sensing devices to detect physical/chemical imbalances and eventually this must lead to changes that serve to restore a former condition. For example, it is essential that the temperature of the human body be within 1 degree of 98.6°. Chemical reactions occurring within cells are temperature dependent, and even small changes in body temperature may affect tissue functioning. The temperature of the external environment may vary by as much as 150°, yet temperature in the core of the body still remains near 98.6°. The brain plays a crucial role in this homeostatic mechanism. The hypothalamus is apprised of changes in core temperature and skin temperature and if body temperature rises, the activity of cells in this portion of the brain leads to dilation of cutaneous blood vessels, sweating, and/ or behavioral changes such as shielding oneself from the sun, turning on an air conditioner, or the slowing of body movements. If body temperature is lowered, cells in the hypothalamus, via the autonomic nervous system, cause a constriction of peripheral blood vessels, and shivering. An increase in body movements, or various behavioral adjustments may also occur.

Regulation of Caloric Intake

Maintaining sufficient nutrients to satisfy tissue needs involves rather complex physiological mechanisms and only a summary of the many factors involved is presented here.

The liver appears to monitor the body's supply of nutrients and probably is the single most important organ in detecting nutritional deficits (Friedman, Rowland, Saller, & Stricker, 1976; Niijima, 1969; Russek, 1971; Russek & Racotta, 1980). It contains receptors that monitor glucose utilization and the amount of stored nutrients. When there is a deficiency of nutrients, afferent neurons originating from the liver convey this information to the brain so that feeding behaviors can be initiated.

The brain also appears to be involved in the monitoring of nutrients. When there are nutritional deficits the brain conveys this information to the adrenal glands via action potentials sent along efferent neurons. Epinephrine is then released by the adrenal glands and this hormone serves to break down stored nutrients (Stricker, Rowland, Saller, & Friedman, 1977).

As for the initiation of feeding behavior, speculations prevail over empirical findings. One such speculation is that nutritional deficits trigger neurons that inhibit interneurons that are themselves inhibitory (Mogenson, 1976). These interneurons are believed to synapse upon programmed neural circuits that control feeding reflexes and other behaviors associated with consumption of food.

The cessation of eating behavior is also only partially understood but a gastrointestinal hormone cholecystokinin appears to be important, as injections of this hormone inhibit feeding. Also, gastric receptors are undoubtedly involved in satiety mechanisms (Deutsch, 1978; Deutsch, Young, & Kalogeris, 1978). Other factors such as oral (the taste of the food) ones are important too.

Reward Mechanisms

The regulation of body temperature and caloric intake and other homeostatic processes constitute a relatively well-defined problem area in the study of the physiological mechanisms of motivation. In modern civilization, however, only a small fraction of one's daily activities are devoted to satisfying bodily needs. Additional motivational concepts must be invoked to account for most of our behavior. Perhaps the most essential of these concepts are reinforcement and punishment. Reinforcement and punishment are forms of feedback from the environment. One way to view these concepts is in terms of their effects on neuronal subsystems within the CNS. Positive feedback occurs when the behavior that precedes the feedback increases the activity within reward areas in the brain— called *positive reinforcement,* or decreases activity within areas that underlie pain—*negative reinforcement.* Punishment is a type of negative feedback. Thus reinforcing stimuli are ones that tend to increase the likelihood of the behavior that precedes the reinforcer and punishing stimuli are ones that decrease the probability that the behavior will occur in the future.

One of the most important discoveries regarding the brain substrates of rein-forcement occurred in 1954 when Olds and Milner were examining the effect of *electrical stimulation of the brain* (ESB) on rats. They were attempting to stimu-late the reticular formation and one of the electrodes missed the target and found its way into an adjacent brain structure (probably the hypothalamus). To their surprise, it appeared that the ESB was functioning as a positive reinforcer. Subsequent studies have demonstrated that rats will press a lever several thousand times per hour, until exhaustion, in order to receive ESB in "reward" areas. These rates are much higher than those resulting from natural rewards like food or sex. In addition to lever pressing, animals will engage in a variety of behaviors like running through a maze or crossing an electrified grid, in order to have portions of their brains stimulated electrically. In a study reported by Routtenberg and Lindy (1965) rats were trained to press two levers, one for ESB and one for food pellets. The animals were allowed to press the levers for 1 hour per day. Some of them spent so much time on the bar that delivered ESB that they starved to death.

A massive set of experiments were conducted in a number of laboratories to map the anatomy of the reward system. Many of the reward sites were found to be in the *limbic system,* a neural subsystem of the brain long associated with emotions and motivation. Self-stimulation could be elicited by electrodes in various locations, including the brainstem and cerebral hemispheres. One of the most reliable sites was a region called the *medial forebrain bundle.* In fact, the reward areas of the brain are often referred to as the medial forebrain system. The medial forebrain bundle is a diffuse system of axons that connects a large number of neural areas in the brainstem and cerebral hemispheres. Many of the axons of neurons of the locus coeruleus and ventral tegmental nucleus (discussed earlier) are found in the medial forebrain bundle.

Neuroscientists have endeavored to determine the synaptic transmitter or transmitters that mediate the rewarding effects of ESB. It appears that at least one of the transmitters is dopamine (Angrist, Sathananthan, Wilk, & Gershon, 1974; Clavier & Gerfen, 1979; Fibiger, 1978; Fuxe, Nystom, Tovi, Smith, & Ogren, 1974; Mora, Sanguinetti, Rolls, & Shaw, 1975). Basically the studies aforementioned demonstrate collectively that drugs that increase dopamine transmission increase response rates to ESB, and drugs that decrease dopamine levels cause a decrease in responding.

It now appears that the mesolimbic dopaminergic system mediates many of the effects of rewarding ESB (Claiver & Gerfen, 1979; Mora et al., 1975; Rolls, Rolls, Kelly, Shaw, Wood, & Dale, 1974). The cell bodies of these neurons are located in the ventral tegmental area of the brainstem and connect to a number of regions in the brainstem and the cerebral hemispheres. Their axons pass through the medial forebrain bundle.

It is important to point out that the mesolimbic dopaminergic system *is not the* reward area of the brain. In general, rewarding ESB of this region stimulates axons that project to a number of regions in the brain, any of which may be involved in reward. Also, experiments that demonstrate the importance of dopamine in reward do not preclude the possibility that other transmitters are involved. Furthermore, as suggested by Carlson (1981), drive induction may be a major component of what is referred to as positive reinforcement. Drive induction refers to the activation of neuronal systems that are associated with specific drives such as thirst, hunger, sex, etc. Drive induction can occur as a result of external stimuli or internal mechanisms such as a deficit in nutritional needs.

Behavioral Disorders Involving Emotions and Motivation

Schizophrenia

Schizophrenia is a behavioral disorder characterized by incoherent speech, a loss of normal associations between ideas, lack of motivation, and either flat or inappropriate affect. Bizarre delusional systems and hallucinations are also associated with the disease.

There is ample evidence for a genetic component to schizophrenia (Kety, 1978), so it is natural to speculate that there is a dysfunction in an information-processing mechanism or mechanisms within the CNS. Two ideas, the *attention hypothesis* and the *anhedonia hypothesis* receive some support from pharmacological, neurophysiological, and histological studies.

The attention hypothesis states that schizophrenia results from an inability of the patient to control his or her attentional processes. Thus dysfunction would occur because of disattention to feedback. A quote from a woman who suffered from numerous schizophrenia episodes summarizes the view: "the mind must have a filter which functions without our conscious thought, sorting stimuli, and allowing those stimuli which are relevant to the situation in hand to disturb consciousness, and this filter must be working at maximum efficiency at all times, particularly when we require a high degree of concentration. What had happened to me. . . was a breakdown in the filter, and a hodge-podge of unrelated stimuli were distracting me from things which should have had my individual attention [McDonald, 1960, p. 218]."

A variation of this hypothesis is the view that a dysfunction in attention mechanisms prevents the appropriate integration of affective information from the right hemisphere and cognitions from the left hemisphere. This view receives support from studies that demonstrate that schizophrenics show right lateral eye movement in response to most visual/spatial and emotional questions (Schweitzer, Becker, & Welsh, 1978). Also, schizophrenics apparently lack the ability to integrate visual information presented to the left hemisphere with visual information presented to the right hemisphere (Beaumont & Dimond, 1973).

Anhedonia is defined as the inability to experience pleasure and is thought to be one of the major symptoms of schizophrenia (Rado, 1964). The anhedonia hypothesis states that there is a neural and/or chemical dysfunction in areas of the brain associated with reward so that feedback from the environment is ineffective in modifying behavior. This view would account for the amotivational component of the syndrome.

It is important to point out that the attention and anhedonia hypotheses are not totally incompatible. If areas in the brain associated with attention are not functioning, feedback from the environment or transhemispheric information may never reach neurons that underlie the effects of reward or behavior. If there is a malfunction in CNS attentional gates or filters that sort information fed from the environment, by memory areas, and regions associated with affect, it could lead to a number of behavioral dysfunctions including, loose associations between thoughts, delusions, flat or inappropriate affect, and anhedonia.

Biogenic Amines and Schizophrenia.   A large body of evidence strongly suggests that synapses that receive dopaminergic input are involved in schizophrenia. Almost all the antischizophrenic drugs, despite differences in their chemical structure, interfere with dopaminergic transmission by blocking dopamine receptors at postsynaptic cells (Carlsson, 1974, 1978; Johnstone, Crow, Frith, Carney, & Price, 1978; Snyder, Burt, & Creese, 1976). Alpha-methyl-paratyrosine, a drug that interferes with the synthesis of dopamine, enhances the effectiveness of antischizophrenic drugs (Walinder, Skott, Carlsson, & Roos, 1976). In addition, drugs that augment dopaminergic transmission have been shown to induce schizophrenic symptoms. The drugs that show this effect are L-dopa (Barchas, Elliott, & Berger, 1977; Goodwin & Murphy, 1974), methylphenidate (Davis, 1974), amphetamine (Angrist et al., 1974; Griffith, Cavanaugh, Held, & Oates, 1972; Johnstone, Crow, Frith, Carney, & Price, 1978), apomorphine (Creese, Burt, & Snyder, 1976) and cocaine (Barchas, Elliott, & Berger, 1977). Many of the drugs that increase dopaminergic transmission have a similar effect on norepinephrine. A study by Angrist et al. (1974), however, provides rather convincing evidence that dopamine, rather than norepinephrine, is involved in schizophrenia. D-amphetamine and L-amphetamine are known to stimulate both dopamine and norepinephrine synapses but d-amphetamine is 10 times more effective in activating norepinephrine synapses. When Angrist et al. injected volunteers with varying dosages of the two drugs they found them to be equally effective in producing psychotic symptoms. If norepinephrine were the most important transmitter in schizophrenia, d-amphetamine should have been considerably more effective. Moreover, they found that they could allay the amphetamine-induced psychosis by injecting drugs that blocked dopaminergic synapses but did not affect norepinephrine synapses.

As suggested by Sachar (1981), there are several explanations that could account for the apparent hyperactivity at dopaminergic synapses of schizophrenics but there is no evidence, however, to support the simplest of the explanations—that more dopamine is secreted at the synapses. If this were the case one would expect an increase in the metabolites of dopamine in the cerebrospinal fluid of schizophrenics. This was found not to be the case for schizophrenics tested in mental hospitals (Bowers, 1974; Post, Fink, Carpenter, & Goodwin, 1975) or recently deceased schizophrenics (Owen, Cross, Crow, Longden, Poulter, & Riley, 1978).

There is some evidence to support the view that there are more dopamine receptors in the brains of deceased schizophrenics (Crow, Johnstone, Longden, & Owen, 1978). Sachar (1981) suggests that this finding may be secondary to long-term treatment with antischizophrenic drugs, but five of the patients that were tested had not received antischizophrenic medication for a year before they died and two patients had never received this type of medication.

Neuroanatomical Substrates of Schizophrenia.   There are five major dopaminergic pathways in the brain (Sacher, 1981). If, indeed, hyperactivity at dopaminergic synapses underlies some or all of the symptoms of schizophrenia, the mesolimbic dopaminergic pathway would be likely to be involved in the disorder. Destruction of neurons in this pathway causes "sensory neglect" (indifference to stimuli), a major side effect of antischizophrenic drugs (Ungerstedt & Pycock, 1974). Also many of the axons of the mesolimbic system pass through the medial forebrain bundle—the axonal system most frequently associated with the rewarding effects of ESB.

It will be recalled that Parkinson's disease results from a deficiency of the transmitter dopamine secreted by cells of the nigrostriatal dopaminergic system. One of the major side effects of the antipsychotic drugs like chlorpromazine is that the schizophrenic patient often shows symptoms resembling Parkinson's disease. One antipsychotic drug that minimizes this side effect (clozapine) has been shown to have a minor effect on dopaminergic synapses in the nigrostriatal system but a strong suppressive effect upon dopamine-secreting cells in the limbic system (Anden & Stock, 1973). These findings thus provide indirect support for the idea that the mesolimbic dopaminergic system is involved in schizophrenia.

One of the limbic regions that receive mesolimbic projections is the nucleus accumbens. Stevens (as cited in Sacher, 1981) has proposed the idea that the nucleus accumbens and its related structures serve as gates or filters for memory and affective information, and that mesolimbic dopaminergic projections modulate the flow of activity through this filter network, thereby implicating dopaminergic neurons in attentional mechanisms.

As discussed earlier, two major hypotheses have been posited that would account for schizophrenia in terms of CNS processing: the attention hypothesis and the anhedonia hypothesis. The findings of psychopharmacological and neuroanatomical studies are consistent with both of these views.

Evidence for Other Factors Involved in Schizophrenia.   Although there is a substantial amount of research implicating dopamine in schizophrenia, several findings indicate that other factors are important. First, improvement in the symptoms of schizophrenia from medication usually are not seen for a week or more, yet the effects of antischizophrenic drugs on dopamine receptors occurs rather rapidly (Cotes, Crow, Johnstone, Bartlett, & Bourne, 1978). Also, about 10% of schizophrenic patients who receive antipsychotic medication suffer from tardive dyskinesia. It will be recalled that this disorder results when the ratio of dopamine to acetylcholine transmission is high. Yet, antischizophrenic medication decreases this ratio. As suggested by Carlson (1981), this side effect may result from the phenomena known as *denervation hypersensitivity*. When the chemical input to a neuron diminishes substantially there may be a compensatory increase in the sensitivity of the neuron—perhaps from an increase in the number of receptors. Thus long-term use of antidopaminergic drugs by schizophrenics may lead to an increase in dopaminergic receptors. Although this is a plausible explanation for the development of tardive dyskinesia, it also suggests that schizophrenic symptoms should return. Perhaps this does not occur because schizophrenics had developed an excess of dopamine receptors before taking the medication or perhaps the fact that different neuronal systems are involved in the two disorders accounts for this finding.

The dopamine issue is complicated further by the fact that schizophrenics have enlarged ventricles, compared to normal individuals of the same age, suggesting that they may suffer from brain damage. Thus it appears unlikely that enhanced dopamine transmission is the only factor involved in schizophrenia.

Affective Psychosis

The primary symptom of the affective psychoses—mania, depression, and manic depression—is distortions in emotions. For these patients affect becomes divorced from reality. Their feelings of extreme elation (mania) or despair (depression) are not justified by events in their lives. Positive and negative affective feedback from the environment is either magnified or attenuated so dysregulation occurs. There is a high risk of suicide in severe cases of psychotic depression.

The most prevalent idea concerning the nature of psychotic depression is that there is a functional deficiency in the transmission of one or both of the mono-amines norepinephrine and serotonin. The two most effective classes of antidepressant drugs, the *monoamine oxidase inhibitors* and the *tricyclic antidepressants*, are known to increase brain monoamine levels (Baldesserini, 1980), a fact that is certainly consistent with the monoamine hypothesis. However, the clinical response to the tricyclics, the more effective of the two types of drugs, takes 2 to 3 weeks, whereas the pharmacologically induced increases in the transmitters takes place very rapidly. Moreover, both cocaine and amphetamines increase norepinephrine and serotonin levels but, in general, are of little therapeutic value. It seems likely that receptor changes must take place before they become effective so that a change in the set point for transmission of one or more transmitters is altered.

Additional evidence for the norepinephrine/serotonin hypothesis comes from studies that show that the effectiveness of monoamine oxidase inhibitors is potentiated by drugs like L-tryptophan, a chemical precursor to serotonin (see Murphy, Campbell, & Costa, 1978). Also PCPA, which inhibits serotonin synthesis, can precipitate symptoms of depression in patients who are in remission (see Murphy et al., 1978). Triiodothyronine is a hormone that is thought to increase the sensitivity of catecholamine receptors. This drug potentiates the effectiveness of tricyclics (Schildkraut, 1978).

Mania. It has been hypothesized that mania results from augmented transmission of norepinephrine. Although there is some evidence that lithium increases the release of norepinephrine at neuron terminals (Fieve, 1979), the mechanism by which lithium alters mood is not understood. Lithium has been used to treat manic depression, so its general effect on behavior is to stabilize the mood of the patient. The effectiveness of lithium may be related to its ability to improve an impaired lithium transport mechanism at the cell membrane (Dorus, Pandey, Shaughnessy, Gaviria, Val, Ericksen, & Davis, 1979).

Speculations Regarding the Relation Between Depression, Sleep, and Aggression. It appears that some depressed patients have a deficiency in serotonin transmission at synapses, whereas others have a deficiency in norepinephrine transmission. The tricyclic antidepressant drugs are the major drugs used to treat the disorder. One class of these drugs has greater effect on serotonin transmission whereas a second class of tricyclics has a greater effect on norepinephrine transmission. One way to test for the appropriate tricyclic antidepressant is to measure urine levels of MHPG (3-methoxy-4-hydroxy-phenylglycol), a metabolite of norepinephrine. If MPHG levels are low, a tricyclic that enhances norepinephrine transmission is given, if the baseline levels of MHPG are within the normal range, a tricyclic that increases serotonin levels are given.

A large body of research (Valzelli, 1981) provides evidence that serotonin is important to the inhibition of aggressive behaviors. Thus it seems reasonable to speculate that patients with depression accompanied by irritability and aggressive behaviors are deficient in serotonergic transmission. Also, the tricyclics that have their greatest effect on serotonin, rather than norepinephrine, have a sedative effect. Many depressed patients show an early onset of dream sleep (Vogel, 1979). Perhaps this is due to a deficiency in serotonin transmission, as this transmitter is involved in the inhibition of dream sleep.

It also seems reasonable to postulate that patients with a retarded depression (where the patient is sluggish rather than agitated) have a deficiency in norepinephrine transmission. It will be recalled that norepinephrine is secreted by neurons of the locus coeruleus. This nucleus is associated with a neural system involved in the control of the general arousal level of the brain. Thus this nucleus may be involved in depression (Weiss, 1983).

Other Transmitters Involved in Affective Disorders. Serotonin and norepinephrine certainly are not the only transmitters involved in depression because some tricyclics have no effect on these biogenic amines. It has now been established that all the clinically effective tricyclics are potent blockers of histamine receptors (Green & Maayani, 1977; Kanof & Greengard, 1978). A study by J. Schwartz (1977) provides evidence that histamine is a neurotransmitter in the brain. Also, there is evidence for a system of histaminergic neurons that connect the brainstem to the cerebral hemispheres. It is well known that some of the antischizophrenic drugs have antidepressive effects. These drugs also block histamine receptors. It will be recalled that cocaine, a drug that increases mono-amine levels, is ineffective in the treatment of depression; this drug does not affect histamine receptors.

The transmitter acetylcholine also appears to be important in the affective disorders. Physostigmine, a drug that increases acetylcholine levels, can briefly reverse the symptoms of mania. Also, symptoms of depression can be induced by increasing acetylcholine levels. All of the tricyclic antidepressant drugs have an anticholinergic effect. Thus the affective disorders may be related to the ratio of transmission of transmitters in the brain. Mania may result when the ratio of norepinephrine to acetylcholine (and/or histamine) is high. Depression may occur when the ratio of norepinephrine or serotonin to acetylcholine (and/or histamine) is too low.

CONCLUSIONS

Man's last great frontier may well be the nervous system. Because of the accelerating pace of insights into its mechanisms of actions there has been a corresponding mushrooming of the application of new discoveries to the treatment of physical and emotional dysfunctions. The use of drugs, behavioral training techniques, and surgical interventions has become essential to the treatment of many disorders, and these methods will become even more common as research leads to further advances in our understanding of the nervous system. As we learn more about various regulatory subsystems within the CNS that are involved in stress, nutrition, immunity, and behavior, our understanding of the role that behavior plays in disease will become clearer.

REFERENCES

Anden, N. E., & Stock, G. Effects of clozapine on the turnover of dopamine in the corpus striatum and in the limbic system. *Journal of Pharmacy and Pharmacology,* 1973, *25,* 346 – 348.

Angrist, B., Sathananthan, G., Wilk, S., & Gershon, S. Amphetamine psychosis: Behavioural and biochemical aspects. *Journal of Psychiatric Research,* 1974, *11,* 13 – 24.

Baldessarini, R. J. Drugs and the treatment of psychiatric disorders. In A. G. Gilman, L. S. Goodman, & A. Gilman (Eds.), *The pharmacological basis of therapeutics.* New York, Toronto, London: MacMillan, 1980.

Barchas, J. D., Elliott, G. R., & Berger, P. A. Biogenic amine hypothesis of schizophrenia. In J. D. Barchas, P. A. Berger, R. D. Ciaranello, & G. R. Elliott (Eds.), *Psychopharmacology: From theory to practice.* London and New York: Oxford University Press, 1977.

Barchas, J. D., Elliott, G. R., & Berger, P. A. In J. D. Barchas, P. A. Berger, R. D. Ciaranello, & G. R. Elliott (Eds.), *Psychopharmacology*. Oxford University Press, 1977.

Beaumont, G., & Dimond, S. Brain disconnection and schizophrenia. *British Journal of Psychiatry*, 1973, *123*, 661−662.

Bloch, V., Hennevin, E., & Leconte, P. Interaction between post-trial reticular stimulation and subsequent paradoxial sleep in memory consolidation processes. In R. R. Drucker-Collin & J. L. McGaugh (Eds.), *Neurobiology of sleep and memory*. New York: Academic Press, 1977.

Bowers, M. B. Central dopamine turnover in schizophrenic syndromes. *Archives of General Psychiatry*, 1974, *31*, 50−54.

Brain, R. *Speech disorders*. London: Butterworth, 1961.

Carlson, N. R. *Physiology of behavior*. Boston, London, Sydney, Toronto: Allyn & Bacon, 1981.

Carlsson, A. Antipsychotic drugs and catecholamine synapses. *Journal of Psychiatric Research*, 1974, *11*, 57−64.

Carlsson, A. Antipsychotic drugs, neurotransmitters, and schizophrenia. *American Journal of Psychiatry*, 1978, *135*, 164−172.

Carroll, D., Lewis, S. A., & Oswald, I. Effects of barbiturates on dream content. *Nature*, 1969, *223*, 865−866.

Cartwright, R. D., Gore, S., & Weiner, L. *Paper presented at the meeting of the Association for the Psychophysiological Study of Sleep*. San Diego: 1973. Cited by Greenberg and Pearlman, 1974.

Clavier, R. M., & Gerfen, C. R. Neural inputs to the prefrontal agranular insular cortex in the rat—horseradish peroxidase study. *Brain Research Bulletin*, 1979, *4*, 347−353.

Cote, L. Basal ganglia, the extrapyramidal motor system, and diseases of transmitter metabolism. In E. R. Kandel & J. H. Schwartz (Eds.), *Principles of neural science*. New York: Elsevier/North Holland, 1981.

Cotes, M., Crow, T. J., Johnstone, E. C., Bartlett, W., & Bourne, R. C. Neuroendocrine changes in acute schizophrenia as a function of clinical state and neuroleptic medication. *Psychological Medicine (London)*, 1978, *8*(4), 657−665.

Creese, I., Burt, D. R., & Snyder, S. H. Dopamine receptor binding predicts clinical and pharmacological potencies of antischizophrenic drugs. *Science*, 1976, *192*, 481−483.

Crow, T. J., Johnstone, E. C., Longden, A. J., & Owen, F. *Life Sciences*, 1978, *23*, 563−568.

Davis, J. M. A two-factor theory of schizophrenia. *Journal of Psychiatric Research*, 1974, *11*, 25−30.

Dement, W. The effect of dream deprivation. *Science*, 1960, *131*, 1705−1707.

Dement, W. C. *Some must watch while some must sleep*. San Francisco: W. H. Freeman & Company, 1974.

Deutsch, J. A. The stomach in food satiation and the regulation of appetite. *Progress in Neurobiology*, 1978, *10*, 135−153.

Deutsch, J. A., Young, W. G., & Kalogeris, T. J. The stomach signals satiety. *Science*, 1978, *201*, 165−167.

Dobelle, W. H., Meadjowsky, M. G., & Girvin, J. P. Artificial vision for the blind: Electrical stimulation of visual cortex offers a hope for a functional prosthesis. *Science*, 1974, *183*, 440−444.

Dorus, E., Pandey, G. N., Shaughnessy, R., Gaviria, M., Val, E., Ericksen, S., & Davis, J. M. Lithium transport across red cell membrane: A cell membrane abnormality in manic-depressive illness. *Science*, 1979, *205*, 932−933.

Drucker-Colin, R. R., & Spanis, C. W. Is there a sleep transmitter? *Progress in Neurobiology*, 1976, *6*, 1−22.

Drucker-Colin, R. R., Spanis, C. W., Cotman, C. W., & McGaugh, J. L. Changes in protein level in perfusates of freely moving cats: Relation to behavioral state. *Science*, 1975, *187*, 963−965.

Ehringer, H., & Hornykiewicz, O. Verteilung von noradrenalin und dopamin (3-hydroxytyramin) im gehirn des menschen und ihr verhalten bei erkrankungen des extrapyramidalen systems. *Klin. Wochenschr*, 1960, *38*, 1236−1239.

Engelman, K., Lovenberg, W., & Sjoerdsma, A. Inhibition of serotonin synthesis by parachlorophenylalanine in patients with the carcinoid syndrome. *New England Journal of Medicine*, 1967, *277*, 1103 – 1108.

Fibiger, H. C. Drugs and reinforcement mechanisms: A critical review of the catecholamine theory. *Annual Review of Pharmacology and Toxicology*, 1978, *18*, 37 – 56.

Fieve, R. R. The clinical effects of lithium treatment. *Trends in NeuroSciences*, 1979, *2*, 66 – 68.

Friedman, M. I., Rowland, N., Saller, C., & Stricker, E. M. Different receptors initiate adrenal secretion and hunger during hypoglycemia. *Neuroscience Abstracts*, 1976, *2*, 299.

Fuxe, K., Nystrom, M., Tovi, M., Smith, R., & Ogren, S. O. Central catecholamine neurons, behavior and neuroleptic drugs: An analysis to understand the involvement of catecholamines in schizophrenia. *Journal of Psychiatric Research*, 1974, *11*, 151 – 162.

Geschwind, N. The organization of language and the brain. *Science*, 1970, *27*, 940 – 945.

Geschwind, N. Language and the brain. *Scientific American*, 1972, *226*, 76 – 83.

Goodwin, F. K., & Murphy, D. L. Biological factors in the affective disorders and schizophrenia. In M. Gordon (Ed.), *Psychopharmacological agents*. New York: Academic Press, 1974.

Green, J. P., & Maayani, S. Tricyclic antidepressant drugs block histamine H2 receptor in brain. *Nature*, 1977, *269*, 163 – 165.

Greenberg, R., Mayer, R., Brook, R., Pearlman, C., & Hartmann, E. Sleep and dreaming in patients with post-alcoholic Korsakoff's disease. *Archives of General Psychiatry*, 1968, *18*, 203 – 209.

Greiser, C., Greenberg, R., & Harrison, R. H. The adaptive function of sleep: The differential effects of sleep and dreaming on recall. *Journal of Abnormal Psychology*, 1972, *80*, 280 – 286.

Griffith, J. D., Cavanaugh, J., Held, N. J., & Oates, J. A. Dextrocemphetamine: Evaluation of psychotomimetic properties in man. *Archives of General Psychiatry*, 1972, *26*, 97 – 100.

Gur, R., & Gur, R. Defense mechanisms, psychosomatic symptomatology, and conjugate lateral eye movements. *Journal of Consulting and Clinical Psychology*, 1975, *43*, 416 – 420.

Heilman, K. M., Scholes, R., & Watson, R. T. Auditory affective agnosia. Disturbed comprehension of affective speech. *Journal of Neurological Neurosurgery of Psychiatry*, 1975, *38*, 69 – 72.

Hendricksen, D., Dement, W., & Barchas, J. The role of serotonin in the regulation of a phasic event of rapid eye movement sleep: The ponto-geniculo-occipital wave. *Advances in Biochemical Psychopharmacology*, 1974, *11*, 169 – 179.

Jacobs, B. L., & Trulson, M. E. Dreams, hallucinations, and psychosis—the serotonin connection. *Trends in Neuro-Sciences*, 1979, *2*, 276 – 280.

Johnstone, E. C., Crow, T. J., Frith, C. D., Carney, M. W. P., & Price, J. S. Mechanism of the antipsychotic effect in the treatment of acute schizophrenia. *Lancet*, 1978, *1*, 848 – 851.

Jones, B. E., Bobillier, P., & Jouvet, M. Effects de la destruction des neurons contenant des catecholamines du mesencephale sur le cycle veille-sommeils du chat. *Comptes Rendus de la Societe de Biologie, Paris*, 1969, *163*, 176 – 180.

Jones, B. E., Harper, S. T., & Halaris, A. E. Effects of locus coeruleus lesions upon cerebral monoamine content, sleep wakefulness states and the response to amphetamine in the cat. *Brain Research*, 1977, *124*, 473 – 496.

Kanof, P. D., & Greengard, P. Brain histamine receptors as targets for antidepressant drugs. *Nature*, 1978, *272*, 329 – 333.

Kelley, J. P. Cranial nerve nuclei, the reticular core and biogenic amine-containing neurons. In E. R. Kandel, & J. H. Schwartz (Eds.), *Principles of neural science*. New York, Amsterdam, Oxford: Elsevier/North-Holland, 1981.

Kety, S. S. The biological roots of mental illness: Their ramifications through cerebral metabolism, synaptic activity, genetics, and the environment. *Harvey Lectures*, 1978, *71*, 1 – 22.

Lucero, M. A. Lengthening of REM sleep duration consecutive to learning in the rat. *Brain Research*, 1970, *20*, 319 – 322.

Mayer, D. J., & Liebeskind, J. C. Pain reduction by focal electrical stimulation of the brain: An anatomical behavioral analysis. *Brain Research*, 1974, *68*, 73 – 93.

McDonald, N. Living with schizophrenia. *Journal of the Canadian Medical Association*, 1960, *82*, 218 – 221.

McFayden, V. M., Oswald, I., & Lewis, S. A. Starvation and human slow wave sleep. *Journal of Applied Physiology,* 1973, *35,* 391 – 394.

McGinty, D. J. Effects of prolonged isolation and subsequent enrichment on sleep patterns in kittens. *Electroencephalography and Clinical Neurophysiology,* 1969, *26,* 332 – 337.

McGrath, M. J., & Cohen, D. B. REM sleep facilitation of adaptive waking behavior: A review of the literature. *Psychological Bulletin,* 1978, *85,* 24 – 57.

Meyers, R. E., & Sperry, R. W. Interhemispheric communication through the corpus callosum. Mnemonic carry-over between the hemispheres. *Archives of Neurology and Psychiatry,* 1958, *80,* 298 – 303.

Milner, B., Branch, C., & Rasmussen, T. Evidence for bilateral speech representation in some non-righthanders. *Transactions of the American Neurological Association,* 1966, *91,* 306 – 308.

Mogenson, G. J. Neural mechanisms of hunger: Current status and future prospects. In D. Novin, W. Wyrwicka, & C. Bray (Eds.), *Hunger: Basic mechanisms and clinical implications.* New York: Raven Press, 1976.

Mora, F., Sanguinetti, A. M., Rolls, E. T., & Shaw, S. G. Differential effects of self-stimulation and motor behavior produced by microintracranial injections of a dopamine-receptor blocking agent. *Neuroscience Letters,* 1975, *1,* 179 – 184.

Morruzzi, G., & Magoun, H. W. Brain stem reticular formation and activation of the EEG. *Electroencephalography and Clinical Neurophysiology,* 1949, *1,* 455 – 473.

Murphy, D. L., Campbell, I., & Costa, J. L. Current status of the indoleamine hypothesis of the affective disorders. In A. DiMascio, & K. F. Killam (Eds.), *Psychopharmacology: A generation of progress.* New York: Raven Press, 1978.

Niijima, A. Afferent impulse discharge from glucoreceptors in the liver of the guinea pig. *Annals of the New York Academy of Science,* 1969, *157,* 690 – 700.

Olds, J., & Milner, P. Positive reinforcement produced by electrical stimulation of septal area and other regions of rat brain. *Journal of Comparative and Physiological Psychology,* 1954, *47,* 419 – 427.

Owen, F., Cross, A. J., Crow, T. J., Longden, M., Poulter, M., & Riley, G. J. Increased dopamine-receptor sensitivity in schizophrenia. *Lancet,* 1978, *2*(8083), 223 – 226.

Penfield, W., & Roberts, L. *Speech and brain mechanisms.* Princeton, N.J.: Princeton University Press, 1959.

Post, R. M., Fink, E., Carpenter, W. T., & Goodwin, F. K. Cerebrospinal fluid amine metabolites in acute schizophrenia. *Archives of General Psychiatry,* 1975, *32,* 1063 – 1069.

Rado, S. Hedonic self-regulation of the organisms. In R. G. Heath (Ed.), *The role of pleasure in behavior.* New York: Harper & Row, 1964.

Rolls, E. T., Rolls, B. J., Kelly, P. H., Shaw, S. G., Wood, R. J. & Dale, R. The relative attenuation of self-stimulation, eating, and drinking produced by dopamine-dopamine-receptor blockade. *Psychopharmacologia,* 1974, *38,* 219 – 230.

Ross, E. D. The aprosodias: Functional – anatomical organization of the affective components of language in the right hemisphere. *Archives of Neurology,* 1981, *42.*

Routtenberg, A., & Lindy, J. Effects of the availability of rewarding septal and hypothalamic stimulation on bar pressing for food under conditions of deprivation. *Journal of Comparative and Physiological Psychology,* 1965, *60,* 158 – 161.

Russek, M. Hepatic receptors and the neurophysiological mechanisms controlling feeding behavior. In S. Ehrenpreis & O. C. Solnitzky (Eds.), *Neurosciences research.* New York: Academic Press, 1971.

Russek, M., & Racotta, R. A. A possible role of adrenaline and glucagon in the control of food intake. *Frontiers in Hormone Research, 1980.*

Sachar, E. J. Psychobiology of schizophrenia. In E. R. Kandel & J. H. Schwartz (Eds.), *Principles of neural science.* Oxford: Elsevier/North-Holland, New York, Amsterdam, 1981.

Sackheim, H. A., Gur, R. C., & Saucy, M. Emotions are expressed more intensely on the left side of the face. *Science,* 1978, *202,* 434 – 436.

Schildkraut, J. J. Current status of the catecholamine hypothesis of affective disorders. In M. A. Lipton, A. DiMascio, & K. F. Killam (Eds.), *Psychopharmacology: A generation of progress.* New York: Raven Press, 1978.

Schrima, L. An etiology of narcolepsy-cataplexy and a proposed cataplexy neuromechanism. *International Journal of Neuroscience*, 1981, *15*, 69 – 86.

Schwartz, G. E. Psychosomatic disorders and biofeedback: A psychobiological model of disregulation. In J. D. Maser & M. E. Seligman (Eds.), *Psychopathology: Experimental models*. San Francisco: W. H. Freeman, 1977.

Schwartz, G. The brain as a health care system. In G. C. Stone, F. Cohen, & N. E. Adler (Eds.), *Health psychology*. San Francisco, Washington, London: Jossey-Bass Inc., 1980.

Schwartz, G. E., Davidson, R. J., & Maer, F. Right hemisphere lateralization for emotion in the human brain: Interactions with cognition. *Science*, 1975, *190*, 286 – 288.

Schwartz, J. C. Histaminergic mechanisms in brain. *Annual Review of Pharmacology and Toxicology*, 1977, *17*, 325 – 339.

Schweitzer, L., Becker, E., & Welsh, H. Abnormalities of cerebral lateralization in schizophrenia patients. *Archives of General Psychiatry*, 1978, *35*, 982 – 985.

Sitaram, N., Wyatt, R. J., Dawson, S., & Gillin, J. C. REM sleep induction by physostigmine infusion during sleep. *Science*, 1976, *191*, 1281 – 1283.

Sitaram, N., Nurnberger, J. I., Jr., Gershon, E. S., & Gillin, J. C. Faster cholinergic REM sleep induction in euthymic patients with primary affective illness. *Science*, 1980, *208*, 200 – 208.

Snyder, S. H., Burt, D. R., & Creese, I. Dopamine receptor of mammalian brain: Direct demonstration of binding to agonist and antagonist states. *Neuroscience Symposia*, 1976, *1*, 28 – 49.

Sperry, R. W. Hemisphere deconnection and unity in consciousness awareness. *American Psychologist*, 1968, *23*, 723 – 733.

Sperry, R. W. Lateral specialization in the surgically separated hemispheres. In F. O. Schmitt, & F. G. Worden (Eds.), *The neurosciences third study program*. Cambridge, Mass.: MIT Press, 1974.

Sternbach, R. A. *Pain: A psychophysiological analysis*. New York: Academic Press, 1968.

Stoyva, J., & Metcalf, D. Sleep patterns following chronic exposure to cholinesterase-inhibiting organophosphate compounds. *Psychophysiology*, 1968, *5*, 206.

Stricker, E. M., Rowland, N., Saller, C. F., & Friedman, M. I. Homeostasis during hypoglycemia: Central control of adrenal secretion and peripheral control of feeding. *Science*, 1977, *196*, 79 – 81.

Tilley, A. J., & Empson, J. A. C. REM sleep and memory consolidation. *Biological Psychology*, 1978, *6*, 293 – 300.

Ungerstedt, U., & Pycock, C. Functional correlates of dopamine neurotransmission. *Bulletin der Schweizewrisschen Akademie der Medizinischen Wissenschaften*, 1974, *30*, 44 – 55.

Valzelli, L. Psychopharmacology of aggression: An overview. *International Pharmacopsychiatry*, 1981, *16*, 39 – 48.

Vogel, G. W. A motivational function of REM sleep. In R. Drucker-Colin, & M. B. Sterman (Eds.), *The functions of sleep*. New York: Academic Press, 1979.

von Bertalanffy, L. *General systems theory*. New York: Braziller, 1968.

Wada, J. A new method for the determination of the side of cerebral speech dominance: A preliminary report on the intracarotid injection of sodium amytal in man. *Medical Biology*, 1947, *14*, 221 – 222.

Walinder, J., Skott, A., Carlsson, A., & Roos, B. Potentiation by metyrosine of thioridazine effects in chronic schizophrenics: A long-term trial using double-blind cross-over technique. *Archives of General Psychiatry*, 1976, *33*, 501 – 505.

Weiss, J. *Neurochemical basis of depression*. Paper presented at the Miami Symposium on Stress and Coping, February, 1983.

Wiener, N. *Cybernetics: Control and communication in the animal and machine*. Cambridge, Mass.: MIT Press, 1948.

Wyatt, R. J. The serotonin-catecholamine dream bicycle: A clinical study. *Biological Psychiatry*, 1972, *5*, 33 – 64.

5 Psychophysiologic Reactions to Stress

Philip M. McCabe

Neil Schneiderman
University of Miami

INTRODUCTION

Stress is a normal part of life. As such, it can be either beneficial or harmful. To the extent that individuals can successfully cope with stressors and then move on to other things, stress may provide enriching experiences and reinforce a sense of competence. In contrast, when stress is too severe and/or too prolonged and/or the individual is too fragile, stress can have harmful effects on a person's physical and/ or mental health. For the purposes of the present chapter stress can be defined as any change or threat of change that demands *adaptation* by an individual. The stimulus for this change is referred to as a *stressor,* and the adaptation can be described in terms of behavioral (e.g., fight, flight, depression) or physiological responses (e.g., increase in plasma epinephrine, depression of lymphoblast transformation). In the present chapter the stressors considered are physical, psychosocial, and sociocultural in nature and the adaptations involve the central nervous, skeletomotor, sympathoadrenomedullary, hypothalamico-pituitary-adrenocortical, immune, and endorphin — enkephalin systems. The organismic variables interposed between the stressors and adaptations involve personality variables (e.g., perceptual and response styles) employed in *active coping* versus *helplessness, hypervigilance, and conservation — withdrawal.* A reasonable understanding of the psychophysiological responses to stress therefore implies the use of a biopsychosocial multisystems approach.

STRESSFUL LIFE EVENTS

Both systematic research studies and anecdotal clinical observations indicate that life events that are perceived as stressful can adversely influence morbidity and mortality (Engel, 1971; Kimball, 1971; Rahe, Bennett, Romo, Seltanen, & Arthur, 1973; Reich, De Silva, Lown, & Murawski, 1981; Theorell & Rahe, 1971). In addition to the objective presence of a stressful life event (e.g., bankruptcy), disease onset can be affected by the individual's: (1) perception of the event; (2) ability to cope or adapt to it psychologically; (3) general physical health status and reserve; (4) genetic or constitutional predisposition to a disease; and (5) exposure to a disease-causing agent (Braunstein, 1981; Rabkin & Struening, 1976). For these reasons the relation of life stress to disease is probably better conceptualized as being part of a multiple risk factor constellation than as being a sole causal agent (Braunstein, 1981; Rahe, 1979).

Several specific diseases, involving diabetes mellitus (Kimball, 1971), infectious mononucleosis (Kasl, Evans, & Niederman, 1979), myocardial infarction (Theorell & Rahe, 1971), rheumatoid arthritis (Solomon, 1981), and tuberculosis (Hawkins, et al., 1957) have been reported to occur more often following stressful life events. Engel (1971) collected 170 cases from newspaper clippings in which a precipitating life event was clearly stated. Sudden cardiac death was related either to the collapse or death of a close person or to a period of acute grief (i.e., within 16 days) in 41% of the cases, whereas personal danger or threat of injury accounted for another 27%. Reunions, triumphs, or "happy endings" were related to sudden cardiac death in only 6% of cases.

In addition to Engel's (1971) anecdotal findings, several retrospective studies have clearly implicated psychosocial emotional stressors as significant postdictors of sudden cardiac death (Meyers & Dewar, 1975; Reich et al., 1981; Rissanen, Romo, & Seltanen, 1978). In each of these three studies, approximately 20% of the victims experienced unusual stress during the day of the fatal or near fatal attacks.

In an attempt to measure the relative stressfulness of life events, several investigators have asked large groups of respondents to provide numerical ratings of stressfulness using lists of life events (Dohrenwend, Krasnoff, Askenasy, & Dohrenwend, 1978; Holmes & Rahe, 1967; Paykel, Prusoff, & Uhlenhuth, 1971). In the first of these efforts, Holmes and Rahe developed a Social Readjustment Rating Scale (SRRS). The SRRS contained 43 items dealing with health, work, family, personal life, social relations, and finances. Included in the list were both pleasant and unpleasant experiences. Thus, for example, death of a spouse received the highest score, 100, marriage was rated at 50, and going on vacation 13.

In one retrospective study using the SRRS, reports of illness during a 1-year period were correlated with the accumulation of life change units recalled for the previous year by 2000 navy employees (Rahe, 1972). Individuals with life change units between 150 and 300 reported significantly more illness than those scoring less. For those scoring more than 300, fully 70% reported becoming ill during the following year.

In a subsequent retrospective study of 88 resident physicians working in a Washington hospital, Holmes and Masuda (1974) found a correlation between the magnitude of life crises and the change in the health status of physicians. A change in health status was reported to have followed a mild life crisis 37% of the time, a moderate life crisis 51%, and a major life crisis 79%.

Although a large number of studies examining life events have related life stress to changes in health status (Holmes & Masuda, 1974; Rahe, 1972), depression and suicide (Paykel, 1974), and schizophrenia (Brown & Birley, 1968), life event checklists have been criticized in terms of their lack of reliability and validity as well as the low correlations actually found between stressful life events and disease (Rabkin & Streuning, 1976). For the most part these studies have been retrospective in nature and subject to distortions due to inaccurate recall by subjects. Thus, the value of these studies is primarily heuristic in nature, raising questions about the specificity of the relationships between stresses and diseases and the putative mechanisms that might mediate these relationships.

THE GENERALITY AND SPECIFICITY OF STRESS

The major pioneer in stress research has been Hans Selye. In his original work Selye defined stress as the nonspecific response of the body to any demand (Selye, 1936, 1946, 1970, 1976a,b). He believed that diverse noxious agents produced a chronological sequence called the *general adaptation syndrome*. This syndrome consists of three phases: (1) *alarm;* (2) *resistance;* and (3) *exhaustion.* During the alarm reaction, Selye noted an increased discharge of adrenocorticotrophic hormone (ACTH), corticoids, catecholamines, and development of thymicolymphatic involution, eosinopenia, and peptic ulcers. Although Selye believed that a stressor of sufficient magnitude could mobilize the general adaptive system of the entire body (i.e., induce intense nervous arousal, with consequent stimulation of the *hypothalamico — pituitary — adrenocortical* [HPAC] and *sympathoadreno-medullary* [SAM] systems), he also believed that specific aspects of a particular stressor can influence the stereotyped stress pattern by suppressing or enhancing some of its manifestations. According to Selye's description of the general adaptation syndrome, the relationship between stress and disease is primarily manifested during the stage of exhaustion.

Selye's (1936, 1946, 1970, 1976a,b) view that stress elicits a nonspecific response was consistent with the neurophysiological (Lindsley, 1951; Magoun, 1958) and psychological (Schachter, 1966) arousal theories of the 1950s and 60s. Lindsley, for instance, linked the *reticular activating system* of the brainstem to a behavioral dimension ranging from drowsiness to excitement and related these neurophysiological and behavioral dimensions to drive theory and autonomic nervous system (ANS) functioning. Schachter treated emotions as generalized forms of arousal that could be distinguished qualitatively by the cognitive label a person attaches to a particular situation. In summary, then, the general theorizing and experimentation of Lindsley and Schachter supported the view that ANS arousal tends to be diffuse and generalized, and that there is little evidence for explicit patterns of arousal that correspond to various emotions.

Although the theoretical positions espoused by Selye, Lindsley, and Schachter have had tremendous impact on the study of stress and emotions, they appear to be in need of modification. It now appears that responses to stress are more specific than was previously supposed.

Mason (1975), for example, examined endocrine profiles of responses to a variety of physical stressors (e.g., heat, cold, exercise, fasting). He found that: (1) a different profile of hormonal response was obtained for each type of stressor; and (2) in the absence of psychological threat, corticosteroid production did not increase.

In terms of the organization of the central nervous system (CNS), it appears that the CNS integrates separate patterns of concomitant ANS responses and behavior. In one study, for example, we found in rabbits that electrical microstimulation of the medial hypothalamus, particularly the ventromedial hypothalamic nucleus, elicited pronounced increases in heart rate (i.e., tachycardia) and blood pressure. These were associated with circling movements, hind-limb thumping, and other responses usually associated with aggressive behavior (Gellman, Schneiderman, Wallach, & Le Blanc, 1981). In contrast, stimulation of an intermediate zone, including the anterior and posterior hypothalamus, elicited pronounced, non-reflexive heart rate slowing (i.e., primary bradycardia) and a blood pressure increase as well as other manifestations of sympathetic arousal (e.g., pupil dilation). The animals tended to show behavioral immobility except for rather slow, orienting-like movements of the head. A third pattern of responses, identi-fied by microstimulation of the lateral hypothalamus, elicited profound bradycar-dia, a small depressor response, and quiet inactivity.

Of particular importance for the present discussion was the finding by Gellman et al. (1981) that microstimulation of the ventromedial hypothalamus produces a pressor response and tachycardia, whereas stimulation of the anterior and pos-terior hypothalamus produces a pressor response and bradycardia. In both in-stances the animals are clearly aroused sympathetically. Stimulation of the ventromedial hypothalamus also *inhibits* the vagal cardioinhibitory motoneurons that mediate bradycardia (Jordan, Khalid, Schneiderman, & Spyer, 1979), whereas stimulation of the anterolateral hypothalamus *activates* cardioinhibitory moto-neurons (Wallach, Ellenberger, Schneiderman, Liskowsky, Hamilton, & Gell-man, 1979).

Just as experiments in our laboratory have indicated that two separate patterns of autonomically mediated cardiovascular responses are associated with sympathetic activation, a similar division of responses has been observed during aversive behavior experiments conducted on animals. The animal behavior literature indi-cates that mammals confronted with an aversive situation generally tend to reveal one pattern of autonomic activity if appropriate *active coping* responses are being attempted, (i.e., fight, flight), but another pattern of ANS activity if coping responses are unavailable. The former pattern, sometimes referred to as the *defense reaction*, is characterized by increased movement, heart rate, cardiac output (i.e., quantity of blood pumped by the heart each minute), and vasodilation in skeletal muscle (Abrahams, Hilton, & Zbrozyna, 1960; Cannon, 1929; Djojosugito, Folkow, Kylstra, Lisander, & Tuttle, 1970; Hess, 1957). The second pattern, which occurs in aversive situations in which an aversive coping response does not seem available, is characterized by extreme vigilance, an inhibition of movement, an increase in *sympathetic nervous system* (SNS) activity, but also a vagally mediated decrease in heart rate (Von Holst, 1972).

Examples of the two basic patterns of response, one associated with active coping and the other with anticipation of aversive consequences, have been demonstrated within individual experiments (Adams, Baccelli, Mancia, & Zanchetti, 1968; Anderson & Tosheff, 1973; Baccelli, Ellison, Mancia, & Zanchetti, 1971; Lawler, Obrist, & Lawler, 1975). In one experiment, for example, Anderson and Tosheff examined the cardiovascular responses of dogs during daily hour-long sessions of unsignaled shock avoidance as well as during the 1 hour preceding the avoidance task when the animals were kept in a restraint harness within the experimental chamber. In terms of the active coping versus helplessness distinction, the avoidance situation can be conceptualized as one in which an active coping mechanism is available, whereas the preavoidance situation does not permit an active coping response to be made.

Anderson and Tosheff (1973) found that the dogs repeatedly placed in a restraint harness for a 1-hour period immediately preceding the avoidance contingency came to show a progressive increase in total peripheral resistance (i.e., constriction of arteries and arterioles) and arterial pressure accompanied by a progressive decrease in heart rate. In contrast, once the avoidance contingency was initiated, heart rate and cardiac output increased while the increase in blood pressure was maintained or augmented.

In a similar manner the differences in cardiovascular response patterns have been described in cats before and during confrontation with other animals (Adams et al., 1968; Baccelli et al., 1971). In general, the period preceding fighting, in which active coping was not possible, was associated with hind-limb vasoconstriction, increased total peripheral resistance, decreased cardiac output, and bradycardia. Conversely, during actual fighting, heart rate, hind-limb blood flow, and cardiac output increased, while total peripheral resistance decreased.

The avoidance-yoke experiment also permits an assessment of the effects of active coping on physiological responses. In this type of experiment the designated "avoidance" animal can make a particular response (e.g., wheel rotation) to prevent an electric shock from occurring. Failure to make the wheel rotation response results in both the "avoidance" animal and its "yoked" partner receiving shock. In one such set of experiments, Weiss (in press) demonstrated that rats permitted to make the "avoidance" response demonstrated less extensive gastric erosions and lower levels of plasma corticosterone than the yoked animals.

Because the physical factor of shocks received was identical for the two groups of rats, the less extensive gastric lesions and lower levels of *plasma corticosterone* in the avoidance animals must have been due to the purely psychological factor of being able to perform a coping response.

In a similar set of experiments Weiss, Stone, and Harrell (1970) found that the level of brain *norepinephrine* (NE) was increased in animals permitted to make a coping response, but was decreased in their yoked partners. Control experiments conducted by Weiss, Glazer, and Pohorecky (1976) clearly indicated that it is the ability to perform a coping response, rather than the level of physical activity, that is responsible for the difference in the level of brain NE.

The differences in physiological responsiveness as a function of coping mechanisms appear to apply also in situations involving psychosocial stress. If one assumes that dominant animals are able to cope, whereas subordinate animals may be subjected to more unavoidable stressors, an experiment by Henry, Ely, and Stephens (1972) may be interpreted in terms of the coping versus relative helplessness framework. Briefly, Henry et al. examined changes that occur in adrenal weight and blood pressure as a function of dominant and subordinate roles assumed by mice in normally socialized colonies.

During early stages of differentiation, the dominant mice in the Henry et al. (1972) study revealed increased release of *catecholamines* relative to subordinates. Conversely, the subordinates revealed a relative increase in adrenocortical activity. These biochemical changes eventually vanished after about 5 months, but were replaced by a chronic increase in blood pressure for the dominant and an increase in adrenal weight for the submissive animals.

The results of research conducted during the past two decades therefore suggest that the response to stressors is more specific than was previously supposed. Schachter's (1966) hypothesis that emotions are generalized forms of arousal that could be distinguished qualitatively by the cognitive label a person attaches to a particular situation, rested rather heavily on an experiment by Schachter and Singer (1962). In this study, several groups were told that they were being given a vitamin injection, when indeed they were being given an injection of epinephrine (E) or a placebo. In one condition a confederate of the experimenter acted euphoric, running around the room, tossing paper airplanes. Subjects in another condition were asked to complete an embarrassing questionnaire and were joined by a confederate who was instructed to act in an angry fashion.

The results of the Schachter and Singer (1962) experiment were interpreted as demonstrating that subjects felt "happiness" or "anger" depending on the cues offered by the confederate, and did not differ in terms of physiological response. Unfortunately, the investigators used heart rate as their sole indicator of physiological response, and this measure, which reflects both sympathetic and parasympathetic activity, is a notoriously poor indicator.

In addition, the experimental procedures and data analyses used by Schachter and Singer (1962) have been criticized on methodological grounds, including the post hoc elimination of 49 of 185 subjects (Maslach, 1979; Plutchick, 1980). It is perhaps also worth noting that injection of E tends to produce anxiety in human subjects when the experimental environment is not intentionally manipulated (Basowitz, Konchin, Oken, Goldstein, & Gussack, 1956). Thus, in spite of the strong impact that the Schachter and Singer experiment had on subsequent research and theory, the evidence is not convincing that emotional responses represent generalized forms of arousal.

Thus far, we have presented evidence that psychological responses to a stressor may differ as a function of stimulus (Mason, 1975), availability of a coping mechanism (Weiss, in press) or individual difference characteristics evidenced in psychosocial situations (Henry et al., 1972). Although these findings indicate that a certain amount of specificity does exist in physiological responses to stressors, the case can also be made that a stereotyped, generalized stress response occurs during the initial presentation of a highly aversive, ambiguous, overwhelming situation in which the availability of a coping mechanism is not apparent. In such situations, organisms tend to respond with pronounced SNS arousal, increases in blood pressure, heart rate, cardiac output, vasodilation in skeletal muscles, and secretion of E and NE from the adrenal medulla, as well as activation of the adrenal cortex (Mason, Mangan, Brady, Conrad, & Rioch, 1961).

As the initial, ambiguous, overwhelming, aversive situation becomes more predictable and subject to control, both E and cortisol tend to diminish in humans as well as monkeys, whereas NE remains involved in maintaining homeostasis under situational stress (Frankenhaeuser, 1980; Mason, 1975). In one experiment, for example, Frankenhaeuser, Sterky, and Jarpe (1962) placed subjects in a human centrifuge. Initially, excretions of both E and NE were markedly elevated. During the course of six weekly sessions, however, progressive decreases were obtained for both self-reported distress and E excretion; NE excretion remained elevated and unchanged. Similarly, during a 72-hour unsignaled avoidance experiment conducted on rhesus monkeys, both E and NE were initially elevated (Mason, Tolson, Brady, Tolliver, & Gilmore, 1969). During the course of the session, E progressively declined while NE increased.

In summary, the data indicate that in the face of a novel, intense, highly aversive stressor, in which a coping response is not readily apparent, mammals, including humans, respond by mobilizing both the SAM and HPAC systems. In less overwhelming situations the nature of the stimulus, the availability or nonavailability of a coping response, and individual difference variables can influence the pattern of physiological responses elicited. In the next sections we look at the manner in which the SAM, HPAC, CNS catecholamine, immune, and endorphin – enkephalin systems are influenced by stress, and examine the manner in which they may mediate relationships between stress and disease. The intent is to provide a basis for comprehending the role of stress in the behavioral contributions to disease (e.g., cancer, coronary heart disease) discussed in subsequent chapters.

Although the distinction is not complete in all respects, it appears to be useful, and we shall therefore contrast the psychophysiological adjustments associated with active coping on the one hand as opposed to those associated with helplessness, aroused vigilance, and conservation – withdrawal on the other.

PSYCHOPHYSIOLOGY OF ACTIVE COPING

The key to the psychophysiology of active coping is the SAM system. This system plays a preeminent role by increasing metabolic activity in response to situations perceived as being stressful. Other systems that may play some role in the psychophysiology of active coping are the HPAC system and the endorphin – enkephalin system.

The HPAC system, which is discussed more extensively in the section on "Helplessness, hypervigilance, and conservation – withdrawal" may also work synergistically with the SAM system, as an energy source during active coping. In emergency situations, for instance, the glucorticoids, primarily cortisol, cause the rapid mobilization of amino acids and fats from cellular stores. These then become available directly as an energy source and as a source for the synthesis of energy-rich glucose.

The endorphin – enkephalin system is an endogenous opiate system (Jaffe & Martin, 1980; Kuhar, Pert, & Snyder, 1973) that may be involved in aversive situations requiring active coping. These endogenous opiates may play a role in reducing fear, inhibiting pain-related withdrawal behaviors, and providing analgesia during fighting and other coping reactions.

Sympathoadrenomedullary (SAM) System

The SAM system is activated during fight, flight, and other active coping behaviors. Typically, but not always, this involves physical exertion. During active coping situations, particularly in those perceived as threatening, the SNS releases NE from sympathetic nerve terminals and NE and E from the adrenal medulla. Although Cannon (1929) suggested that activation of the SNS was accomplished as a unitary mass discharge, this is actually not the case. Plasma NE is preferentially released during exercise (Dimsdale & Moss, 1980), whereas plasma E is preferentially released during SNS activity associated with emotional behavior (Dimsdale & Moss, 1980; Glass, Krakoff, Contrada, Hilton, Kehoe, Mannucci, Collins, Snow, & Elting, 1980). Differential SNS activity is also seen during active coping versus aroused helplessness.

During behavioral stress that elicits active coping (e.g., the defense reaction) the heart increases its rate and force of contraction. The venous side of the circulation decreases its volume, thereby increasing the return of venous blood to the heart. Cardiac output is increased. The arterioles in the skin and gut constrict, increasing resistance to blood flow. This is at least partially offset, however, by increased flow of blood to skeletal muscle. Activation of the SNS during the defense reaction also stimulates: (1) adipose tissue to mobilize free fatty acids; (2) the liver to release glucose; and (3) the kidney to release renin and to decrease the excretion of sodium and water. The increases in free fatty acids and glucose provide increased energy resources and the effects upon the kidney increase arterial blood pressure.

In contrast to the defense reaction, which is elicited in situations involving active coping, another pattern of SNS activation occurs in aversive situations in which active coping is not perceived as being possible. In this situation increases in blood pressure are largely due to an increase in peripheral resistance associated with vasoconstriction in the skin, gut, and skeletal muscles. Heart rate and cardiac output are actually decreased.

Before considering hypotheses relating SAM activity to pathological processes, *we should recognize that sympathetic activation can be highly adaptive in challenging situations.* The performance of the skilled athlete during competition, the fireman rescuing someone from a burning building, and the individual hurrying to an appointment are all aided by activation of the SNS. However, if the challenge is too severe, too prolonged, or perhaps too often repeated, or if the individual is in poor physical condition, activation of the SNS can aggravate existing disorders or initiate new pathology. Thus, although Selye's (1936) general adaptation syndrome was originally conceptualized in terms of HPAC activity, it has also become a useful concept in terms of SNS function.

Behavioral stress, related to SNS activation, has been implicated in hypertension (Graham, 1945; Harburg, Erfurt, Havenstein, Chape, Schull, & Schork, 1973), atherosclerosis (e.g., Bassett & Cairncross, 1977; Lang, 1967), angina pectoris (Nestel, Verghese, & Levell, 1967), arrhythmias (Lown, Verrier, & Corbalan, 1973), myocardial ischemia and infarction (Raab, 1966; Russek, 1973), thrombosis (Haft & Fani, 1973), and sudden cardiac death (Lown, 1979). In addition, injections of even modest concentrations of catecholamines have been shown to produce arrhythmias (Guideri, Barletta, Chau, Green, & Lehr, 1975), myocardial ischemia and necrosis (Eliot, Todd, Clayton, & Pieper, 1978; Rona, Chappel, Balasy, & Caudry, 1959), and atherosclerosis (Friedman, Oester, & Davis, 1955).

There are a large number of ways in which SNS activity may mediate relationships between behavioral stress and cardiovascular pathology. These include: (1) induction of myocardial ischemia due to an increased need for myocardial oxygenation in conjunction with a reduced blood supply resulting from coronary atherosclerosis; (2) precipitation of life-threatening arrhythmias; (3) increased heart work in pumping blood at elevated arterial blood pressure; (4) increased resistance to blood flow through the arterioles; (5) deposition and incorporation into coronary artery plaques of thromboembolitic components of the blood; and (6) facilitation of necrosis, calcification, and rupture of plaques, which could, in turn, produce thrombosis and myocardial infarction.

At this point it may be of some value to distinguish between SNS activity occurring during emotional stress (e.g., the defense reaction) not necessarily involving pronounced exertion, and SNS activity occurring during aerobic exercise. When catecholamines are released during either exertion or emotional stress they mobilize lipid stores from adipose tissues (Heindel, Orci, & Jeanrenaud, 1975), which are hydrolized to free fatty acids for energy production in muscular activity (Zieler, Maseri, Klassen, Rabinowitz, & Burgess, 1968). In this way, SNS activation related to exercise demands leads to the effective utilization and rapid clearance of free fatty acids from the circulation. In contrast, when lipid mobilization induced by emotional stress is not accompanied by vigorous physical activities, the free fatty acids are not cleared as rapidly, and some of them become converted to triglycerides by the liver. These are then circulated as a component of *very low density lipoproteins* (VLDLs) in the blood (Schonfeld & Pfleger, 1971). Remnants of these VLDLs become converted into *low density lipoproteins* (LDLs) by the liver and are then returned to the circulation (Sigurdsson, Nicoll, & Lewis, 1975). It is the LDLs that are the source of most lipids in atherosclerotic plaques (Miller, 1980).

Other important differences in SNS activity can be seen as a function of aerobic exertion versus sedentary emotional stress. These include differences in the preferential release of E and NE and in the innervation of beta-adrenergic receptors at the heart. As previously mentioned, most experimental evidence is consistent with the view that NE is preferentially released during exercise (Dimsdale & Moss, 1980) and that E is preferentially released during emotional stress (Dimsdale & Moss, 1980; Glass et al., 1980).

The release of NE at the heart during exercise occurs via nerve terminals primarily at the sinoatrial (SA) and atrioventricular (AV) nodes, with some limited innervation also occurring at the ventricles. Interestingly, most beta-adrenergic receptors in the heart are not found in the vicinity of the SA and AV node, but are found in the left ventricle (Baker & Potter, 1980). Moreover, most of these receptors in the ventricle cannot be activated by the release of NE by sympathetic nerves. Instead, these receptors appear to be activated by circulating E released by the adrenal medulla in life-threatening situations (e.g., hemorrhage, severe acidosis) or during emotional stress. In hearts compromised by myocardial ischemia, circulating E could sensitize the myocardium and lead to potentially lethal arrhythmias. The means by which excessive SNS activity may contribute to neurogenic hypertension and coronary heart disease is addressed elsewhere in this volume by Schneiderman and Hammer (Chapter 17).

The Endogenous Opiates

Findings that the CNS contains receptor sites for binding opiates (Kuhar et al., 1973) provided a major puzzle for neuropharmacology. After all, the administration of heroin, morphine, and other opiates is a particularly human enterprise, but the development of opiate receptors follows an evolutionary course. What functional significance could these receptors have unless the brain contains endogenous opiates? The answer to the puzzle came when Hughes and associates (Hughes, Smith, Kosterlitz, Fothergill, Morgan, & Morris, 1975) isolated and characterized two pentapeptides, *met-* and *leu-enkephalin.* Subsequent work identified other, larger polypeptides such as *alpha-, beta-, and gamma-endorphins.*

All the amino acid sequences of enkephalins and endorphins are found in the pituitary prohormone, beta-lipotropin, which comes from the same precursor as adrenocorticotropic hormone (ACTH). Interestingly, manipulations that cause the release of ACTH in the rat, including behavioral stress, also lead to the release of beta-endorphin (Guillemin, 1978). Stimulation of the adrenal medulla also results in the secretion of met-enkephalin and leu-enkephalin into the circulation (Wilson, Chang, & Viveros, 1982). The secretion of opiate peptides and catecholamines is proportional to the cell content of these substances, which are both stored in the same cells.

Endogenous opiates also appear to be important in regulating the secretion of pituitary hormones during stress. Naloxone, for example, which is an opiate antagonist, can attenuate the stress release of prolactin (Rossier, French, Rivier, Shibaski, Guillemin, & Bloom, 1980) and corticosteroids (Gibson, Ginsberg, Hall, & Hart, 1979). The corticosteroid response may be mediated through endogenous action upon ACTH or upon the adrenal cortex.

The enkephalins and endorphins appear to be morphologically and functionally distinct systems. *Enkephalins* are widely distributed in the brain. Their location in nerve terminals, calcium-dependent release, and rapid destruction are consistent with the view that they are either neurotransmitters or neuromodulators at central synapses (Jaffe & Martin, 1980). In contrast, the *endorphins,* which seem to be localized in the hypothalumus and pituitary, are suspected of being neurohormones due to their longer duration of action. Another endogenous opiate, *dynorphin,* has also been localized in the pituitary.

The distribution of the endogenous opiates follows closely the distribution of the opiate receptors. As discussed elsewhere in this volume by Winters (Chapter 20), these compounds are particularly prevalent in regions of the CNS that mediate pain. In addition, endogenous opiates have been localized in areas such as the globus pallidus and locus coeruleus, which are brain structures related to movement and mood.

Acute or chronic stress appears to produce an activation of specific CNS and pituitary pools of endogenous opiates (Millan & Emrich, 1981). Foot shock in rats, for example, has been found to lead to release of beta-endorphin in the hypothalamus, septum, and periaqueductal gray (Millan, Przewlocki, Jerlicz, Gramsch, Hollt, & Herz, 1981). This is accompanied by increased levels of plasma beta-endorphin and an increase of pituitary beta-endorphin. These changes suggest that pituitary beta-endorphin is mobilized into the systemic circulation. Hypothalamic leu-enkephalin has also been found to be released following foot shock (Rossier,

Guillemin, & Bloom, 1978). In addition, stressed rats show increased plasma dynorphin and depletion of pituitary dynorphin (Millan, Tsang, Przewlocki, Hollt, & Herz, 1981). Chronic stress, such as arthritis (Cesselin, Montastrue, Gros, Bourgoin, & Hammon, 1980), postnatal stress (Torda, 1978), and being reared in isolation (Bonnett, Miller, & Simon, 1976) have been reported to be accompanied by elevation of endogenous opiates and an increase in the number of opiate receptors in the CNS.

Bolles and Fanselow (1982) have suggested that the primary function of the endogenous opiates is to provide analgesia and inhibit pain-motivated withdrawal responses when defensive behavior is necessary. In this respect, it is interesting that increased SNS activity associated with baroreceptor activation in the rat is associated with decreased shock avoidance behavior (Dworkin, Filewich, Miller, Craigmyle, & Pickering, 1979), which could be due to the release of endogenous opiates. Administration of morphine in humans not only eliminates pain itself, but also alleviates anxiety and the anticipation of pain in aversive situations (Millan & Emrich, 1981).

In summary, it would appear that in stressful situations in which active coping is required, the SAM system becomes mobilized and increases metabolic activity. HPAC activity can also help to increase this metabolic activity. The endorphin – enkephalin system appears to act in concert with the SAM and HPAC systems to provide analgesia and inhibit pain-motivated withdrawal responses.

HELPLESSNESS, HYPERVIGILANCE, AND CONSERVATION – WITHDRAWAL

During highly stressful situations in which a coping response is not evident, a large number of behavioral and physiological reactions may occur. The behavioral responses include poor performance in tasks requiring active motor behavior (Seligman & Maier, 1967; Weiss & Glazer, 1975), loss of normal aggressiveness or competitiveness (Henry & Stephens, 1977), as well as decreased sleep (Weiss, in press) and appetite (Ritter, Pelzer, & Ritter, 1978). Physiological responses include increased SNS activity associated with decreased cardiac output and heart rate (von Holst, 1972), increased ACTH and adrenocortical secretions (Selye, 1936, 1946), decreased levels of brain NE (Weiss et al., 1976), and suppression of the immune system (Riley, 1981). The ANS changes have already been discussed in detail. Let us now turn our attention to the HPAC system.

Hypothalamico-Pituitary-Adrenocortical (HPAC) System

A wide variety of physical, neurogenic, and behavioral stressors can activate the HPAC system. These include intense heat or cold, infection, surgery, physical restraint, or administration of sympathomimetic drugs. Emotional stress associated with novelty, uncertainty, and unpredictability are potent stimuli for both catecholamine and corticosteroid release (Mason, 1975). As previously mentioned, the HPAC system is also activated in response to emotionally stressful situations in which an active coping mechanism is not available (Henry & Meehan, 1981; Schneiderman, 1983). The resulting behavior is characterized by extreme vigilance, inhibition of movement, SNS activation, but also bradycardia mediated by the parasympathetic nervous system. This "conservation-withdrawal pattern" (Selye, 1946, 1970, 1976a,b) has been associated with suppression of the immune system, peptic ulceration, clinical depression, and various cardiovascular disorders (Henry & Stephens, 1977).

Several studies have contrasted SAM and HPAC activity during behavioral experiments in humans. In one of these studies Lundberg (1980) found that a vigilance task, which was interpreted to be stressful, produced excretion of cortisol. In contrast, a self-paced reaction time task elicited the preferential excretion of catecholamines. Both Lundberg (1980) and Frankenhaeuser (1980) have interpreted results such as these as evidence that effort without distress leads to activation of the SAM system; whereas, distress without effort elicits activation of the HPAC system. Furthermore, they suggest that distress without effort, and the concomitant release of cortisol, are associated with feelings of helplessness and passivity.

The mechanism by which the HPAC system becomes activated has been traced to parvocellular neurons in the medial basal hypothalamus. Thus, the system is actually under the control of the CNS. In response to stimulation, the neurons in the medial basal hypothalamus secrete *corticotropin-releasing factor* CRF. The chemical structure of CRF is presently unknown although most hypothalamic-releasing and inhibiting hormones appear to be small peptides. In any event, the CRF is transported to the anterior pituitary (i.e., adenohypophysis) via the hypothalamicohypophyseal portal system, which consists of a network of small blood vessels. In the adenohypophysis, CRF stimulates secretion of ACTH into the systemic circulation. The target organ, which is the adrenal cortex, is then activated by ACTH to release adrenocorticosteroids such as cortisol and corticosterone. Humans and other primates primarily release cortisol (hydrocortisone), whereas rodents primarily release corticosterone.

The HPAC system appears to have several important negative feedback aspects. One of these is for the control of corticosteroid secretion. The major aspect of this control involves the excitation of the hypothalamus by various stressors. These activate the system, causing the release of corticosteroids within minutes. The release of corticosteroids, in turn, initiates metabolic effects directed at relieving damage caused by the stressor (e.g., reduction of fever or inflammation). In addition, corticosteroids have direct negative feedback effects: (1) on the hypothalamus to decrease formation of CRF; and (2) on the adenohypophysis to decrease the formation of ACTH. This feedback serves to stabilize the concentration of corticosteroids in the circulation when the body is not experiencing stress. However, the stabilizing feedback is disrupted when a stressor does appear.

Elevated cortisol secretion is frequently seen in clinically depressed human patients (Sachar, 1976) and in persons experiencing bereavement (Carroll, 1976). In the latter case administration of dexamethasone, which normally suppresses cortisol release through negative feedback, is ineffective. It thus appears that bereavement and perhaps clinical depression may override the normal cortisol feedback mechanism.

Elevations in cortisol are seen in highly stressful situations in which active coping responses do not seem readily available. Clinically depressed people often express a sense of hopelessness, and bereaved individuals a sense of powerlessness. Squirrel monkeys separated from their mothers prematurely also reveal elevated levels of cortisol, becoming apathetic and depressed (Coe & Levine, 1981).

Animal behavior experiments have provided evidence that increases in the release of the adrenocorticosteroids are closely associated with a lack of control over the environment. Weiss (1972), for example, found that rats receiving inescapable electric shocks revealed significantly higher levels of corticosterone than rats who were able to avoid shocks. Similarly, Hanson, Larson, and Snowden (1976) found that monkeys subjected to unavoidable, intense noise showed elevations in plasma cortisol, whereas this did not occur in monkeys having control over the noise.

The relationship between environmental control and adrenocorticosteroid levels can also be extended to dominance hierarchies. Candland and Leshner (1974), for instance, measured urinary 17-hydroxycorticosterone in squirrel monkeys, shortly after the monkeys had been placed together and formed their order of dominance. They found that the *subordinate* monkeys revealed greater amounts of 17-hydroxycosticosterone than the *dominant* animals. Similarly, Chamove and Bowman (1978) measured plasma cortisol levels as a function of position in dominance hierarchies of monkeys and found that cortisol levels varied inversely with rank.

The relationship between dominance and adrenocortical function is also seen in mice. Victorious mice do not reveal elevated plasma corticosterone following a fight, but defeated, subordinate mice do (Louch & Higginbotham, 1967). The causal role of corticosterone is strongly suggested by the finding that following injection of corticosterone, mice display a submissive posture when attacked by other mice (Leshner & Politch, 1979). Leshner and Politch also found that injection of ACTH reduced aggressiveness, but did not lead specifically to submissive displays.

Although there is some evidence that both ACTH (e.g., short-feedback loop) and corticosteroids (long-feedback loop) can influence behavior by means of feedback to the HPAC system, there is also evidence that CNS influences upon the hypothalamus can influence other parts of the system. Sachar, Anis, Nathan, Halbreich, and Halpern, (1980), for example, found that stimulation of catecholamine activity with dextroamphetamine suppressed plasma cortisol to normal levels in depressed human patients. This finding is consistent with the hypothesis that decreased noradenergic tone disinhibits CRF secretion in the hypothalamus, thereby contributing to cortisol hypersecretion.

The negative feedback aspects of the HPAC system appear also to be important in terms of other behaviors besides depression and subordination. One such behavioral – endocrine loop has been suggested by Christian (1971). According to Christian, increased population density in rodents produces behavioral stress associated with mobilization of the HPAC system. Feedback from this system to the hypothalamus then results in decreased gonadotropin release. This impairs reproductive capacity, thereby decreasing natality and ultimately reducing the population. Christian's (1971) hypothesis is supported by findings that: (1) corticosterone levels become elevated in subordinate mice during intense social interaction (Ely, Henry, & Ciananello, 1974); and (2) gonadotropic hormones of subordinated male mice are decreased during fights to establish social order (Bronson, 1973).

Aside from its role in clinical depression, cortisol hyperresponsivity may play some contributary role in the pathogenesis of both coronary atherosclerosis and acute coronary events. This could occur specifically because of the synergistic relationship that exists between the SAM and HPAC systems under novel stress or emergency conditions. Cortisol, for example, has been shown to: (1) increase the sensitivity of adrenergic receptors to a given level of neurotransmitter; (2) stimulate catecholamine-synthesizing enzyme; and (3) and inhibit catechol-O-methyltransferase, which is a major catecholamine-degrading enzyme (Kvetnansky, 1980). The finding among air force personnel that elevated serial plasma corticol levels during an oral glucose tolerance test is associated with increased severity of angiographically documented atherosclerosis is consistent with the view that cortisol hyperresponsivity may contribute to atherogenesis (Troxler, Sprague, Albanese, Fuchs, & Thompson, 1977).

In terms of more acute effects upon the heart, Selye (1970) reported that rats pretreated with glucocorticoids and mineral corticoids were extremely susceptible to myocardial necrosis in response to a stressful situation such as forced exercise, restraint, or a cold bath.

In Chapter 16 of this volume, Carver, Diamond, and Humphries review evidence that the Type A behavior pattern is a risk factor for coronary heart disease. Interestingly, a recent study by Williams, Lane, Kuhn, Melosh, White, and Schlanberg (1982) indicates that during a mental arithmetic task, Type A (coronary prone) men showed enhanced secretions of cortisol, N, and E, relative to Type B men.

In summary, it would appear that the HPAC and SAM systems can work synergistically in stressful situations, and this may contribute to atherosclerotic coronary heart disease and to acute coronary events in susceptible individuals. The HPAC system seems to become particularly active in stressful situations in which coping responses are not readily available. Elevated cortisol levels are associated in animals with defeats in fighting and being forced to assume a subordinate role. Increased cortisol release is also seen in humans subjected to aversive tasks over which they have little control. Cortisol hyperresponsivity also occurs in humans experiencing bereavement or clinical depression. Both cortisol and ACTH have been implicated in the regulation of behavior, but cortisol elevation can also reflect NE depletion in parts of the brain.

Brain Catecholamines, Stress, and Depression

Relationships among hypothalamic function, pituitary — adrenocortical activities, and clinical depression were long suspected because: (1) clinical depression is often associated with changes in mood, appetite, sex drive, sleep, ANS activity, and circadium rhythms that are suggestive of hypothalamic disturbances; and (2) neuroendocrine activity is regulated by the same biogenic amines in the hypothalamus that have been implicated in affective disorders (Sachar et al., 1980).

Cortiscosteroid secretion follows a *circadian* rhythm. This rhythm is at least in part under the control of the *suprachiasmatic nucleus* of the hypothalamus. Lesions of this structure in the rat, for example, abolish the circadian adrenal corticosterone rhythm (Moore & Eichler, 1972). The normal circadian rhythm of cortisol secretion in humans peaks at about 8:00 A.M. with afternoon and evening values at relatively low levels (Sachar, 1981). In contrast, profoundly depressed people exhibit hypersecretion of cortisol in the afternoon and evening hours as well as during the morning. As previously mentioned, Sachar et al. (1980) have found evidence consistent with the view that depletion of NE in the CNS disinhibits CRF secretion in the hypothalamus thereby contributing to the cortisol hypersecretion observed in clincal depression.

The most widely held theory concerning the role of the CNS in depression is that it involves a depletion of NE, although other neurotransmitters and neuromodulators may also be involved (Cooper, Bloom, & Roth, 1978). This NE depletion theory first developed from observations made in clinical psychopharmacology. Administration of reserpine, for example, was found to lead to depressive episodes in psychiatric patients who were prone to affective disorders (Schaffer, Pandey, Noll, Killian, & Davis, 1981); reserpine causes a depletion of NE, dopamine, and serotonin in the brain. In contrast to the effects of reserpine, symptoms of depression were found to improve following administration of monoamine oxidase (MAO) inhibitors. The enzyme MAO degrades biogenic amines, so that its inhibition causes the level of amines (i.e., neurotransmitters) to rise. Tricyclic medications have proven even more effective as antidepressants. These compounds block the presynaptic uptake of NE and serotonin, thereby leaving greater amounts of these transmitters in the synaptic cleft (Maas, 1972).

Within the brain NE is metabolized into 3-methoxy-4-hydroxy-phe-nethyleneglycol (MHPG), which is then excreted in the urine. Clinically depressed patients excrete significantly less MHPG than control subjects (Mass, 1972). Studies such as these have linked the depletion of brain NE to clinical depression. As pointed out by Winters in the previous chapter, however, the issue is actually more complex, and there may be some depressed patients with primarily NE deficiency and others with mostly serotonin deficiency.

Studies conducted on animal models have linked depression to: (1) specific kinds of behavioral stress; and (2) depletion of NE in specific regions of the brain. In an early experiment Overmier and Seligman (1967) found that animals exposed to uncontrollable electric shocks subsequently were unable to acquire and perform a shuttle-box avoidance-escape response that animals normally learn and perform quite readily. Subsequent experiments have clearly established that it is the lack of control over the stimulus that leads to the behavioral deficit, as experience with controllable shocks do not lead to the deficit (Seligman & Maier, 1967; Weiss & Glazer, 1975).

The aforementioned findings are of interest for the development of an experimental model of depression, because depressed persons commonly report that they feel helplesss and unable to cope or control events. It is also of interest that several of the treatments that are effective in relieving depression in humans, such as administration of MAO inhibitors and tricyclic antidepressive drugs, are able to: (1) counteract the effects of uncontrollable shocks; or (2) prevent the occurrence of the behavioral deficits initially (Glazer, Weiss, Pohorecky, & Miller, 1975; Leshner, Remler, Biegon, & Samuel, 1979; Petty & Sherman, 1980). These deficits can also be reversed by *electroconvulsive shocks,* which are also used in the treatment of severe depression. Electroconvulsive shocks appear to provide their therapeutic effects by inducing *tryosine hydroxylase,* which is the rate-limiting enzyme in the biosynthesis of NE (Masserano, Takimoto, & Weiner, 1981; Musacchio, Jolou, Kety, & Glowinski, 1969).

Weiss (in press) has further pointed out that some of the behavioral disturbances observed in animals following uncontrollable shock are similar to those observed in clinically depressed people. These include deficits in motor activity, appetitive behavior, grooming, and sleep. The failure of animals to make escape – avoidance responses in the shuttle box after first receiving unavoidable shocks was initially attributed to "learned helplessness" (Seligman, 1974). Further studies, however, have indicated that the decrease in performance is actually due to a motor activation deficit related to a decrease in brain NE (Weiss et al., 1976).

Evidence has been presented that stress-induced depression of motor activity correlates highly with regional changes of NE in the brainstem (Weiss, Bailey, Pohorecky, Korzeniowski, & Grillone, 1980). More recently Weiss (in press) has suggested that stress-induced depression is due to a fall of NE level within the locus coeruleus. Based upon experiments in which he and his colleagues have infused various adrenergic agonists and antagonists into the locus coeruleus, Weiss suggests that stress-induced behavioral depression is related to a functional blockade of alpha 2 receptors in the locus coeruleus.

Caveats.   The literature reviewed in this section suggests: that (1) uncontrollable stress can precipitate severe depression; and (2) the depression is associated with a decrease in the level of brain NE, possibly in the locus coeruleus. Although these findings may be correct, the story is undoubtedly incomplete. Genetic factors also appear to play an important role in the development of depression, and other neurotransmitters in the CNS besides NE have been implicated in depression.

As fas as the genetic predisposition for depression is concerned, Kety (1979) has reported that the biological parents of adopted depressive patients have a higher rate of depression that the adopted parents of control adoptees. Also with regard to depression, monozygotic twins have a concordance rate of 69%; whereas, dizygotic twins and siblings have a rate of about 13% (Sachar, 1981). Thus, behavioral stress may play an important precipitating role in clinical depression, but genetic factors may have an important predisposing influence in many instances.

Although NE appears to be an important mediator of stress-induced depression, the phenomenon has also been linked to systemic changes in brain acetylcholine (Anisman, 1975) and serotonin (Sherman & Petty, 1980). These findings are not mutually exclusive with the NE findings, however, because serotonergic neurons are known to synapse upon NE neurons in the locus coeruleus (McRae-Degueurce & Pujol, 1979) and NE neurons originating in the locus coeruleus influence cholinergic activity in the neocortex (Vizi, 1980). In summary, it appears that: (1) uncontrollable stress can precipitate severe depression, but genetic factors are also important; and (2) severe depression is associated with a decrease in the level of brain NE, but other neurotransmitters also appear to be involved.

Behavioral Stress and the Immune System

A substantial body of research indicates that behavioral stressors may alter immune responses and thereby increase disease susceptibility. One pathway by which behavioral stress has been shown to affect immunity is through the HPAC system (Borysenko & Borysenko, 1982; Riley, Fitzmaurice, & Spackman, 1981). A second pathway involves bidirectional communication between the CNS and lymphoid organs (Locke, 1982). In general, the research that has related behavioral variables to immune deficiencies has supported the view that exposure to intense, unavoidable stress may increase susceptibility to illness.

The Immune System.   In order to understand the relationships among behavior, immune deficiencies, and disease it is important to have some understanding of the immune system, which represents our protection against foreign bodies. The immune system's functions are carried out primarily by white blood cells (i.e., leukocytes) and their derivatives. One distinction that can be made is between *innate* and *acquired* immunity. Innate immunity is conveyed by *phagocytes*. The phagocytes are capable of ingesting and destroying: (1) bacteria; (2) small foreign cells; or (3) degenerating tissue. Phagocyte cells are electronegatively charged and therefore repel other electronegative objects. Most normal particulates in the extracellular fluid are also negatively charged. In contrast, most damaged tissues as well as foreign bodies that have been attached to antibodies acquire positive charges and therefore can be phagocytized (Kaplan, 1979).

In contrast to innate immunity, acquired immunity is conveyed by *lymphocytes*. There are two kinds of acquired immunity: *humoral immunity* and *cellular immunity*. Humoral immunity consists of the formation of antibodies, which circulate in the blood and attach to an invading substance. This humoral immunity is based on the function of B cells, which mature in the bone marrow. When activated by invading proteins called *antigens,* B cells are responsible for transformation into tissue plasma cells, which secrete protein *antibodies* called *immunoglobulins*. These antibodies attack the invading agent.

Cellular immunity differs from humoral immunity in that whole *sensitized lymphocytes* are released into the lymph instead of antibodies. The acquired cellular immunity is based on the function of T cells, which mature in the *thymus* gland. Unlike humoral immunity, in which antibodies persist for only a few months, cellular immunity has an indefinite time span. This long duration system of sensitized lymphocytes is activated in response to slow developing bacterial diseases (e.g., tuberculosis), cancer cells, tissue transplants, and some viruses.

The body must be able to recognize its own tissue in order to prevent the immune system from destroying the host. This process is known as *tolerance*. During the development of the fetus, the thymus gland destroys lymphocytes that are specific for the body's own tissue. Failure of this system can lead to autoimmune diseases such as rheumatic fever and myasthenia gravis (Sampter, 1978).

Stress, Endocrines, and Immune Responses.   It has been known for many years that acute stress can cause involution of the thymus gland (Dougherty, 1952). Thymic involution can also be mimicked by administration of corticosteroids (Claman, 1977). Corticosteroids lyse lymphocytes in the thymic cortex of mice, rats, and rabbits, and inhibit lymphocyte metabolism and proliferation in monkeys and humans. Following prolonged stress there are fewer circulating lymphocytes. Existing pools of mature cells are subject to inhibition both by circulating epinephrine and by corticosteroids (Borysenko & Borysenko, 1982). In addition, circulating catecholamines and corticosteroids can also apparently inhibit the functions of macrophages, mast cells, neutrophils, and eosinophils, which are known to interact with the immune system.

In a comprehensive series of experiments, Riley (1981) examined relationships among stress, immunity, and corticosteroid function. He found that mice living in standard laboratory animal quarters had corticosterone levels that were 10 to 20 times higher than those of mice housed in low-stress environments. Riley found that mice, stressed either by living in the standard vivarium or exposed to mild rotation, consistently showed increases in tumor growth following tumor implants. These results could be mimicked by injection of natural or synthetic cortico-steroids into the animals. In contrast, other experiments reviewed by Borysenko and Borysenko (1982) suggest that the effects of stress on tumor progression can be abrogated when coping mechanisms are made available to experimental animals.

Although there is some evidence linking stress to increased disease suscep-tibility by the corticosteroid-mediated suppression of antibody production, the evidence is not overly convincing. Support for the hypothesis has actually been unequivocal only when high levels of exogenous steroids are administered.

Several studies conducted upon humans have shown positive relationships between behavioral stress and suppression of immune responses, but have failed to relate the immune deficiencies to corticosteroid production. Moreover, these studies emphasize the time-dependent nature of the immune changes. In one study Bartrop, Luckhurst, and Lazarus (1977) compared lymphoblast transformation in 33 bereaved spouses with lymphoblast transformation in control subjects matched in terms of age, sex, and race. Lymphoblast transformation is a measure of lymphocyte responsivity to mitogens. Bartrop et al. found that blast transforma-tion was depressed among bereaved spouses at 8 weeks but not at 2 weeks postbereavement. In a similar study, Schleifer, Keller, McKegney, and Stein (1980) found a depression of lymphoblast transformation 5 to 7 weeks postbereavement in a sample of husbands whose wives had died from breast cancer. In neither case could the immune suppression be readily explained by concomitant measures of neuroendocrine function. In both studies, however, the sample sizes were small, and no attempt was made to examine neuroendocrine changes as a function of disturbances in circadian pattern. Nevertheless, the findings are of considerable interest in view of: (1) bereavement being an example of a stressful experience in which an obvious coping mechanism is not available; and (2) the increased disease susceptibility and mortality reported for recently bereaved individuals (Jacobs & Ostfeld, 1977).

Another stressful experience, prolonged sleep deprivation, has been used by Palmblad and his collaborators to examine the effects of stress upon immune competence and neuroendocrine responsiveness in human experimental subjects. In the first study, neutrophils exhibited a decreased ability to phagocytize *Sta-phlyococcus aureus* as a consequence of 72 hours of sleep deprivation (Palmblad, Cantell, Strander, Froberg, Karlsson, Levi, Granstrom, & Unger, 1976). Neu-trophils, which are part of the innate immune system, are mature cells that attach bacteria and viruses in the blood.

In a subsequent experiment Palmblad, Petrini, Wasserman, and Akerstedt (1979) found that the synthesis of blood lymphocytes was reduced after 48 hours of sleep deprivation. The findings by Palmblad and his collaborators suggest that diminished host defense occurs during sleep deprivation. However, within a very few days, after the end of deprivation, lymphocyte depression regressed and interferon production and phagocytosis were enhanced.

In both studies by Palmblad and his coworkers (Palmblad et al., 1976, 1979) thyroid hormone activity increased during sleep deprivation. However, serum cortisol and urinary catecholamine output was increased in the first study but decreased in the second. Thus, in the human studies just reviewed (Bartrop et al., 1977; Palmblad et al., 1976, 1979; Schleifer et al., 1980), evidence of stress-induced immune suppression was obtained in each case, but adrenocortical response was reported to be either increased, decreased, or unchanged. Therefore, links between endocrine function and immune suppression in such human studies appears to be as yet unconfirmed.

Individual Differences and Immune Suppression. Kasl et al. (1979) studied the effects of academic stress upon the development of infectious mononucleosis as a function of psychosocial risk factors. In this study 1327 entering cadets at the West Point Military Academy were screened for the presence of Epstein – Barr virus antibody to infectious mononucleosis. Kasl et al. found that two-thirds of the entering cadets arrived immune, 20% of the susceptibles became infected (seroconverted) each year, and of these, 25% contracted infectious mononucleosis. Psychosocial risk factors were predictive of both seroconversion and the development of clinical infectious mononucleosis. The risk factors were: (1) having a high level of motivation for a military career; (2) doing relatively poorly academically; and (3) having fathers perceived as being "overachievers."

In another experiment described by Locke (1982), 108 college undergraduates underwent psychometric and immunologic assessment before and after influenza immunization. Immunologic assessment included natural killer cell activity, which is a type of cell-mediated cytotoxicity. Locke found that those individuals who reported they have extensive psychologic symptoms under stress had significantly diminished natural killer cell activity in comparison to their reportedly "better coping counterparts."

Temporal Relations and Immune Suppression. Although evidence suggests that unavoidable stressors (e.g., rotation of mice, loss of a spouse, sleep deprivation) and poor coping mechanisms (Kasl et al., 1979; Locke, 1982) may lead to immune suppression, evidence of stress-induced enhancement has also been reported. Much of the apparent conflicting evidence appears to be related to the timing of the stress exposure in relationship to measurement of the host defense. In general, depressed immune function and increased morbidity and mortality seem to occur if the infectious agent or antigen is administered prior to or during the stress exposure (Bartrop et al., 1977; Hill, Greer, & Felsenfeld, 1967; Palmblad et al., 1976; Solomon, 1969). In contrast, increased resistance may occur if exposure to the stressor precedes antigen administration or the determination of immune function (Palmblad et al., 1976, 1979; Solomon, Merigan, & Levine, 1967). Thus, it would appear that exposure to a stressor may initially depress a host defense, but that this may be followed by enhanced resistance.

Comment. An extensive body of research knowledge supports the view that acute stress induces an increase in steroid hormones known to be lympholytic, and that this results in lessened immune responses. This in turn has been linked to increased susceptibility to infection and to increased likelihood of the spread of tumors. In addition to the involvement of the HPAC system, changes in immune capability can be influenced directly by the CNS.

Although progress has been made in understanding relationships between behavioral stress and immune responses there are many complexities inherent in the relationship. One of these is that an initial alarm reaction may be reflected in a depressed host response, whereas a subsequent resistance phase may be reflected in an enhanced host response. In some cases, psychosocial challenge imposed prior to pathogenic challenge may lower resistance to a particular virus while increasing resistance to a parasite (Friedman, Glasgow, & Ader 1969). In any event, an understanding of the systematic relationships among psychosocial stress, immune suppression, and disease will require: (1) better characterization of stressors; (2) improved understanding of species (host) differences; (3) broader evaluation of immune competence; (4) more systematic categorization of immune responses (e.g., humoral versus cellular immunity) in relation to specific stressors and behavioral responses (e.g., active coping versus helplessness); and (5) a more comprehensive understanding of putative immune mechanisms.

COPING WITH STRESS

The literature reviewed in this chapter indicates that individual stress can elicit physiological adjustments, and that these physiological changes may, under certain conditions, contribute to the development of physical disorders. A distinction was made between the physiological responses associated with active coping on the one hand and with helplessness, hypervigilance, and conservation – withdrawal on the other. We suggested that activation of the SAM system, and particularly the defense reaction, is associated with active coping in response to threats ranging from mild to extreme. This pattern of response, which includes an increase in heart rate, cardiac output, and sympathetic vasodilation in skeletal muscle can readily be elicited during challenging behavioral tasks ranging from mental arithmetic and video arcade games to full-blown fight or flight reactions.

The physiologic responses involved in active coping are closely linked to physical exertion in nonhuman species, as they were also for our primitive human forebears. In twentieth-century America, however, a distinction needs to be made between the physiologic changes involved in exercise and those that are involved in emotional coping. Although both emotional behavior and aerobic exercise may both mobilize the SAM system, these two activities often can be differentiated in terms of oxygen utilization. Thus, although considerable SNS activation may occur in angry altercations between employee and employer, customer and merchant, etc., these episodes only rarely end in violent confrontations. In the absence of confrontation, the mobilization of the SAM system results in the relatively slow clearance of free fatty acids and their sequelae.

In the present chapter we have provided some evidence that mobilization of the SAM system during the defense reaction lead to the concomitant activation of the endorphin − enkephalin system. The release of endogenous opiates by this sytem may provide analgesia and inhibit withdrawal responses during aversive situations requiring active coping. Although this is an attractive hypothesis, it must be conceded that relatively little is presently known about the detailed relationships between the endorphin − enkephalin system and behavioral stress.

In contrast to the physiologic responses associated with active coping, stressful situations in which an obvious coping response is not apparent may lead behaviorally to hypervigilance and psychologically to feelings of helplessness and hopelessness. A different pattern of SNS activation is elicited than that seen during active coping, and depletion of brain NE, activation of the HPAC system, and/or suppression of the immune system may also occur.

In view of the differences in behavioral circumstances, psychologic processes, and physiologic responses associated with active coping on the one hand and helplessness, hypervigilance, and withdrawal-conservation on the other, the means for dealing with these two forms of stress are likely to be different. Nevertheless the methods for dealing with both kinds of stress need to focus on modifying: (1) the stressful environment; (2) maladaptive perceptual and response styles characteristic of the individual; and/or (3) the physiologic responses evoked by the stressor.

In the case of persons exposed to high stress environments, where time pressures are real, decisions continually have to be made, and there is little time for reflection during daily living, the individuals can: (1) accept the stress; (2) look for "time-outs" in the form of vacations and/or daily recreational activities; and/or (3) restructure their lives to follow an alternative course. Sometimes physical symptoms (e.g., essential hypertension), disease (e.g., angina pectoris, myocardial infarction [M.I.]), consequences of the highly stressful life-style on the family, or the death or illness of a close associate can set the stage for establishing environmental changes.

Although changing the environment provides one means of coping with stress, an alternative or supplementary strategy is to change perceptions and consequent behaviors. This may involve modifying assumptions, attributions, and beliefs and/ or substituting assertiveness for aggressiveness.

Another method for dealing with behavioral stress is to alter psychologic and physiologic responses. Administration of propranolol (Inderal) or diazepam (Valium) reflect a pharmacologic approach. Relaxation training, which we shall discuss further, offers a behavioral approach. Before discussing the specifics of relaxation training, let us briefly examine a study that aimed to reduce mortality by restructuring the environment, altering perceptual and response styles, and changing the responsiveness of Type A individuals who were recovering from M.I. (Friedman, Thoresen, Gill, Ulmer, Thompson, Powell, Price, Elek, Rabin, Breal, Piaget, Dixon, Bourg, Levy, & Tasto, 1982). Some of the procedures used in the study are summarized in Table 5.1.

Details of the study are described elsewhere in this volume by Schneiderman and Hammer (Chapter 17). Comprehensive discussion of the Type A coronary-prone behavior pattern is presented by Carver, Diamond, and Humphries (Chapter 16) and details of some of the specific interventions used are described by Tapp (Chapter 9).

At this point our specific interest in the Friedman et al. (1982) study is that it attempted to prevent recurrent M.I.'s and reduce premature mortality in persons whose life-styles may have been excessively preoccupied with active coping. According to Friedman and Rosenman (1974), Type A individuals are high in competitive achievement, time urgency, and hostility. Glass (1977) has suggested that these characteristics reflect an attempt by the Type A individual to cope actively with a world perceived as threatening. Schneiderman (1978, 1983) and Herd (1978, 1981) have related Type A behavior to excessive SAM activity. The

TABLE 5.1
Altering Behavior After Myocardial Infarction
(Based upon Friedman et al., 1982)

A. Restructuring of Environment

    1. Elimination of excess daily activities.
    2. Modification of work and social environments.
    3. Renewal of old friendships.
    4. Acquisition of new hobbies.

B. Altering Perceptual and Response Styles

    1. Cognitive-affective learning.
      a. Modification of assumptions, attributions, and beliefs.
      b. Reassessment of personal qualities.
    2. Self-instruction and self-management.
      a. Substitution of assertiveness for aggression.
      b. Role playing.
      c. Avoidance of polyphasic thinking and activity.
      d. Self-reinforcement.

C. Altering Responsiveness

    1. Recognition and modification of exaggerated arousal reactions.
    2. Progressive muscle relaxation.
    3. Mental relaxation (e.g., meditation).

Western Collaborative Group Study has identified Type A behavior as a risk factor for coronary heart disease (Rosenman, Brand, Jenkins, Friedman, Straus, & Wurm, 1975).

In the Friedman et al. (1982) study, which successfully reduced the incidences of recurrent M.I. and premature mortality by altering behavior, attempts to restructure the environment included modification of work and social environments (Table 5.1). Efforts to modify perceptual and response styles focused on changing assumptions, attributions, and beliefs, with the aim of making the subjects less time-urgent and hostile in their behaviors. Both progressive muscle relaxation and mental relaxation (e.g., meditation) procedures were used. Although the 5-year prospective study by Friedman et al. has not yet been completed, the results thus far indicate that the rate of nonfatal infarction is significantly lower among those receiving both behavioral interventions and cardiologic counseling than among those receiving only cardiologic counseling.

Among the procedures used in the Friedman et al. (1982) study was relaxation training. According to Benson, Greenwood, and Klemchuk (1977) a basic relaxation response can be elicited by meditational procedures. The common ingredients of techniques used in eliciting the relaxation response are said to be: (1) a constant mental stimulus repeated silently or audibly; (2) a passive attitude; (3) decreased muscle tonus; and (4) a quiet environment. Elicitation of the relaxation response is typically associated with decreased SNS activity associated with decreased oxygen consumption, heart rate, and blood lactate (Wallace, Benson, & Wilson, 1971).

Although the exact mechanisms by which relaxation training attenuates the physiologic changes elicited by active coping in an aversive environment are not known, the functional organization of the hypothalamus provides some reasonable clues. Stimulation of the ventromedial hypothalamus in the rabbit, for instance, elicits the defense reaction, whereas stimulation of the lateral hypothalamus elicits a depressor response, bradycardia, and quiet inactivity (Gellman et al., 1981). Preliminary data from our laboratory further indicate that stimulation of the ventromedial hypothalamus elicits a preferential release of E, whereas stimulation of the lateral hypothalamus evokes a decrease in the release of E and NE. Also, when stimulation of the posterior lateral hypothalamus is used as the unconditioned stimulus in a Pavlovian conditioning experiment, the conditioned response includes a decrease in blood pressure (Brickman & Schneiderman, 1977). It would therefore be interesting to determine whether stimulation of the lateral hypothalamus or presentation of a stimulus previously paired with lateral hypothalamic stimulation could attenuate the cardiovascular and catecholamine components of an elicited defense reaction.

Concomitant studies conducted upon humans should examine the physiological and hormonal changes that occur when an individual uses learned relaxation techniques to counter the effects of known behavioral stressors. In any event, the use of relaxation techniques with humans has thus far been successful in the treatment of several physical disorders, including hypertension (Patel & North, 1975), migraine (Blanchard, Theobald, Williamson, Silver, & Brown, 1978), and Raynaud's disease (Keefe, Surwit, & Pilon, 1980).

The methods required for dealing with stresses associated with helplessness, hypervigilance, and conservation – withdrawal are likely to be somewhat different from those used upon individuals already engaged in active coping behaviors. For those who perceive themselves as being helpless, depression is likely to be a problem. Merely removing the individual from the overwhelming situation (i.e., environmental change) may be useful, but is certainly not a panacea for the clinically depressed individual. Such a person is likely to emit few behavioral responses that can be reinforced, and the usual reinforcers that may normally shape behavior (i.e., affectionate responses from others; a sense of self-satisfaction for accomplishment) may lack effectiveness. Pharmacologic treatment with tricyclic medication may be useful.

Depression tends to follow a phasic course, however, and the opportunity to change perceptions and response styles with a view toward developing more adequate coping behaviors and enhancing self-esteem may occur once the depression begins to wane. Positive results may be obtained by means of cognitive psychotherapy, behavior modification, and/or self-initiated behavior changes. Frequently, assertiveness training and life-style changes that increase personal and interpersonal activity levels are helpful. This is particularly the case for spinal cord injury, stroke, and pain patients. Procedures that improve coping skills in the aged and those with chronic diseases are also likely to be useful. In conclusion, more and better research is needed to: (1) recognize and classify stress and stressors; (2) identify relationships among behavioral stress, pathophysiology, and disease; (3) improve our abilities to use adequate coping behaviors in stress situations; and (4) assesses the effectiveness of improved coping in combatting disease and promoting wellness.

REFERENCES

Abrahams, V. C., Hilton, S. M., & Zbrozyna, A. Active muscle vasodilation produced by stimulation of the brain stem: Its significance in the defense reaction. *Journal of Physiology (London)*, 1960, *154*, 491–513.

Adams, D. B., Baccelli, G., Mancia, G., & Zanchetti, A. Cardiovascular changes during naturally elicit fighting behavior in the cat. *American Journal of Physiology*, 1968, *216*, 1226 – 1235.

Anderson, C. E., & Tosheff, J. Cardiac output and total peripheral resistance changes during preavoidance periods in the dog. *Journal of Applied Physiology*, 1973, *34*, 650–654.

Anisman, H. Time-dependent variations in adversity-motivated behaviors: Nonassociative effects of cholinergic and catecholaminergic activity. *Psychological Review*, 1975, *82*, 359–385.

Baccelli, G., Ellison, G. D., Mancia, G., & Zanchetti, A. Opposite responses of muscle circulation to different emotional stimuli. *Experientia*, 1971, *27*, 1183–1184.

Baker, S. P., & Potter, L. T. Biochemical studies of cardiac-beta-adrenoceptors, and their clinical significance. *Circulation Research*, 1980, *46*, (Supplement I), 34–42.

Bartrop, R. W., Luckhurst, E., & Lazarus, L. et al. Depressed lymphocyte funtion after bereavement. *Lancet*, 1977, *1*, 834–836.

Basowitz, H., Konchin, S. J., Oken, D., Goldstein, M. S., & Gussack, H. Anxiety and performance changes with a minimal dose of epinephrine. *Archives of Neurology and Psychiatry,* 1956, *76,* 98–108.

Bassett, J. R., & Cairncross, K. D. Changes in the coronary vascular system following prolonged exposure to stress. *Pharmacology, Biochemistry, and Behavior,* 1977, *6,* 311–318.

Benson, H., Greewood, M., & Klemchuk, H. The relaxation response: Psychophysiologic aspects and clinical applications. In Z. J. Lipowski, D. R. Lipsitt, & P. C. Whybrow (Eds.), *Psychosomatic medicine.* New York: Oxford University Press, 1977.

Blanchard, E. B., Theobald, D., Williamson, P., Silver, B., & Brown, B. Temperature feedback in the treatment of migraine headaches. *Archives of General Psychology,* 1978, *35,* 581–588.

Bolles, R. C., & Fanselow, M. S. Endorphins and behavior. *Annual Review of Psychology,* 1982, *33,* 87–101.

Bonnett, K. A., Miller, J. M., & Simon, E. J. The effect of chronic opiate treatment and social isolation on opiate receptor in the rodent brain. In Kosterlitz (Ed.), *Opiates and endogenous opioid peptides.* Amsterdam: Elsevier, 1976.

Borysenko, M., & Borysenko, J. Stress, behavior, and immunity: Animal models and mediating mechanisms. *General Hospital Psychiatry,* 1982, *4,* 59–67.

Braunstein, J. Reactions to stress. In J. J. Braunstein & R. P. Toister (Eds.), *Medical applications of the behavioral sciences.* Chicago: Year Book Medical Publishers, Inc., 1981.

Brickman, A., & Schneiderman, N. Classically conditioned blood pressure decreases induced by electrical stimulation of posterior hypothalamus in rabbits. *Psychophysiology,* 1977, *14,* 287–292.

Bronson, F. H. Establishment of social rank among grouped male mice: Relative effects on circulating FSH, LH, and corticosterone. *Physiological Behavior,* 1973, *10,* 947–951.

Brown, G. W., & Birley, J. L. T. Crises and life changes and the onset of schizophrenia. *Journal of Health and Social Behavior,* 1968, *9,* 203–214.

Candland, D. K., & Leshner, A. I. A model of agonistic behavior: Endocrine and autonomic correlates. In L. V. DiCara (Ed.)., *Limbic and autonomic nervous systems research.* New York: Plenum, 1974.

Cannon, W. R. *Bodily changes in pain, hunger, fear, and rage* (2nd ed.). New York: Appleton, 1929.

Carroll, B. J. Limbic system-adrenal cortex regulation in depression and schizophrenia. *Psychosomatic Medicine,* 1976, *38,* 106–121.

Cesselin, F., Montastrue, J. L., Gros, C., Bourgoin, S., & Hammon, M. Met-enkephalin levels and opiate receptors in the spinal cord of chronic suffering rats. *Brain Research,* 1980, *191,* 289–293.

Chamove, A. S., & Bowman, R. E. Rhesus plasma cortisol response at four dominance positions. *Aggressive Behavior,* 1978, *4,* 43–55.

Christian, J. J. Population density and reproductive efficiency. *Biological Reproductions,* 1971, *4,* 248–294.

Claman, H. N. Corticosteroids and lymphoid cells. *New England Journal of Medicine,* 1977, *287,* 388–397.

Coe, C. L., & Levine, S. Normal responses to mother-infant separation in nonhuman primates. In D. F. Klein, & J. G. Rabkin (Eds.), *Anxiety: New research and changing concepts.* New York: Raven Press, 1981.

Cooper, J. R., Bloom, F. E., & Roth, R. H. *The biochemical basis of neuropharmacology.* New York: Oxford University Press, 1978.

Dimsdale, J. E., & Moss, J. M. Plasma catecholamines in stress and exercise. *Journal of the American Medical Association,* 1980, *243,* 340–342.

Djojosugito, A. M., Folkow, B., Kylstra, P., Lisander, B., & Tuttle, R. S. Differentiated interaction between the hypothalamic defense reaction and baroreceptor reflexes. I. Effects on heart rate and regional flow resistance. *Acta Physiologica Scandinavica,* 1970, *78,* 376–383.

Dohrenwend, B. S., Krasnoff, L., Askenasy, A. R., & Dohrenwend, B. P. Exemplification of a method for scaling life events: The PERI Life Events Scale. *Journal of Health and Social Behavior,* 1978, *19,* 205–229.

Dougherty, T. F. Effects of hormones on lymphatic tissue. *Physiological Review,* 1952, *32,* 397–401.

Dworkin, B. R., Filewich, R. J., Miller, N. E., Craigmyle, N., & Pickering, T. G. Baroreceptor activation reduces reactivity to noxious stimulation: Implications for hypertension. *Science*, 1979, *205*, 1299–1301.

Eliot, R. S., Todd, G. L., Clayton, F. C., & Pieper, G. M. Experimental catecholamine-induced acute myocardial necrosis. In V. Manninen & P. I. Halonen (Eds.), *Advances in cardiology* (Vol. 25). Basel: S. Karger AG, 1978.

Ely, D. L., Henry, J. P., & Ciananello, R. D. Long-term behavioral and biochemical differentiation of dominant and subordinate mice in population cages. *Psychosomatic Medicine*, 1974, *36*, 463

Engel, G. L. Sudden and rapid death during psychological stress, folklore or folk wisdom? *Annals of Internal Medicine*, 1971, *74*, 771–782.

Frankenhaeuser, M. Psychobiological aspects of life stress. In S. Levine & H. Ursin (Eds.), *Coping and health*. New York: Plenum Press (Nato Conference Series), Series III: Human Factors, Vol. 12, 1980.

Frankenhaeuser, M., Sterky, K., & Jarpe, G. Psychophysiological relations in habituation to gravitational stress. *Perceptual and Motor Skills*, 1962, *15*, 63–72.

Friedman, M. & Rosenman, R. H. *Type A behavior and your heart*. New York: Knopf, 1974.

Friedman, S. B., Glasgow, L. A., & Ader, R. Psychosocial factors modifying host resistance to experimental infections. *Annals of the New York Academy of Science*, 1969, *164*, 381–393.

Friedman, S. B., Oester, V. T., & Davis, O. F. The effect of arterenol and epinephrine on experimental arteriopathy. *Archives Internationales de Pharmcodynamie et de Therapie*, 1955, *102*, 226–234.

Friedman, M., Thoresen, C. E., Gill, J. J., Ulmer, D., Thompson, L., Powell, L., Price, V., Elek, S. R., Rabin, D. D., Breal, W. S., Piaget, G., Dixon, T., Bourg, E., Levy, R. A., & Tasto, D. L. Feasibility of altering Type A behavior pattern after myocardial infarction. Recurrent coronary prevention project study: Methods, baseline, results and preliminary findings. *Circulation*, 1982, *66*, 83–92.

Gellman, M., Schneiderman, N., Wallach, J., & Le Blanc, W. Cardiovascular responses elicited by hypothalamic stimulation in rabbits reveal a medio-lateral organization. *Journal of the Autonomic Nervous System*, 1981, *4*, 301–317.

Gibson, A., Ginsberg, M., Hall, M., & Hart, S. L. The effects of opiate receptor agonists and antagonists on the stress-induced secretion of corticosterone in mice. *British Journal of Pharmacology*, 1979, *65*, 139–146.

Glass, D. C. *Behavior patterns, stress and coronary disease*. Hillsdale, N.J.: Lawrence Erlbaum Associates, 1977.

Glass, D. C., Krakoff, L. R., Contrada, R., Hilton, W. F., Kehoe, K., Mannucci, E. G., Collins, C., Snow, B., & Elting, E. Effect of harassment and competition upon cardiovascular and plasma catecholamine responses in Type A and Type B individuals. *Psychophysiology*, 1980, *17*, 453–463.

Glazer, H. I., Weiss, H. M., Pohorecky, L. A., & Miller, N. E. Monamines as mediators of avoidance–escape behavior. *Psychosomatic Medicine*, 1975, *37*, 535–543.

Graham, J. D. P. High blood pressure after battle. *Lancet*, 1945, *248*, 239–240.

Guideri, G., Barletta, M., Chau, R., Green, M., & Lehr, D. Method for the production of severe ventricular dysrhythmias in small laboratory animals. In P. Roy & G. Ronal (Eds.), *The metabolism of contraction*. Baltimore: University Park Press, 1975.

Guillemin, R. Control of adenohypophysial functions by peptides of the central nervous system. *Harvey Lecture*, 1978, *71*, 71–131.

Haft, H. I., & Fani, K. Intravascular platele and aggregation in the heart induced by stress. *Circulation*, 1973, *48*, 164–169.

Hanson, J. P., Larson, M. E., & Snowden, C. T. The effects of control over high intensity noise on plasma cortisol levels in rhesus monkeys. *Behavioral Biology*, 1976, *16*, 333–340.

Harburg, E., Erfurt, J. C., Havenstein, L. S., Chape, C., Schull, W. J., & Schork, M. A. Socioecological stress, suppressed hostility, skin odor, and black-white male blood pressure: Detroit. *Psychosomatic Medicine*, 1973, *35*, 276–296.

Hawkins, N., et al. Evidence of psychosocial factors in the development of pulmonary tuberculosis. *American Review of Tuberculosis and Pulmonary Disease*, 1957, *75*, 768.

Heindel, J. J., Orci, L., & Jeanrenaud, B. Fat mobilization and its regulation by hormones and drugs in white adipose tissue. In E. J. Masoro (Ed.), *International encyclopedia of pharmacology and therapeutics: Pharmacology of lipid transport and atherosclerotic processes*. Oxford: Pergamon, 1975.

Henry, J. P., Ely, D. L., & Stephens, P. M. Changes in catecholamine-controlling enzymes in response to psychosocial activation of the defence and alarm reactions. In *Physiology emotion and psychomatic illness, Ciba Foundation Symposium 8*. Amsterdam: Associated Scientific Publishers, 1972.

Henry, J. P., & Stephens, P. M. *Stress, health and the social environment: A sociobiologic approach to medicine*. New York: Springer-Verlag, 1977.

Henry, J. P., & Meehan, J. P. Psychosocial stimuli, physiological specificity, and cardiovascular disease. In H. Weiner, M. A. Hofer, & A. J. Strunkard (Eds.), *Brain, behavior, and bodily diseases*. New York: Raven Press, 1981.

Herd, J. A. Behavioral factors in the physiological mechanisms of cardiovascular disease. In S. M. Weiss, J. A. Herd, & B. H. Fox (Eds.), *Perspectives on behavioral medicine*. New York: Academic Press, 1981.

Herd, J. A. Physiological correlates of coronary prone behavior. In T. M. Dembroski, S. M. Weiss, J. L. Shields, S. G. Haynes, & M. Feinlieb (Eds.), *Coronary prone behavior*. New York: Springer-Verlag, 1978.

Hess, W. R. *Functional organization of the diencephalon*. New York: Grune & Stratton, 1957.

Hill, C. W., Greer, W. E., & Felsenfeld, O. Psychosocial stress, early response to foreign proteins, and blood cortisol in vervets. *Psychosomatic Medicine*, 1967, *29*, 279 – 283.

Holmes, T. H., & Masuda, M. Life change and illness susceptibility. In B. S. Dohrenwend & B. P. Dohrenwend (Eds.), *Stressful life events*. New York: John Wiley & Sons, 1974.

Holmes, T. H., & Rahe, R. H. The social readjustment rating scale. *Journal of Psychosomatic Research*, 1967, *11*, 213 – 218.

Hughes, J., Smith, T. W., Kosterlitz, H. W., Fothergill, L. A., Morgan, B. A., & Morris, H. R. Identification of two related pentapeptides from the brain with potent opiate agonist activity. *Nature*, 1975, *258*, 577 – 580.

Jacobs, S., & Ostfeld, A. An epidemiological review of bereavement. *Psychosomatic Medicine*, 1977, *39*, 344 – 357.

Jaffe, J. H., & Martin, W. R. Opioid analgesks and antagonists. In A. G. Gilman, L. S. Goodman, & A. Gilman (Eds.), *The pharmacological basis of therapeutics*. New York: Macmillan Publication Company, 1980.

Jordan, D., Khalid, M., Schneiderman, N., & Spyer, K. M. The inhibitory control of vagal cardiomotor neurons. *Journal of Physiology (London)*, 1979, *301*, 54p.

Kaplan, J. G. *The molecular phagocytosis basis of immune cell function*. New York: Elsvier/North-Holland, 1979.

Kasl, S. V., Evans, A. S., & Niederman, J. C. Psychosocial risk factors in the development of infectious mononucleosis. *Psychosomatic Medicine*, 1979, *41*, 445 – 466.

Keefe, F. J., Surwit, R. S., & Pilon, R. N. Biofeedback, autogenic training and progressive relaxation in the treatment of Raynaud's disease. *Journal of Applied Behavior Analysis*, 1980, *13*, 3 – 11.

Kety, S. S. Disorders of the human brain. *Scientific American*, 1979, *241*, 202 – 214.

Kimball, C. P. Emotional and psychosocial aspects of diabetes mellitus. *Medicine of Clinicians in North America*, 1971, *55*, 1007 – 1018.

Kuhar, M. J., Pert, C. B., & Snyder, S. H. Regional distribution of opiate receptor binding in monkey and human brain. *Nature*, 1973, *245*, 447 – 450.

Kvetnansky, R. In E. Usdn, R. Kvetnansky, & I. J. Kopin (Eds.), *Catecholamines and stress: Recent advances*. Amsterdam: Elsevier/North Holland, 1980.

Lang, C. M. Effects of psychic stress on atherosclerosis in the squirrel monkey (*Saimiri sciureus*). *Proceedings of the Society of Experimental Biology and Medicine*, 1967, *126*, 30 – 34.

Lawler, J. E., Obrist, D. A., & Lawler, K. A. Cardiovascular function during preavoidance, avoidance, and postavoidance in dogs. *Psychophysiology*, 1975, *12*, 4 – 11.

Leshner, A. I., & Politch, J. A. Hormonal control of submissiveness in mice: Irrelevance of the androgens and relevance of the pituitary – adrenal hormones. *Physiological Behavior*, 1979, *22*, 531 – 534.

Leshner, A. I., Remler, H., Biegon, A., & Samuel, D. Effect of desmethylimipramine (DMI) on learned helplessness. *Psychopharmacology*, 1979, *66*, 207 – 213.

Lindsley, D. B. Emotion. In S. S. Stevens (Ed.), *Handbook of experimental psychology*. New York: Wiley, 1951.

Locke, S. E. Stress, adaptation and immunity: Studies in humans. *General Hospital Psychiatry*, 1982, *4*, 49 – 58.

Louch, C. D., & Higginbotham, M. The relation between social rank and plasma corticosterone levels in mice. *General Comparative Endocrinology*, 1967, *8*, 441 – 444.

Lown, B. Sudden cardiac death: The major challenge confronting contemporary cardiology. *American Journal of Cardiology*, 1979, *43*, 313 – 328.

Lown, B., Verrier, R. L., & Corbalan, R. Psychologic stress and threshold for repetitive ventricular response. *Science*, 1973, *132*, 834 – 836.

Lundberg, U. Catecholamine and cortisol excretion under psychologically different laboratory conditions. In E. Usdin, R. Kvetnansky, & I. J. Kopin (Eds.), *Catecholamines and stress*. New York: Elsevier/North Holland, 1980.

Maas, J. Adrenocortical steroid hormones, electrolytes and the disposition of the catecholamines with particular reference to depressive states. *Journal of Psychiatric Research*, 1972, *9*, 227 – 241.

Magoun, H. W. *The waking brain*. Springfield, Ill.: Thomas, 1958.

Maslach, C. Negative emotional biasing of unexplained arousal. In C. Izard (Ed.), *Emotion, personality and psychopathology*. New York: 1979.

Mason, J. W. A historical view of the stress field. Part I. *Journal of Human Stress*, 1975, *1*, 6 – 12.

Mason, J. W., Mangan, G. F., Brady, J. V., Conrad, D., & Rioch, D. M. Concurrent plasma epinephrine, norepinephrine, and 17-hydroxycorticosteroid levels during conditioned emotional disturbances in monkeys. *Psychosomatic Medicine*, 1961, *23*, 344 – 353.

Mason, J. W., Tolson, W. W., Brady, J. V., Tolliver, G. A., & Gilmore, L. I. Urinary epinephrine and norepinephrine responses to 72-hour avoidance sessions in the monkey. *Psychosomatic Medicine*, 1969, *31*, 300 – 309.

Masserano, J. M., Takimoto, G. S., & Weiner, N. Electroconvulsive shock increases tyrosine hydroxylase activity in the brain and adrenal gland of the rat. *Science*, 1981, *214*,(6) 662 – 664.

McRae-Degueurce, A., & Pujol, J. F. Correlation between the increase in tyrosine hydroxylase activity and the decrease in serotonin content in the rat locus coeruleus after 5, 6-dihydroxytryptamine. *European Journal of Pharmacology*, 1979, *5*, 2139 – 2144.

Meyers, A., & Dewar, H. A. Circumstances attending 100 sudden deaths from coronary artery disease with coroner's necropsies. *British Heart Journal*, 1975, *37*, 1133 – 1143.

Millan, M. J., & Emrich, H. M. Endorphinergic systems and the response to stress. *Psychotherapy and Psychosomatics*, 1981, *36*, 43 – 56.

Millan, M. J., Przewlocki, R., Jerlicz, M. Gramsch, C., Hollt, V., & Herz, A. Stress induced release of brain and pituitary beta-endorphin: Major role of endorphins in generation of hyperthermia, not analgesia. *Brain Research*, 1981, *308*, 325 – 338.

Millan, M. J., Tsang, V. F., Przewlocki, R., Hollt, V., & Herz, A. The influence of stress upon brain, pituitary, and spinal cord pools of immunoreactive dynorphin. *Neuroscience Letters*, 1981, *24*, 75 – 79.

Miller, G. J. High density lipoproteins and atherosclerosis, *Review of Medicine*, 1980, *31*, 97 – 108.

Moore, R. H., & Eichler, V. B. Loss of a circadian adrenal corticosterone rhythm following suprachiasmatic nucleus lesions in the rat. *Brain Research*, 1972, *42*, 201 – 206.

Musacchio, J. M., Jolou, L., Kety, S., & Glowinski, J. Increase in rat brain tyrosine hydroxylase activity produced by electroconvulsive shock. *Proceedings of the National Academy of Sciences, USA.*, 1969, *63*, 1117 – 1119.

Nestel, R. J., Verghese, A., & Levell, R. R. Catecholamine secretion and sympathetic nervous system responses to emotion in men with and without angina pectoris. *American Heart Journal,* 1967, *73,* 227 – 234.

Overmier, J. B., & Seligman, M. E. P. Effects of inescapable shock on subsequent escape and avoidance learning. *Journal of Comparative and Physiological Psychology,* 1967, *63,* 23 – 33.

Palmblad, J., Cantell, K., Strander, H., Froberg, J., Karlsson, C. G., Levi, L., Granstrom, M., & Unger, P. Stressor exposure and immunological response in man: Interferon-producing capacity and phagocytosis. *Journal of Psychosomatic Research,* 1976, *20,* 193 – 199.

Palmbald, J., Petrini, B., Wasserman, J., & Akerstedt, T. Lymphocyte and granulocyte reactions during sleep deprivation. *Psychosomatic Medicine,* 1979, *41,* 273 – 278.

Patel, C. H., & North, W. R. S. Randomized controlled trial of yoga and biofeedback in management of hypertension. *Lancet,* 1975, *7925,* 93 – 95.

Paykel, E. S., Prusoff, B. A., & Uhlenhuth, E. H. Scaling of life events. *Archives of General Psychiatry,* 1971, *25,* 340 – 347.

Paykel, E. S. Life stress and psychiatric disorder: Application of the clinical approach. In B. S. Dohrenwend & B. P. Dohrenwend (Eds.), *Stressful life events: Their nature and effects.* New York: John Wiley & Sons, Inc., 1974.

Petty, F., & Sherman, A. D. Reversal of learned helplessness by imipramine. *Community Psychopharmacology,* 1980, *3,* 371 – 373.

Plutchick, R. *Emotion: A psychoevolutionary synthesis.* New York: Harper & Row, 1980.

Raab, W. Emotional and sensory stress factors in myocardial pathology. *American Heart Journal,* 1966, *72,* 538 – 564.

Rabkin, J. G., & Streuning, E. L. Life events, stress, and illness. *Science,* 1976, *194,* 1013 – 1020.

Rahe, R. H. Life change events and mental illness: An overview. *Journal of Human Stress,* 1979, 2 – 10.

Rahe, R. H., Bennett, L., Romo, M., Seltanen, P., & Arthur, R. S. Subject's recent life changes and coronary heart disease in Finland. *American Journal of Psychiatry,* 1973, *130,* 1222 – 1226.

Rahe, R. H. *Annals of Clinical Research,* 1972, *4.*

Reich, P., DeSilva, R. A., Lown, B., & Murawski, J. Acute psychological disturbances preceding life-threatening ventricular arrhythmias. *Journal of the American Medical Association,* 1981, *246,* 233 – 235.

Riley, V. Biobehavioral factors in animal work on tumorigensis. In S. M. Weiss, J. A. Herd, & B. H. Fox (Eds.), *Perspectives on behavioral medicine.* New York: Academic Press, 1981.

Riley, V., Fitzmaurice, M. A., & Spackman, D. H. Psychoneuroimmunologic factors in neoplasia: Studies in animals. In R. Ader (Ed.), *Psychoneuroimmunology.* New York: Academic Press, 1981.

Rissanen, V., Romo, M., & Seltanen, P. Premonitory symptoms and stress factor preceding sudden death from ischemic heart disease. *Acta Medica Scandinavica,* 1978, *204,* 389.

Ritter, S., Pelzer, N. L., & Ritter, R. C. Absence of glucoprivic feeding after stress suggests impairment of noradrenergic neuron function. *Brain Research,* 1978, *149,* 399 – 411.

Rona, G., Chappel, C. I., Balasy, T., & Caudry, R. An infarct-like myocardial lesion and other toxic manifestations produced by isoproterenol in the rat. *Archives of Pathology,* 1959, *67,* 443 – 455.

Rosenman, R. H., Brand, R. J., Jenkins, C. D., Friedman, M., Straus, R., & Wurm, M. Coronary heart disease in the Western Collaborative Group study: Final follow-up experience of 8 1/2 years. *Journal of the American Medical Associaton.* 1975, *233,* 872 – 877.

Rossier, J., Guillemin, R., & Bloom, F. Foot shock-induced stress decreases leu-enkephalin immunoreactivity in rat hypothalamus. *European Journal of Pharmacology,* 1978, *48,* 465 – 466.

Rossier, J., French, E., Rivier, C., Shibaski, J., Guillemin, R., & Bloom, F. E. Stress-induced release of prolactin: Blockade by dexamethasone and naloxene may indicate beta-endorphin mediation. *Proceedings of the National Academy of Sciences USA,* 1980, *77,* 666 – 669.

Russek, H. I. Emotional stress as a cause of coronary heart disease. *Journal of American College Health Associaton,* 1973, *22,* 120 – 123.

Sachar, E. J. Neuroendocrine abnormalities in depressive illness. In E. J. Sachar (Ed.), *Topics in psychoendocrinology.* New York: Grune & Stratton, 1976.

Sachar, E. J. Psychobiology of affective disorders. In E. R. Kandel, & J. H. Schwartz (Eds.), *Principles of neural science*. New York: Elsevier/North-Holland, 1981.

Sachar, E. J., Anis, G., Nathan, R. S., Halbreich, U., & Halpern, F. Recent studies in the neuroendocrinology of major depressive disorders. *Psychiatric Clinics of North America*, 1980, *3*, 313–326.

Sampter, M. *Immunological diseases*. Boston: Little Brown, 1978.

Schachter, S. The interaction of cognitive and physiological determinants of emotional state. In C. D. Spielberger (Ed.), *Anxiety and behavior*. New York: Academic Press, 1966

Schachter, S., & Singer, J. E. Cognitive, social and physiological determinants of emotional state. *Psychological Review*, 1962, *69*, 379–399.

Schaffer, C. B., Pandey, G. N., Noll, K. M., Killian, G. A., & Davis, J. M. Introduction and theories of affective disorders. In G. C. Palmer (Ed.), *Neuropharmacology of central nervous system and behavioral disorders*. New York: Academic Press, 1981.

Schleifer, S. J., Keller, S. E., McKegney, F. P., & Stein, M. *Bereavement and lymphocyte function*. Paper given at American Psychiatric Association meeting (unpublished). Department of Psychiatry, Mt. Sinai School of Medicine, New York, 1980.

Schneiderman, N. Animal models relating behavioral stress and cardiovascular pathology. In T. M. Dembroski, S. M. Weiss, J. L. Shields, S. G. Haynes, & M. Feinleib (Eds.), *Coronary prone behavior*. New York: Springer-Verlag, 1978.

Schneiderman, N. Behavior, autonomic function and animal models of cardiovascular pathology. In T. M. Dembroski, T. H. Schmidt, & G. Blümchen (Eds.), *Biobehavioral bases of coronary heart disease*. Basle: Karger, 1983.

Schonfeld, G., & Pfleger, B. Utilization of exogenous free fatty acids for production of very low density lipoprotein triglyceride by livers of carbohydrate-fed rats. *Journal of Lipid Research*, 1971, *12*, 614–621.

Seligman, M. E. P., & Maier, S. F. Failure to escape traumatic shock. *Journal of Experimental Psychology*, 1967, *74*, 1–9.

Seligman, M. E. P. Depression and learned helplessness. In R. J. Friedman & M. M. Katz (Eds.), *The psychology of depression: contemporary theory and research*. Washington, D.C.: V. H. Winston, 1974.

Selye, H. A syndrome produced by diverse nocuous agents. *Nature (London)*, 1936, *138*, 32.

Selye, H. The general adaptation syndrome and the diseases of adaptation. *Journal of Clinical Endocrinology*, 1946, *6*, 117.

Selye, H. The evolution of the stress concept: Stress and cardiovascular disease. *American Journal of Cardiology*, 1970, *26*, 289.

Selye, H. *Stress in health and disease*. Reading, Mass.: Butterworths, 1976. (a)

Selye, H. *The stress of life*. New York: McGraw-Hill, 1976. (b)

Sherman, A. D., & Petty, F. Neurochemical basis of the action of antidepressants on learned helplessness. *Behavioral and Neurology and Biology*, 1980, *30*, 119–134.

Sigurdsson, G., Nicoll, A., & Lewis, B. Conversion of very low density lipoprotein to low density lipoprotein. *Journal of Clinical Investigation*, 1975, *56*, 1481–1490.

Solomon, G. F. Stress and antibody response in rats. *International Archives of Allergy and Applied Immunology*, 1969, *35*, 97–104.

Solomon, G. F. Emotional and personality factors in the onset and course of autoimmune disease: Particularly rheumatoid arthritis. In R. Ader (Ed.), *Psychoneuroimmunology*. New York: Academic Press, 1981.

Solomon, G. F., Merigan, T., & Levine, S. Variation in adrenal cortical hormones within physiological ranges: Stress and interferon production in mice. *Proceedings of the Society for Experimental Biology and Medicine*, 1967, *126*, 74.

Theorell, T., & Rahe, R. Psychosocial factors and myocardial infarction. I. An inpatient study in Sweden. *Journal of Psychosomatic Research*, 1971, *15*, 25.

Torda, C. Effects of recurrent postnatal pain-related stressful events on opiate receptor – endogenous ligand system. *Psychoneuroendocrinology,* 1978, *3,* 85 – 91.

Troxler, R. G., Sprague, E. A., Albanese, R. A. Fuchs, R., & Thompson, A. J. The association of elevated plasma corticol and early atherosclerosis as demonstrated by coronary angiography. *Atherosclerosis,* 1977, *26,* 151 – 162.

Vizi, E. S. Modulation of cortical release of acetylcholine by nor-adrenaline released from nerves arising from the rat locus coeruleus. *Neuroscience,* 1980, *5,* 2139 – 2144.

Von Holst, D. Renal failure as the cause of death in *Tupaia belangeri* (tree shrews) exposed to persistent social stress. *Journal of Comparative Physiology,* 1972, *78,* 236 – 273.

Wallace, R. K., Benson, H., & Wilson, A. F. A wakeful hypometabolic physiologic state. *American Journal of Physiology,* 1971, *221,* 795 – 799.

Wallach, J., Ellenberger, H., Schneiderman, N., Liskowsky, D., Hamilton, R., & Gellman, M. Preoptic-anterior hypothalamic area as mediator of bradycardia responses in rabbits. *Neuroscience Abstracts,* 1979, *5,* 52.

Weiss, J. M., Stone, E. A., & Harrell, N. Coping behavior and brain norepinephrine level in rats. *Journal of Comparative Physiological Psychology,* 1970, *72,* 153 – 160.

Weiss, J. M. Influence of psychological variables on stress induced pathology. *Physiology, Emotion and Psychosomatic Illness, Ciba Foundation Symposium,* 1972, *8,* 253 – 265.

Weiss, J. M., & Glazer, H. I. Effects of acute exposure to stressors on subsequent avoidance – escape behavior. *Psychosomatic Medicine,* 1975, *37,* 499 – 521.

Weiss, J. M., Glazer, H. I., & Pohorecky, L. A. Coping behavior and neurochemical changes: An alternative explanation for the original "learned helplessness" experiments. In G. Serban & A. Kling (Eds.), *Animal models in human psychobiology.* New York: Plenum Press, 1976.

Weiss, J. M., Bailey, W. H., Pohorecky, L. A., Korzeniowski, D., & Grillone, G. Stress-induced depression of motor activity correlates with regional changes in brain norepinephrine but not in dopamine. *Neurochemical Research,* 1980, *5,* 9 – 22.

Williams, R. B., Lane, J. D., Kuhn, C. M., Melosh, W., White, A. D., & Schlanberg, S. M. *Physiological and neuroendocrine response patterns during different behavioral challenges: Differential hyperresponsivity of young type A men.* In press.

Williams, R. B., Lane, J. D., Kuhn, C. M., Melosh, W., White, A. D., & Schanberg, S. M. Type A behavior and elevated physiological and neuroendocrine responses to cognitive tasks. *Science,* 1982, *218,* 483 – 485.

Wilson, S. P., Chang, K. J., & Viveros, O. H. Proportional secretion of opioid peptides and catecholamines from adrenal chromaffin cells in culture. *Journal of Neuroscience,* 1982, *2,* 1150 – 1156.

Zieler, K. L., Maseri, A., Klassen, D., Rabinowitz, D., & Burgess, J. Muscle metabolism during exercise in man. *Transcripts of the Association of American Physicians,* 1968, *81,* 266 – 268.

III ASSESSMENT AND TREATMENT IN BEHAVIORAL MEDICINE

6   Psychological Assessment in Medical Settings

Catherine J. Green
University of Miami

INTRODUCTION

In traditional medicine the goal of clinical diagnosis is the identification of the ongoing disease process and the formation of a plan to deal with the disease. When psychosocial factors are added to the medical symptomatology, the patient cannot be seen simply as a vessel, so to speak, who carries a group of predictable or constant symptoms available for evaluation. Rather, the psychosocial events and the patient's premorbid personality covary to create a changing constellation. Under these circumstances clinical analyses must not only systematically evaluate these varied elements but must also elucidate their interrelationships and dynamic flow. Current behaviors and attitudes must be interpreted in conjunction with the physical basis of the presenting problem. The premorbid background of the patient must be delineated in an effort to clarify the historical context or pattern of the syndrome. Moreover, personality and environmental circumstances must be appraised to optimize therapeutic recommendations. Ultimately, the goal of psychological assessment is the development of a preventive or remedial plan.

As in other settings, problems occur when this assessment relies solely on the evaluation skills and impressions of the clinician involved. Clinicians often see what they anticipate. It is unlikely that the data obtained will be at variance with these expectancies. Moreover, questions likely to unearth unanticipated information are rarely asked. It is in this regard that objective psychological assessment is so important; these tools serve to standardize clinical evaluations and to ensure comprehensive coverage. Moreover, it seeks to appraise the patient's present status within the context of the past and within his or her larger social framework or environment, including both current physical and psychosocial stressors. Although the clinician evaluates a patient caught at one point in time, it is necessary to trace the sequence of events preceding and leading to that point. This knowledge allows the formulation of a remedial plan that is based on understanding the interface between the patient's illness and the resources available to manage the problem successfully. Clinical psychological analysis with medical patients is both an abbreviated and more extensive evaluation than for the psychiatric patient as characterized by Millon (1969). The first task is the description of the current clinical picture. The presenting medical problem is often the most obvious aspect of this picture; however, it often serves as a precipitant of difficulties of a more extensive or long-lasting nature. The impact of this physical problem must be evaluated both in its effects on the physiology of the individual as well as in the impact on the patient's emotions and those who surround the patient. Throughout the evaluation process various levels are observed, including the overt behaviors and stated reports of feelings, along with the inferred intrapsychic processes, as well as the biophysical processes.

As stated, the patient is caught at one point in time, and yet the analysis must consider and attempt to elucidate the developmental influences on the presenting problems. Here again the physical and emotional, along with current stressors, may be relevant to etiology. This information, combined with the clinical picture, may allow for the construction of a clinical syndrome. Rather than labeling, the effort here is to clarify the complex interactive roles of medical concerns, the feelings of the patient, and the individuals surrounding the patient. This, hopefully, will be helpful in prognosis and the formulation of therapeutic management. All these issues must be evaluated to assess a patient optimally; however, psychological assessment in medical settings did not generally assume so comprehensive an approach.

Assessment Trends in Medical Settings

Initially, psychologists employed traditional psychometric instruments that could answer specific questions regarding problems of psychopathology but often did not illuminate questions posed in requests for nonpsychiatric psychological services. New instruments designed to assess the general medical patient developed very slowly, many by clinicians unfamiliar with psychometric theory. Consequently, these new tests often were poorly grounded in theory and gave minimal evidence of validity or reliability. The following sections of this chapter serve as a guide to the evaluation and use of selected objective self-report instruments. These tools have been chosen because of the ease with which they can be employed in medical settings. Although the list is by no means exhaustive, it does encompass a variety of approaches, theoretical stances, and issues found significant for medical patients.

The instruments selected have been evaluated in terms of general psychological test criteria and their relevance to medical-psychological issues specifically. If an instrument fails to meet general psychometric consideration, its value as a medical diagnostic instrument is seriously compromised.

General Criteria for Test Evaluation

The first criteria for evaluating a psychometric instrument are whether it addresses a characteristic relevant to a target population, is tailored to gauge some specific trait or behavior through the parsimonious use of questions, and displays simplicity of administration and economy of time. Brevity, clarity, and minimal intrusiveness maximize patient compliance and minimize fatigue.

Although different methods have been employed in the development of the following tests, the same criteria of test construction must be applied. These include evaluating reliability (test-retest, reliability across forms of the test, and internal consistency) and validity (construct, content, and empirical) as well as the completeness of the manual and instructions for interpretation.

Further evaluation criteria must be applied to those instruments that are utilized in medical settings. First, are the behaviors, traits, and attitudes addressed relevant to the patient's problem and to treatment planning? Another major criterion relates to the predictive value of the instrument. What is the likelihood of illness occurring in a patient who is otherwise asymptomatic, or what is the likely course or reaction to treatment of an ongoing disease process?

The following sections detail evaluations of a number of instruments utilizing these criteria. A description of the test and what it seeks to measure is given. Administration and scoring information are then followed by an evaluation of construction and postconstruction empirical data. The instrument is next evaluated in terms of its use and relevance to medical populations.

INSTRUMENTS DEVELOPED PRIMARILY FOR RESEARCH PURPOSES

State-Trait Anxiety Inventory (STAI)

This inventory was originally developed as a research instrument for investigating anxiety in normal adults (Spielberger, Gorsuch, & Lushene, 1970) and is composed of two questionnaires of similar format, one asking the subject to indicate how he or she feels *right now,* the other how the individual *generally* feels. The subject's choices are either "almost never," "sometimes," "often," or "almost always." This instrument was specifically developed to evaluate feelings of tension, nervousness, worry, and apprehension. It was posited by the test developers that it could serve as either a clinical tool for evaluating anxiety proneness or, in the case of state scores, the evaluation of level of anxiety or anxiety change.

Administration, Scoring, and Development of Norms. The STAI was designed to be self-administered and may be given individually or in groups; complete instructions are printed on the test form. College students generally require less than 15 minutes to complete both questionnaires, whereas disturbed or less educated individuals often take 30 minutes or more.

Subjects respond to each STAI item by rating themselves on a 4-point scale. The scoring weights for items relate to anxiety; these figures are then converted to T-scores or percentiles. Templates and machine scoring are available.

Normative data are available for large samples of college and high school students. The sample of general medical patients is both small ($N = 161$) and all male. Given the difference between male and female responses on this inventory with high school and college samples, caution should be used in viewing the medical sample as a comparison group.

Interpretation is straightforward; higher scores on A-Trait indicate higher levels of anxiety proneness. High A-State scores are conceptualized as transitory or characterized by subjective or consciously perceived feelings of apprehension. The instrument is not intended to be used for individual evaluation, but for assessment of group differences.

Construction.   The instrument was developed from the item pool of the IPAT Anxiety Scale, the Taylor Manifest Anxiety Scale, and the Welsh Anxiety Scale. Items that correlated with all three full scales were then rewritten to reflect both trait and state anxiety. The 177 items were critiqued for clarity and content by advanced undergraduate psychology students, reducing the item number to 124. Administered to another group of students for state and trait ratings, items were retained if they held for state and trait and were seen applicable by students. Further item-validation procedure, including administration for state and trait under imagined A-State, relax, and examination condition, reduced the form to 23 items. Form A of the STAI represented 20 of these 23 items. It was at this point that the developers turned to the idea of separate but parallel state-trait questionnaires, reaching through further additions and reductions to Form X. Despite the extensive revisions and refinements, the test authors' own dissatisfaction with these approaches indicates that they share concerns regarding whether the STAI was the best possible product of sequential construction methodology. Although a variety of student groups were utilized in various stages of construction, the normative samples are extremely narrow in scope, including very few noncollege or clinical populations.

Postconstruction Empirical Evaluation.   As would be expected, test-retest reliability for state was low, .20 to .40 regardless of time elapsed. Trait anxiety test-retest was higher at about .80; KR_{20}s ranged from .83 to .92. Not surprisingly, the A-Trait correlates highly with IPAT Anxiety Scale (.75) and the Taylor Manifest Anxiety Scale (.80), from which its items were drawn, while correlating less strongly with the Affect Adjective Checklist (.57). A-State, as would be expected, varies considerably across conditions. Content validity and empirical validity of the instrument are two critical issues. At no point was the score obtained on these inventories compared to any nontest evaluation of anxiety, although item selection sometimes employed hypothetical stress situations. In fact, the STAI was built solely on the belief that the initial item pool covered the full domain of anxiety and that further selection on the basis of internal consistency would not distort this circumstance. (The bridge from construct to instrument to the "real world" was, therefore, never satisfactorily completed.)

Criteria for Utilization with Medical Patients.   It is possible to see how both state and trait anxiety can contribute to an ongoing disease process, or complicate its management. Additional validation studies with medical patients would be desirable.

Life Experiences Survey (LES)

The Life Experiences Survey, developed by Sarason, Johnson, and Siegel (1978) was formulated to assess an individual's perception of the life stresses experienced during the preceding 12 months. The notion that life stresses lead to an increase in the frequency of illness is well entrenched in medical literature. Holmes and Rahe (1967) were the first to address this issue in their early Schedule of Recent Experience (SRE), an objective self-report measure of significant events that may have occurred in the subject's life. They posited that each life event, regardless of its positive or negative impact, requires adaptive coping on the part of the individual. Events were chosen for the SRE because their advent required adaptation on the part of the individual. Standardized weights were then determined for each event, reflecting the amount of social readjustment they appeared to require. This absolutist approach to events contrasts with that of Lazarus (1977), who states that the individual's perception of the meaning of the event is of critical importance.

Sarason et al. developed the LES as a means of gauging both the occurrence of an event and its perceived significance. The 57-item LES self-report inventory has two sections. The first, completed by all respondents, contains 47 specific events plus three blank spaces where individuals can add unlisted events. These events cover a wide range of experiences. The second section is designed primarily for use with students. In both sections, the respondent is asked to indicate which events were experienced during the past year and, in addition: (1) whether they viewed the event as positive or negative on a 7-point scale; and (2) the perceived impact of the event at its time of occurrence on a 7-point scale.

Administration, Scoring, and Development of Norms.   The inventory is self-administered, with instructions printed on the first page of the form. Individuals are asked to check which events have occurred, when in the last year these took place, and then indicate the type and extent of impact the event may have had. The LES takes approximately 20 minutes to complete.

The respondents themselves provide weights for each event. A positive change score is obtained by summing the impact ratings of events designated as positive;

negative change scores are derived by summing the impact of negative events. The total change score is the sum of these.

Normative studies involved the administration of the instrument to 345 Introduction to Psychology students (females, $N = 171$; males, $N = 174$). No significant differences were obtained between males and females on any of the three life change measures.

The most useful scores appear to be the negative and total change scores. A negative life change score is often significantly related to several stress-related dependent measures. The higher these scores, the greater the likelihood of future physical and/or psychological problems (Yunik, 1979).

Construction and Postconstruction Empirical Evaluation.   The LES items were chosen to represent life changes frequently experienced by individuals in the general population. Thirty-four of the 57 items are similar in content to those of the SRE. Specific items were clarified or reworded so as to be applicable to both male and female respondents. No further details are given as to the development of the item pool.

As stated, the underlying construct is that stress requires adaptation and that this adaptation will in part rest upon the individual's perception of the event. It is further assumed that this level of adaptive behavior will be related to illness events. Although efforts were made to be representati ͮe, it was impossible to tap the entire domain of potentially significant life events. Leaving a section of blanks to be filled in addresses this problem, but recall is likely to be a less adequate process than recognition as a means of identifying events. There was no indication that external criteria were utilized in the construction of the instrument, although numerous correlational studies were employed to evaluate the relationship between LES scores and relevant personality indices. One hopes that a formal manual, when published, will address a number of these issues.

Test − retest data with two samples show that positive change scores correlate .19 and .53 for 5 to 6 weeks, whereas negative scores correlated .56 and .88, and total change scores .63 and .64; the N's were 34 and 58 respectively. It must be noted that test − retest reliability is underestimated, as changes in events will occur with the passage of time.

LES scores were correlated with a number of other instruments. Negative scores correlated .29 with Trait Anxiety on the STAI and .46 with State; an almost zero correlation was found between positive scores and State or Trait Anxiety. Crowne − Marlowe Social Desirability correlations were also in the zero range, suggesting that the LES is free of social desirability bias. Employing the Psychological Screening Inventory, correlations of .28 between Extraversion and positive LES scores were found. From these data it would appear that personal maladjustment is marginally associated with negative change scores. Another modest correlation was found between the I − E Scale (.32) and negative LES changes. No studies were reported on the relationship of these scores and illness onset, the posited sequel to life stress.

Applications of Medical Criteria.   This instrument proposes to address the issue of life events only. It is posited that these have an impact on the incidence of illness and psychological difficulties. Although no construction validity studies have been reported on the efficacy of this instrument in making such predictions, research (Yunik, 1979) indicates that negative weighted events tend to have a high correlation with future illness; negative impact scores correlated .42 with the total number of illness problems reported. On the basis of this preliminary study, it appears that the LES may prove to be useful in predicting illness behavior.

INSTRUMENTS DEVELOPED PRIMARILY FOR INDIVIDUAL ASSESSMENT

The following instruments were developed for utilization in diagnosis of patients, rather than in the assessment of group differences.

Symptom Check List – 90 (SCL – 90)

This 90 item self-report symptom inventory was based on the Hopkins Checklist and was designed to reflect psychological symptom patterns of psychiatric patients. Derogatis (1977), the developer of the test, suggests that it also has utility for assessment of medical patients. Each item is rated on a 5-point scale of distress from "not at all" to "extremely." These responses are then interpreted along nine primary symptom dimensions: somatization, obsessive – compulsive, interpersonal sensitivity, depression, anxiety, hostility, phobic anxiety, paranoid ideation, psychoticism. In addition, three global indices of distress are calculated: global severity, positive symptom distress index, positive symptom total. The SCL – 90 is intended as a measure of current psychiatric symptom states, not as a measure of personality. It is designed to be interpreted on three levels. The first level is the global, and the "global severity index" (GSI) is employed as the gauge. The primary symptom dimensions address the patient's level of psychopathology. Individual items are used to relate the presence or absence of specific symptoms.

Administration, Scoring, and Development of Norms.   Instructions are simple and written on the test form. There is a note that asks the patient to record how much discomfort a particular problem has caused during the last X number of days. Most patients take 15 – 30 minutes to complete the task.

Scoring requires either templates or transferring the 90-item scores from the test paper to profile sheet, where weighted scores are summed to arrive at distress scores for each of the nine symptom dimensions. The global severity index, positive symptom total, and symptom distress index are also calculated. Raw scores are transformed into T-scores, utilizing nonpsychiatric patient norms.

The non-psychiatric normative group (females, $N = 80$; males, $N = 493$) was a stratified random sample drawn from one county in a mid-Atlantic state. No determination was made as to their status as medical patients. Brief descriptions of the clinical significance of each scale and global indices are provided. The GSI is considered an indicator of overall distress, whereas the nine primary symptom dimensions provide a profile of the patient's status in psychological terms. Discrete symptoms may also be noted. Small-sample profiles are provided as guides.

Construction. The SCL−90 was constructed to serve as a checklist of psychiatric symptomatology. It was developed through a combination of clinical/ rational and empirical/analytic procedures. The original item pool was drawn from the Hopkins Symptom Checklist (Derogatis, Lipman, Rickels, Uhlenhuth, & Covi, 1974a, 1974b), which, in turn, can be traced back to the CMI item pool (Wider, 1948). Core items of the Hopkins checklist were retained, some were dropped, and 45 new items were added to create four new symptom dimensions. The distress continuum was expanded to a 5-point scale. The method of developing these new items is not detailed in the manual, nor is the method for the initial reduction of the Hopkins checklist. In developing the instrument, Derogatis states that he chose to look only at those constructs that lend themselves to the self-report mode. Relying on factor analysis to establish construct validity, he arrived at an internal consistency measure of .77 to .90 for scales. Although this high measure of internal consistency may indicate a true homogeneity of scale dimensions, closer examination suggests that it may simply be the product of items that appear to restate the same concept in slightly different words. One-week test-retest reliability ranges from .78 to .90.

In an effort to evaluate the empirical validity of the instrument the concurrence of physicians' and patient-reported levels of psychological distress have been compared (Derogatis, Abeloff, & McBeth, 1977). Concurrent validity studies have proved somewhat disappointing. Of course, scales with the same name may not measure the same construct; thus, if the correlation of two similarly named scales proves to be low, it may be a function of tapping different constructs. MMPI correlations with similarly labeled scales were in the .50 to .60 range although the full matrix of MMPI correlations is not presented.

Applications of Medical Criteria. The SCL − 90 includes both medical and psychiatric symptoms, but is geared primarily to the level and nature of psychopathology present. Although a brief cataloging of psychiatric distress is of value, the majority of nonpsychiatric medical patients will vary along such a narrow band of differences that the results will be of minimal value. Furthermore, the information obtained from the SCL − 90 is unlikely to contribute very much to treatment planning among general medical patients. Although profile scores are presented to discriminate among various medical and psychiatric groups, these profiles merely represent the mean scores obtained for selected patient groups. Turning to other criteria, the SCL − 90 does not attempt to gauge prognosis or probable occurrence of later illness; rather, it calculates the presence of current feelings and behaviors.

Its major utility in patient management is in relation to psychiatric complications. The problems of utilizing a test developed for psychiatric patients in a non-psychiatric setting is a serious one. Even a well-designed psychiatric instrument is likely to provide information that is distorted, when applied to a medical population. Problems arise because of the unsuitability of norms, the questionable relevance of clinical signs, and the consequent inapplicability of interpretations. In brief, a standard interpretation of results obtained with a medical sample on a diagnostic test that was developed and designed to assess a psychiatric population runs hard against every major principle of sound test use.

Beck Depression Inventory

The Beck Depression Inventory (Beck, 1972) is an instrument that seeks to approximate clinical judgments of depression intensity. Efforts were made also to clearly differentiate depressed from nondepressed psychiatric patients. The inventory is composed of 21 multiple-choice items reflecting specific behavioral signs of depression, which were weighted in severity from zero to 3.

Depression was defined by Beck (1972) as: "an abnormal state of the organism manifested by signs and symptoms such as low subjective mood, pessimistic and nihilistic attitudes, loss of spontaneity and specific vegetative signs. This construct could be identified in many diverse types of patients who differ vastly in terms of other characteristics, such as degree of conceptual disorganization, presence of anxiety, prognosis [p. 201]." It should be noted that the inventory was designed for research purposes and was conceived as appropriate for discriminating levels of depression only in psychiatric populations.

Administration, Scoring, and Development of Norms.   Originally designed to be administered by a trained interviewer who read each statement and asked the patient to select the statement that fit best, the instrument is now often presented as a self-administered inventory. No information is given regarding the possible impact upon norms and scores of this modification to a self-administered format.

The total score is obtained by adding the weighted values for each response endorsed by the patient. No attempt is made to transform raw scores. Scores of $0-9$ are considered normal, the $10-15$ range is seen as representing mild depression, $16-19$ represents mild to moderate severity, $20-29$ judged as moderate to severe, and $30-63$ as severe depression.

Two patient samples were utilized in the development of the inventory. Both groups of patients were drawn from routine admissions to the psychiatric outpatient department of a university hospital and to the psychiatric outpatient department and psychiatric inpatient service of a metropolitan hospital. Patients were usually seen the day of their first visit, or at a later appointment within a few days. The majority of patients were white, of lower socioeconomic class, and ranging in age from 15 to 44. Patients were excluded if they had organic brain damage or mental deficiency. Major diagnostic categories represented included psychotic disorder (41%), psychoneurotic disorder (43%), and personality disorder (16%).

Construction and Postconstruction Empirical Evaluation.   The test developer sought to develop explicit, rather than inferred behavioral criteria for evaluating depression. To accomplish this, items were selected from the literature and clinical experience. Each subcategory describes a specific behavioral manifestation of depression and consists of a graded series of self-evaluative statements. The items were chosen on the basis of their relationship to overt behavioral manifestations of depression and do not reflect a particular theory regarding etiology or viewpoint concerning the psychological processes underlying depression.

Two methods for evaluating the internal consistency of the instrument were used. Two hundred cases were analyzed, with the score for each category compared to the total score on the Depression Inventory. It was found that all categories showed a significant relationship to the total inventory score. In a later study the subcategories also correlated positively with the total score (range .31 to .68). Split-half reliability results in a coefficient of .86.

Test – retest was not employed in the traditional manner due to the assumption that change would be occurring and that this would significantly alter the interpretation of results. Indirect methods were utilized to assess change scores over time; in general, total depression tended to parallel clinical changes.

Concurrent validity was addressed by comparing scores with clinical assessment of levels of depression (correlations between test scores and clinical judgments averaged .66). It is of some note that prediction of clinical change was accurate in 85% of the cases. At the same time it was seen that the instrument was capable of discriminating between anxiety and depression, correlating .59 with clinical ratings of depression and only .14 with clinical ratings of anxiety.

Application of Medical Criteria.   The total depression score seeks only to address level of severity among psychiatric patients, having been developed expressly for this purpose. It can serve a function with medical patients in this regard if clinical levels of depression are suspected, and may help direct the health team to psychotherapeutic or pharmacologic intervention.

Jenkins Activity Survey (JAS)

The Jenkins Activity Survey (Form C), developed by Jenkins, Zyzanski, and Rosenman (1979), is the latest version, a 52-item self-report questionnaire designed to measure the Type A behavior pattern. This pattern is characterized by extreme competitiveness, impatience, haste, restlessness, and feelings of being challenged and under the press of time. The behavior pattern is not conceived as a personality trait, or a standard reaction to a challenging situation, but rather the reaction of a predisposed person to a situation that challenges him or her. A large body of research has been built around the significance of this pattern in the development and persistence of coronary heart disease (CHD). Although the instrument is actively marketed to be utilized for individual diagnostic assessment, the test developers recommend that the instrument be used primarily for research into group differences, and given the multifactorial pathogenesis of CHD, they state that the test should not be used by itself to predict individual risk. The instrument proposes to tap three factors within Type A: speed and impatience, job involvement, and hard-driving competition.

Administration, Scoring, and Development of Norms. The JAS is easily administered to individuals and groups and is suitable for use with currently or recently employed adults who can read at eighth-grade level or better. The majority of subjects complete the instrument in 15 − 20 minutes.

Each response is assigned numerical points based on an optimal scaling weight for that response. The sum of the points for all items constitutes the raw score. Hand-scoring templates are available, but machine scoring is encouraged.

Normative data are based on a 2588 male sample drawn exclusively from individuals in middle and upper echelon jobs. Scores were normalized with the mean set of 0 and each standard deviation equal to 10 points. Scores on the plus side indicate Type A behavior; minus scores signify a Type B inclination. Percentile rankings are also provided. One serious flaw in this area of evaluation is the total absence of female subjects in both the development and normative stages of test construction. This compounds the narrow socioeconomic group employed for building norms.

JAS scores and the factors they comprise are briefly described in the Manual and are conceived as contributing independently to the total Type A behavior pattern.

Construction. The JAS was constructed over an 8-year period; four earlier editions were developed. Previous to this instrument Rosenman, Friedman, Straus, Wurm, Kositchek, Hahn, and Werthessen (1964) designed a structured interview protocol to assess the Type A behavior pattern. Items for the JAS were derived from this interview, as well as Jenkin's observations of interview behavior and the theory of Type A behavior. This early form of the instrument was administered to 120 males who had also been rated on the structured interview. Forty items, found to correlate with these ratings, were retained and 21 new questions were devised and added to comprise the 1965 edition. No information is given in the manual as to the basis for these new questions, nor the specific purpose for adding them. This form was then taken by a sample of 2951 males. Discriminant function analysis was employed to select items that might best differentiate between independently assessed Type A and Type B groups. The 19 best items made only 73% valid identification. In the following year a new sample of 844 men were tested on a second edition in which several new items were deleted and added. At this time 26 items produced optimal discrimination. Not all 19 items from the previous year's analysis entered this form. This time only 71% valid identifications were made with the construction sample. Factor analysis of the second form produced three derived factors: S—Speed and Impatience; J—Job Involvement, H—Hard-Driving and Competitive. A 64-item third edition of the instrument utilized earlier test forms as criterion measures. Discriminant functions sought to reduce the total item pools to subsets based on their presumed predictive accuracy and brevity. No cross-validation steps were taken after the item list had been reduced. Efforts to remove sex biases resulted in Form B; Form C consists of the best discriminatory 52 items from Form B.

A major flaw in the development sequence of the JAS was the use of discriminant function as the prime tool of scale construction. Each successive form of the test was changed substantially insofar as specific item content. Without adequate data on cross-validation, items were dropped, whereas others, retained on the basis of discriminant utility, had to be dropped later when new samples were employed. Discriminant function always separates construction sample groups, these discriminations may not hold up on further cross-validation work.

Postconstruction Empirical Evaluation.   Test-retest reliabilities at 4- to 6-month intervals ran from .65 to .82 on the four factors, with internal consistency ranging from .73 to .85.

Turning to validity, the construct underlying the test has some intuitive logic as well as empirical support. Initially developed to maximize its correlation with the structured interview, the JAS attempts to adhere closely to its major features. As development progressed, however, particularly in later stages, it became uncertain as to whether the original Type A domain was still being fully addressed; that is, the items selected and the factors produced may have become a product of statistical manipulation and sample idiosyncracies. Each step in the construction phase appeared to move the instrument further away from the original base in the structured interview.

Criteria for Utilization With Medical Populations.   The JAS was specifically developed to address the issue of Type A behavior, a pattern that is strongly implicated in coronary heart disease. Although the developers recommend that it be primarily for research in group differences, it can be and has been utilized for assigning individuals to preventive intervention groups. It has been employed as a predictor of CHD with some success, although recent literature shows that it does not improve on the predictive accuracy of the structured interview itself. (Brand, Rosenman, Jenkins, Stoltz, & Zyzanski, in press.) The instrument does not propose to provide information on the progress and management of ongoing disease processes.

PERSONALITY INVENTORIES

The following instruments deal with the realm of personality functioning and not with single traits or dimensions. They represent different conceptions of personality and different procedures. The instruments included are the 16 Personality Factor Inventory, the Minnesota Multiphasic Personality Inventory, and the Millon Behavioral Health Inventory.

16 Personality Factor Inventory (16PF)

The 16PF (Cattell, Eber, & Tatsouka, 1970), one of the oldest personality tests currently in use, was first published in 1949. It is composed of a multidimensional set of 16 scales arranged in omnibus form. If the supplement is used it is supposedly capable of tapping 23 personality dimensions. The most commonly used form, comprised of 187 trichotomous items, is designed to tap what Cattell terms "source traits" rather than syndromes. The traits evaluated are said to have withstood critical examination of over 30 years of factor-analytic research. Because the scales are claimed to be factorially pure, there is no item overlap; consequently, each scale score is gauged by responses to between only 10 and 13 items. Each of its several forms is geared to a seventh grade reading level and has been translated into numerous foreign languages. Standardized on a stratified sample of 15,000 normal adults, it has been used in a variety of research studies, as well as in clinical assessment in both psychiatric and medical settings.

Administration, Scoring, and Development of Norms.   A paper and pencil self-report inventory, the 16PF takes generally less than 45 minutes for the subject to complete and requires no assistance from the individual administering the test.

Hand-scoring templates, as well as machine-scoring and computer-generated narratives are available. Raw scores are transformed into sten scores for the 16 traits.

A variety of normative samples have been developed over the years. As mentioned earlier, standardization of the instrument involved a sample of 15,000 normal adults; however, it is unclear from the manual as to the nature and size of the original construction samples.

The traits are viewed as bipolar and scores are evaluated in terms of their location on the trait continuum. A variety of publications are available to help in interpreting scores (Karson & O'Dell, 1976), including a book specifically addressing the issue of the medical patient (Krug, 1977).

Construction.   A significant body of literature has been developed utilizing the 16PF; the meaning of many of the results is often unclear. Regarding initial construction, Rorer (1972) states that the scales are of indeterminate origin and unknown significance. Data gathered in support of the instrument often employ samples selected in an unknown way and the manual is not very specific as to which form, developmental stage, or population was employed in many of the reported studies. One of the continuing difficulties in evaluating this instrument is the atypical manner in which data are presented in the Handbook (Cattell, Eber, & Tatsouka, 1970). Although large quantities of data are presented, they are not comparable to standard psychometric evaluation techniques.

Postconstruction Evaluation.   Test — retest reliabilities are reported to be in the .70 to .90 range short term and drop to .50 to .80 at 2 months. Split-half reliabilities have indicated considerable within-factor heterogeneity. There is a high likelihood that several of the supposedly pure factors subsume a number of different traits. This finding is especially troublesome, as the instrument rests on the factorial purity of the 16 traits. No effort is made to provide correlation data with instruments purported to measure similar traits. Furthermore, the factoring method that Cattell has used is but one of the many available, each of which might have produced different results. Correlations between identical scales on different forms of the test are sometimes very low, ranging from .15 to .82; in fact, some scales correlate more highly with other scales than with their matched scales. This puts into question the meaning and reliability of these scales; at the very least, it makes comparison across forms impossible.

Applications of Medical Criteria.   The 16PF has been proposed as suitable for assessing the personality of medical patients. If it is valid at all, it may actually be more suitable with so-called normals than with general psychiatric populations, for whom it has also been claimed to be useful. The edited volume *Psychological Assessment in Medicine* (Krug, 1977) is devoted exclusively to the 16PF, but it provides largely anecdotal information on how to interpret the test.

One is left in reviewing this instrument with a sense of considerable methodological sophistication. At the same time, one is struck by the idiosyncratic conception of personality and the reluctance to compare this instrument and its results with anything other than itself. The use of esoteric proofs and the absence of more widely employed techniques seriously hamper the outsider in efforts to evaluate the instrument. These deficits and idiosyncrasies seriously compromise the confidence one may have in the 16PF's construct validity and consequent usefulness.

Minnesota Multiphasic Personality Inventory (MMPI)

The MMPI is an empirically derived instrument that was constructed by Hathaway and McKinley in 1939 to serve as an objective aid in a psychiatric case work-up and as a tool for determining the severity of specific psychiatric conditions. In its original development the MMPI had little to do with personality traits. As stated by Dahlstrom, Welsh, and Dalhstrom (1972), the MMPI was developed and validated as a psychiatric nosologic categorizing device leading to dichotomous discrimination between psychiatric patients and normals. They wrote:

> Although the content covered in the MMPI item pool included by far a larger array of personological topics than in any other instrument available, subsequent studies have indicated that—while some areas of emotional maladjustment may be overrepresented—items referring to values, to primary group relationships, and to mood, temperament, and various special attitudes are probably too scarce to provide a well-balanced coverage of the domain of personality (p. 6).

The final 566-item true – false questionnaire had 10 clinical scales: hypochondriasis, depression, hysteria, psychopathic deviance, male sexual introversion, paranoia, psychasthenia, schizophrenia, hypomania, and social introversion, along with the following validity scales: cannot say, lie scale, confusion scale or straight validity, K or suppressor factor.

Administration, Scoring, and Development of Norms. The test was developed so that those 16 years old or above with 6 years of school would be able to complete the inventory. Booklets are available for group testing, or for the patient to complete independently. Card sort format is also available, and if required, the test can be administered orally. The instrument takes on the average of 1 to 1 1/2 hours to complete, although there are no limits to the time alloted to complete the inventory.

Hand-scoring templates are available, as are machine-scoring; these scores may be transformed into profiles or computer generated narratives. Raw scores are converted to T-scores with separate norms for males and females. A T-score of 50 is the mean score for the normative construction sample and 10 represents one standard deviation. T-score scaling assumes normal distribution, an unlikely assumption given the highly variable prevalence rates of the syndromes involved.

The original normative group was drawn from samples of Minnesota adults, with male and female groups. Most lived in rural or semirural areas, worked in skilled or semiskilled trades, and had an eighth grade education. The test itself has not been renormed since this 1940 sample; numerous local norms have been developed for a variety of settings and special populations.

Originally, only single-scale elevations were interpreted. Over the years extensive clinical data have led to its increased utility. A number of codebooks have been written to aid in profile interpretations. (Gilberstadt & Duker, 1965; Good & Brantner, 1974; Marks & Seeman, 1963).

Construction. The original item pool of over 1000 items was drawn from other inventories, clinical reports, interviews, and clinical experiments. It was reduced to 504 to eliminate duplication and maximize readability. Fifty-five items dealing with male sexual inversion (MF) were added at a later date. The original

504-item form was given to subjects in a card sort task in which subjects were asked to describe themselves as accurately as possible. Construction criterion groups were selected from adult psychiatric clinics and wards of the University of Minnesota hospitals; "normal" subjects were families and visitors of the patients. Items were selected for inclusion in a scale based on their capacity to discriminate between normals and each of the criterion groups. No effort was made at that time to examine scale overlap or to develop a rationale for item selection. Cross-validation samples were employed to evaluate the stability of the obtained separation and the generality of initial scale findings. Three hundred and fifty-one of the 550 items (16 are repeated) are utilized in scoring the initial 10 clinical scales.

Postconstruction Empirical Evaluation. The MMPI is without doubt the most thoroughly researched personality instrument available. One problem in evaluating the inventory is that its manual has not been updated since 1967, and vast quantities of information on the test's empirical utility and validation reside in hundreds of journal articles often beyond the reach of all but the most diligent students. However, a significant amount of data are published concisely in the two-volume Handbook (Dahlstrom et al. 1972).

Test — retest reliability in one sample at 3 to 4 days ranged from .56 to .88 with the majority in the low 80s. College student test — retest scores at 8 months yielded correlations of .44 to .73. Psychiatric patients show 1-week test — retest ranging from .59 to .86 with the majority in the high 70s. At 1 year, correlations drop to .36 to .72. Test — retest can be difficult to interpret because it is not possible to discriminate real change from reliability error, particularly in the case of psychiatric patients undergoing treatment for extended periods of time. Kuder — Richardson internal consistency estimates are reported on a sample employing the KR_{21} formula. These ranged from .36 to .93 with a median of .70.

Validity data are best summarized in the MMPI Handbook (Dahlstrom et al. 1972). As one reads through reviews of the MMPI chronologically, one is struck by the response of individuals utilizing the test clinically. In 1945, reviews such as those by Benton and Probst (1945) state that there is a significant agreement on ratings and test scores on only Psychopathic deviate, Paranoia, and Schizophrenia, but not the other scales. Schmidt (1945) wrote that psychiatric patients can be distinguished from normals, but it is difficult to distinguish among different abnormal populations. Rotter (1945), in his review, thoughtfully notes that reliability and validity are dependent on the reliability and validity of the criterion disease groups themselves, which appear to have been much less than might be desired. For example, those diagnosed as belonging to one disease group were more likely than not to have their highest score on a scale other than the expected one. Ellis (1959) stated that the individual diagnostic utility of the instrument was still in question, but that it was useful for purposes of group discrimination. Adcock (1965) noted that the instrument failed to demonstrate discriminative validity regarding those who do and those who do not need help in a normal population. He went on to note that most clinicians assume the validity of the instrument rather than evaluate it as critically as one should. This acceptance often led to misinterpretations of the meaning of scores. Lingoes (1965) continued in his review to note difficulties in discriminating among groups of psychiatric patients. Undoubtedly the best instrument of its generation, it has assumed an almost mystical impregnability as a function of its age. For its time and purpose, its excellence of construction was unmatched.

Applications of Medical Criteria.   The MMPI has been employed in a variety of medical settings with rather equivocal results. Most frequently it has been used to differentiate psychosomatic from organic disease, to delineate psychological factors associated with psychosomatic disorders, and to predict the outcome of surgery or recovery from illness (Dahlstrom et al., 1972). As Butcher and Owens (1978) note, however, the MMPI does not appear to successfully differentiate psychosomatic types, and the commonly noted $1 - 3/3 - 1$ elevation may indicate a general neurotic overlay that does not preclude the diagnosis of organic disease (Schwartz, Osborn, & Krupp, 1972). Although utilized in a number of studies with medical patients, the MMPI appears to serve as an aid only if psychiatric issues are prominent.

Millon Behavioral Health Inventory (MBHI)

The MBHI was developed specifically with physically ill patients and medical – behavioral decision-making issues in mind (Millon, Green, & Meagher, 1982). A major goal in constructing the MBHI was to keep the total number of items comprising the inventory small enough to encourage use in all types of medical diagnostic and treatment settings, yet large enough to permit the assessment of a wide range of clinically relevant behaviors. Geared to an eighth-grade reading level, it contains 150 items.

Diagnostic instruments such as the MBHI have increased usefulness if they are linked systematically to a comprehensive clinical theory or are anchored to empirical validation data gathered in their construction (Loevinger, 1957). The eight basic "coping styles" comprising the first eight scales of the MBHI are derived from a theory of personality (Millon, 1969). The six "psychogenic attitude" scales were developed to reflect psychosocial stressors found in the research literature to be significant precipitators or exacerbators of physical illness. The final six scales comprising the present form were empirically derived for the MBHI either to appraise the extent to which emotional factors complicate particular psychosomatic ailments or to predict psychological complications associated with a number of diseases.

Administration, Scoring, and Development of Norms.   Self-administered, with instructions printed on the questionnaire; the great majority of patients can complete the inventory in 20 to 25 minutes.

Machine scoring and computer-generated narratives are available. The raw scores on the 20 scales are transformed into base rate scores.

There are some conditions for which the traditional method of transforming raw scores into standard scores is inappropriate. Standard scores by definition assume "normal" distributions or comparable frequency spreads of the traits or variables being measured. This assumption is not met when a set of scales represents coping styles, as these are not normally or equally distributed in the populations. Furthermore, it is not the primary purpose of a clinical instrument to locate the relative position of a patient on a frequency distribution, but rather to identify or calculate the probability that a patient is or is not a member of a particular class. On both grounds, differential base rates and optimal classificatory efficacy, it would be useful to employ transformation scores that are more meaningful and useful than standard scores (Meehl & Rosen, 1955).

For the MBHI, these base rate conversions were determined by known or estimated prevalence data and by utilizing cutting lines that maximize correct classifications; that is, calculated in term of optimal valid positive to false positive ratios.

Norms for the MBHI are based on several groups of nonclinical subjects and numerous samples of medical patients involved in diagnosis, treatment, or follow-up. The nonclinical groups involved in the construction phases of test development consisted of subjects drawn from several settings (e.g., colleges, health maintenance organizations, nursing schools, medical schools, factories, etc.) and was composed of 212 males and 240 females; the test construction patient group, drawn from diverse clinical populations (e.g., surgical clinics, pain centers, dialysis units, cancer programs, etc.) consisted of 1019 males and 1094 females.

Interpretation is based on both profile configurations and single-scale elevations. The first eight scales, the basic coping styles, characterize patients regarding interpersonal and personality traits. For most patients, these characteristics blend with other features in a configural pattern of several scales.

The psychogenic attitude scales represent the personal feelings and perceptions of the patient regarding different aspects of psychological stress presumed to increase psychosomatic susceptibility or aggravate the course of a current disease. Scores are gauged by comparing these attitudes to those expressed by a cross-section of both healthy and physically ill adults of the same sex. Some details concerning these six scales may be useful.

The Chronic Tension Scale gauges level of stress, a factor that has repeatedly been found to relate to the incidence of a variety of diseases. More specifically, qualitative studies of chronic stress, such as persistent job tensions or marital problems, have been carried out with particular reference to their impact on heart disease, often addressed as Type A-Type B behavior (Friedman & Rosenman, 1974; Gersten, Frii, & Lengner, 1976; Jenkins, 1976; Rahe, 1977). Constantly on the go, they live under considerable self-imposed pressure and have trouble relaxing.

The Recent Stress Scale addresses the patient's perception of events in the recent past that were experienced as stressful. This is a phenomenological assessment similar to the Social Readjustment Rating Scale (Holmes & Rahe, 1967) and Sarason et al.'s Life Experience Survey (1978). High scorers on this scale are assumed to have an increased susceptibility to serious illness for the year following test administration. The occurrence of recent marked changes in their lives predicts a significantly higher incidence of poor physical and psychological health than in the population at large (Andrew, 1970; Head, 1979; Yunik, 1979).

The *Premorbid Pessimism Scale* represents a dispositional attitude of help-lessness — hopelessness that has been implicated in the appearance or exacerbation of a variety of diseases such as multiple sclerosis, ulcerative colitis, and cancer (Mei-Tal, Meyerowitz, & Engel, 1970; Paull & Hislop, 1974; Schmale, 1972; Stavraky, Buch, Lott, & Wanklin, 1968). It differs from other "depression" indices by noting characterologic tendencies toward viewing the world in a negative manner. High scorers on this scale are disposed to interpret life as a series of troubles and misfortunes and are likely to intensify the discomforts they experience with real physical and psychological difficulties (Levine, 1980; Yunik, 1979).

The *Future Despair Scale* focuses on the patient's willingness to plan and look forward to the future (Engel, 1968; Wright, 1960). This is more likely than the previous scale to tap the patient's response to current difficulties and circumstances rather than a general or lifelong tendency to view things negatively. High scorers do not look forward to a productive future life and view medical difficulties as seriously distressing and potentially life threatening.

Social Alienation looks at level of familial and friendship support, both real and perceived, which appears to relate to the impact of various life stressors (Cobb, 1977; Rabkin & Struening, 1976). This sense of aloneness had been detailed in sociological literature (Berkman, 1967; Comstock & Partridge, 1972; Moss, 1977). High scorers are prone to physical and psychological ailments. A poor adjustment to hospitalization is also common. These patients perceive low levels of family support and social support and may not seek medical assistance until illness is extremely discomforting.

All the aforementioned stressors seem to be significantly modulated upward or downward by the preoccupations and fear that patients may express about their physical state, a characteristic addressed in the *Somatic Anxiety Scale*. Studies of what may be called somatic anxiety reflect the general concerns that patients have about their bodies (Lipsitt, 1970; Lowy, 1977; Lucente & Fleck, 1972; Mechanic & Volkart, 1960). High scorers on this scale tend to be hypochondriacal and susceptible to various minor illnesses. They experience an abnormal amount of fear concerning bodily functioning and are likely to overreact to the discomforts of surgery and hospitalization.

The next set of three scales was derived empirically. They have been labeled the "Psychosomatic Correlates" Scales and are designed for use only with patients who have previously been medically diagnosed as exhibiting one of the following specific disease syndromes: allergy, gastrointestinal problems, cardiovascular difficulties. The scores of each scale gauge the extent to which the patient's responses are similar to comparable diagnosed patients whose illness has been judged substantially psychosomatic or whose course has been complicated by emotional or social factors.

The last three of the empirically derived scales, those labeled "Prognostic Indices," seek to identify future treatment problems or difficulties that may arise in the course of the patient's illness. The scores of each scale: *Pain Treatment Responsivity; Life Threat Reactivity;* and *Emotional Vulnerability,* gauge the extent to which the patient's responses are similar to patients whose course of illness or treatment has been more complicated and unsatisfactory than is typical.

Construction.   The MBHI was developed following procedures recommended by Loevinger (1957) and Jackson (1970). They contend that validation should be an ongoing process involved in all the phases of test construction, rather than a procedure for assessing or corroborating an instrument's accuracy following completion. The three aspects of this validation procedure are theoretical-substantive, internal-structural and, external-criterion.

Theoretical-Substantive Validation Stage.   Over 1000 items were gathered from numerous sources, including other psychological tests, abnormal and personality texts, as well as written specifically for item pool purposes. Items were developed so as to cover the full range of characteristics to be tapped by both the personality and psychogenic scales. At this stage the number of items in the personality style scales ranged from 60 to 135. The psychogenic attitude scale items ranged in number from 37 to 57. The item set for the six empirically derived scales was drawn entirely from the final pool based on the 14 personality and psychogenic scales; they were not subject to initial theoretical-substantive analysis. Items were balanced at this stage so that the response "true" signified the style or attitude in half, and half in which the response "false" would do so; balance of this type was done to attempt to correct for "acquiescent" bias (Jackson & Messick, 1960).

Items were deleted according to the following general criteria: too complicated for patient understanding; obvious desirability bias; lack of clarity in phrasing; probable extreme endorsement frequency. Items were retained if they exemplified the traits of the scale for which they were written, and efforts were made to cover the full range of behaviors and attitudes typified by a given scale. To achieve this, 10 health professionals with knowledge of the personality theory and with experience in psychological traits among medical patients were asked independently to sort these items into their theoretically appropriate personality and psychogenic categories. The criteria for inclusion required that the item be sorted in the "correct" scale by at least seven of the judges.

Internal-Structural Validation State.   To accord with the theoretical model, items should give evidence not only of substantial within-scale homogeneity, but selective overlap within the MBHI was both expected and constructed in line with theoretical consideration; this contrasts with other instruments, such as the MMPI, where overlap among items on different scales is solely a function of empirically obtained covariations. A detailed explanation of this rationale may be found in the MCMI manual (Millon, 1982).

According to the theory underlying both the MCMI (Millon, 1969) and the MBHI, no personality style or psychogenic attitude is likely to consist of entirely homogeneous and discrete psychological dimensions. Rather, they comprise complex characteristics, sharing many traits, as well as distinctive features. Items are expected to exhibit their strongest, but not their only association with the specific scale for which they were developed. The ultimate test of an item's or scale's efficiency is not a statistical one, but a discriminatory or predictive one; procedures that enhance high item-scale homogeneity through studies of internal consistency are the best methods for optimizing, rather than maximizing discriminations among scales.

The initial items had been chosen to accord with theoretical − substantive validation data and were reduced on preliminary internal-consistency and structural validation grounds to the 289 "best." The 289-item "personality" form was administered to over 2500 persons in a variety of settings, somewhat over the majority being students at urban universities; medical populations were not included in this evaluation phase.

Several procedures were followed after this form had been administered to these subjects. Most importantly, item − scale homogeneities were again calculated using measures of internal consistency; additionally, true and false endorsement frequencies were obtained. Point − biserial correlations (corrected for overlap) were calculated between each item and each personality scale. To maximize scale homogeneity, only items that showed their highest correlation with the scale to which they were originally assigned were retained for further evaluation. Items showing a correlation of lower than .30 were eliminated, with few exceptions. The median biserial correlation for all items retained for inclusion in the MBHI from the provisional 289-item inventory was .47. The final number of items retained for inclusion in the MBHI from the provisional 289-item inventory was 64; these comprised the core group of coping style items for the final 150-item inventory.

Items for the six psychogenic attitude scales were developed on theoretical − substantive grounds, following the development of the core 64 personality items. Lists of approximately 35 to 60 items were developed for each of the six scales on the basis of previous research by other investigators into the characteristics to be measured. These item lists were then rated by clinicians with experience in assessing the role of psychological influences upon physical illness. Items "correctly" placed by more than 75% of the raters were the only ones considered for inclusion in the inventory. Efforts were made to include some representation of the several diverse traits comprising each scale. Eighty-three items were added in total by this procedure to the core group of 64 personality items; an additional three "correction" items were also included, resulting in a final form of 150 items.

External-Criterion Stage. The final 150 item form of the inventory was administered in a large number of medical settings to develop a series of empirically derived scales. The central idea behind this step, both as a construction approach and as a method of validation, is that items comprising a test scale should be selected on the basis of their empirically verified association with a significant and relevant criterion measure. The procedure by which this association is gauged is also direct. Preliminary items are administered to two groups of subjects that differ on the criterion measure. The "criterion" group exhibits the trait with which the item is to be associated, the "comparison" group does not. In the case of the MBHI all subjects were patients with a given diagnosis, but who varied according to clinical judgments regarding the degree to which various psychological or social complications were involved. After administration, true – false endorsement frequencies obtained with each group were calculated on every item. Items that statistically differentiated the criterion group from the comparison group were judged "externally valid." This was the approach followed in attempting to construct empirical scales that would either identify (correlate) or predict (prognose) certain clinically relevant criteria.

Point – biserial correlations between each of the 150 items and all scales were recalculated and reexamined. Items that showed high correlation (usually .30 or more) with any scale other than a theoretically incompatible one were added as an item to that scale.

At 4 1/2 months the coping style scales showed reasonably high test – retest reliabilities, with most in the range of .77 to .88 and a mean of .82. The psychogenic attitude scales also show high reliabilities, averaging around .85, as do the empirically derived scales at about .80, with the single exception of emotional vulnerability.

KR_{20} s were calculated as the optimal method for addressing internal consistency. The coefficients for all scales ranged from .66 to .90, with a median of .83.

Correlational data have been obtained employing a variety of different and often homogeneous patient and nonpatient samples. Among the inventories used were the MMPI, the SCL – 90, I – E Scale, Beck's Depression Inventory, the Personal Orientation Inventory, the Life Events Survey, the Webber–Johansson Temperament Survey and the California Personality Inventory, and are reported at length in the MBHI manual (Millon, Green, & Meagher, 1979).

Applications of Medical Criteria. The MBHI addresses interpersonal style, attitudes shown to be sufficient to the management of health concerns, likelihood of psychological components of medical problems, and specific prognostic issues. It uses this information to make probabilistic statements about the patient's behavior in relation to illness, its management, and health-care personnel. Directly addressing specified disease processes and their management, it provides the basis for making recommendations across a variety of medical problems regarding the likelihood of illness occurring and probable progress as well as optimal management of the disease process.

Although the MBHI was specifically designed for use in medical settings, full acceptance of the instrument will depend on: (1) future validation studies that are reported in refereed journals; (2) research clearly demonstrating the inventory's usefulness; and (3) its judged efficacy by clinicians in medical settings. As a new instrument, it has not yet had the widespread use of the MMPI or even the Cattell 16PF. As the first comprehensive psychological assessment instrument specifically designed for use with medical patients, however, it would appear to have considerable potential.

DISCUSSION

The process of evaluating the medical patient is currently evolving from a strictly medical – diagnostic approach to one encompassing an examination of the presenting symptoms along with events, actions, reactions, and personality interactions occurring in an everchanging situation. Psychologists employing interview and diagnostic testing procedures contribute to this evaluation by delineating psychological aspects of the patient's life as well as by developing diagnostic and prognostic statements.

This review of self-report inventories widely used with medical patients provides the practitioner with an overview of the state of the art. Ranging from simple checklists to single-trait assessments and multidimensional personality inventories, these instruments provide a variety of diagnostic options for the clinician. Unfortunately, even within this selected group, construction and postconstruction validation results have often proved disappointing. It is critical that the clinician utilizing a given instrument demonstrate caution, in both application and interpretation. Employing tests developed and normed with psychiatric populations may fit old habits and be expedient, but only rarely have such instruments proved useful in nonpsychiatric health-care settings. Psychological assessment is new to the nonpsychiatric medical world and instruments must be carefully evaluated regarding not only their construction, but their suitability to provide answers to the diagnostic and decision-making requirements of the medical staff.

REFERENCES

Adcock, C. J. *Review in the 6th mental measurements yearbook.* Highland Park, N.J.: The Gryphon Press, 1965.

Andrew, J. M. Recovery from surgery, with and without preparatory instruction, for three coping styles. *Journal of Personality and Social Psychology,* 1970, *15*(3), 223 – 226.

Beck, A. T. *Depression: Causes and treatment*. Philadelphia: University of Pennsylvania Press, 1972.

Benton, A. L., & Probst, K. A. A comparison of psychiatric ratings with MMPI scores. *Journal of Abnormal and Social Psychology*, 1945, *41*, 75 – 78.

Berkman, P. L. Spouseless motherhood, psychological stress, and physical morbidity. *Journal of Health and Social Behavior*, 1967, *10*, 323 – 334.

Brand, R. J., Rosenman, R., Jenkins, C., Stoltz, R., & Zyzanski, S. Comparison of coronary heart disease prediction in the WCGS using the structured interview and the JAS assessments of the coronary-prone Type A behavior pattern. *Journal of Chronic Diseases*, in press.

Butcher, J. N., & Owens, P. L. Objective personality inventories: Recent research and some contemporary issues. In B. Wolman (Ed.), *Clinical diagnosis of mental disorders: A handbook*. New York: Plenum Press, 1978.

Cattell, R. B., Eber, H. W., & Tatsouka, M. M. *Handbook for the Sixteen Personality Factor Questionnaire (16PF)*. Champaign, Ill.: Institute for Personality and Ability Testing, Inc., 1970.

Cobb, S. Epilogue: Meditation on psychosomatic medicine. In Z. J. Lipowski, D. R. Lipsitt, & P. C. Whybrow (Eds.), *Psychosomatic medicine: Current trends and clinical applications*. New York: Oxford Press, 1977.

Comstock, G. W., & Partridge, K. B. Church attendance and health. *Journal of Chronic Disease*, 1972, *25*, 665 – 672.

Dahlstrom, W. G., Welsh, G. S., & Dahlstrom, L. E. *An MMPI handbook* (Vol. 1 and 2). Minneapolis: University of Minnesota Press, 1972.

Derogatis, L. R. *SCL–90R (revised) version manual-I*. Baltimore, 1977.

Derogatis, L. R., Abeloff, M., & McBeth, C. Cancer patients with their physicians in the perception of psychological symptoms. *Psychosomatics*, 1977, *18*.

Derogatis, L. R., Lipman, R. S., Rickels, K., Uhlenhuth, E. H., & Covi, L. The Hopkins Symptom Checklist (HSCL): A measure of primary symptom dimensions. In P. Pichot (Ed.), *Psychological measurements in psychopharmacology*. Basel: Karger, 1974. (a)

Derogatis, L. R., Lipman, R. S., Rickels, K., Uhlenhuth, E. H., & Covi, L. The Hopkins Symptom Checklist (HSCL): A self-report symptom inventory. *Behavioral Science*, 1974, *19*, 1 – 15. (b)

Ellis, A. *Review of the MMPI 5th mental measurements yearbook*, Oscar Buros (Ed.). Highland Park, N.J.: The Gryphon Press, 1959.

Engel, G. L. A life setting conducive to illness: The given-up – giving-up complex. *Bulletin of the Menninger Clinic*, 1968, *32*, 355 – 365.

Friedman, M., & Rosenman, R. H. *Type A behavior and your heart*. New York: Knopf, 1974.

Gersten, J. C., Frii, S. R., & Lengner, T. S. Life dissatisfaction and illness of married men over time. *American Journal of Epidemiology*, 1976, *103*, 333 – 341.

Gilberstadt, H., & Duker, J. *A handbook for clinical and actuarial MMPI interpretation*. Philadelphia: W. B. Saunders, 1965.

Good, P., & Brantner, J. *A practical guide to the MMPI*. Minneapolis: University of Minnesota Press, 1974.

Head, R. *The impact of personality on the relationship between life events and depression*. Unpublished doctoral dissertation. University of Miami, 1979.

Holmes, T. H., & Rahe, R. The social readjustment rating scale. *Journal of Psychosomatic Research*, 1967, *11*, 213.

Jackson, D. N. A sequential system for personality scale development. In C. D. Spielberger (Ed.), *Current topics in clinical and community psychology* (Vol. 2). New York: Academic Press, 1970.

Jackson, D. N., & Messick, S. Acquiescence and desirability as response determinants in the MMPI. *Educational and Psychological Measurement*, 1960, *21*, 771 – 790.

Jenkins, C. D. Psychologic and social precursors of coronary disease. *New England Journal of Medicine*, 1976, *284*(6), 307 – 317.

Jenkins, C. D., Zyzanski, S. J., & Rosenman, R. H. *Jenkins activity survey manual*. New York: The Psychological Corporation, 1979.

Karson, S., & O'Dell, J. *Clinical use of the 16PF*. Champaign, Ill.: Institute for Personality and Ability Testing, 1976.

Krug, S. E. *Psychological assessment in medicine*. Champaign, Ill.: Institute for Personality and Ability Testing, 1977.

Lazarus, R. Cognitive and coping processes in emotion. In A. Monat & R. Lazarus (Eds.), *Stress and coping*. New York: Columbia University Press, 1977.

Levine, R. *The impact of personality style upon emotional distress, morale, and return to work in two groups of coronary bypass surgery patients*. Unpublished thesis, University of Miami, 1980.

Lingoes, J. C. *Review of the MMPI 6th mental measures yearbook*, Oscar Buros (Ed.). Highland Park, N.J.: The Gryphon Press, 1965.

Lipsitt, D. R. Medical and psychological characteristics of "Crocks." *International Journal of Psychiatry in Medicine*, 1970, *1*, 15 – 25.

Loevinger, J. Objective tests as instruments of psychological theory. *Psychological Reports*, 1957, *3*, 635 – 694.

Lowy, F. H. Management of the persistent somatizer. In Z. J. Lipowski, D. R. Lipsitt, & P. C. Whybrow (Eds.), *Psychosomatic medicine: Current trends and clinical applications*. New York: Oxford Press, 1977.

Lucente, F. E., & Fleck, S. A study of hospitalization anxiety in 408 medical and surgical patients. *Psychosomatic Medicine*, 1972, *34*, 304 – 312.

Marks, P., & Seeman, W. *The actuarial description of abnormal personality*. Baltimore: The Williams & Wilkins Co., 1963.

Mechanic, D., & Volkart, E. H. Stress, illness behavior and the sick role. *American Sociological Review*, 1960, *26*, 51.

Meehl, P. E., & Rosen, A. Antecedent probability and the efficiency of psychometric signs, patterns or cutting scores. *Psychological Bulletin*, 1955, *52*, 194 – 216.

Mei-Tal, V., Meyerowitz, S., & Engel, G. L. The role of psychological process in a somatic disorder: Multiple sclerosis. I. The emotions of illness onset and exacerbation. *Psychosomatic Medicine*, 1970, *32*, 67 – 86.

Millon, T. *Modern psychopathology*. Philadelphia: Saunders, 1969.

Millon, T. *Millon clinical multiaxial inventory manual* (2nd ed.). Minneapolis: National Computer Systems, Inc., 1982.

Millon, T., Green, C., & Meagher, R. *Millon behavioral health inventory manual*. Minneapolis: National Computer Systems, Inc., 1982.

Moss, E. Biosocial resonation: A conceptual model of the links between social behavior and physical illness. In Z. J. Lipowski, D. R. Lipsitt, & P. C. Whybrow (Eds.), *Psychosomatic medicine: Current trends and clinical applications*. New York: Oxford Press, 1977.

Paull, A., & Hislop, I. G. Etiological factors in ulcerative colitis: Birth, death and symbolic equivalents. *International Journal of Psychiatry in Medicine*, 1974, *5*, 57 – 64.

Rabkin, J. C., & Struening, E. L. Life events, stress and illness. *Science*, 1976, *194*, 1013 – 1020.

Rahe, R. H. Subjects' recent life changes and their near future illness susceptibility. *Advances in Psychosomatic Medicine*, 1977, *8*, 2 – 19.

Rorer, L. G. *Review of the 16PF 7th mental measurements yearbook*. Oscar Buros (Ed.). Highland Park, N.J.: The Gryphon Press, 1972.

Rosenman, R.H. , Friedman, M., Straus, R., Wurm, M., Kositchek, R., Hahn, W., & Werthessen, N. T. A predictive study of coronary heart disease: The Western Collaborative Group Study. *Journal of the American Medical Association*, 1964, *189*, 15 – 22.

Rotter, J. B. In O. Buros (Ed.), *Review of the MMPI* (3rd ed.) *mental measurements yearbook*. Highland Park, N.J.: Gryphon Press, 1945.

Sarason, I. G., Johnson, J. H., & Siegel, J. M. Assessing the impact of life changes. *Journal of Consulting and Clinical Psychology*, 1978, *46*, 932 – 949.

Schmale, A. H. Giving up as a final common pathway to changes in health. In Z. J. Lipowski (Ed.), *Psychological aspects of physical illness*. Basel, Switzerland: Karger, 1972.

Schmidt, H. O. Test profiles as a diagnostic aid: The MMPI. *Journal of Applied Psychology*, 1945, *29*, 115 – 131.

Schwartz, M. S., Osborne, D., & Krupp, N. E. Moderating effects of age and sex on the association of

158 GREEN

medical diagnoses and 1 − 3/3 − 1 MMPI profiles. *Journal of Clinical Psychology,* 1972, *28,* 502 − 505.

Speilberger, C. D., Gorsuch, R. L., & Lushene, R. *The state − trait anxiety inventory manual.* Palo Alto, Calif.: Consulting Psychologists Press, 1970.

Stavraky, K. M., Buch, C. N., Lott, J. S., & Wanklin, J. M. Psychological factors in the outcome of human cancer. *Journal of Psychosomatic Research,* 1968, *12,* 251 − 259.

Wider, A. *The Cornell medical index.* New York: The Psychological Corporation, 1948.

Wright, B. A. *Physical disability: A psychological approach.* New York: Harper, 1960.

Yunik, S. *The relationship of personality variables and stressful life events to the onset of physical illness.* Unpublished doctoral dissertation, University of Miami, 1979.

7 Behavioral Assessment in Medical Settings

David M. Schwartz
University of Miami

Jack T. Tapp
University of Miami and Nova University

Bernard Brucker
University of Miami

INTRODUCTION

Assessments of physical disorders are designed to fulfill several objectives: (1) they clearly delineate the conditions and subconditions that are contributing to the disorder; (2) they provide a degree of predictability about the future course of the disorder; (3) they provide some direction to the practitioner in the course of planning and implementing a program of intervention that will regulate the course of the pathological condition; and (4) they provide a common language facilitating the communication between the specialists who treat or otherwise respond to the disorder.

In physical diagnosis the clinician works from a theoretical system that specifies the parameter and ranges of "normal" functioning. Deviations from these parameters define the signs of disease. When coupled with symptoms, and a knowledge of the probability of prevalent disorders, the diagnostician can assess the potential for disease (Elstein, Shulman, & Sprafka, 1978). The language used to describe the disease condition communicates to others who are similarly schooled; it delineates between subconditions of the disorder, it provides a degree of predictability about the course of the disorder, and in most instances there is an implicit course of intervention (i.e., return the parameters of dysfunction to normal range and alleviate the symptoms).

Behavioral assessments are generally consistent with this model of diagnosis. Normal ranges of behavioral functioning are identified and deviations from these reflect the "disease" condition. These are assessed by a variety of methods outlined in the following pages including the assessment of the subjective symptoms of the behavioral abnormality. Behavioral assessments within a health care setting typically occur within the context of a health problem. The symptoms of the disease or the behavioral manifestations of the emotional sequelae associated with the disease are the "targets" of the treatment. The objective of behavioral assessment is to gather sufficient data to develop a plan for intervention. When pronounced pathophysiology is involved, such as in stroke, myocardial infarction, or postsurgery, behavioral assessments and interventions are constrained by the limits imposed by the physiological condition of the disease.

Behavioral assessments also present a somewhat different set of problems to the diagnostician. The parameters of the disease (i.e., the behavioral deviations from "normal" ranges) are often difficult to define in as precise terms as the parameters of physiological functioning. There is often (but not always) a greater emphasis on the subjective report and experiences of the patient than in physical diagnosis. These are subject to distortions via denial or exaggeration. There is frequently a confusion in the significance of behaviors for a person with a behavioral problem that is associated with a disease process.

When considered in light of the process of diagnosis as a problem-solving task, the similarities between behavioral assessments and physical diagnosis outweigh the differences.

In this chapter we review the theory underlying behavioral diagnosis, some of the schemes that are employed in formulating these assessments, and the particular methods that are used in their application to specific problems.

BEHAVIORAL AND PSYCHOLOGICAL ASSESSMENT

The development and utilization of psychometric instruments reflects a history of psychological measurement grounded in personality theory. It is presumed that the self-reported descriptions or the projected aspects of personality will allow inferences to be made about how the person is likely to behave in diverse situations. This prediction follows from the elucidation of drives, needs, motives, cognitions, and attitudinal orientations that reflect the individual's characteristics as shown on the tests. Such information is of considerable value in the design of a treatment plan.

Behavioral approaches to diagnosis differ from these more traditional approaches to psychological assessment in a number of ways:

1. Methodologically, psychological assessment strategies have traditionally relied on the subjective report of patients in structured (or semistructured) situations. The patients are given an opportunity to respond to a class of stimuli that are presented as questions on a test and/or amorphous situations that require interpretations. Based on these samples of verbal behavior, inferences are made about how the patients respond to other situations and their general modes of behavior. These are called "traits" or attributes of personality.

Behavioral assessments focus on the actions of the individuals as reflected in their performance. These measurements may be taken in simulated situations where performance is stressed or they may be based on a combination of observations made by others and verbal reports made by the patient. In all of these instances the behavioral assessment focuses on identifiable behaviors or actions of the patient as they are related to the situation or the symptoms, and inferences about the total pattern of behavior are limited.

2. Specificity is essential to behavioral assessment. The behavior that is being examined is defined as precisely and as operationally as possible. There is minimal attempt to relate the behavior to attributes of the person who exhibits it. The manifest expression of the act or the associated symptoms are identified as the behavior to be measured and it is assessed in terms of its frequency of appearance and/or its amplitude.

In behavioral medicine this strategy is applied within the context of the physical diagnosis of the relevant diseases. Once the potential for underlying pathology has been examined and critical diseases have been ruled out, the symptom is viewed as "the problem." The symptom is not seen as an expression of an unconscious conflict or a repressed desire, but it reflects a learned response that has identifiable consequences for the patient.

Psychological assessments frequently focus on generalities about the person. It is presumed that behavior is the expression of underlying attributes of character and that the samples of behavior taken from self-reported descriptions can allow one to make inferences about how that individual will behave in diverse situations. These predictions about future behavior follow from the understanding of the underlying meaning and motives for that behavior as reflected in the psychological assessments.

3. Theoretically, psychological assessments are based on the view that specific traits or aspects of personality such as dependency, aggressiveness, or Type A behaviors will manifest themselves in a characteristic manner that will impact on all the life experiences of that individual. Because these aspects of behavior are general and cut across situations, they will certainly reflect themselves in how the individual responds to disease.

Behavior assessment assumes that behavior is under the control of identifiable factors in the person's environment. Specifically, the situations within which one finds oneself are the strongest influences on how the individual will behave. If there have been rewards for certain performances in the situation in the past, those behaviors that reflect those performances will be repeated at a high rate. The individual has cognitive and behavioral influence over the situation, in that certain behavioral and environmental contingencies can be arranged to alter and reinforce behaviors.

In recent years there has been an increased recognition that cognitive factors are critical determinants of behavior beyond, but not exclusive of their situational manifestations. This has resulted in an increased utilization of cognitive assessments in a form that keeps them tied to the specific behaviors that are being analyzed. In other words, the form of cognitive testing may resemble other psychological tests, but the function is related to an analysis of the presenting problems as seen through the patient's eyes.

From this discussion of psychological and behavioral assessment, it is apparent that both points of view have their scientific and theoretical legitimacy and that neither is more "correct" than the other. Both meet the pragmatic criteria for diagnosis offered here. The differences lie in emphasis and in the application of underlying purposes of assessment. They supplement one another and in many instances they are mutually necessary (e.g., the management of chronic pain, or cardiac rehabilitation, as both forms of "diagnosis" can provide a much more comprehensive view of the individual and his or her behavior than either one alone).

FOUNDATIONS OF BEHAVIORAL ASSESSMENT

Conditioning Models

Historically, behavioral assessment has its roots in classical studies of learning. This historical tradition has evolved from the scientific study of the factors that influence changes in the behavior of individual organisms. Beginning with Thorndike's (1913) observations of the behavior of cats in a puzzle box and Pavlov's (1927) studies of classical conditioning in dogs, the assessment of behavior change has followed a tradition that has emphasized quantitative precision and scientific observation. These early investigations led to the assertion that behavior could be "explained" by understanding the factors in the environment that influenced the particular expressions of behavior. Accordingly, there was no need to postulate "conscious or unconscious processes" to account for behavior. All that was needed to predict and control behavior was the capacity to control environmental stimuli and the consequences of behavior on the environment. This viewpoint describes the Stimulus-Response model of behavior.

A historical influence of direct relevance to assessment in behavioral medicine developed from research on interoceptive conditioning. The Nobel Prize-winning studies of Pavlov on the gastric secretions of the stomach led him to the investigation of the acquired associations between environmental stimuli and smooth muscle responses. By pairing previously neutral stimuli such as a light or a buzzer with puffs of food powder applied to the tongues of dogs, he was able to show that neutral stimuli would elicit salivation in much the same manner as the food powder. This paradigm, known as *classical* or *respondent conditioning*, became a working model for the acquisition of emotionally laden "meaning." Anxiety or learned fear was the result of interoceptive visceral cues that were elicited in situations where fear had been experienced. These cues were subject to the laws of learning (i.e., they could *generalize* to new situations, they could be *differentially conditioned* to different classes of stimuli, and, most importantly, they could be *habituated* by repeated presentations or *extinguished* by changing the stimulus environment).

The observation that a behavior pattern that was followed by a reward would increase in frequency was the basis for studies of another type of learning called *instrumental learning* or *operant conditioning*. The importance of instrumental learning has also been well established as a means for controlling and directing behavior. In institutional settings this method, known as *behavior modification,* has repeatedly established itself as an efficient and humane way of effecting improved functioning in self-care and social behavior. By rewarding "good" behavior with tokens and/or approval, great strides have been made in improving the lives of retarded individuals and hospitalized patients with psychiatrically defined illnesses. The development and the judicious application of these methods to a variety of situations that require the extinction of old learning and the acquisition of new behaviors is one of the major contributions made by the behavior sciences to society.

For theoretical and practical reasons it became important to determine if interoceptive responses were subject to the laws of instrumental conditioning (i.e., could they be influenced by rewards in the same manner as other behaviors?). Over the period of the last two decades research has demonstrated that these response patterns can be *reinforced* and strengthened when they are followed by desirable consequences. It has become a well-established fact that internal stimuli such as changes in heart rate or blood pressure or gastric motility can be brought under stimulus control and used as responses in learning studies. If these responses are made discriminable to the learner this facilitates the procedure. It is not our purpose to elaborate the specific parameters of these phenomena, but suffice it to point out that any visceral response that has been monitored has been conditioned and that most of these can be reinforced and strengthened by an appropriate arrangement of environmental contingencies.

Subsequent research and theory development pointed to the limitations of the Stimulus-Response (S-R) model. Work by Hull (1952) and Spence (1956), for example, demonstrated that certain classes of stimulus events that were presumed to be internal to the organism, such as drives, could improve the predictive power of the S-R model. Bandura (1977) pointed to the importance of social events as determinants of behavior patterns. As a result, the model was expanded to include organismic variables and social consequences as determinants of behavior. The S-O-R-K-C model of Kanfer and Phillips (1970) was offered as an acronym for assessing the Stimulus (S), Organismic (O), Response (R), Contingencies (K), and Consequences (C) of behavior. This model expanded the learning concepts and offered a more comprehensive view of the variables that control behavior.

Social Learning

The importance of the social environment as an influence on the learning behaviors of human beings was also repeatedly demonstrated by scientific
investigation. Not only were the contingencies of *social rewards* established as
extremely powerful reinforcers, but human imitation or *modeling* was established
as a significant source of human learning. Bandura (1977) pointed to three major
influences of modeling on learning: (1) observational learning in which the
observer acquires new patterns of behavior that did not exist as integrated response
patterns prior to the experience; (2) the strengthening or weakening of response
inhibitions previously existent in the observer's repetoire; and (3) response facilitation in which the behavior of others serves as discriminative stimuli to facilitate the
behavior of the observer. These effects were obvious in numerous studies, particularly with children. Their influence as a potential source of behavioral expression is obvious as is their implication for behavioral assessment. Research on the
effects of modeling in medical settings is virtually nonexistent, yet it affords a
potentially powerful set of variables for learned expressions of disease symptomatology.

Cognitive Learning

Cognitive factors in behavior have been introduced relatively recently as an area of
assessment and treatment. The theoretical roots of this perspective can be traced to
the sign learning theories of Tolman (1932). He postulated that the units of learning
were composed of both cognitive and behavioral factors. Organisms learned that
certain cues were "signs" that signified consequent events, and that these led to the
formulation of hypotheses that were tested out as behaviors. Those sign-signifi-
cant-behavior sequences that were reinforced led to the formulation of learned
expectations. Unlearning requires the disconfirmation of a previously learned
hypothesis.

Rotter (1970) provided a more contemporary elaboration of this viewpoint.
Like Tolman, he saw behavior as goal directed. An individual's behaviors, needs,
and goals are a functionally related system developed from a reinforcement history
that has satisfied needs. These are particularly important systems for the satisfaction of social needs. From this perspective the assessment questions focus on
"What ends are being achieved by a particular form of behavior?".

This cognitive-expectancy model has been elaborated as an extension of the
more traditional behavioral analysis. Seligman (1975) has used the model to
explain depression from the standpoint of learned expectations of helplessness.
The organism learns that the probability of an outcome is independent of performance (i.e., rewards are not contingent on any particular response). This generates
the expectation that behavior is not dependent on any particular response with the
associated belief that there is little or no control over environmental contingencies.

These expectancies generalize to new situations with the associated loss in control and self-esteem that characterizes depression.

The application of these cognitive-behavioral concepts to emotional and stress-related disorders has been developed and elaborated by a number of authors (Bandura, 1977; Beck, 1976; Ellis & Harper, 1975; Mahoney & Arnkoff, 1979; Meichenbaum, 1977). They represent one of the most significant recent developments in behavioral assessment (Meichenbaum & Cameron, 1981), and their application to issues of emotional control and management has been well established (Davidson, 1976).

As behavioral medicine has developed, there has been a natural and logical extension of the conditioning, social, and cognitive learning concepts into this field. The S-O-R-K-C model can be easily extended to the analysis of physical symptoms. Stimuli from a variety of sources including social stimuli can serve to elicit organismic reactions in the form of visceral and autonomic responses and/or cognitions and expectations. These in turn produce behaviors that have their environmental contingencies and consequences. Over a period of time the behaviors associated with symptoms have consequences that satisfy individual needs and are thereby reinforcing. This history results in the development of "secondary gains" from the expression of symptoms, which in turn reinforces cognitive expectations and beliefs about the symptoms. Thus stimuli have eliciting properties for a number of behaviors that can be variously observed as actions, cognitions, emotions, visceral and/or autonomic responses, all of which occur simultaneously (more or less) within the same human being. The consequences determine the course of these behaviors.

Stress and Behavioral Assessment

Claude Bernard's assertion that the constancy of the internal environment was necessary for the maintenance of the free and independent life, reflects a fundamental attribute of living systems (viz. the activity of organisms is conducted to maintain internal environmental stability in the face of physical entropy). Over an extended period of time the human organism has evolved neurally controlled systems that are intended to regulate this state of constancy or homeostasis. These systems are dependent on behavior to achieve these ends.

Thus the human organism is constantly under stress. Though there will be varying degrees and qualities to the stressful existence, entropy will ultimately prevail. The challenge of living is to maintain the systemic balance for as long as possible.

Beginning with Selye's (1956) classic work on the stress reactions of the body, there has been an increasing awareness of the role of stress factors in the etiology of disease. It is now widely recognized that there are a multitude of sources of stress stemming from environmental, psychological, and social sources, as well as from pathological deficiencies in organ structure and infectious agents of disease. The general adaptation syndrome describes the manner in which organisms adapt to stress regardless of its source. The alarm reaction, the stage of resistance, and the state of exhaustion are predictable sequences in the stress syndrome, each with characteristics that define their effects on the organism (see Chapter 5).

Selye (1956) defines stress as "the state manifested by the specific syndrome which consists of all the nonspecifically induced changes within a biologic system [p. 54]." By this definition it is reaction of the body with definite parameters of response. This reaction can be produced by stimuli from a number of sources: environmental conditions such as noise, cold, and heat; living conditions such as crowding; excessive and demanding work; lack of adequate financial resources; social conflicts with significant persons; ineffective role behaviors; social isolation; changes in social networks and supports; excessive emotional strain; disease onset; chronic health problems; and, in general, changes in living status that can arise from a number of sources (moving, being promoted, graduation from school, going to jail, losing a loved one, etc.).

Though negative changes generally have a greater probability of producing stress reaction, to a large extent the consequences of these events are determined by how they are perceived and cognitively interpreted (Sarason & Sarason, 1979). For assessment purposes, optimistic perspectives and denial have potential for mitigating against stress responses, whereas negative expectations and perceived helplessness augment stressful reactions (Cohen & Lazarus, 1979). Thus cognitions play a significant role in affecting the outcomes of sources of stress.

Physiological reactions to stress have been discussed in Chapter 5. The clinical manifestations of stress take a variety of forms. Fatigue, irritability, symptom exacerbation, excessive muscle tension, anxiety, lack of sleep, inability to concentrate, nausea, diarrhea, excessive concern about physical health, loss of appetite, withdrawal, preoccupation with self doubts, interpersonal tensions, changes in sexual habits, increased alcohol consumption, increased eating, decreased work productivity, feelings of pressure, and absence from work, are but a few of the potential physical, behavioral, and cognitive expressions of stress. These symptoms of stress, along with disease presentations discussed in Chapter 9, have made stress reactions critical to assessment in behavioral medicine.

Cybernetic Models

Within the past few years there have been some notable attempts to develop cybernetic models of behavioral control that extend behavioral analysis further and relate it to general systems theory. Though these theories have not been extended into the clinical realm to the same degree as the models for assessment reviewed thus far, they do offer a conceptual point of view that is significant for future assessment theory. Carver and Scheier (1983) outline a control theory approach to human behavior based on the work of Powers (1973) that affords a scheme for interrelating cognitions with behaviors. A similar scheme has been outlined by Glasser (1981) though with a somewhat different emphasis.

According to the model there are multiple levels of control that are hierarchically organized and lead to the integration of the principles used to define the self with the behavioral acts that carry out these principles. The cognitions that represent the definition of the self require principles of behavior that are consistent with this definition. Programmed acts (scripts) are followed that are consistent with the relationship defined by the principles. These behavior sequences are made up of transitional acts that have a defined configuration with feedback via the sensations and intensity of the movement of muscles. Each level in this hierarchy is subject to the feedback from every other level and all of them interact to control the behavior of the actor.

It is not our intention to elaborate all the parameters of the model. Suffice it to say that the model points to the close interconnectedness of the organization of cognitions and behaviors and the feedback systems that serve to regulate these interrelationships. What is particularly important about this model is its potential for analyzing the diverse ramifications of cognitive factors in disease. The particular behaviors that are elicited as a consequence of symptoms will depend on the belief (health beliefs) that the patient has about the symptoms. How the patient responds to symptoms will depend on the programs that accompany these beliefs. In the area of psychosomatic diseases, this model affords an analysis of "the choice of symptoms" and the cognitive factors in the development of particular diseases. These applications await further refinement and research before they become integrated into an assessment scheme. They do represent a direction for future exploration and development.

Multisystems Theory

The multisystems perspective on disease asserts that biological, psychological, and social systems are interrelated levels of organization and that disease reflects a disruption of equilibrium within one or more levels of this organized hierarchy. This perspective has demanded an expanded view of behavioral assessment. The application of these concepts to clinical problems is imminent.

The model is based on a biopsychosocial conception of disease offered by Engel and Schmale (1977) as an alternative to the traditional biomedical view. In essence the model suggests that biological, psychological, and social factors interplay in the specific expression of disease for any individual. Without postulating cause and effect relationships in this interrelatedness, the model suggests that all facets of the disease should be investigated and "diagnosed" in order to comprehensively respond to the needs of the patient.

Leigh and Reiser (1980) propose a "patient model" that incorporates the three levels of assessment as biological, personal, and environmental. They further suggest that assessment be made against three time contexts reflecting the current, recent, and background history of the patient. This grid as outlined in Table 7.1, they call the Patient Evaluation Grid. It is a relatively comprehensive assessment scheme and would provide a great deal of information about the patient that would

TABLE 7.1
Patient Evaluation Grid (PEG). Form used by biopsychosocially
oriented clinicians to organize diagnostic information in biological,
personal (psychological), and environmental (primarily social)
dimensions. (From H. Leigh & M. F. Reiser, *Biological, Psychological
and Social Dimensions of Medical Practice*. New York: Plenum Press,
1980. Copyright 1980 by Plenum Press. Reprinted by permission.)

	Contexts		
Dimensions	*CURRENT* (*Current States*)	*RECENT* (*Recent Events and Changes*)	*BACKGROUND* (*Culture, Traits, Constitution*)
Biological	Symptoms Physical examination Vital signs Status of related organs Medications Disease	Age Recent bodily changes Injuries, operations Disease Drugs	Early nutrition Constitution Predisposition Early disease
Personal	Chief complaint Mental status Expectations about illness and treatment	Recent illness, occurrence of symptoms Personality change Mood, thinking, behavior	Developmental factors Early experience Personality type Attitude to illness
Environmental	Immediate physical and interpersonal environment Supportive figure, next of kin Effect of help-seeking	Recent physical and interpersonal environment Life changes Family, work, others Contact with ill persons Contact with doctor or hospital	Early physical environment Cultural and family environment Early relations Cultural sick role expectation

transcend the traditional biomedical data. Its major limitations are: (1) it is historical in focus and not oriented to facilitate designed interventions such as those that relate to behavioral treatments; (2) it is not behaviorally refined, analyzing for cause-effect relationships that would aid in understanding specific behavioral needs; and (3) it does not reflect a specific viewpoint that ties the model into a theory of disease. It might also be criticized on the grounds that it is too comprehensive to be workable except in hospital settings.

Schwartz (1981) has expanded the theory underlying this model in a direction that ties it to theories of cybernetic control from a multisystems perspective. The mechanisms of feedback within a system are used to regulate and support the autonomy of the system, a state that maintains and promotes health in living systems. Biological, psychological, and social systems all have their feedback mechanisms (Miller, 1978), which self-regulate the state of the system. Schwartz

(1979) suggests that the brain acts as a "health care system" regulating the internal workings of the organ systems within the body. When the nervous system cannot correctly respond to negative feedback, the resulting "disregulation" promotes disorder and disease. Under these conditions higher order systems must be brought into play to correct the disregulation.

Edelstein, Ross, and Schultz (1982) exemplify how such an intervention might work in clinical situations. Particularly they review a number of cases referred to a consultation-liaison service in a department of psychiatry. Assessments focus on data collected from multiple sources: the physical exam and medical history, laboratory tests, medications, nurses' observations, an interview with the patient, discussions with the patient's physician and family. Intervention is then designed according to the needs identified from the data.

Another system of assessment that integrates with the multisystems concepts at a pragmatic level has been developed by Ireton and Cassata (1976) and elaborated by Howe, Tapp, and Jackson (1982). Termed a "psychosocial systems review" the scheme was advanced as an extension of the "review of systems" that is normally incorporated into a physical examination conducted in an office setting. In the Ireton and Cassata model it was assumed that the physician was gathering data on the physiological parameters of system functioning for appropriate biological systems. They expanded this to include an assessment of emotional status; life situation with regard to job, family, supports, intimate relationships; personality; coping resources; daily living pattern; and a family diagram. They offered the model to physicians as a "systematic means for understanding and dealing with his patient's emotional and social problems as an essential element in the provision of comprehensive care." p. 159

Howe et. al. (1982) expanded this assessment system from a functional perspective. From the multisystems model, health requires biopsychosocial integration. Therefore functional assessments must be made that determine the relative degree of equilibrium in all levels of functioning. Furthermore, from a behavioral perspective, assessment should provide a means for directing the course of treatment when dysfunction was assessed. Thus in addition to assessing the function of biological systems, the assessment of psychosocial function should recognize the sources of healthy functioning as well as determine the potential for dysfunctions in these spheres of living.

They designed a structured interview that was intended to assess system functioning in the three areas of a person's life: (1) the intrapersonal or self-system; (2) the interpersonal social system; and (3) the sociocultural-environmental system.

The self-system was presumed to function for the purpose of self regulation. To evaluate intrapersonal functioning, questions were designed to: (1) determine the individual's personal value system particularly in regard to the ideal self; (2) assess the capacity for thought and problem-solving skills; and (3) evaluate the person's emotional status and capacity to cope with the stresses and strains of normal living.

Interpersonal-social functioning was assessed in terms of: (1) the capacity to develop and maintain intimate relationships with others, including sexual intimacy; (2) the availability of social supports and skills that allowed the individual to utilize them; and (3) the performance of social role functions in work, family, and other social relationship spheres.

Sociocultural-environmental functioning was determined in areas of: (1) work-finances; (2) living conditions and self-support skills; and (3) utilization of leisure time and recreational activities.

The Psychosocial Systems Review, PSR, in this format provided a relatively efficient scheme for determining a number of aspects of the patient's behavior and resources. It was used and evaluated in a setting where family medicine residents were being trained. It was helpful in a number of respects: (1) in identifying resources for medical treatment; (2) in identifying potential sources of stress that might result in health risk; (3) for determining needs for further investigation and evaluation for services to help with problems that might arise; and (4) assessing attributes of the relationship between the physician and the patient.

This assessment scheme can be integrated with other perspectives on the biopsychosocial model. It appears to offer a systematic, goal-oriented assessment scheme for determining the needs of the patient and projecting behaviorally oriented treatment interventions that are responsive to those needs. A summary of the model is presented in Table 7.2.

Principles of Behavioral Assessment

Behavioral assessments are based on some specific and identifiable principles that apply regardless of the scheme employed. These cut across all levels of analysis and represent those elements of diagnosis that differentiate a behavioral perspective from other, more traditional diagnostic frameworks.

1. The first principle of behavioral assessment is: *Define the behavior or symptom precisely so that it can be quantitatively assessed either in terms of the frequency or the amplitude of its occurrence.* Behavioral assessment is an empirical method of collecting data about behavior. The focus is therefore on defining the behavior or the symptom in a way that allows it to be quantified either in terms of its frequency, its amplitude, or both. When the behavior is objectifiable, such as is the case with smoking or eating, the task is relatively simple. The number of cigarettes smoked/unit of time or the number of bites of food taken are quantifiable measures that can be recorded and assessed by impartial observers.

When the behavior is more diffuse more precision is needed. For example, pain behaviors are those that accompany the experience of pain. They may be more complex and diverse response patterns that differ at different times and under different circumstances, reflecting, for example, grimacing, bending over slightly, holding the lower back, and crying out with some verbal display indicat-

TABLE 7.2
Psychosocial Systems Review: General Background

I. The Psychosocial Systems Review is used to *assess three major systems:* the intrapersonal (self-system), interpersonal (relations with others) and the social-cultural systems.

Each of these general systems can be broken into three important areas:

   A. Intrapersonal (self-system)
   Mood-feeling: level and type of everyday emotional reactions.
   Thought-speech: patterns of attention, thinking, clarity in speaking.
   Values-meaning: personal beliefs, standards, codes of conduct.

   B. Interpersonal (relations with others)
   Intimacy-belonging: relationships characterized by emotional closeness.
   Support-help: availability of other people for aid, support.
   Boundaries of self—Roles: appropriate definition of social roles (e.g. parenthood, professional roles, etc.)

   C. Social-Cultural
   Economic: having adequate and predictable sources of income.
   Leisure-recreation: having and making adequate use of recreational, relaxing resources.
   Community-place: knowing the general resources of one's community; having a sense of belonging to a community.

II. Four general *types of skills* are needed for a person to function well in the above areas. These are:

   A. *Awareness:* Being able to perceive one's effect on others, the status of one's relationships, the availability of options for action.

   B. *Control-management:* Ability to manage one's time, energy and resources to handle daily problems; includes self-control in necessary areas.

   C. *Problem-solving:* Strategies for looking at life problems, searching for alternatives, dealing with obstacles, testing various actions; includes handling emotional stress, social problems, etc.

   D. *Negotiation:* Skills of asserting one's own rights and wants while recognizing and respecting those of others. Using discussion, confrontation and support to come to mutually beneficial agreements whenever possible.

ing pain. Such response patterns are still objectifiable and could be counted by an independent observer.

When the behavior or the symptom is more subjective such as with tension headaches or emotional experiences like anger, it becomes even more difficult to pinpoint the symptom with precision because much of it is not observable. The behavior displays that accompany these symptoms may be countable (e.g., instances of verbal reports of headaches, aggressive acts toward others), but only the patient can record the subjective experience of the symptom. For this the assessment must rely on self-report as the primary means of gathering data. For a diversity of reasons, most of them related to unreliability and inaccuracy, self-report is less than desirable as a method for collecting data.

On the other hand, most therapeutic interventions depend on the patients to change their behaviors and rearrange the contingencies of their environment with respect to the symptomatology they present. From this perspective, self-report is an important part of the therapeutic process. In order to understand the environmental events that are related to particular symptoms, the patient must be taught to be an objective observer of behavior. The process of defining the symptoms and the associated behavior with precision and monitoring those subjective experiences enhances awareness of the behavior and the contingencies that contribute to it and reinforce its presence.

2. The second principle of behavioral assessment is: *Keep written records.* Perhaps it goes without saying that data need to be recorded. But the implementation of assessment is often limited by the demands of time, and record keeping is relegated to memory. The scientific model of intervention demands that the data base be recorded with the precision that will allow the determination of the success of the intervention. Graphing and charting behaviors over time gives visual feedback about behavior and establishes the base line from which successful therapy can be determined. Just as the parameters of physiological diseases are monitored and recorded, the parameters of behavioral treatments need to be documented consistently to evaluate therapeutic effectiveness.

3. The third principle of behavioral assessment is: *Sample the behavior under a variety of circumstances to assess its generality.* Because many aspects of behavior are situationally determined, it is important to determine when and where the behavior occurs. The social aspects of a behavior are of considerable importance in this regard. Frequently, behaviors have a modeling or socially rewarding component that supports maladaptive responses and potentially mitigates against behavior change strategies. This process brings the behavior into focus and further promotes an understanding of its functional attributes.

In addition, this sampling process defines a base line against which intervention strategies can be evaluated. The process of measuring the behavior becomes a part of the means used to treat it. By bringing the behavior into perspective and by understanding more precisely those situations under which it occurs, the behavior becomes more manageable and less overwhelming. In all aspects, this sampling procedure makes the process of intervention manageable.

4. The fourth principle of behavioral assessment is: *Analyze the causes and consequences of the symptoms and/or the target behavior.* This principle involves determining the stimulus events that elicit the behavior and the contingencies and consequences that sustain it. The S-O-R-K-C model provides the framework for such an analysis. The behavior or symptom being evaluated (R) is frequently elicited by some stimulus (S) that is antecedent to the appearance of the behavior. This S is a cue that has a high degree of association with the R. Having a cup of coffee prior to a cigarette is a classic example of an instance when a stimulus is antecedent to a response. It is not unusual to find that some state of the organism will also be a stimulus that is antecedent to the behavior. Boredom is a subjective

state characterized by anxiety and an associated restlessness. It frequently leads to exploratory behaviors that result in open refrigerator doors, where the organism stands staring wistfully into the cold, white interior in search of a source of stimulation and relief of the boredom. For a patient who has experienced a heart attack, a paraventricular contraction can be a stimulus that elicits anxiety or subjectively experienced fear.

Similarly, the consequence of behaviors and symptoms can reinforce the behavior and sustain it. In pain behaviors, the expressions that accompany pain are cues to others to respond with sympathy and support that might not be available under other circumstances. A headache can be an excuse for avoiding a difficult social situation. Ingesting food gives pleasure and reduces anxiety.

Relatively standard procedures have developed for monitoring or "charting" behaviors. The differences in procedure depend on who is doing the charting and the definition of the target behavior. Most procedures will define the behavior and monitor: (1) the time it occurs; (2) where it occurs; (3) who else is present when it occurs; (4) preceding stimulus events or actions; (5) preceding thoughts or self-talk; (6) the intensity of the behavior; (7) subsequent events or actions; (8) subsequent thoughts or self-talk; (9) the reactions of others; and (10) comments. In those instances where the patient is the observer, the monitoring is done in the form of a daily diary. In hospital, home, or school settings the monitoring is done by a trained observer.

Such data, collected over a period of time, provide the basis for dissecting the event sequences that are antecedent and consequent to the behavior. The S-O-R-K-C model can be applied to determine the critical aspects of the environmental events that trigger and support the behavior when it occurs.

The fifth principle of behavior assessment is: *Analyze the reinforcing consequences of the behavior or symptoms*. Those stimuli that are repeated at a high frequency are being maintained because they satisfy some need. Though this may not account for all the variance in behavior, it is a good working principle. When the symptoms persist there is reason to seek help to change the consequences of the symptoms unless the benefits of the symptoms outweigh the costs of having them. Physical, psychological, and social well being are desirable consequences of behavior. Health and happiness are reasonable end products of activity. Unfortunately, illness behaviors can result in consequences that approximate these more desirable states and achieve limited ends that are "relatively" beneficial. Against this background the reinforcers that sustain symptoms are relative to the needs that are being satisfied.

The analysis of rewards is based on determining the manner in which the consequences of a behavior are satisfying to some need. Cognitive analysis of self-talk and an examination of the social consequences of events will frequently reveal those elements that are being processed as "desirable" in the sense of providing a level of need gratification. The rearrangement of these response consequences, in a manner that is consistent with the healthy gratification of needs, is the goal of therapeutic intervention.

BASIC METHODS IN BEHAVIORAL ASSESSMENT

Comprehensive assessment in behavioral medicine utilizes data from multiple sources organized in a consistent and meaningful manner. The sources of these data were from medical records, psychological tests, interviews with the patient, questionnaires relevant to the problem, the reports of others who have the opportunity to observe the patient, and, most importantly, direct observations of the patient's performance under a variety of circumstances. This information is integrated to provide a comprehensive picture of the patient's behavioral assets and liabilities. The purpose is to design an intervention that will capitalize on the assets and correct the liabilities.

Medical Records

Medical records provide information about the physiological condition of the person in varying degrees of detail. The history of the disease presentation is an indicator of the cause, course, and severity of the disease. Laboratory tests, X-rays, computerized tomography (CT Scan), and position emission tomography (PET Scan) assist in delineating the nature and the extent of the physical disorder. Planning for intervention will be made against this information as a determinant of physiological limitations and functional capacities.

Bjorn and Cross (1971) have developed a method for gathering medical information and organizing it in a systematic manner. It is a problem-oriented medical record system that focuses on systematic data gathering for functional biological systems (e.g., the eyes, ears, nose, mouth, endocrine, and skin) and organizing the data to facilitate the medical problem solving process. The root of the method consists of identifying the objective signs of disease and the subjective symptoms and using this information to assess the problem and formulate a plan that will expedite further problem solving and treatment. The acronym for this process is the SOAP system, where S is subjective data from the patient, O is objective data from laboratory tests, A is assessment, and P is the plan for further intervention.

When a health problem is identified, it is listed on a master sheet of problems and a process is initiated to identify it precisely and delineate the steps to its solution. The problem can be variously defined and may include behavioral problems. The process works toward the goal of restoring normal functioning. The method helps to organize the response to the problem. When physical diagnosis is conducted within this context it easily is expandable into the realms of behavioral assessment.

Psychological Tests and Questionnaires

The questionnaires reviewed in Chapter 6 provide information about patients' perceptions of themselves and their reactions to diverse situations. The personality profiles derived from such tests as the Minnesota Multiphasic Personality Inventory or the Millon Clinical Multiaxial Inventory provide information about the manner in which individuals will respond to disease presentations. For example, the "neurotic triad" or the "conversion-V" pattern of the MMPI, characterized as high scores on the hysteria and hypochondriasis scales and somewhat lower scores on the depression scale (forming V pattern for the first three clinical scales) has been related to unsuccessful medical treatments for low back pain. Though this work has been challenged by several investigators (see Long, 1981) there is sufficient evidence to indicate that responses on personality measures such as this predict patient's reactions to diseases. These forms of questionnaires do provide information about the patient's characteristic response to disease.

Questionnaires that are more specific to emotional conditions are of more use in assessing the emotional concomitants of disease. Depression scales such as the Beck Depression Inventory, anxiety scales such as the Spielberger State-Trait Anxiety Scales, and hostility measures such as the Buss-Durkee Anger Inventory provide specific information about the emotional accompaniments of the disease. These instruments also give a direction to both symptom monitoring and planning interventions that are responsive to the patient's needs for emotional management.

Standardized intelligence tests have an application in behavioral medicine with children and with adults. In conjunction with other information, these tests provide information about functional capabilities, particularly in the assessment of neurological deficits. Other neurological assessment methods are reviewed in Chapter 8.

There are also questionnaires specific to the presenting problem that aid in identifying the relative contributions of different cognitive and behavioral factors to the problem under treatment. Some of these are discussed later. In general these methods analyze the components of the individual's need structure that are being satisfied by the particular behavior pattern. For example, in the management of chronic pain, the McGill Pain Questionnaire is an aid in determining the operant and respondent components of the pain, the antecedents and consequences of the pain behaviors, the specific locations and duration of the pain episodes, and the cognitive components of the pain experience. Similar questionnaires and checklists are available for a variety of dysfunctions and behavior patterns including arthritis, cancer, hypertension, asthma, pain, headaches (Cautela, 1981b), smoking (Frith, 1971), eating (Plutchik, 1976), and sexual behaviors (Cautela, 1981a). These questionnaires are specific to the presenting problem and provide an assessment that helps in pinpointing the behavioral/emotional components of the presenting condition. In this they are useful adjuncts to intervention.

Interviews

The clinical interview has two objectives: building rapport and trust with the patient and gathering information relevant to the presenting symptoms and/or disease. Though the interview lacks some of the psychometric precision of other methods of data collection, it is the most important and widely used method for gathering information in behavioral medicine. The process of gathering information should implicitly express a concern for the patient's welfare and be conducted with compassion and empathic understanding.

Interviews come in a variety of forms and their use depends on the nature of the problem and the purposes of the information that is being collected. There are several standard interview methods, the most notable being the Mental Status Examination. This interview is intended to provide information on the functional mental status of the patient with regard to his or her psychiatric condition. It collects data on general appearance including mood, behavior, attitude and interpersonal contact; speech and mentation, emotional state, affect, and appropriateness of emotional displays; mental organization and thought content; and orientation to time and space and general intelligence.

The Psychosocial Systems Interview (Howe et al., 1982) is based on a structured interview that assesses assets and liabilities within a medical setting. Such information can be used as an adjunct to treatment planning as well as to identify potential for stress-induced physical reactions.

Other interview methods are more specialized for the particular problems that they are addressing. For example, the Type A interview of Friedman and Rosenman was designed to assess attributes of personal characteristic styles of responding that were predictive of coronary heart disease. (Chapters 16 and 17) The Hackett-Cassem denial measure (Hackett, Cassem, & Wishnie, 1969) is intended to provide information about patients' reactions to heart disease that indicate denial of the anxiety associated with heart disease. Standardized methods for taking a sexual history have developed that are intended to pinpoint the origins and the extent of sexual problems.

Observational Methods

Direct observations of symptomatic behaviors and their pattern is probably the most direct and accurate diagnostic procedure. This is possible in all settings, though more difficult in outpatient settings than in the hospital. When the symptom behavior is clearly identified, the patient can be asked to demonstrate the behavior pattern associated with the symptom. These demonstrations provide a model means of assessment and a mechanism for demonstrating corrective actions.

In an inpatient setting, the nursing staff provides a vital role in monitoring specific symptom-related behaviors. Because the nurses are available on a 24-hour basis, they are in the best position to provide a time sample of symptoms. It should be recognized that nurses are not trained as behavioral observers, therefore, education in the precision and methods of observation is frequently necessary to define the problem.

Significant others are also an important source of observational information. Again, structuring the assessment procedures in detail facilitates the recording of accurate information.

One of the major innovations in behavioral observation techniques can be found in the literature on the interrelationships between behavioral factors and cardiovascular diseases (See Chapter 17). Research in this area has identified the phenomenon that indicates that cardiovascular reactivity can be induced by psychological challenges and that these expressions of cardiovascular behavior are related to such psychological or behavioral characteristics as Type A personality and hostility. Furthermore, these patterns of behavior are "risk factors" for cardiovascular diseases. By combining physiological measures with behavioral and psychological stressors, it appears possible to diagnose those individuals who are at some higher degrees of risk for coronary heart disease.

Other methods such as assessing sleep patterns of insomniacs using the electroencephalograph, measuring nocturnal penile tumescence as an assessment of sexual dysfunction (Karacan, 1969, 1978), and electromyographic measurement of muscle reactivity following stroke, are examples of the use of physiological measures to assess functional capacity.

Self-Report via "Charting"

One of the most widely used methods of assessment in behavioral medicine is self-reported monitoring of the presenting symptoms. These methods are intended to make the patient his or her own observer and to aid the clinician in identifying the pattern of symptom expression, its antecedents, and its consequences. This is an important aspect of intervention in that it focuses the patient on the particular aspects of his or her behavior that relate to the symptoms and the disease. It combines behavioral and cognitive methods into an assessment procedure and provides the basis for the development of a scientific (empirical) and systematic intervention strategy aimed at developing self-control skills in the patient.

The S-O-R-K-C method outlined previously provides a generic framework for this form of data collection. The patient is asked to write down, in a prepared format, those elements of the symptom presentation that are related to the disease. These methods can be applied to behaviors such as smoking or eating, or to symptoms such as headaches, stomach aches, or angina. Prior to intervention, these methods define the base rate of the presenting problem in terms of its frequency of occurrence. During treatment they give the patient a means of monitoring his or her progress. After treatment they are the measure of the success of the intervention.

If there is an essential strategy for the development of an effective, accountable intervention it is embodied in the application of self-monitoring procedures. Through self-monitoring the patient begins to recognize those aspects of his or her behaviors that relate to symptom presentations and intensity. This form of understanding develops the groundwork necessary for the applications of cognitive and behavioral control mechanisms leading to successful interventions.

APPLICATIONS IN BEHAVIORAL MEDICINE

The transition from theory to practice is often a difficult process. Table 7.3 presents an outline intended to facilitate the transition from a theoretical model to application of behavioral assessment practices. The organization suggested by the outline may not fit every problem but it provides a framework for data gathering.

The initial step in organizing clinical information is the identification of the primary presenting problem and the secondary problems associated with it. For example a patient with a spinal cord injury at the C5-6 level with loss of sensation and motor function below the shoulders has the spinal cord injury as the primary presenting problem. A secondary physiological problem such as a neurogenic bladder resulting from the loss of neural control of the bladder would potentially have a psychological concomitant problem related to fear of voiding in public. Difficulties in self-care and other activities of daily living might also be secondary problems along with limitations in social support systems. For comprehensive treatment planning these must be addressed along with the therapy for the spinal cord injury.

The next step in assessment involves developing a functional analysis of the behaviors involved to identify the behavioral assets and liabilities. Assets are those behaviors that are strong and useful in the patient's current or past behavioral repetoire. Behavioral deficits are those aspects of behavior that are lacking or inadequate at the time of assessment that might reflect chronic disabilities or that might be altered through a program of intervention.

In this section we review a few specific strategies and assessment methods as they relate to particular behavioral-disease entities. There is no attempt to be exhaustive or to delineate the particular form of intervention. Rather, the examples are intended to acquaint the reader with the methods available for assessments that aid in the development of multisystems intervention strategies.

Smoking

Smoking behaviors appear to be relatively simple yet the eliciting stimuli that provoke smoking and the reinforcement contingencies that maintain it can be quite complex. Nellis, Emurian, Brady, and Ray (1982) analyzed smoking patterns and found them to be relatively individualistic. There was a strong dependency

TABLE 7.3
Behavioral Assessment Outline

I. Problem Identification

A. Primary Presenting Problem
B. Secondary Problems

II. Problem Definition and Description

A. Primary Presenting Problem
   1. Pertinent history
      a. Onset
      b. Duration
      c. What makes it better
      d. What makes it worse

   2. Determine response characteristics
      a. Response precisely defined
      b. Frequency
      c. Intensity—Magnitude
      d. Duration
      e. Degree of appropriateness

   3. Identification of controlling variables
      a. Antecedents
      b. Consequences
      c. Family support system
      d. Existing social support system (Extrafamilial)

B. Secondary Problems
   1. Obtain pertinent history
   2. Determine response characteristics
      a. Frequency
      b. Intensity—Magnitude
      c. Duration
      d. Degree of appropriateness

III. Functional Analysis

A. Primary Problem and Secondary Problems
   1. Behavioral assets
      a. Consequences in terms of gains
      b. Short and long range benefits
   2. Behavioral deficits
      a. Consequences in terms of losses
      b. Short and long range costs

between the occurrence of smoking and coffee drinking, and within any subject there was a cyclicity to the smoking pattern that was time dependent and differed from subject to subject. Smoking in this laboratory situation was comparable to smoking outside the laboratory.

Assessment for the treatment of smoking will necessarily focus on the identification of the contingencies for each smoker that are antecedent and consequent to the behavior. Traditional behavioral assessment procedures for intervention have targeted the behavior per se. A typical assessment program would have the smoker chart his or her behavior over some time period and then design interventions to alter the behavior. These have met with varying successes. (See Chapter 13.)

Questionnaires can be used to analyze the situations that contribute to smoking. These allow the further delineation of the conditions that promote the behavior. Frith (1971) analyzed a smoking situation questionnaire and identified two main factors that related to high and low stress situations. People who smoke in high stress situations smoke to calm themselves down. Smoking in low stress situations is tended to increase stimulation.

Horn (1982) has developed a questionnaire for the National Institutes of Health that allows a self-assessment of the reinforcing attributes of smoking (e.g., stimulation, handling, relaxation, tension reduction, addiction, and habit). These "motivations" help the smoker identify those needs that are being satisfied by the smoking behaviors. Suggestions for alternative behavioral strategies that will resolve the need by substitution of other nonsmoking behaviors are suggested. This work reflects a pragmatic approach to examining the choice behaviors reflected in the decision to smoke. It is an extension of earlier work by the author on the study of personal choice in health behavior (Horn, 1976).

O'Connor (1980) identified three factors that contribute to smoking: an activity factor, an emotional factor, and an attentional factor. Introverts tended to smoke under conditions where high attention was demanded. O'Connor and Stravynski (1982) used this typology to develop specific treatment programs to meet the requirements of the smoker. This form of intervention was highly successful at 8-month follow-up.

Behavioral assessments of smoking behavior include: (1) an interview to assess the motivation of the patient to stop and the particular patterns of self-perceived smoking; (2) questionnaires to determine the beliefs about smoking, the needs that are being satisfied by smoking, and the situational determinants of smoking; and (3) charting to analyze the frequency and environmental antecedents and consequences of smoking. From these data it becomes possible to design a treatment intervention that is individualized for the patient. The methods described in Chapter 9 could be implemented against these findings to alter the behavior pattern. Such a multiple-intervention strategy would enhance the potential efficacy of treatment (Elliott & Denny, 1978).

Obesity

Given the variety of health problems that are related to obesity, intervention into this condition is an important part of the treatment armamentarium of the behavior medicine specialist.

Obesity is defined as an excess of ideal body weight by more than 20% (Katahn, 1980). It is measured by a comparison of the weight of the patient against standards of normal body weight for height and body frame for the sex of the patient (Benn, 1971), or by measures of skin fold thickness (Durnin & Womersley, 1974), which provides an estimate of percentage of body fat (Keys, Fidanza, Karvonen, Kimura, & Taylor, 1972). Obesity is the result of a combination of energy intake in the form of food and energy expenditure in the form of metabolism during rest and exercise. Though there are a number of intervening conditions that will influence this equation, when energy expenditure exceeds energy intake, the individual loses weight; when energy expenditure is less than energy intake the individual gains weight (Powers, 1980).

From a conceptual perspective it is not possible to develop a behavior program to treat obesity (i.e., obesity [weight] cannot be treated directly; only the behaviors that influence weight can be treated). The modification of energy intake and output are the target behaviors in the management of obesity. The treatment of obesity must regulate this flow of energy in a way that will make output exceed input until the ideal weight range is reached, then stabilize the balance of energy expenditure (Garrow, 1978). Katahn (1982) argues that burning 200 calories a day in excess of usual food intake by exercise will lead to longer range weight loss than dieting, though the combination of dieting and exercise will obviously produce more weight loss than either method alone.

Long-range planning and persistence are the essential ingredients of weight control. Patterns of dieting contribute to overeating. Low and Orleans (1981) have shown these obese individuals tend to vacillate between strict dieting and overeating. Many obese individuals experience frustration when they skip meals and wind up not losing weight. They suggest that strict dieting and fasting set the stage for extreme hunger, feelings of self-deprivation, and depression related to low blood sugar and prolonged self denial. When these feelings reach a particular threshold the individual may overeat to achieve relief. This is reinforcing and over an extended period the pattern of behavior is repeated (Rosenthal & Marx, 1979).

Mischel (1968) pointed out that behavioral analysis should focus on situation-specific behaviors rather than on the behaviors an individual might exhibit in a variety of situations. This includes an analysis of the duration, frequency, pervasiveness, and intensity of caloric intake and output as they are related to specific eating behaviors. Katell, Callahan, Fremouw, and Zitter (1979) have monitored specific eating behaviors including bites, sips, utensil drops, and utensil down time. These patients kept detailed daily calorie intake logs that included information about the antecendents to eating such as location, time, subjective ratings of hunger, emotional state, presence of others and so on. These were correlated with other forms of eating behaviors to show the specific interrelationships to caloric consumption.

A detailed analysis of eating can aid in modifying specific patterns of intake and in developing alternative strategies of behavior change to reinforce behaviors that aid in the regulation of caloric intake. The assessment of these patterns of behavior is usually done by a structured charting analysis in which the individual keeps detailed records of the pattern of food intake. From the analysis of these eating patterns, programs designed to regulate food intake can be developed to produce weight loss.

Emotional factors relevant to eating must also be assessed. Boredom, anxiety, frustration, depression, and their associated subjective states are often the cues for eating. Eating becomes an instrumental behavior that will alter these undesirable feelings. Developing alternative ways of reacting to these emotional states can aid in regulating food intake.

Cognitive expectations and evaluations are a part of the total response to food intake. For example body image and beliefs about food are determinants of the pattern of eating. These can be manipulated to aid in the restructuring of the cognitive set relevant to food.

In effect, all aspects of the eating pattern need to be addressed in developing a structured plan for overeating. These include: (1) eating and dieting patterns; (2) physical activity patterns; (3) emotional antecedents and consequences of eating; (4) cognitive control variables; (5) physiological and biochemical effects, and finally long-term consequences and plans for follow-up to insure successful maintenance of the controlled pattern of energy expenditure.

Sexual Assessments

The examination of sexual dysfunction is conducted primarily by interview, though there are questionnaires that are helpful. Structured interviews are published in the literature, but in essence they consist of three parts: (1) determination of the precise nature of the presenting problem and the circumstances under which it occurs by questioning the couple; (2) evaluation of the potential for medical problems related to drug use, disease, or gonadal difficulties; and (3) an in depth exam to assess psychopathology, sexual history, and the relationship quality of the couple including sexual feelings and interactions.

The interview will necessarily focus on an analysis of the details of the behavioral sequence, the cognitive and emotional topology that accompanies the sequence, and the stimulus conditions under which the sexual behaviors occur. This will include signaling cues for both partners, self-talk, anticipatory excitement, anxieties, frustrations, and before, during, and after interchanges.

Paper and pencil measures are available to assess knowledge (Leif & Reed, 1972), experience (Bentler, 1978), attitude, arousal, and reinforcements (Cautela, 1981a). Asking both partners to fill out such questionnaires and discuss them together can open up communications and facilitate the flow of interaction and exchange.

Physiological assessment procedures are emerging as measures of arousal level. This methodology has obvious applications in research. Bancroft, Jones, and Pullan (1966) have described a plethysmograph for measuring penile enlargement that can be used as a measure in treating erectile dysfunctions (Kockott, Dittmar, & Nusselt, 1975). These techniques have been reviewed recently by Caird and Wincze (1977). Their clinical applications are still relatively rare except in research reports. One interesting innovative method is the use of a tape recorder to investigate human sexual response (Sarrel, Foddy, & McKinnon, 1977). EKG, EEG, and vaginal photoplethysmography can be recorded during sexual behavior.

These methods aid in the delineation of the specific identification of the sources and expressions of sexual dysfunctions and in particular in the development of interventions that alter the associated behaviors.

Sleep Disorders

There are four categories of sleep disorders: (1) disorders of initiating and main-taining sleep (insomnias); (2) disorders of excessive somnolence; (3) disorders of sleep-wake schedule; and (4) dysfunctions associated with sleep, sleep stages, or partial arousals. Each of these has associated subgroups. As a category, sleep disorders are common complaints that accompany physical and mental health problems.

Assessments for the sleep disorders consist of interviews to identify the particular pattern of difficulty and the patient's expectations about sleep disturb-ances. Questionnaires are also available that help delineate the disturbance pattern (Cautela, 1981b). Rating scales have been developed to analyze dream content (Karle, Carriere, Hart, & Woldenberg, 1980) and patterns of sleep behaviors (Kazarian, Howe, & Csapo, 1979).

Sleep logs that are filled out immediately on waking have become a standard procedure to provide daily records of the sleep behaviors and subjective evaluation of the sleep experience. Though such logs do not provide a complete cure for sleep problems, there is evidence to suggest that such self-monitoring will provide a behavior change in sleep onset for insomniacs (Jason, 1975; Shealy, 1979).

The difficulties associated with the development of direct observations of sleep patterns has led to the development of sleep laboratories to assess these patterns of behavior. Three basic measures of physiological behavior are used in these settings: electrooculography (EOG) to measure eye movements to distinguish REM sleep from non-REM sleep; electroencephalography (EEG) to measure brain activity; and electromyography (EMG) to measure movement patterns. The com-bination of these procedures with behavioral observations and self-report mea-sures provides a comprehensive picture of the sleep disturbance. Because there are large individual differences in sleep disturbance patterns a comprehensive assess-ment substantially aids in the diagnosis and the subsequent design of a treatment for sleep disturbances.

Neurological Disorders

Cerebral vascular accidents, spinal cord injuries, palsies, epilepsies, and other neurological disorders present complex problems in assessment that require a combination of procedures to delineate clearly the total extent of the secondary problems that accompany these disorders. In addition to psychosocial assessments that might be applied to other disorders, these dysfunctions will require measurements of functional capacities that incorporate neuropsychological assessments (Chapter 8) and electromyographic (EMG) measurements to elaborate the extent and type of muscular involvements. For example, a right hemiparesis must be analyzed into the components of muscular dysfunction. The measurement of EMG activity in the bicep, tricep, deltoid, and trapezius muscles would provide an evaluation of the pattern of firing in these muscles. Spasticity resulting from the cocontraction of incompatible muscle groups such as the biceps and triceps could be assessed and biofeedback treatment designed accordingly.

Similarly, in spinal cord injuries EMG recordings will pick up the firing of those motor neuron units that are intact, even though they may be of limited function. These assessments provide the basis for developing treatments that incorporate this information into the rehabilitation process. In the analysis of palsies the use of EMG can aid in determining the extent of involuntary contractions. Through biofeedback some of these patterns can be modified to improve functioning (Harris, Speleman, & Hymer, 1974).

Though radiographic techniques such as Computerized Tomography (CT Scan) can provide information on the location and extent of the damage to an area of the brain, it does not provide information on the extent of functional damage. The use of neuropsychological testing is an important source of information about the functional limitations of neurological damage.

Cancer

The diagnosis of cancer is a precipitant of an individual crisis. Of all the diseases of contemporary society, this one carries more stigma and fear than any other. As Sontag (1977) has said: "the disease itself arouses thoroughly old-fashioned kinds of dread. Any disease that is treated as a mystery and acutely enough feared will be felt to be morally, if not literally, contagious. Thus a surprisingly large number of people with cancer find themselves being shunned by relatives and friends and are the object of practices of decontamination by members of their household [p. 10]." Against this backdrop, behavioral assessments of the individual with cancer must take place.

Approximately 50% of all cancerous diseases are cured. When the disease is detected early the number of successful cures is over 80%. Prevention rates by early diagnosis are thus very high.

The biological treatment of cancer is generally intended to destroy the cancer cells via surgery, radiology or chemotherapy. The effectiveness of these interventions depends on the cancer type, the stage of its development within the individual, and the response of the patient to treatment. The interventions are themselves stressful. Surgery is frequently an unknown entity to the patient, and like any form of intervention it carries its risks. The unknown quality of surgery is exacerbated by the fact that some cancer surgery is conducted to explore the limits of the developing neoplasm before it is excised. All of these factors contribute to the mystique and the associated anxiety. Finally there is often a lack of definitive result that occurs following surgery that in most instances contributes to the continued feelings of dread.

The assessment interviews with cancer patients should explore these feelings and expectations and identify sources of anxiety. The methods are similar to those used in preparing patients for surgery in a more general sense. They differ in that the focus must include a discussion of the implications of the intervention for the specific disease, cancer. Questionnaires and psychological assessments can be useful in delineating the knowledge and beliefs about cancer. Care must be exerted to retain an element of human contact in these procedures that is responsive to the patient's need for interpersonal involvement and acceptance. The assessment system should be designed to promote: (1) the alleviation of anxiety that occurs as a response to the unknown elements of surgical intervention; (2) the patient's coping skills and his or her internal resources that can serve as a therapeutic; and (3) the psychosocial environment and the supportive quality of its fabric and behavioral interactive patterns regarding hospitalization and surgery.

Radiation therapy and chemotherapies are frequently accompanied by side effects that sometimes make the treatment worse than the cure. Loss of hair, nausea and vomiting, weakness, and other signs of cellular damage make the patient feel as if it would be better to accept the inevitable death than endure the horrors of treatment. The discomfort of nausea and vomiting after chemotherapy can cause the patient to miss appointments, avoid the clinic, and "hate" the doctor, nurse, or technician who administers the treatment.

Again the assessment strategies focus on the identification and management of the discomforts and anxieties associated with the intervention. The S-O-R-K-C model is useful in identifying the environmental stimuli that elicit the nausea, the cognitive and other internal cues that contribute to the nausea, the contingencies and consequences of the illness behaviors. The analysis of the sequence can lead to the development of the alternative strategies in intervention that will reformulate and restructure the sequence. Relaxation and hypnosis have been shown to be effective in altering these events (Chapters 9 and 16).

Psychological assessment of the cancer patient undergoing chemotherapy should also assess the social network of the patient and its capacity to respond supportively to the patient's needs. Full disclosure of the treatment, its effects, and the consequences to the patient's family can be helpful in anticipating the effects of treatment. Frequently it is helpful to instruct the family on the anticipated stresses to family members and direct supportive behaviors among family members. Disclosure and assistance in planning for the emotional consequences of the disease on the patient's support network are the "ounces of prevention" that can facilitate "pounds of cure" for the psychosocial consequences of the disease.

Pain

Weisenberg (1977) referred to pain as follows: "In some respects it is a sensation, in other respects it is an emotional-motivational phenomenon that leads to escape and avoidance behavior [p. 1008]." The dual nature of the pain experience makes it difficult to manage, and in patients with severe and chronic pain the difficulty is exacerbated by the anxiety-depression sequelae that accompany a pain career. When there is a lack of identifiable pathological tissue the management of pain becomes even more difficult.

Behavioral assessment techniques used with chronic pain are designed to identify and measure the diversity of the behaviors and experiences that accompany pain, including subjective, behavioral, and physiological reactions to the pain. Self-report inventories like the Visual Analogue Scales (Joyce, Zutshi, Hrubes, & Mason, 1975) and Magnitude Estimation Scales (Greenhoot & Sternbach, 1974; Swanson, Swenson, Maruta, & McPhee, 1976) focus on subjective responses. These are structured around the psychophysics of estimation and ask the patient to evaluate the magnitude and intensity of the pain. Pain maps are used in localizing the pain (Keefe, 1948). The McGill Pain Questionnaire incorporates all these procedures into a common test (Melzack, 1975).

Personality inventories have been used to measure the individual characteristics of pain patients. The MMPI, the SCL-90, the Millon Behavior Health Inventory, and the Middlesex Hospital Questionnaire (Crown & Crisp, 1966) appear to be useful supplements to evaluation of the chronic pain patient.

Behavioral responses may be assessed through self-observation and direct behavioral observation. In self-observation, the patient is given a recording sheet and has the target behavior defined. Next, instruction is given on keeping accurate records of the target behaviors, and the importance of record keeping throughout the treatment program is stressed. Finally, the patient is asked to summarize his or her data and to contribute to the evaluation of the treatment plan. Self-observation according to such a protocol increases the patient's awareness of the target behavior and potentially contributes to the therapy (Fordyce, 1976).

Direct observation is another approach to behavioral assessment of chronic pain. This can take place in a number of settings and can involve significant others: hospital staff, visiting nurses, physical therapists, friends, and others involved with the patient. Training these individuals in the identification of the target behavior and the nature of the recording procedure is essential; such procedures enhance the overall accuracy of the information collected and consequently a better understanding of the context of the behavior.

Electromyographic (EMG) recordings are another assessment procedure for measuring musculoskeletal responses to pain. Holmes and Wolff (1952) found that generalized overactivity of the skeletal muscle was characteristic of back pain patients. This was evident under conditions of emotional stress and physical activity. The utility of EMG measurements varies with the individual cases

(Basmajian, 1978), and therefore the relevance of the EMG use should be evaluated on an individual basis.

It is the total assessment that reflects the response of the pain patient to the multiple-stimulus aspects of pain. This information can be used to provide a complete profile of the patient and thus develop a comprehensive intervention strategy designed to be responsive to the physiological, cognitive, behavioral, emotional, and social aspects of pain experiences.

ISSUES IN BEHAVIORAL ASSESSMENT

The issues in behavioral assessment are the same as those that accompany the development of any diagnostic scheme. Namely, does the method reliably reflect critical aspects of the disease process and can it aid in the development of an intervention that will facilitate the treatment of the condition?

Reliability issues are rarely systematically addressed in behavioral assessment in clinical settings and too frequently are ignored in research. It is often assumed that because of the relatively concrete and defined nature of the behavior, the assessment can be repeated. This assumption can be tested within the clinic setting by utilizing procedures for determining the agreement among observers used in laboratory settings, by repeating the application of questionnaires, by comparing the consistency of responses to items within questionnaires, and by repeating physiological and behavioral tests. In brief, each clinical setting has some responsibility to assure that the measurements that are incorporated into the assessment procedures meet the criteria of reliability that would be imposed on other measurement procedures.

Validity in behavioral assessment is also not systematically addressed. Behavioral assessment is intended to provide measures of an individual's performance in situations outside the assessment situation. It is generally assumed that the interview or the questionnaire is accurately reflecting these behaviors, but there is rarely a concurrent measurement that will substantiate the patient's self-report. The validity of specific methods of assessment needs to be addressed both in the development of the method and in its utilization.

The major issues facing the evolution of behavioral assessments are their ultimate integration with the pragmatic and scientific aspects of health and disease. At the pragmatic level, behavioral assessments must be integrated into the patterns of medical management. It is clearly possible to assess aspects of cognitive, emotional, and social behavior in medical situations. It is equally possible to develop assessment procedures that will aid in altering behavior patterns that contribute to the onset and course of diseases. The remaining chapters of this volume testify to the fact and utility of this process. However the use of this information as the basis for interventions that will enhance the quality of life for people with illnesses is in a very preliminary stage of evolution.

Traditionally, disease has been viewed as a biologically based dysfunction. As the pattern of disease has shifted to include the recognition of its psychosocial causes and consequences, there has been an inertia in developing and utilizing this information in quantitative, reproducable forms as an integral part of the treatment process. The study cited earlier by Howe et. al., (1982), and other work by Pinkerton, Tinnanoff, Willms, and Tapp (1980) demonstrated the difficulties in altering the established behavior patterns of physicians in training to get them to incorporate the new information into their practice habits. In both studies, family practice residents were given information and told what to do with it to enhance the care given to their patients. In the former study they were told to assess aspects of the patient's behavior to determine potential sources of stress; in the latter they were told to prescribe the correct amount of fluoride for children based on a determination of their location of residence in areas with or without fluoridated water. In both studies there was no measurable change in the residents' behavior as reflected in the information recorded in their charts.

At still another level, there is a need to integrate the process of behavioral assessments to include assessments of multiple levels of system functioning. The development of cognitive assessment procedures and the recognition that cognitions operate according to the principles that regulate other forms of behavior, opens up another level of behavioral analysis for inclusion into the data gathering process (Meichenbaum & Cameron, 1980). Karoly has addressed some of these issues, pointing out that the addition of cognitive assessments is intended to expand the functional analysis of behavior to integrate cognitions along with the other forms of behaviors (Karoly, 1982). However these methods of assessment are just beginning to be included as part of behavioral medicine. Though they offer promise for application in behavioral analysis, the limitations of trait and analytic models in their application to psychosomatic and medical treatment suggests that some caution is indicated in the inclusion of cognitive aspects of behavior in disease management. Karoly proceeds to address expectancy effects and other aspects of cognitive assessment that would impact on problems within behavior medicine. The scientific contribution of these measurements to the management of disease processes awaits further study.

Finally there is the need for integrating behavioral assessments into meaningful scientific theories that consider the biopsychosocial context of disease and its effects on the individual. The theories of control as offered by Carver and Scheier (1983) and Glasser (1981) provide the skeleton of such a theoretical framework. From slightly different vantage points these authors build on Powers' (1973) model of perceptual control to integrate cognitions and cognitive information processing into a heirarchical control scheme that expresses itself in individual behaviors. The operational assessments of these theories and their application to studies of health and illness appears to offer a quantum leap into the understanding of the interrelationships among cognitions, behaviors, and physiological processes. This theoretical development may offer the response to the challenge of the biopsychosocial model as described by Schwartz (1982) and pave the way for meaningful and comprehensive multisystems integration.

REFERENCES

Bancroft, J. H. J., Jones, H. G., & Pullan, B. R. A simple transducer in measuring penile erection, with comments on its use in the treatment of sexual disorders. *Behavioral Research and Therapy*, 1966, *4*, 239 – 241.

Bandura, A. *Social learning theory*. Englewood Cliffs, N.J.: Prentice Hall, 1977.

Basmajian, J. V. Muscle spasm in the lumbar region and the neck: Two double-blind controlled clinical and laboratory studies. *Archives of Physical Medicine and Rehabilitation*, 1978, *59*, 58 – 63.

Beck, A. T. *Cognitive therapy and the emotional disorders*. New York: International Universities Press, 1976.

Benn, R. T. Some mathematical properties of weight-for-height indexes used as measures of adiposity. *British Journal of Preventive Social Medicine*, 1971, *25*, 42 – 50.

Bentler, P. Heterosexual behavior assessment I. Males; II. Females. *Behavior Research and Therapy*, 1978, *6*, 21 – 30.

Bjorn, J. C., & Cross, H. D. *Problem-oriented practice*. Chicago: Modern Hospital Press, 1971.

Bray, G. A. *The obese patient*. Philadelphia: Saunders, 1976.

Caird, W. K., & Wincze, J. P. *Sex therapy: A behavioral approach*. Hagerstown, Ma: Harper & Row, 1977.

Carver, C. S., & Scheier, M. F. A control theory approach to human behavior and implications for problems in self-management. In P. C. Kendall (Ed.), *Advances in cognitive-behavioral research and therapy*, New York: Academic Press, 1983.

Cautela, J. R. *Organic dysfunction survey schedules*. Champaign, Ill: Research Press, 1981. (b)

Cautela, J. R. *Behavioral analysis forms for clinical intervention (Vol.2)*. Champaign, Ill: Research Press, 1981. (a)

Cohen, F., & Lazarus, R. S. Coping with the stresses of illness. In, C. G. Stone, F. Cohen, & N. E. Adler & Associates (Eds.) *Health psychology-A handbook*. San Francisco: Jossey-Bass, 1979.

Crown, S., & Crisp, A. H. A short clinical diagnostic self-rating scale for psychoneurotic patients: The Middlesex Hospital questionnaire. *British Journal of Psychiatry*, 1966, *112*, 917 – 923.

Davidson, P. O., Ed. *Behavioral management of anxiety. Depression Pain*. New York: Brunner/Mazel, 1976.

Durnin, J. V. G. A., & Womersley, J. Body fat assessed from total body density and its estimation from skinfold thickness: Measurements on 481 men and women aged from 16 – 72 years. *British Journal of Nutrition*, 1974, *32*, 77 – 97.

Edelstein, P., Ross, W. D., & Schultz, J. R. The biopsychosocial approach: Clinical examples from a consultation-liason service, Part I. *Psychosomatics*, 1982, *23*, 15 – 19, 141 – 151, 233 – 242.

Elliott, C. H., & Denny, D. R. A multiple component treatment approach to smoking reduction. *Journal of Consulting and Clinical Psychology*, 1978, *46*, 1330 – 1339.

Ellis, A. & Harper, R. A. *A new guide to rational living*. Englewood Cliffs, N.J.: Prentice Hall, 1975.

Elstein, A. S., Shulman, L. S., & Sprafka, S. A. *Medical problem solving: An analysis of clinical reasoning*. Cambridge, Ma.: Harvard University Press, 1978.

Engel, G. L., & Schmale, A. The need for a new medical model: A challenge for biomedicine. *Science*, 1977, *196*, 126 – 136.

Fordyce, W. E. *Behavioral methods for chronic pain and illness*. St. Louis, Mo.: C. V. Mosby, 1976.

Franzini, L. R. & Grimes, W. B. Skinfold measures as the criterion of change in weight control studies. *Behavior Therapy*, 1976, *7*, 256-260.

Frith, C. D. Smoking behavior and its relation to the smoker's immediate experience. *British Journal of Social and Clinical Psychology*, 1971, *10*, 73 – 78.

Garrow, J. S. *Energy balance and obesity in man* (2nd ed.). Amsterdam: Elsevier/North Holland Biomedical Press, 1978.

Glasser, W. *Stations of the mind.* New York: Alfred Knopf, 1981.

Greenhoot, J. H., & Sternbach, R. A. Conjoint treatment of chronic pain. *Advances in Neurology,* 1974, *4,* 595 – 603.

Hackett, T. P., Cassem, N. H., & Wishnie, H. A. Detection and treatment of anxiety in the coronary care unit. *American Heart Journal,* 1969, *78,* 727 – 730.

Harris, F. A., Speleman, F. A., & Hymer, J. W. Electronic sensory aids as a treatment for cerebral palsied children: Inapproprioception, Part II. *Physical Therapy,* 1974, *54,* 354 – 365.

Holmes, T. H., & Wolf, H. G. Life situations, emotions, and backache. *Psychosomatic Medicine,* 1952, *14,* 18 – 33.

Horn, D. A model for the study of personal choice health behavior. *International Journal of Health Education,* 1976, *19,* 3 – 12.

Horn, D. H. *Why do you smoke?* National Institutes of Health Publication No. 82 – 1822, 1982.

Howe, G. W., Tapp, J. T., & Jackson, M. Training family physicians in behavioral aspects of primary care: The psychologist's role. *Professional Psychology,* 1982, *13,* 806 – 813.

Hull, C. L. *A behavior system.* New Haven, Cn.: Yale University Press, 1952.

Ireton, H. E., & Cassata, D. A psychological systems review. *The Journal of Family Practice,* 1976, *3,* 155 – 159.

Jason, L. A. Rapid improvement in insomnia following self-monitoring. *Journal of Behavior Therapy and Experimental Psychiatry,* 1975, *6,* 349 – 350.

Joyce, C. B., Zutshi, D. W., Hrubes, V., & Mason, R. M. Comparison of fixed interval and visual analog scales for rating chronic pain. *European Journal of Clinical Pharmacology,* 1975, *8,* 415 – 420.

Kanfer, F. H., & Phillips, J. S. *Learning foundations of behavior therapy.* New York: John Wiley & Sons, 1970.

Karacan, I. Advances in the psychophysiological evaluation of male erectile impotence. In J. LoPiccolo, & L. LoPiccolo (Eds.), *Handbook of sex therapy.* New York: Plenum Press, 1978.

Karacan, I. A simple and inexpensive transducer for quantitative measurements of penile erection during sleep. *Behavior Research Methods and Instrumentation,* 1969, *1,* 251 – 252.

Karle, W., Carriere, R., Hart, J., & Woldenberg, L. The functional analysis of dreams: A new theory of dreaming. *Journal of Clinical Psychology,* 1980, *36,* 5 – 78.

Karoly, P. Cognitive assessment in behavioral medicine. *Clinical Psychology Review,* 1982, *2,* 421 – 434.

Katahn, M. Obesity. In R. M. Woody (Ed.). *Encyclopedia of clinical assessment.* San Francisco: Jossey-Bass, 1980.

Katahn, M. *The 200 calorie solution.* New York: W. W. Norton & Co., 1982.

Katell, A., Callahan, E. J., Fremouw, W. J., & Zitter, R. E. The effects of behavioral treatment and fasting on eating habits and weight loss: A case study. *Behavior Therapy,* 1979, *10,* 579 – 587.

Kazarian, S. S., Howe, M. G., & Csapo, K. G. Development of the sleep behavior self-rating scale. *Behavior Therapy,* 1979, *10,* 412 – 417.

Keefe, K. D. The painchart. *Lancet,* 1948, *2,* 6 – 8.

Keys, A., Fidanza, F., Karvonen, M. J., Kimura, N., & Taylor, H. L. Indexes of relative weight and obesity. *Journal of Chronic Disease,* 1972, *25,* 329 – 343.

Kockott, H. G., Dittmar, F., & Nusselt, H. Systematic desensitization of erectile impotence: A controlled study. *Archives of Sexual Behavior,* 1975, *4,* 493 – 500.

Leif, H. & Reed, D. *Sexual knowledge and attitude test (SKAT).* University of Pennsylvania, School of Medicine; Division of Family Study, Department of Psychiatry, 2nd ed., 1972.

Leigh, H. & Reiser, M. F. *The patient: Biological, psychological, and social dimensions of medical practice.* New York: Plenum Press, 1980.

Long, C. J. The relationship between surgical outcome and MMPI profiles in chronic pain patients. *Journal of Clinical Psychology,* 1981, *37,* 744 – 749.

Low, A. D., Jr., & Orleans, C. S. Binge eating in obesity: Preliminary findings and guidelines for behavioral analysis and treatment. *Addictive Behaviors*, 1981, *6*, 155 – 166.

Low, A. D., Jr., & Orleans, C. S. Behavioral assessment of obesity. In F. J. Keefe & J. A. Blumenthal (Eds.), *Assessment strategies in behavioral medicine*. New York: Grune & Stratton, 1982.

Mahoney, M. J., & Arnkoff, D. B. Self-management. In O. F. Pomerleu, & J. P. Brady (Eds.), *Behavioral medicine: Theory and practice*. Baltimore, Md.: William & Wilkins, 1979.

Meichenbaum, D. *Cognitive behavior modification: An integrative approach*. New York: Plenum Press, 1977.

Meichenbaum, D., & Cameron, R. Cognitive behavior modification: Current issues. In C. Franks & T. Wilson (Eds.), *Handbook of behavior therapy*. New York: Guilford Press, 1980.

Meichenbaum, D., & Cameron, R. Issues in cognitive assessment: An overview. In T. Merluggi, C. Glass, & M. Genest (Eds.), *Cognitive assessment*. New York: Guilford Press, 1981.

Melzack, R. The McGill Pain Questionnaire: Major properties and scoring methods. *Pain*, 1975, *1*, 277 – 299.

Metropolitan Life Insurance Company. Frequency of overweight and underweight. *Statistical Bulletin*, 1960, *41*, 4 – 7.

Metropolitan Life Insurance Company. New weight standards for males and females. *Statistical Bulletin*, 1959, *40*, 2 – 3.

Miller, J. G. *Living Systems*, New York, McGraw Hill Book Co., 1978.

Mischel, W. *Personality and assessment*. New York: Wiley, 1968.

Nellis, M. J., Emurian, H. H., Brady, J. U., & Ray, R. L. Behavior analysis of cigarette smoking. *Pavlovian Journal of Biological Sciences*, 1982, *17*, 140 – 149.

O'Connor, K. P., Individual differences in situational preferences amongst smokers. *Personality and Individual Differences*, 1980, 1249 – 1258.

O'Connor, K. P., & Stravynski, A. Evaluation of a smoking typology by use of a specific behavioral substitution method of self-control. *Behavior Research and Therapy*, 1982, *20*, 279 – 288.

Pavlov, I. *Conditioned reflexes*. London: Oxford University Press, 1927.

Pinkerton, R. E., Tinnanoff, N., Willms, J. L., & Tapp, J. T. Resident physician performance in a continuing education format. Does newly acquired knowledge improve patient care? *Journal of the American Medical Association*, 1980, *244*, 2183 – 2185.

Plutchik, R. Emotions and attitudes related to being overweight. *Journal of Clinical Psychology*, 1976, *32*, 21 – 24.

Powers, P. S. *Obesity: The regulation of weight*. Baltimore, Md: Williams & Wilkins, 1980.

Powers, W. T. *Behavior: The control of perception*. Chicago: Aldine, 1973.

Rodin, J. Current status of the internal-external hypothesis for obesity: What went wrong? *American Psychologist*, 1981, *26*, 361 – 372.

Rosenthal, B. S., & Marx, R. D. *A comparison of standard behavioral and relapse prevention weight reduction programs*. Paper presented at the 13th Annual Association for the Advancement of Behavior Therapy convention. San Francisco, California: December 1979.

Rotter, J. B. Some implications of social learning theory for the practice of psychotherapy. In D. J. Levis (Ed.), *Learning approaches to therapeutic behavior change*. Chicago: Aldine, 1970.

Sarrel, P. M., Foddy, J., & McKinnon, J. B. Investigation of human sexual response using a cassette recorder. *Archives of Sexual Behavior*, 1977, *6*, 341 – 348.

Sarason, I. G., & Sarason, B. R. *The importance of cognition and moderator variables in stress*. Office of Naval Research Technical Report, No. N00014-75-C-0905, NR 170 – 804. Arlington, Va., 1979.

Schwartz, G. E. A systems analysis of psychobiology and behavior therapy: Implications in behavioral medicine. *Psychotherapy and Psychosomatics*, 1981, *36*, 159 – 184.

Schwartz, G. Testing the biopsychosocial model: The ultimate challenge facing behavioral medicine. *Journal of Consulting and Clinical Psychology*, 1982, *50*, 1040 – 1053.

Schwartz, G. The brain as a health care system. In G. Stone, N. Adler, & F. Cohen (Eds.), *Health Psychology*. San Francisco: Jossey-Bass, 1979.

Seligman, M. E. P. Helplessness: On depression, development and death. San Francisco: W. H. Freeman, 1975.

Selye, H. *The stress of life* (Rev. ed.). New York: McGraw-Hill, 1956.

Shealy, R. C. The effectiveness of various treatment techniques on different degrees and durations of sleep-onset insomnia. *Behavior Research and Therapy,* 1979, *17,* 541 – 546.

Sontag, S. *Illness as metaphor.* New York: Random House, 1977.

Spence, K. W. *Behavior theory and conditioning.* New Haven: Yale University Press, 1956.

Swanson, D. W., Swenson, M. W., Maruta, T., & McPhee, M. C. Program for managing chronic pain: I. Program description and characteristics of patients. *Mayo Clinic Proceedings,* 1976, *51,* 401 – 408.

Thorndike, E. L. *The psychology of learning.* (Educational Psychology). New York: Teachers College, 1913.

Tolman, E. C. Purposive behavior in animals and men. New York: Appleton, 1932.

Weisenberg, M. Pain and pain control. *Psychological Bulletin,* 1977, *84,* 1008 – 1044.

8   Clinical Neuropsychology

Elbert W. Russell
Veterans Administration Medical Center
Miami, Florida

INTRODUCTION

Neuropsychology has been variously defined as "the field of brain – behavior relations" (Reitan & Davison, 1974, p. 1); the study of the "role of individual brain systems in complex forms of mental activity" (Luria, 1973, p. 17); or "the study of the neural mechanism underlying human behavior" (Hecaen & Albert, 1978, p. 1). It is thus a field that relates behavior to neurology, neurosurgery, and the other clinical neurosciences. Whereas neurology and physiological psychology study the actions of the entire central nervous system, neuropsychology is generally restricted to examining the functions of the cerebral cortex.

Divisions of Neuropsychology

Neuropsychology has several subdivisions, described in Fig. 8.1. Experimental neuropsychology is primarily concerned with the relationship between the brain and intellectual and emotional functions. Linguistic neuropsychology, sometimes called aphasiology, studies the effects of brain damage on speech mechanisms. Clinical neuropsychology is the application of psychometric methods to assess the effects of pathological brain conditions on psychological functioning. This contrasts with the neurological approach, which utilizes brief tests in a manner similar to that used by neurologists (Walsh, 1978, p. 289). The Russian neuropsychologist, Luria (1973), exemplifies this approach. Neurologists are now calling this specialty *behavioral neurology*.

In the metric form of clinical neuropsychology, traditional psychometric methods are applied to the assessment of organic conditions. The abilities tests are

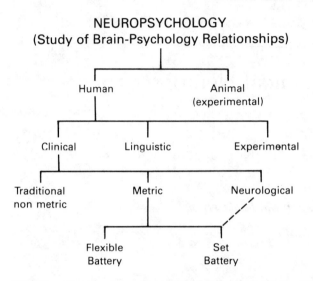

FIG. 8.1.   Neuropsychology (Study of Brain-Psychology Relationships).

applied in either a flexible (Lezak, 1983) or a set manner (Russell, Neuringer, & Goldstein, 1970), such as the Halstead – Reitan Battery (HRB). The Luria – Nebraska Battery (LNB), which attempts to combine the neurological approach and the set psychometric approach (Golden, 1981), does not appear to have succeeded (Spiers, 1981).

Theoretical and Historical Basis for Clinical Neuropsychological Testing

In a recent article, Luria (Luria & Majovski, 1977) compared clinical neuropsychology as practiced in the United States (Halstead, 1947; Reitan, 1974; Russell et al., 1970) with the Russian methods. Luria (Luria & Majovski, 1977) thought that American neuropsychological testing: "lacks grounding in a theoretical formulation of the brain's functional organization governing psychological processes affecting behavior [p. 961]." In contrast he thought that there was a strong theoretical basis for the Russian or European clinical neuropsychological examination as exemplified by Luria's own works.

In contrast to Luria's argument, the basis of the American approach to neuropsychology is to be found in: (1) the psychometrics of intellectual abilities that reflect cortical functions; and (2) clinical lore. A large body of concepts and principles, which have seldom been made explicit, have been utilized successfully in evaluation of patients (Reitan, 1964). Part of this lore is based on effects of brain damage that are only apparent through use of a set battery of psychometric tests that have graded scales.

Historical Issues

The primary issue in human neuropsychology is the localization of brain dysfunction. The "narrow localization" conception (Luria, 1973) was begun by Broca when he demonstrated that expressive aphasia is related to the inferior portion of the second frontal gyrus. His work was soon followed by that of Fritz and Hitzig (Luria, 1980, p. 13), who found through electrical stimulation that certain areas of the cortex are related to types of body movements.

A more holistic attitude toward brain functioning was begun by the work of Florenz, who found that in animals, the more of the cortex that was removed the more impairment there was to the animal's functioning. Other neurologists followed this route, such as Von Monkow, Head, and Kurt Goldstein. Goldstein thought that brain damage produced a general effect—impaired abstract thinking (Walsh, 1978, p. 118 – 122).

During the early 1900s to the 1950s the concept of "wholism," that the brain operates as a whole, dominated physiological psychology. In the experimental field, Lashley's (1929) concepts of equipotentiality and mass action explained brain functioning. The concept of *equipotentiality* postulated that each area of the brain could perform the same function as other areas. *Mass action* reflected the belief that the amount of impairment was dependent on the amount of tissue destroyed.

In the area of neurology and in neuropsychological testing, Kurt Goldstein's idea of organistic functioning was a major concept. His associate, Martin Scheerer, brought Goldstein's concepts into psychology through the development of the Goldstein-Scheerer Neuropsychological tests (Goldstein & Scheerer, 1941). These utilized Goldstein's notion that any damage to the brain impaired abstract thinking, so the brain damaged person shifted to a concrete mode of thinking. This deficit was tested by presenting problem-solving tasks and watching for this shift in thinking. These tests were used in psychology to assess brain damage until about 1950.

The psychometric approach to brain functioning in the form of intelligence testing had, of course, been well developed. In the 1940s psychometric methods began to be applied in the experimental area to brain damage by such people as Teuber (1955) and Milner (1970). In the clinical area Benton, Wepman, and Halstead (1947) began this application. The approach by Benton and Wepman is best presented by Lezak (1983).

The most common approach in clinical neuropsychology was pioneered by Halstead and Reitan. Halstead (1947) investigated the effect of brain damage on a large number of psychological tests that were in existence during the 1940s. From these investigations he developed a battery of 10 tests that became the basis for the Halstead – Reitan Battery (HRB).

Following Halstead other neuropsychologists continued to develop his method of testing. Ralph Reitan applied some neurological principles to Halstead's battery and added new tests. This permitted a sophisticated pattern analysis of the battery (Reitan & Davison, 1974). Reitan's interpretations are largely based on an "intuitive" or inferential understanding of these patterns. One of Halstead's and Reitan's students, Philip Rennick, began transforming the battery into a more complete psychometric instrument. Based on unpublished studies, Rennick established preliminary scale scores for the HRB. Subsequently, work by Russell and Goldstein (Russell et al., 1970) applied Rennick's scales to the development of neuropsychological keys. A *"key"* is a biological taxonomic method of determining to which of several classes an organism or object belongs. In this study it was used to distinguish normal subjects from subjects with right, left, and diffuse damage and to separate acute, static, and congenital damage.

In the 1950s, Reitan (1955) began a research program that demonstrated that lateralized lesions will differentially affect scores on the WAIS. Along with the work by experimental neuropsychologists this has shifted the paradigm away from "holism" to the study of localized effects. The emphasis since the 1960s has been on localizing functions in a manner that is more sophisticated than that of the early narrow localization school.

THEORETICAL PRINCIPLES

The primary contribution of American neuropsychology is found in the application of psychometrics to neuropsychological testing and the clinical lore of those engaged in that testing. Part of this lore consists of the relationship of various tests to different areas of the brain. These relationships are available in published works (Hecaen & Albert, 1978; Walsh, 1978). Although largely unpublished, other principles used in this lore are fairly well known, at least to the followers of Reitan. These principles that underlie neuropsychological test interpretation are reviewed in the following section.

Principle of Complexity

A function is complex when it contains a number of elementary functions necessary for the operation of that function. The complexity of the function is equal to the number of elementary functions of which it is composed. Although it is now accepted (Luria, 1980) that a particular function of an organism is the product of a whole system of brain actions and that many areas of the brain are involved in any function, a judicious application of testing methods can isolate the particular contribution of each component in a functional system. Luria's own work (1973, 1980) demonstrates how this can be accomplished. Tests can thus be constructed that will measure either an elementary function, or the complex functioning of many elementary functions. Research demonstrates that simple and complex functions can be separated (Satz, 1966; Teuber & Weinstein, 1958).

This principle provides a way of separating functions into three types according to complexity: (1) elementary; (2) complex; and (3) general. An *elementary function* may be defined as: a function that is primarily dependent on a single relatively small area of the cortex. An example of a relatively simple function with a known location is that of the Digit Span Forwards Test. The area related to this test, according to a study by Warrington, Logue, and Pratt (1971) is that of the supermarginal and angular gyrus of the left hemisphere.

A *complex function* is a function that is composed of two or more elementary functions. Thus it is related to many areas of the cortex. If any of those areas are damaged the function as a whole will be impaired. Inasmuch as, according to Luria's (1980, p. 23 – 28) concepts, there is often a certain interchangeableness among the elements of a functional system, the usual finding is that complex functions are impaired but not eliminated by limited damage. The total function may be reorganized and performed at a lower level of the brain. The number of complex functions is limited only by the number of possible combinations of elementary functions. Complex functions can be classified by the types of component elementary functions they include.

A *general function* is defined as a function that is related to all areas of the cortex. Acute damage anywhere in the cortex will affect a general function. Also the impairment of a general function will affect most activities of the brain, as general functions underlie other functions. The two most commonly accepted general functions are mental speed and attention.

This principle of complexity has several major implications. Tests of elementary functions will provide information about focal lesions. However, tests of more complex and general functions are more sensitive to widespread diffuse damage. As such, they are useful in screening for the existence of all forms of brain damage. A fully balanced neuropsychological examination battery should include tests of general, complex, and simple functions.

Principle of Localization

The principle of localization states that each elementary function is related to a single separate area of the cortex. The problem of localizing damage involves both analyzing complex functions into their component elementary functions and determining areas to which the elementary functions are related. Most of the present work in neuropsychology is concerned with the localization of functions. As such, it is extensively covered in other writings (Hecaen & Albert, 1978; Walsh, 1978).

All-or-None Effect

The all-or-none effect principle (Russell, 1980b) states that some mental functions tend to be impaired by brain lesions either completely or not at all, whereas other functions are impaired in a graduated manner.

All-or-none functions appear to be related to specific projection areas of the cortex, tracts, and subcortical nuclei. Graduated functions appear to be located in the cerebral cortex association areas outside the projection areas. For instance, damage to the visual tracts or visual projection areas produces a scotoma, or area without any vision, while vision in the surrounding areas may be normal.

This all-or-none effect has been demonstrated for pure tactile sensation as well as the visual pathways. In a study by Russell (1980b) the control subjects had no impairment on a test of the amount of tactile sensation in the person's hands. The organic patients were either unimpaired or severely impaired with almost no cases in the middle range. By contrast, several cognitive tests, such as the WAIS Block Design, formed a skewed but continuously graded distribution of scores extending from the normal range to complete impairment. All-or-none functions produce extremely good evidence for the existence and location of damage when they are present because the impairment is directly related to a limited area.

Almost all the functions tested in most of the usual neurological examination are all-or-none functions that reflect impairments from damage to tracts, subcortical nuclei, or projection areas of the cortex. The neurological examination using brief all-or-none tests can cover the entire body and the cranial nerves rapidly and effectively. This would be difficult if the functions that were being examined were continuous functions that required long graded scales.

The mental status part of a neurological examination deals with cognitive or association area functions that operate in a graded manner rather than an all-or-none manner. However, the mental status examination uses brief questions rather than scales. These items can be designed to fit graded functions by selecting items in the borderline range of intelligence (Russell, 1980b). If by history the examiner knows that the patient previously had normal intelligence but cannot now pass these items, the examiner can be fairly certain that there has been a drastic reduction in intellectual ability.

This method of approaching continuous functions is adequate as a screening test to determine the existence of fairly gross neurological pathology. However, when dealing with borderline cases or when a detailed pattern analysis of cortical functioning is desired, tests that utilize a graded continuous distribution are required. Clinical neuropsychological testing is almost entirely confined to the cerebral cortex in which only the projection areas contain all-or-none functions. Thus the neuropsychologist is dealing, in most cases, with graduated continuous functions that require utilizing graded homogeneous scales for an adequate measure of the deficit.

Principle of Fluidity

This principle is derived from Cattell's (1943) distinction between fluid and crystallized intelligence. The concept of fluidity states that *fluid intelligence* is the type of ability used in novel situations and problem solving. It is closely related to the basic intellectual ability of an individual. In contrast, *crystallized intelligence* is composed of intellectual abilities that have been well learned and are strongly affected by culture. Horn (1976) points out that both of these require learning but that in the case of fluid ability the proportionate use of unlearned processes is much greater. As such, fluid ability represents the active processing of material by the brain to produce new concepts or solutions, whereas crystallized ability is simply the retrieval of previously learned material.

Because fluid ability requires a more active processing by the brain it is more vulnerable to any kind of damage or lesion. As such, the principle of fluidity states that crystallized intelligence is more resistant to the effects of brain lesions than fluid intelligence.

Since the late 1950s the concept of two types of intelligence has tended to fade from view as neuropsychology began to emphasize localization of intellectual abilities. Although originally a holistic concept, this concept of fluid and crystallized abilities can be reformulated to be compatible with the localization of functions. In the reformulization, different areas of the brain are related to different functions, which may be either crystallized or fluid.

According to this concept, then, one would expect that certain abilities would be affected by both localization and fluidity. Several studies and papers lend support for this concept without using the term "fluidity" (Finlayson, 1977; Reed & Reitan, 1963; Reitan, 1972). Recently Russell (1979, 1980a) related this concept to the Wechsler Adult Intelligence Scale. In the 1979 study both fluidity and localization affect the WAIS. Four groups of 40 patients, each matched on age and education, took the WAIS. These consisted of a slowly progressive diffuse damage group, an acute right hemisphere lesion group, an acute left hemisphere lesion group and a control group of non-brain damaged patients. For the diffuse group the verbal abilities remained relatively near the normal level, whereas the performance scales, with the exception of Picture Completion, deteriorated strongly. This follows, as the verbal tests are crystallized ability tests, whereas the performance tests tend to be fluid ability tests (Horn, 1976).

The results of right hemisphere damaged patients were very similar to those of the diffusely impaired group. They showed impairment in Block Design, Picture Arrangement, and Object Assembly, which are more impaired by right hemisphere damage, and in the Digit Symbol, which is apparently impaired by almost all types of brain damage regardless of lateralization. Thus, apparently, the same tests that are sensitive to right hemisphere lateralized damage are also the tests of fluidity.

By contrast, patients with left hemisphere damage showed only a slight reduction in their verbal scores as compared to the Block Design, Picture Arrangement, and Object Assembly scores. Apparently the verbal tests on the WAIS are both left hemisphere tests and crystallized abilities tests. Consequently, the lateralization and fluidity effects counteracted each other and canceled out the expected effects of lateralization.

This research then both supports the concept of fluidity and has important implications for neuropsychological testing. The most obvious implication is that there appears to be no one pattern for the WAIS related to brain damage. The WAIS does not measure fluid verbal abilities, though measures of such abilities exist (Reitan, 1972). Furthermore, measures that are most sensitive to brain damage are tests of fluid ability. Thus tests that have been particularly designed to indicate brain damage are simply fluid ability measures. As such, this principle is the foundation for much of psychometric neuropsychology.

Distant Effects

The effects of a lesion in the cortex often extend beyond the boundaries of the lesion itself. This "distant effect" of a lesion was first described in detail by Von Monakow (Smith, 1975), who called this effect "diaschisis." Recently Aaron Smith (1975, p. 70−73) has discussed this phenomenon in considerable detail. The distant effect may be due to the generalized effects produced by such conditions as increased intercranial pressure, edema, or compression, though diaschisis is considered to be a distinct type of distant effect (Smith, 1975, p. 70).

The distant effect principle states that a brain lesion may effect functions in an undamaged area of the cortex at a distance from the lesion. The pattern of spread is not known but it appears to decrease in strength with distance (Luria, 1973, p. 136). Because lesions may affect functions in distant areas of the brain, this effect may have produced some of the confused results of previous neuropsychological interpretation and experimentation.

Another implication is an interaction effect that was exemplified in Russell's (1979) study of the WAIS. Because the performance tests, which are right hemisphere tests, are more fluid than the verbal tests (Horn, 1976; Russell, 1979), they are more easily impaired by damage in the opposite or left hemisphere than are the verbal tests by damage in the right hemisphere. Thus, in this study the Performance IQ was lower than the Verbal IQ in 40% of the subjects with *left* hemisphere lateralized brain damage.

Chronicity Effect

Clinical experience indicates that as distance effects resolve, these effects are gradually reduced such that there is a return of those functions that are not related to the damaged areas. The chronicity effect principle states that the strength of distant effects decreases with the chronicity or the age of a nonprogressive lesion. A corollary of this principle is that the elementary functions related to the area of cortex that was destroyed will remain permanently impaired.

According to this principle, if a battery of tests is repeatedly administered to a patient with an acute focal nonprogressive lesion, those tests that are not directly related to the area of damage will gradually return to normal while functions directly related to the area that was destroyed will remain impaired. The length of time for maximum return of functions appears to be approximately 2 years.

However, there is a decelerating return of functions; functions return rapidly at first and then more slowly with increasing time. Most of the return of functions will have occurred within the first year, according to our clinical experience.

Although as yet no formal research has been done on the chronicity effect, a single case study (Russell, 1981) illustrates this effect. This was a case study of a 30-year-old male who became ill with viral encephalitis that was concentrated in the left temporopatietal area of his cortex. This localization of the disease was determined by a series of four radioisotope brain scans and two EEGs. In addition he was given neuropsychological testing using the Halstead-Reitan Battery four times over a period of 2 years after his illness and then again 6 years later.

The encephalitis left this patient with a permanent dyslexia that was documented both by the neuropsychological testing and his inability to read material required by college courses. In accordance with the chronicity effect concept, the tests that were related to areas of this patient's brain not directly affected by the damage returned to normal in approximately 16 months, whereas his reading ability, which is related to the area of the brain that was damaged, never returned to normal. The return of functions followed a generally decelerating course such that much of the recovery had occurred by 6 months.

This concept of a chronicity effect helps explain the long-standing finding that the Wechsler Intelligence Test is lateralized with acute lesions but not for chronic lesions (Fitzhugh, Fitzhugh, & Reitan, 1962). If it is assumed that the lateralization impairment on the WAIS is largely a reflection of distant effects rather than the effect of a direct lesion, then the test scores would return to the normal range as the lesion ages (Russell, 1981). This of course would not occur if the lesion is directly in an area that is producing aphasia.

The chronicity effect supplies one method of distinguishing between chronic and acute focal brain damage on the basis of a correctly designed neuropsychological battery. In acute focal damage one would expect to find not only more severe impairment but also a mixture of focal and diffuse impairments due to remote effects. In static damage only the focal effects for elementary functions would be found. This produces what may be called a "punch card effect." The measured functions of an individual with static damage tend to look like a computer punch card in which most of the elementary functions are normal, whereas the few elementary functions that are directly related to the area of damage are punched out or impaired. Functions that are complex and consequently cover many areas of the brain will obviously be affected by damage to any of the component elementary functions.

Although most of the previous research in clinical neuropsychology has been that related to localization of functions, these additional principles such as all-or-none, fluidity, distance, and chronicity effects should help to provide a more complete neuropsychological assessment. The effects of brain damage are not simply those of localization. Depending upon such factors as the type of function, the distance from the lesion, and the age of the lesion, different test results may be derived from lesions in the same area.

NEUROPSYCHOLOGICAL ASSESSMENT ISSUES

The area of neuropsychology involves more effects and is richer than one would expect from simply examining the concepts of localization. For this reason a neuropsychologist must be trained in a more extensive manner than would be expected if the only problem were that of a one-to-one relationship between a single test and an area of the brain.

Among specialists in neuropsychology there is general agreement that advanced training beyond the doctoral degree is necessary for neurological assessment (Meier, 1981). The growth of knowledge in the area of neurology led psychologists to recognize that there was no such entity as "brain damage" in general, but that the effects of brain damage were quite complex (Boll, 1981). Consequently what was needed for the assessment of brain pathology was not a single test but a relatively large battery designed to tap various psychological abilities. These reveal patterns related to different locations and types of brain damage. The amount of knowledge a psychologist needed in order to assess brain functioning became quite extensive because it was necessary to have a working knowledge of neurology as well as psychology. Neuropsychological testing was no longer an easily learned part of clinical psychology but an extensive field in its own right.

Today the general clinical psychologist should be able to screen patients for organic difficulties. Then, if there is evidence of an organic problem, the patient should be referred to a neurologist or a neuropsychologist for more extensive specialized testing.

Qualitative Versus Quantitative Approach

The controversy between qualitative and quantitative assessments was best described by Luria in his article comparing American and Russian neuropsychology (Luria & Majovski, 1977). He characterizes Russian psychology as "qualitative" whereas American psychology is considered to be "quantitative."

The qualitative approach to clinical neuropsychology involves an intensive study of an individual patient and the pattern of his or her impairments, whereas the quantitative approach makes use of group norms and a statistical comparison to describe a particular case. The qualitative examination utilizes many brief pass/fail tests selected from a very large group of tests. Luria's genius in part involves the development of literally hundreds of these brief tests (Luria, 1980).

The quantitative description involves an assessment based on graded scales with statistical norms. This examines a wide range of functions in terms of level ability or deficit. The "qualitative" approach describes more functions but only as to whether each is severely impaired or not impaired. The quantitative approach enables the examiner to determine the amount of impairment to each area and function of the brain.

The quantitative approach has numerous advantages. It is quite as applicable to diffuse and scattered damage as it is to focal damage, whereas the qualitative method is primarily designed to study the effects of focal lesions. The quantitative approach enables a wider spectrum of brain damage to be described. In clinical practice over half the cases seen are diffuse or multifocal in nature. In questions of rehabilitation or patient management, the quantitative approach provides a far more useful description than the qualitative approach (Lynch, 1981), as it describes the amount of both the deficits and assets of the patient.

A Flexible Versus a Set Battery

A central controversy within psychometric neuropsychology relates to the method of test selection. In the flexible approach, tests are selected to fit a particular problem. Alternatively, the set battery approach utilizes the same battery of tests with each patient. In the set battery approach the tests in the ideal battery are standardized so that a scale score on one test will be equivalent to a scale score on the other tests.

The flexible approach has been described most completely by Lezak (1983). The set approach is used by the Halstead — Reitan Battery (HRB) and more recently with the Luria Nebraska Battery (LNB). Although many neuropsychologists such as A. Smith (1975) have their own set battery that is different from the Halstead — Reitan Battery, most of the people who do not use the Halstead — Reitan Battery tend to favor the flexible approach.

The entire controversy between the set and the flexible approach hinges on a single rather obvious principle that is axiomatic to neuropsychology and to a certain extent to all of psychology. This principle is that one cannot determine whether a certain function is impaired unless that function is tested.

The primary advantage of a flexible battery is adaptability. Variations in the types and severity of impairment can be taken into consideration and the tests can be related to the consultation problem. A set battery may not be exactly appropriate for a specific problem.

Although a flexible battery enables the examiner to adapt tests to a particular problem, it also means that the neuropsychologist's function is largely confined to that of confirming or disconfirming the existence of a particular problem presented by the neurologist or referring service. No new problems or any unexpected areas of damage would in most cases be uncovered. Because a good set battery is designed so that all areas of the brain and all basic mental processes are covered, the neuropsychologist may be able to contribute information about the patient's brain functioning that was not previously suspected.

The main advantage of a set battery is that the tests can be compared to each other in order to obtain patterns. Because the tests are standardized on the same population, the scores on one test can be directly compared with scores on another test. This is the great advantage of the WAIS, which is essentially a battery of tests.

The meaning of the differences between tests and patterns cannot be known on a battery except through extensive experience and research in which the tests are utilized *with each other* under a wide variety of conditions. Such experience and research is necessarily lacking for a flexible battery, as the same tests are not repeated. It is the fact that the subtests in the Halstead-Reitan Battery are given as a group that enables Reitan and his followers to read the patterns that occur on a battery (Reitan, 1964).

Another advantage of a set battery is that it can be utilized to answer many problems, some of which may not have been posed by the original consultation. The same report can be utilized by people other than the original requester. As such, a set battery of tests may require less total time than it would take for a neuropsychologist to give a series of flexible batteries each designed to answer different specific questions.

The administration of a set battery does not require knowledge of a wide range of tests. Rather it requires consistency. Thus a trained technician is able to administer a set battery and may often provide more consistent and accurate data than a professional neuropsychologist. The greatest advantage, however, is efficiency, in that the time of a neuropsychologist is not utilized in giving routine tests. Although the entire HRB requires approximately 5 to 7 hours of testing time, the time utilized by the neuropsychologist to write his or her report may be less than an hour.

Although it appears that the flexible and set batteries are incompatible they are in fact quite complementary. Once the tests in a large set battery have been standardized together or standardized on a normal population, the tests can be selected from the battery in order to answer specific questions with greater efficiency. Such a selection from a large set battery provides the psychologist with a reliable flexible battery to meet unusual conditions.

BASIC TOOLS—TESTS AND TEST BATTERIES

In clinical neuropsychological assessment, the basic tools are in most circumstances various neuropsychological tests. There are now in existence quite a large number of tests that are related to the assessment of organic conditions (Lezak, 1983).

Single Tests of Organicity

Probably the best known single test for organic brain conditions is the Bender – Gestalt Test (Bender, 1938; Lezak, 1983). Of the several scoring systems for the Bender – Gestalt the best known are those of Pascal and Suttle (1951) and Hutt and Gibby (1970). It probably obtains its ability to diagnose brain damage from the fact that it reflects a fluid type of intelligence and that, being primarily a test of right hemisphere functions (Russell, 1976), it tests areas of the brain that are not obvious in a verbal examination. Left hemisphere damage often produces aphasia which is generally fairly obvious.

The use of the Bender – Gestalt alone as an indication of brain damage has recently come under heavy attack (Bigler & Ehrfurth, 1981; Russell, 1976) due to its inaccuracy. These criticisms, it should be noted, apply to all "brain damage" tests when used alone.

The Benton Visual Retention Test (Benton, 1963) consists of a series of simple design drawings that the patient is required to draw from memory. This test also appears to be a right hemisphere test. Another memory test for brain damage is the Memory-for-Designs Test by Graham and Kendall (1960). This test appears to be as accurate as the Bender – Gestalt (Brilliant & Gynther, 1963; Quattlebaum, 1968) and also more affected in right hemisphere lesions than left (McFie, 1960). The three major individual tests for brain damage—Bender – Gestalt, Benton Visual Retention and Memory-for-Design Test—appear to be roughly equivalent in their ability to separate brain damage from non-brain damage patients, and all three appear to be right hemisphere fluid ability tests.

The Rorschach and the Wechsler Adult Intelligence Scale have been used to indicate brain damage. Several scoring systems for brain damage have been proposed (Exner, 1974) but the most widely accepted method is that created by Piotrowski (1937; Lezak, 1983). All clinical psychologists using the Rorschach should be able to recognize these "organic" patterns in order to screen for brain damage while testing emotional factors and to prevent them from making errors in interpretation.

The Wechsler Adult Intelligence Scale was never designed to measure brain damage yet it has become the only test that is universally utilized for this purpose. It appears to have two advantages: The IQ of a person is needed in order to determine their level of intellectual functioning, whether or not they have brain damage; and the pattern of test results gives an indication of the existence and type of damage. The utilization of the WAIS and subtest patterns is discussed in several places (Lezak, 1983; Russell, 1979).

Test Batteries

Individual test batteries have been described by Benton (1975), Lezak (1983, pp. 107 – 110, 560 – 575), and A. Smith (1975). In fact even the major set batteries such as the Halstead – Reitan Battery are modified to some extent by various psychologists (Matthews, 1981, pp. 645 – 685). Nevertheless, two batteries presently dominate the field of neuropsychology.

Standardized Luria – Nebraska Battery (LNB).   In the last few years a new neuropsychological battery, the Luria – Nebraska Battery (LNB) has been introduced into clinical practice. The basic items in this battery, which were originally developed by Luria, were placed into a test format by Anne-Lise Christensen (1975). In this country, Golden (1981) took Anne-Lise Christensen's tests and grouped them into heterogeneous scales in an attempt to force her neurological approach into a psychometric format. The LNB has 269 test items scored fail/pass or pass well, which are collected into 14 heterogeneous scales.

The originators of the LNB have been extremely prolific as well as enthusiastic in their publications (Golden, 1981) and as a result they have flooded the field with their own results. Only recently have articles appeared by psychologists outside the original supporters of the LNB. These have found that the LNB has many drawbacks in design (Crosson & Warren, 1982; Delis & Kaplan, 1982), in theory (Adams, 1980; Spiers, 1981) and even in the experimental research that was used to support its attributes (Adams, 1980).

However, the primary problem with this battery is that the scales are heterogeneous and as such the items do not all measure the same function (Nunnally, 1978, p. 254). Consequently it is difficult to determine what a particular scale is measuring (Spiers, 1981). Christensen and Luria did not assume that the items were measuring the same functions and consequently they did not place them into categories or scales (Spiers, 1981). The validation procedures are also questionable (Adams, 1980; Spiers, 1981) for these scales, and it is dubious that pass/fail/ nominal scales are appropriate for cortical functions (Russell, 1980b).

Finally, the LNB appears to be somewhat inadequate in the coverage of some brain areas and functions (Russell, 1980c). The LNB devotes 36% of the subtests to sensory impairment, 19% to motor impairment, 46% to aphasia, and only 13% to intellectual processes. Thus the LNB does not adequately cover the higher cognitive processes (Russell, 1980c).

The basic coverage of aphasia in the LNB is more comprehensive than the brief aphasia screening test in the HRB. However, if one is attempting to measure aphasia, the Boston Aphasia Examination (Goodglass & Kaplan, 1972) and Western Aphasia Examination (Kertesz, 1979) are more accurate (Crosson & Warren, 1982; Delis & Kaplan, 1982) and have considerably greater coverage than the LNB.

Halstead – Reitan Battery (HRB).   The Halstead – Reitan (HRB) (Boll, 1981; Reitan, 1974) is the oldest and most popular of the set batteries. Its basic tests were originally constructed by Halstead (1947) and subsequently transformed by Reitan (1974) into a highly sophisticated instrument that could be utilized to assess not only the existence of brain damage but the kind and location of the damage. More recently, work by Russell et al. (1970), utilizing the unpublished work of Phillip Rennick, modified this battery into a more thoroughly psychometric battery. A neurological key or algorithm demonstrated that, using complete psychometric principles, the lateralization and the chronicity of a lesion could be determined with acceptable accuracy. Utilization of this scoring system permits not only the determination of the existence of brain damage, but also the amount of impairment of intellectual abilities. As such, the amount of overall impairment as well as the amount of impairment of separate functions can be assessed.

The HRB utilizes tests related to the different principles that were discussed earlier. Fluid tests such as the Category, Form Board, and Trail-Making tests determine the existence of damage and amount of overall deficits. They also indicate how a person will function in high-level complex cognitive activities. A person with intact speaking ability may give an impression of a lack of impairment. However, such impairment may be found when active processing or fluid abilities are measured.

Finally, a large number of different types of functions are measured (Russell, 1975, 1976; Russell et al., 1970). These are summarized in Table 8.1 as used in Russell's laboratory at present.

TABLE 8.1
Halstead–Reitan Battery
Areas of Mental Functioning That are Measured

Function	Tests
A. Cognitive functions	
1. General	
a. Problem solving, abstract thinking	Category test
b. Mental flexibility (Ability to shift)	Trails B
2. Verbal	
a. Logical and arithmetic	WAIS Arithmetic
b. Abstract verbal	WAIS Similarities
c. Conceptual thinking	WAIS Vocabulary
d. Practical thinking	WAIS Information
	WAIS Comprehension
3. Figural (spatial relations)	WAIS Block Design
	WAIS Object Assembly
	Trails A
	Drawing Cross
	Form Board (TPT)
4. Nonverbal sequence and understanding social situations	WAIS Picture Arrangement
B. Complex sensorimotor coordination	Form Board (TPT)
C. Aphasia and verbal learning	
1. Aphasia	Aphasia Screening Test
2. Verbal coding	Speech Perception
3. Verbal understanding	WAIS Verbal Tests
4. Verbal fluency	H Words
5. Reading	WRAT
	Speech Perception
D. Rhythm	Rhythm Test
E. Attention	Speech Perception
	Rhythm

(Continued)

TABLE 8.1
(Continued)

Function	Tests
F. Mental speed	WAIS Digit Symbol
	Trails A and B
G. Memory	
1. Immediate	WAIS Digit Span
2. Recent verbal	Revised Wechsler
	Memory Scale/(RWMS)
	Logical Memory
3. Recent figural	RWMS Figural Memory
4. Figural learning	Form Board (TPT)
	Memory
	Form Board, Location
5. Verbal storage	WAIS Vocabulary
	WAIS Information
H. Motor	
1. Pure motor speed	Tapping
2. Strength	Grip Strength
3. Complex motor performance	Groove Peg Board
I. Perceptual	
1. Pure sensory	
a. Tactile	Single Stimulation
b. Auditory	Single Stimulation
c. Visual	Visual Fields
2. Complex perceptual	
a. Tactile	Suppression, Tactile
	Figuretip Writing
	Finger Agnosia
b. Auditory	Suppression, Auditory
c. Visual	Suppression, Visual
I. Dominance	Dominance Test
K. Emotional condition	MMPI
L. History of problem	Questionnaire

ABILITIES AND LIMITATIONS OF NEUROPSYCHOLOGICAL TESTING

As with any test or method, neuropsychological measures have their abilities and limitations. The neuropsychologist, as well as persons requesting neuropsychological testing, should be well aware of these abilities and limitations.

Some of the primary abilities of neuropsychological tests are:

1. Detection of brain damage, especially subtle diffuse conditions.
2. Location of a lesion in the brain.
3. Determining the age of the lesion.

4. Helping estimate the expected amount of return of functions.
5. Helping to separate an organic from a functional mental condition.
6. Determining the severity of a schizophrenic process.
7. Helping detect a hysterical basis for impairment.
8. In some cases helping determine the diagnosis of a brain lesion.
9. Setting a base line for determining improvement or deterioration of a brain condition.
10. Measuring the amount of deficits as an aid to rehabilitation of an organic condition.
11. Measuring past trauma and stroke patients' abilities to determine whether they can continue in their occupation.
12. Determining impairment related to compensation and litigation.
13. Helping determine what activities a brain damaged person is capable of doing (e.g., driving a car).
14. Providing information to help a family deal with a brain injured member.
15. Providing research data concerning the way in which the brain operates.

A few comments might be made concerning some of these abilities. In the past the primary function of neuropsychological testing was to detect and determine the location of a brain lesion. The recent development of the computerized tomography (CT scan) has made this function largely obsolete, as the CT scan is more accurate. However, a growing function of neuropsychological testing is that of assessing a brain injured person for rehabilitative, management and compensation purposes. These require a knowledge of the amount of deficits that a patient has. Neurological procedures generally can tell the area of physical destruction to the brain but this does not directly determine the amount of deficits that has accrued. Neuropsychological methods directly measure deficits and assets, and as such they provide the most accurate evaluation of a patient's mental functioning. This is invaluable information in planning a patient's rehabilitation and care, and it is necessary information in settling compensation and litigation claims.

Limitations

There are many limitations in the application of neuropsychological testing that require caution. In neurology each test is judged according to the types of information it can and cannot provide. For instance, plain skull X rays have an overall hit rate that is generally very poor, but with some conditions they are highly accurate. On the other hand, procedures that generally have a "high hit rate" like the CT scan will miss some types of damage. The neurologist knows which tests produce the relevant information and consequently pays attention only to the results of certain tests.

Neuropsychologists have not paid sufficient attention to this type of evaluation. Studies have not been done to know what the different neuropsychological tests can do and, importantly, what they cannot do. Nevertheless, some limitations are known.

The first important limitation is that all neuropsychological batteries are applicable only to cerebral cortical functions. As such, it is of little use when the lesion is in the brainstem or cerebellum.

The second limitation of neuropsychological testing is that tests have not yet been developed that will cover all areas of the cortex. The HRB will not adequately cover the occipital and inferior temporal areas and it is somewhat limited in the frontal areas. Also, there are a number of neurological conditions that may be quite serious or potentially life threatening that will not effect neuropsychological tests because they do not produce impairment of mental functions, such as aneurysms and vascular malformations.

Thirdly, the ability of a neuropsychologist to make diagnoses is quite limited and highly dependent on experience. The neuropsychological examination is not a duplication of the neurological examination, and a psychologically trained neuropsychologist is not a neurologist. Thus in this area a neuropsychologist's function is to provide some information that may be helpful to the neurologist in making diagnoses.

Another limitation of neuropsychological testing is the length of time it takes to administer a battery of tests. One of the principles of test construction is that, in general, the longer the scale, the more accurate it is. Although there is a point of diminishing returns, nevertheless a good scale will contain many homogeneous items. This means that an adequate battery of tests will take a considerable amount of time. The LNB has attempted to avoid this difficulty by having items that use only two or three points (nominal scales). The "scales" are composed of heterogeneous groups of such items. It loses accuracy in its attempt to use heterogeneous scales composed of such brief items (Spiers, 1981).

Although the HRB is longer, most of the examiners have utilized technicians to do the testing (Matthews, 1981). This means that the amount of time actually used by the neuropsychologist is relatively short, as it is only the amount of time that it takes to interpret the results and write a report. Of course, psychologists who have no technician must administer the entire battery themselves, which is an inefficient use of professional time.

Finally, there is the important limitation common to all psychology testing, that testing requires patient cooperation. A patient who has poor motivation or who wishes to look bad may provide examination scores that are far below his or her actual ability. Although there are some ways to check for these motivation effects (Heaton, Smith, Lehman, & Vogt, 1978; Lezak, 1983, pp. 618-622), it remains a difficult problem.

REHABILITATION

In the last few years clinical neuropsychologists have become involved in the rehabilitative aspect of brain injury (Diller & Gordon, 1981). Their particular background, which includes psychometrics, education methods, personality studies, and neurology, is an ideal foundation for rehabilitation activities. As psychologists they are familiar with personality and social variables and testing procedures. To this, their added training in neurology provides an understanding of medical issues. They are in a position of not only testing patients but also interpreting the results and utilizing the results to construct rehabilitation programs. In this they often work closely with speech therapists and other physical rehabilitation specialists.

The neuropsychological examination is a vital part of this program in determining the areas of deficit and the assets of the patient with which the therapist can work (Diller & Gordon, 1981; Lynch, 1981). Various programs have been designed to help specific problems (Diller & Gordon, 1981), including the use of electronic games (Lynch, 1981).

Another aspect of rehabilitation has been that of counseling families of brain injured persons (Lezak, 1978a). Brain damage such as head trauma or stroke can have terrible disruptive effects on a family. The change in the mental status of a member, especially a parent, may require a reorganization of family patterns. Clinical neuropsychologists with training in psychotherapy may be extremely helpful in counseling and administering psychotherapy to the families of such patients (Lezak, 1978a). The effects of brain damage may be obvious and disruptive, or more subtle but just as damaging to social relations (Lezak, 1978b). Neuropsychological testing becomes important as a basis for such counseling (Small, 1980).

Although rehabilitation and counseling activities of neuropsychologists are in their infancy, they undoubtedly will grow in importance for neuropsychologists because there is great need for them (Lezak, 1978a), and the training of clinical neuropsychologists fits them to fulfill this need.

EXAMPLES

Among the many functions that the neuropsychological examination serves, the determination of the severity of impairment in various functions is probably the most important, as this has implications for the rehabilitation and care of patients.

In the first example, which does not require presentation of the patient's actual test scores, there is an older patient who became rather paranoid. He accused his wife of cheating on him and wasting his money. A neuropsychological examination indicated a moderate to severe organic impairment and a pattern consistent with a slowly progressive organic condition such as Alzheimer's disease. As such the paranoia was secondary to the organic problem. Nevertheless, a social worker intern who had not read the patient's record initiated a couples therapy program in order to deal with this patient's "psychological problem." There were no positive results from the therapy, as might be expected. Luckily, the intern's error was discovered by his supervisor, who had read the record. The treatment was changed to counseling the patient's wife as to the effects of brain damage and how to deal with the emotional effect of her husband's organic condition. In this case neuropsychological testing was of crucial importance in the patient's treatment. A book by Small (1980) discusses such problems in detail.

A second example of the importance of such findings is provided by the following case of a 42-year-old male (C0033), who had been a telephone lineman. He had received a severe head injury in an automobile accident 7 months prior to testing. He was unconscious for 2 weeks after the accident and had bloody cerebral spinal fluid. At the time of the neuropsychological examination his neurological examination had almost returned to a normal level. There was only a mild ataxia and a slight wide base gate. The isotope brain scan and EEG were normal (he was not given a CT scan because at the time of this examination they were not in wide use).

This patient's neuropsychological examination scores are summarized in Table 8.2. The scale scores were obtained using the norms created by Rennick (Russell et al., 1970). One is normal, two borderline, and the higher the score the greater the impairment. The Average Brain Damage score (Average B.D.) is the mean of the 12 index scale scores presented immediately below the average. An Average B.D. scale score of more than 1.50 is considered to indicate the beginning of the brain damage range. Only the raw impairment scores are given for the perceptual tests. Any score on these tests indicates some impairment. This patient's score indicates an overall moderate impairment.

However, this score only begins to tell the story. The tests of aphasia, sensory functions (Finger Agnosia, Fingertip Writing), and even motor test (tapping) are in or near the normal range. Consequently there are few physical indications of impairment, and the neurological examination would be expected to appear almost normal, which it was. Inasmuch as the WAIS, Vocabulary, Comprehension, and Information were average, his speaking and thinking would also superficially appear normal. In other words, it would be quite possible for a neurologist to say that his functioning had returned to normal.

The other tests indicate how deceiving was this superficial appearance. All his fluid functions are strongly impaired. His thinking is slow (Digit Symbol and Trails A) and he cannot deal with complex material (Trails B and TPT). He cannot deal very effectively with spatial relations (Block Design, Object Assembly, Trails A). (The specific Spatial Relations test in the index is a hold test and is in the normal range.) Probably, functions in the right hemisphere are more impaired than the left but the primary impairment is of fluid abilities in both hemispheres. (Fluid left hemisphere functions are: Trails B and Speech Perception.)

In regard to disposition, this man could not return to his previous work as a lineman though superficially he might appear able to do so. Because the lesion is 7 months old only mild improvement can be expected. Thus, his disability will undoubtedly be permanent and he will probably need a disability retirement.

He will be able to take care of himself at home as long as he has help for tasks

TABLE 8.2
Neuropsychology Summary

Subject: PF C0033
Age 42 Ed 4
R X L ___ Hand   *Occupation: Telephone Lineman*

	Raw	Scale			Raw	Scale
AVERAGE B.D.	2.71	3	Trails A		145	5
Category	116	4	Trails B		420	5
Trails B	460	5				
Tapping R.L.	37	3	TPT R B1 3 (10.0)	T	17	3
Digit Symbol	0	6	TPT L B1 5 (10.0)	T	15	3
TPT (Time) BL12 T	48	3	TPT B B1 4 (10.0)	T	16	4
TPT (Memory)	6	2				
TPT (Location)	1.5	4				
			MOTOR TESTS			
Rhythm	5	1	Tapping R		37	3
Speech	19	3	Tapping		26	3
Aphasia	12	2	Grip (kilo) R		37	
Spatial Relations	2	1	Grip (kilo) L		29	
Perceptual Errors	9	1				

			PERCEPTUAL TESTS		Raw	
WAIS SCORES	Scale	Age			R	L
Verbal IQ	53	93	Tactile Sup (12)		0	0
Performance IQ	24	71	Auditory Sup (4)		0	0
F S IQ	77	83	Visual Sup (12)		0	0
Information	11	11	F. Agnosia (20)		0	6
Comprehension	13	13	F T W (20)		2	1
Arithmetic	6	6				
Similarities	6	6				
			MEMORY			
Digit Span	7	6	Verbal:	Raw	Scale	%
Vocabulary	10	10	Immed.	NT ___	___	
Digit Span	0	2	1/2 hr.	NT ___	___	
Picture Completion	7	7	Figural:			
Block Design	6	6	Immed.	NT ___	___	
Picture Arrangement	6	7	1/2 hr.	NT ___	___	
Object Assembly	5	6				

that require complex judgment. However, he will no longer be able to be an effective head of the household though his wife may allow him to be the head in name. He may not even be able to drive an automobile safely. His wife may need to go to work if she had not done so previously. Thus, head trauma will have a devastating effect on the family, which will require major reorganization of their duties and their way of dealing with problems. The wife, older children, and any psychologist or social worker who is working with the family should be aware of these potential effects and understand their consequences. As such the neuropsychological examination findings will be of utmost importance.

A second example is that of a 22-year-old white female (C0545), who had a history of dyslexia beginning in grade school. There was no history of head trauma or neurological disease. She has had special training in reading and at one point had psychotherapy with the idea that the dyslexia was functional. She had recently attempted to hold a job as a waitress but had failed. Her neuropsychological test results are given in Table 8.3.

These results of this person's testing are generally within the normal range and in fact the Average B.D. (Average Brain Damage) score 1.30 does not reach the brain damage range of 1.50. Examination of the overall test pattern does however demonstrate an area of decreased function. Almost all tests related to the left temporoparietal area were impaired. Her verbal IQ was 88, whereas her performance IQ was 110. She did especially poorly on Information, Arithmetic, and Vocabulary. Although this might conceivably be due to poor reading ability, the Verbal or "Logical" Memory on the Revised Wechsler Memory Scale (Russell, 1975), which used an auditory presentation, was also rather strongly impaired. At the end of a half hour she retained only about 25% of the amount of material that is normally retained. (The percentage score for this memory test is the percentage retained compared to a normal person, i.e., the control group for the original study, Russell, 1975.)

These findings would be consistent with an area of congenital damage or brain agenesis in the left temporoparietal area. Thus, there appeared to be an organic origin for her dyslexia.

In regard to future planning, she had already had a great deal of remedial training in reading and she was beyond school age. Consequently, the impairment would not be much improved by further remediation. The problem was thus to find an appropriate occupation for her. She had already failed as a waitress, which was quite understandable, as her verbal recent memory was so poor. The recommendation was to seek vocational guidance in order to place her in a job that did not require a large verbal component. This was done and she was able to lead a normal life.

These examples demonstrate the manner in which neuropsychological testing can be of benefit to patients who have brain damage and may help professionals and family members cope with the problems involved in the care of people with brain damage. Modern medicine is enabling a far higher proportion of people who sustain head injury to survive. As a consequence, the number of people with lifelong brain damage is increasing. Adequate care requires the kind of evaluation that a neuropsychological examination can provide. Neuropsychological work in the rehabilitation of such patients is increasing. Thus, neuropsychology will become an increasingly important branch of medical psychology as this area develops.

TABLE 8.3
Neuropsychology Summary

Subject: CK C0545
Age 22 Ed 12
R X L ___ Hand   *Occupation:* _____

	Raw	Scale				Raw	Scale
AVERAGE B.D.	1.30	1	Trails A			25	1
Category	64	2	Trails B			80	1
Trails B	80	1					
Tapping R.L.	51	0	TPT R B1 10	T	7.9	1	
Digit Symbol	58	1	TPT L B1 10	T	4.2	1	
TPT (Time) BL30 T	14.5	1	TPT B B1 10	T	2.4	1	
TPT (Memory)	7	1					
TPT (Location)	2	3					
			MOTOR TESTS				
Rhythm	NT	—	Tapping R			51	0
Speech	NT	—	Tapping L			46	0
Aphasia	11	2	Grip (kilo) R			NT	—
Spatial Relations	2	1	Grip (kilo) L			NT	—
Perceptual Errors	9	1					

			PERCEPTUAL TESTS		*Raw*	
WAIS SCORES	*Scale*	*Age*			R	L
Verbal IQ (prorated)	47	88	Tactile Sup (12)		0	1
Performance IQ	58	110	Auditory Sup (4)		0	0
F S IQ	105	97	Visual Sup (12)		1	0
Information	7	7	F. Agnosia (20)		0	2
Comprehension	NT	—	F T W (20)		1	2
Arithmetic	5	5				
Similarities	11	11				

			MEMORY			
Digit Span	9	9	Verbal:	*Raw*	*Scale*	*%*
Vocabulary	7	7	Immed.	13	4	56
Digit Symbol	11	11	1/2 hr.	6	4	29
Picture Completion	10	10	Figural:			
Block Design	10	10	Immed.	10	1	96
Picture Arrangement	11	11	1/2 hr.	6	3	66
Object Assembly	16	15	WRAT R. Gr.	8.7	Scale	3.4

REFERENCES

Adams, K. M. In search of Luria's battery: A false start. *Journal of Consulting and Clinical Psychology,* 1980, *48,* 511−512.

Bender, L. A visual motor gestalt test and its clinical use. *American Orthopsychiatric Association Research Monographs, No. 3,* 1938.

Benton, A. L. *The revised visual retention test (3rd ed.)*. New York: Psychological Corp., 1963.

Benton, A. L. Psychologic testing. In A. B. Baker & L. H. Baker (Eds.), *Clinical Neurology* (Vol. 1). New York: Harper & Row, 1975.

Bigler, E. D., & Ehrfurth, J. W. The continued inappropriate singular use of the Bender Visual Motor Gestalt Test. *Professional Psychology*, 1981, *12*, 562 – 569.

Boll, T. J. The Halstead – Reitan Neuropsychology Battery. In S. B. Filshov & T. J. Boll (Eds.), *Handbook of clinical neuropsychology*. New York: Wiley – Interscience, 1981.

Brilliant, P. J., & Gynther, M. O. Relationship between performance on three tests of organicity and selected patient variables. *Journal of Consulting Psychology*, 1963, *27*, 474 – 479.

Cattell, R. B. The measurement of adult intelligence. *Psychological Bulletin*, 1943, *3*, 153 – 193.

Christensen, A. Luria's neuropsychological investigation. New York: Halstead, 1975.

Crosson, B., & Warren, R. L. Use of the Luria – Nebraska Neuropsychological Battery in aphasia: A conceptual critique. *Journal of Consulting and Clinical Psychology*, 1982, *50*, 22 – 31.

Delis, D. C., & Kaplan, E. The assessment of aphasia with the Luria – Nebraska Neuropsychological Battery: A case critique. *Journal of Consulting and Clinical Psychology*, 1982, *50*, 32 – 39.

Diller, L., & Gordon, W. A. Rehabilitation and clinical neuropsychology. In S. B. Filshov & T. J. Boll (Eds.), *Handbook of clinical neuropsychology*. New York: 1981.

Exner, J. E. *The Rorschach: A comprehensive system*. New York: Wiley, 1974.

Finlayson, M. A. Text complexity and brain damage at different educational levels. *Journal of Clinical Psychology*, 1977, *33*, 221 – 223.

Fitzhugh, K. B., Fitzhugh, L. C., & Reitan, R. M. Wechsler – Bellevue comparisons in groups with "chronic" and "current" lateralized and diffuse brain lesions. *Journal of Consulting Psychology*, 1962, *26*, 306 – 310.

Golden, C. J. A standardized version of Luria's Neuropsychological evaluation. In S. B. Filshov & T. J. Boll (Eds.), *Handbook of clinical neuropsychology*. New York: Wiley, 1981.

Goldstein, K., & Scheerer, M. Abstract and concrete behavior: An experimental study with special tests. *Psychological Monographs*, 1941, *53*, 2, Whole No. 239.

Goodglass, H., & Kaplan, E. *The assessment of aphasia and related disorders*. Philadelphia: Lea & Febiger, 1972.

Graham, F. K., & Kendall, B. S. Memory-for-designs test: Revised general manual. *Perceptual and Motor Skills*, 1960, *11*, 147 – 188.

Halstead, W. C. *Brain and intelligence*. Chicago: University of Chicago Press, 1947.

Heaton, R. K., Smith, H. H., Lehman, R. A. W., & Vogt, A. T. Prospects for taking believable deficits on neuropsychological testing. *Journal of Consulting and Clinical Psychology*, 1978, *46*, 892 – 900.

Hecaen, H., & Albert, M. L. *Human neuropsychology*. New York: Wiley – Interscience, 1978.

Horn, J. L. Human abilities: A review of research and theory in the early 1970s. *Annual Review of Psychology*, 1976, *27*, 437 – 485.

Hutt, M. L., & Gibby, R. G. *An atlas for the Hutt adaptation of the Bender – Gestalt test*. New York: Grune & Stratton, 1970.

Kertesz, A. *Aphasia and associated disorders: Taxonomy, localization and recovery*. New York: Grune & Stratton, 1979.

Lashley, K. S. *Brain mechanisms and intelligence*. Chicago: University of Chicago Press, 1929.

Lezak, M. D. *Neuropsychological assessment* (2nd ed.). New York: Oxford University Press, 1983.

Lezak, M. D. Living with the characterologically altered brain injured patient. *Journal of Clinical Psychiatry*, 1978, *39*, 592 – 594. (a)

Lezak, M. D. Subtle sequelae of brain damage: Perplexity, distractibility and fatigue. *American Journal of Physical Medicine*, 1978, *57*, 9 – 15. (b)

Luria, A. R. *The working brain*. New York: Basic Books, 1973.

Luria, A. R. *Higher cortical functions in man (2nd rev. ed.)*. New York: Basic Books, 1980.

Luria, A. R., & Majovski, L. V. Basic approaches used in American and Soviet clinical neuropsychology. *American Psychologist*, 1977, *32*, 959 – 968.

Lynch, W. J. *Program description of a brain injury rehabilitation unit*. Unpublished, 1981, VA Medical Center, Menlo Park, Palo Alto, Calif. 94304.

Matthews, C. G. Neuropsychology practice in a hospital setting. In S. B. Filskov & T. J. Boll (Eds.), *Handbook of clinical neuropsychology*. New York: Wiley, 1981.

McFie, J. Psychological testing in clinical neurology. *Journal of Nervous and Mental Disorders*, 1960, *131*, 383 – 393.

Meier, M. INS task force on education, accreditation and credentialing. *The INS Bulletin*, 1981, 5 – 10.

Milner, B. Memory and the medial temporal regions of the brain. In K. H. Pribram & D. E. Broadbent (Eds.), *Biology of memory*. New York: Academic Press, 1970.

Nunnally, J. C. *Psychometric theory* (2nd ed.). New York: McGraw – Hill, 1978.

Pascal, G. R., & Suttell, B. J. *The Bender – Gestalt test: Quantification and validity for adults*. New York: Grune & Stratton, 1951.

Piotrowski, Z. The Rorschach inkblot method in organic disturbances of the central nervous system. *Journal of Nervous and Mental Disease*, 1937, *86*, 525 – 537.

Quattlebaum, L. F. A brief note on the relationship between two psychomotor tests. *Journal of Psychology*, 1968, *27*, 281.

Reed, H. B. C., & Reitan, R. M. Changes in psychological test performance associated with the normal aging process. *Journal of Gerontology*, 1963, *18*, 271 – 274.

Reitan, R. M. Certain differential effects of left and right cerebral lesions in human adults. *Journal of Comparative and Physiological Psychology*, 1955, *48*, 474 – 477.

Reitan, R. Psychological deficits resulting from cerebral lesions in man. In J. M. Warren & K Akert (Eds.), *The frontal granular cortex and behavior*. New York: McGraw – Hill, 1964.

Reitan, R. M. Verbal problem solving as related to cerebral damage. *Perceptual and Motor Skills*, 1972, *34*, 515 – 524.

Reitan, R. M. Assessment of brain – behavior relationships. In P. McReynolds (Ed.), *Advances in psychological assessment* (Vol. 1. 30). San Francisco: Jossey – Bass, 1974.

Reitan, R. M., & Davison, L. A. *Clinical neuropsychology: Current status and applications*. New York: John Wiley, 1974.

Russell, E. W. A multiple scoring method for the assessment of complex memory functions. *Journal of Consulting and Clinical Psychology*, 1975, *43*, 800 – 809.

Russell, E. W. The Bender – Gestalt and the Halstead – Reitan Battery: A case study. *Journal of Clinical Psychology*, 1976, *32*, 355 – 361.

Russell, E. W. Three patterns of brain damage on the WAIS. *Journal of Clinical Psychology*, 1979, *35*, 611 – 620.

Russell, E. W. Fluid and crystallized intelligence: Effects of diffuse brain damage on the WAIS. *Perceptual and Motor Skills*. 1980, *51*, 121 – 122. (a)

Russell, E. W. Tactile sensation—An all-or-none effect of cerebral damage. *Journal of Clinical Psychology*, 1980, *36*, 858 – 864. (b)

Russell, E. W. *Theoretical bases of Luria – Nebraska and Halstead – Reitan batteries*. Paper presented at the 88th Annual Convention of the American Psychological Association, Montreal, Canada, 1980. (c)

Russell, E. W. The chronicity effect. *Journal of Clinical Psychology*, 1981, *37*, 246 – 253.

Russell, E. W., Neuringer, C., & Goldstein, G. *Assessment of brain damage: A neuropsychological key approach*. New York: Wiley – International, 1970.

Satz, P. Specific and nonspecific effects of brain lesions in man. *Journal of Abnormal Psychology*, 1966, *71*, 65 – 70.

Small, L. *Neuropsychodiagnostics in psychotherapy (Rev. ed.)*. New York: Brunner/Mazel, 1980.

Smith, A. Neuropsychological testing in neurological disorders. In W. J. Friedlander (Ed.), *Advances in neurology* (Vol. 7). New York: Raven Press, 1975.

Spiers, P. A. Have they come to praise Luria or to bury him? The Luria – Nebraska Battery controversy. *Journal of Consulting Psychology,* 1981, *49,* 331 – 341.

Teuber, H. L. Physiological psychology. *Annual Review of Psychology,* 1955, *6,* 267 – 296.

Teuber, H. L., & Weinstein, S. Equipotentiality versus cortical localization. *Science,* 1958, *127,* 241 – 242.

Walsh, K. W. *Neuropsychology: A clinical approach.* New York: Churchill Livingstone, 1978.

Warrington, E. K., Logue, V., & Pratt, R. T. C. The anatomical localization of selective impairment of auditory verbal short-term memory. *Neuropsychologia,* 1971, *9,* 377   387.

9   Multisystems Interventions in Disease

Jack T. Tapp
University of Miami and Nova University

INTRODUCTION

Disease is the product of disruption at one or more levels of multiple interacting control systems that are organized hierarchically. Health reflects the relative equilibrium at all these levels of the hierarchy. In this model of disease, diagnosis should assess specific dysfunctions at each level of the hierarchy and, where possible, specify the genetic, environmental, and experiential contributions to the disease process.

The functions of intervention are to: (1) prevent disequilibrium; (2) restore equilibrium in these systems; and (3) improve the capacity of the individual to adapt and grow to a healthier level of functioning. Treatment is thus predicated on restoring function at all levels of the hierarchy. Rehabilitation would enhance the functional state of the organism and minimize the probability of the recurrence of disease. All forms of intervention require the identification of measurable end-points that define systemic equilibrium.

The multisystem model is in its developmental stages in health care. Engel (1980) and Schwartz (1982) have outlined similar concepts, and work by Edelstein, Ross, and Schultz (1982) has shown how particular interventions reflect its application. Research on interventions in behavioral medicine has focused primarily on the evaluation of different levels of intervention and the issues that affect the efficacy of treatment at each level.

This chapter reviews some of the techniques of intervention that involve the behavior of individual patients. The intention is to examine research that has investigated different forms of treatment and to arrive at pragmatic directions in asserting those principles of intervention that appear to be effective. Research in these areas is still in its developmental stages. Extensive evaluation studies are needed to document and establish the efficacy of these methods.

The Behavioral Medicine Perspective

The Yale conference on behavioral medicine was explicit in directing the intervention of behavioral sciences into the application of knowledge and techniques relevant to physical health and illness to the treatment and rehabilitation of physical disorders. The roles of biological, psychological, and social factors in disease were clearly acknowledged as appropriate areas for research application (Schwartz & Weiss, 1978). Although mental illness, substance abuse, retardation, and social welfare are of course, important areas for behavioral intervention, the conference suggested that they be considered outside the usual scope of behavioral medicine except as they might influence the etiology and course of disease. Against this background, intervention strategies necessitate the recognition that the manifestations of disease are reflected in the biopsychosocial context of human existence.

It is imperative to effective intervention to understand that disease processes have a biological basis that may reflect tissue damage and/or organ dysfunctions that are not amenable solely to behavioral interventions. Knowledge of the particular disease and its physiological basis are therefore important considerations in planning and implementating behavioral medicine interventions. The therapist must know and understand the ramifications of the disease for the patient and the consequences of the treatment on the patient's life-style. These factors set limits on the interventions that are feasible and possible. For example, implementing an exercise program for a diabetic patient will have consequences on the use of insulin for the control of diabetes (Skyler, 1979). Ulcers may be produced by excitation of the vagus nerve, which increases gastric motility and hypersecretion of acid into the stomach. This is a physiological response that may be exacerbated by psychological stress and have a greater probability in those individuals who have unresolved conflicts between their needs of dependence and independence (Alexander, 1950). Nevertheless, the bleeding ulcer must be treated along with interventions intended to resolve the behavioral manifestations of stress and/or the unresolved conflicts. The assessment of Type A behavior pattern described by Rosenman and Friedman predicts an increased probability of a reoccurrence of a myocardial infarction (MI) over those who have MI's and who are Type B. Although behavioral treatment may be useful for modifying manifestations of the Type A behavior pattern and reducing the risk of coronary heart disease, care must be expended to insure that the behavioral interventions do not conflict with the medical constraints of the situation.

In these examples, behavioral interventions might be a part of the total treatment plan for the patient. For other diseases, behavioral interventions may reflect the only source of treatment that is effective in the disease. In Raynaud's disease, for example, temperature biofeedback reduces the incidence of attack. There is no physiological treatment available for this disease (Keefe, Surwit, & Pilon, 1979). Irritable bowel syndrome is similarly responsive to behavioral interventions and there are few medical treatments that will produce the same effective results (Latimer, 1981).

The present perspective assumes that interventions into the behavioral manifestations of the disease process require an understanding of the pathophysiology of disease. Behavioral perspectives must recognize the variations in disease presentations (sign, symptom) as well as the idiosyncratic aspects of the person's behavior and social patterns of adjustment. Thus sound intervention should reflect a well-grounded view of physiological, behavioral, and social systems perspectives on the disease process.

Physiological Events as Stimuli and Responses

Psychophysiological and biofeedback research has clearly indicated that many of the internal actions of the body can be monitored as sensory events and brought under stimulus and/or response control. In other words, the actions and reactions of physiological systems are subject to the laws of learning. This principle, as obvious as it might be, has profound implications for preventive, treatment, and rehabilitative interventions. It suggests that the stimulus properties of the pain of infections, angina, tissue damage, muscular ruptures, etc. can serve as discriminative stimuli for the initiation of operant behaviors, or as the unconditioned stimuli for respondent adaptations. It is the recognition that these physiological mechanisms are subject to the "laws of learning" that gives legitimacy to the understanding of the behavioral antecedents and consequences of disease.

The behaviors that an individual engages in also determine the particular manifestations of diseases. The linkage between smoking cigarettes and the incidence of pulmonary and cardiovascular disease is a well-known and valid example of behavior contributing to diseases via physiological manifestation. There are numerous similar examples of behavioral patterns that exacerbate and/or dispose the individual to identifiable diseases.

Disease as a Life Crisis

From the social-psychological perspective, the sudden onset of disease affords the potential for a life crisis. The stress to living imposed by the onset of illness is foreign to the usual experience of a healthy life. Disease onset demands behavioral and life-style adjustments that are often severe in their emotional consequences and in their impact on the individual's psychosocial environment. Depending on the person's coping style, supports, and previous history of adaptation to stress, the onset of disease can precipitate a crisis. Similarly, social stresses may serve as precipitants of biological disease. Studies by Engel (1971), Lindemann (1944),

Rahe and his associates (Rahe, 1972; Rahe, Mahan, & Arthur, 1970), and others are strongly suggestive of this phenomenon (see Chapters 1 and 5).

The rise in emotional tension accompanying a life change, followed by failure of the usual methods of coping, are the first two stages of crisis development. Without resources, tension increases further until a full crisis emerges (Caplan, 1964; Hoff, 1978). The source of the life change that precipitates the crisis can originate from a number of specific events, any of them requiring alterations in behavior to produce a responsive, successful outcome.

The interactive phenomena just described argue strongly for multisystems intervention in disease. When viewed from a holistic perspective, disruption at any level of systemic control can produce alterations in healthy functioning as a consequence and precipitate a crisis. The analysis of these alterations requires examination of the biological, behavioral, and social phenomena reflecting the disease. A comprehensive multisystem treatment plan requires attention to all these areas of functioning simultaneously and to the development of management strategies that achieve definable health goals as the endpoints of treatment.

The Role of the Behavioral Medicine Specialist

The increasing involvement of behavioral scientists in health care has expanded their role into new realms of treatment. These roles are still being defined, although attempts are increasingly being made to delineate them with more precision (Budman & Wertlieb, 1979).

Zimmerman (1981) has outlined three levels of intervention by the behavioral medicine specialist that correspond roughly to the primary, secondary, and tertiary care that delineates the tasks of the therapist. At the level of primary care, behavioral medicine specialists focus on risk reduction, using techniques of behavioral and cognitive interventions. The therapist serves as a teacher or consultant to the patient and assists in developing plans for specific behavioral changes that will lower risk for disease by altering self-destructive behavior patterns. The intervention focuses less on personality alterations or total life-style modification than it does on habit change. Prescriptive treatments are used.

At the level of secondary care, intervention requires a potentially greater degree of alteration in behavior. The individual who has disease and is seeking help is more in need of treatment that will require complex intervention and a high level of motivation to change behaviors that are conducive to the attainment of health. Intervention at this level necessitates cognitive restructuring that goes beyond prescriptive changes to include alterations in belief systems and perceptual set. The relationship to the patient is defined as that of a psychotherapist or counselor, with active, collaborative intervention required. Rapport and the relationship with the patient are an integral part of the treatment paradigm to facilitate motivation of the patient.

At the tertiary level, the behavioral medicine specialist is a part of a total treatment team. The behavioral management of disease at this level potentially requires extensive interventions in altering beliefs, life-styles, contingencies, life goals, relationships, work adjustments, role behaviors, etc. More comprehensive and systematic planning are a necessary part of the treatment.

In all these areas of intervention, Zimmerman (1981) suggests that the critical therapist variables in treatment and those that promote the attainment of therapeutic goals are variables that reflect a quality of emotional involvement with the patient. Such relationships can promote learning and influence persuasion and the healing process. He suggests that the role of "behavioral coach" defines the level of involvement and the methods of persuasion needed to work with people to effect health outcomes. Coaches are instructors, teachers, interpersonal relationship developers, directors, urgers, suggestors, inducers. And probably other things as well. They motivate individuals through a variety of techniques that include cheerleading and prodding, techniques that Zimmerman describes as push – pull methods. In addition, they possess the knowledge and skills about the response repertoires that are necessary to effect behavior changes that lead ultimately to the "success" of the player and the team.

Zimmerman's (1981) orientation offers a great deal of merit in defining the role of the behavior change – behavioral medicine specialist. It deviates from the more traditional role of the psychotherapist and offers an exciting alternative to a passive nondirective approach to intervention. It also reframes the concept of behavior change into a constructive viewpoint—that of winning, achieving goals, and striving for mastery of one's self—and one's health. Overall, it reflects a *positive* strategy with an emphasis on health attainment and self-control through commitment and directed effort.

TREATMENT METHODS

Biofeedback, Relaxation, and Physiological Interventions

Biofeedback as a research and clinical tool for control of muscular and autonomic activity heralded a new perspective on psychological control systems. In effect, biofeedback methods have focused attention on the role of conscious regulation of the body's physiological reactions. Numerous evaluations of these methods and their applications to treatment of a diversity of problems have been reviewed in a number of sources (Burish, 1981; Gaarder & Montgomery, 1977; Holmes, 1981; Katkin & Goldband, 1979). For our purposes, we need only examine prototype procedures, their applications, and limitations.

The endpoint of biofeedback is symptom removal and control of physiological responses. The feedback provided by an instrument that amplifies biological signals is used as a device to: (1) bring the biological signals that are related to stress reactions into the patient's awareness; (2) demonstrate to the patient that control is possible; and (3) provide a criterion for conscious change that will remove or alleviate the symptoms. These methods give salience to physiological stimuli and thereby aid in developing control over these stimuli via regulated responses.

Biofeedback has been used in the study of a great many physiological events. The instrumentation varies depending on the biological system being monitored, but all the devices consist of a transducer that detects the physiological signal and a display device that gives the patient feedback about the signal. The patient is told to control the display in some manner that is presumed therapeutic for alleviation of the symptoms.

Blood pressure, heart rate, vasodilation, muscle tension, skin temperature and electroencephalographic rhythms have all been demonstrated to be controllable when feedback is given. Furthermore, biofeedback techniques have been used for treating the variety of associated disorders to which they are applicable (e.g., some cardiac arrythmias, Raynaud's disease, migraine headaches, tension headaches, and skeletal muscular disorders). In most instances when the patient is motivated to comply and is persistent in practice outside the clinic, these techniques can be demonstrated to be effective in the control and removal of the symptoms that are monitored. Biofeedback has established itself as a useful clinical tool (Blanchard & Young, 1974; Simkins, 1982).

Biofeedback also has direct and important application in the area of skeletal – muscle reeducation. It provides patients with a means of relearning even when some aspects of the feedback system are nonfunctional (e.g., sensory nerve damage). This application has been demonstrated for spinal cord injuries, lower-back spasms, peripheral nerve damage, cerebral palsy, stroke, spasmodic torticollis, and a great number of other muscular problems. Some of this work is reviewed in more detail elsewhere in this volume (see Chapters 8 and 20.)

Neuromuscular reeducation may be the single most important area in the application of biofeedback devices. Electromyographic feedback has been shown to have successful application to hemiplegias following stroke. In these studies, electrodes are inserted or attached to an area of paralysis (e.g., the muscles of the arm), and the patient is taught to increase the signal provided by the feedback unit by moving the muscle. Repeating this process by contracting the muscles leads to enhanced strength in the muscle group. The patient ultimately gains a sense of voluntary control over the limb. With visualization of the limb movement, the patient develops a capacity to regulate movement through feedback. After preliminary training, implanted electrodes are removed and surface electrodes are used with a portable unit for home practice. This application of EMG biofeedback has been reported repeatedly as producing successful recovery to the point where it is a standard procedure in many stroke rehabilitation programs.

Another application of biofeedback neuromuscular reeducation is in a study reported by Engel, Nikoomanesch, & Schuster (1974). In six patients, they were able to teach control of severe fecal incontinence by training the simultaneous contraction of the external anal sphincter along with relaxation of the internal sphincter.

The specific applications of biofeedback to stress-related symptoms has been the subject of theoretical argument and empirical investigation. Research has examined whether it is necessary to use a specific biological response to get the results attributable to biofeedback. Katkin and Murray (1968) studied the response patterns of subjects who were successful in controlling feedback from autonomic activity. Their results indicated that a combination of somatomotor and cognitively mediated behaviors was initiated to produce the observed effects. Subsequent research has repeatedly confirmed these findings. Those studies that have compared biofeedback to other forms of relaxation training have consistently failed to demonstrate any differences in their effectiveness (Burish, 1981; Qualls & Sheehan, 1981). Long-term follow-up studies also show no differences between biofeedback and relaxation although these studies indicate that continued practice is necessary for the effects of biofeedback or relaxation to endure over the long run (Burish, 1981; Lavallee et al., 1977; Reinking & Hutchings, 1976).

Relaxation techniques have been used extensively for their effects on biological and psychological reactivity. The most widely applied and investigated procedure is the technique developed by Jacobsen (1938) and used by Wolpe (1969) in the treatment of phobias and other anxiety-related symptoms. The technique involves training the patient in deep breathing, then alternately tensing and relaxing groups of muscles that usually include all the major muscle groups of the body. The focus of these instructions is on the contrast between the subjective feeling of tension and the feeling of relaxation. The aim of the treatment is to develop a response (relaxation) that is incompatible with the response (tension) that typifies reactions to stress. In the process, the patient becomes more aware of bodily tensions and the stimuli that produce them. The capacity to relax in tension-producing situations is used as a method of treatment and in training self-control of the symptoms. In addition, continued daily practice of relaxation lowers the base line of bodily tension, removing some of the skeletal – muscular responses to stress.

Meditation has also been used as a method of inducing a state of controlled relaxation. Benson (1975) has demonstrated the effectiveness of relaxation techniques in the treatment of hypertension. Benson suggests that there are four elements that cut across methods of relaxation. They are: (1) a quiet environment free from distractions and interruptions; (2) a comfortable position that can be maintained for 20 to 30 minutes without distress; (3) a mental device that is the focal point of attention, such as a mantra, a sound, an object to look at, or some mental image; and (4) a passive attitude in which thoughts, feelings, and other distractions can be cleared from the mind by ignoring them or letting them pass unnoticed. The uses of meditation techniques have been evaluated in numerous studies by their advocates and a variety of conditions have been reported to have been successfully treated.

Hypnosis offers another technique for inducing relaxation and controlling symptoms. It has a very long history of use as an analgesic and in pain control (Crasilneck & Hall, 1975). The method differs from other relaxation procedures in that there is less emphasis on the feelings of relaxation and more direction toward cognitive control and imagery. The instructions to the patient focus on the manipulation of the awareness of and reaction to the perception of the symptoms against which the therapy is being directed. According to Hilgard (1975), the critical components of the process are mental relaxation, a heightened state of suggestibility, and a narrowing of attention. In this state the patient is instructed to perceive the symptom in a manner that is incompatible with the previous perception of the symptom. Instructions might focus on "clear, healthy lungs" for a smoker who wishes to quit or "relaxed, open blood vessels" for someone being treated for hypertension. The procedures used in hypnosis progressively train the patient in the use of their attention as directed in this manner. Typically, patients are taught hypnosis procedures by the therapist until there is mastery of self-hypnosis or autosuggestion. These methods are then used for the relief of symptoms or to effect the behavioral alterations that are desired (e.g., not smoking).

The suggestibility of the subject is a critical factor of hyponosis. It is generally recognized that not all individuals can experience the altered states of consciousness that characterize the hypnotic state. Susceptibility to this state appears to be a critical factor influencing the successful application of hypnosis to behavior change (Wadden & Anderton, 1982).

There are similar attributes to biofeedback, induced relaxation, direct relaxation training, meditation, and hypnosis that are noteworthy. All involve an induced state of relaxation through deep breathing and suggestion. All have a focal point of concentration through feedback and/or verbal self-talk. They differ primarily in the degree to which there is cognitive involvement in the instruction, with hypnosis reflecting the highest level of cognitive input through the use of imagery and cognitive structuring.

Research that directly compares these methods is limited and there is little work that evaluates which of the components of any single method are essential. Surwit, Shapiro, and Good (1978) compared blood pressure biofeedback, EMG biofeedback, and meditation and found no differences among procedures in the reduction of blood pressure. All three conditions were equally effective. Throll (1981) systematically contrasted the effects of transcendental meditation with progressive relaxation over a 4-month time period on a number of variables. Meditators spent more time (4 hours a week) and were most consistent in the home practice exercises over the time period. They also paid money to an organization that reinforced the practice. These factors are of interest in themselves and suggest that the groups were self-selected for differing qualities of motivation. In spite of the fact that there were no differences between groups on any variable at pretest, the meditators showed lower reported anxiety, drug use, neuroticism, and improved health than the relaxation group. The results are generally consistent with other studies of the effects of meditation. It is of some interest that the subjects who practiced progressive relaxation reported that it was boring to use on a daily basis.

In a systematic comparison of the effects of thermal biofeedback, alpha biofeedback, and hypnosis on headache pain, Andreychuk and Schriver (1975) report that all methods decreased the number of incidents of headache. There was no differential effect of one method over the others, but patients who scored high on a measure of suggestibility had a better outcome than those who had low scores on this measure.

Wadden and Anderton (1982) have recently reviewed the effects of hypnosis on particular target behaviors such as eating and smoking. They conclude that: "hypnotic induction does not enhance bodily relaxation, clarity of visual imagery or suggestibility to a greater degree than do waking techniques [p. 240]." Although smoking, overeating, and alcoholism were not responsive, hypnosis did affect pain, warts, and asthma to the extent that the patient was suggestible. They speculate that these findings may reflect the way in which the experience is cognitively restructured via the hypnotic induction.

The involvement of the patient with the therapist is of considerable importance as a factor in the use of these procedures. A study by Beiman, Israel, & Johnson (1978) reported that live relaxation training with a therapist present was superior to taped relaxation, biofeedback, or self-relaxation in decreasing physiological measures of muscle tension, galvanic skin resistance, and respiration rate. All methods reduced self-reported anxiety and all methods produced some reduction in physiological arousal measures.

Exercise, as a form of behavioral intervention, has been prescribed for its health benefits since Hippocrates. Its value for enhancing physical and psychological health are now being established by scientific investigation. Epidemiological studies suggest that exercise may be a preventative measure for heart disease by increasing high density lipoproteins (Wood & Haskell, 1982). Exercise is preventative to the development of obesity and a useful adjunct to obesity treatment (Thompson, Jarvie, Lahey, & Cureton, 1982).

In contrast to the relaxation methods, *exercise* is a form of stress induction. The physiological effects of any single prolonged period of exercise mimics the effects of stress on the body; cardiac output increases; glycogen increases the release of glucose by the liver and its utilization in muscle; oxygen consumption increases via increased breathing rate; corticosteroids are released by the adrenal cortex; catacholamine levels rise in the blood; gastric motility decreases. If this form of stress is prolonged, extreme fatigue follows and the organism approaches a state of exhaustion.

Repeated exercise that is regulated to produce exertion without exhaustion appears to have physiological and psychological benefits for a number of minor chronic diseases. An exercise program that increases heart rate to 150 beats per minute for 15 to 30 minutes and that demands respiratory increases to produce prolonged oxygen consumption will increase physical fitness. After 6 weeks at three to five times per week, such a program will produce demonstrable changes in physiological functioning (Pollock, 1978). Specifically there is an increase in the oxygen utilization capacity of the body, a decrease in body fat, and a decrease in resting heart rate (Pollock, Wilmore, & Fox, 1978).

Simonelli and Eaton (1978) reviewed the cardiovascular and metabolic effects of exercise at a more molecular level. Serum triglycerides decrease and fats are mobilized from adipose tissue. Plasma insulin decreases while glycogen increases, with the consequent mobilization of glucose. The mitochondria in muscles increase as the muscles strengthen. The muscles in the heart strengthen, increasing the volume of blood ejected from the ventricles at a single stroke and enhancing the heart's capacity to contract. Simonelli and Eaton suggest that the effects of exercise may be mediated by hormonal factors. Growth hormone, cortisol, glucagon, and catecholamines are secreted in response to exercise (Sheppard & Sidney, 1973). These substances act to mobilize glucose and fatty acids for energy use.

The effects of exercise appear to be beneficial to improved physiological functioning. Research has shown that regular exercise is beneficial in the regulation of hypertension (Choquette & Ferguson, 1973), obesity (Thompson, Jarvie, Lahey, & Cureton, 1982), diabetes (Skyler, 1979), depression (Greist, Klein, Eischeus, & Faris, 1978) and anxiety (Morgan & Horstman, 1976).

Comparison studies suggest that relaxation training, meditation, hypnosis, biofeedback, and exercise may be useful in prevention, treatment and rehabilitation programs for a variety of health disorders. Rigorous comparative studies, followed by field trials with clinical populations, will be necessary to pinpoint the most efficacious use of these treatment modes. Several of these intervention techniques have been shown to alter the responses of biological systems that mediate the physiological reactions to stress (see Chapter 5 for a more detailed discussion). Relaxation training, for example, reduces the levels of plasma catecholamines (Mathew, Ho, Taylor, & Semchuk, 1981), as has transcendental meditation (Bujatti & Riederer, 1976). This latter finding has not been replicated (Lang, Dehof, Meuver, & Jaufman, 1979). More investigations of the interrelationships among intervention techniques and physiological changes of this type are needed.

Cognitive Methods

Changes in cognitive and emotional reactions have been the focus of all forms of psychotherapeutic interventions since their inception. Though the theories describing the manifestations and meanings of symptoms vary from one form of therapy to another, the communalities in the goals of psychotherapeutic interventions outweigh the means by which they are achieved. "The healthy, happy, full functioning individual who is in control of his/her life and able to accept self and others as imperfect human beings" has defined the endpoints in psychoanalytic, person-centered, gestalt, Adlerian as well as more cognitive behavioral therapies. As in the kingdom of Lilliput, the debate is not over the shape of the egg or its use as food but over how the egg gets broken in order to eat it. The debate in psycho-therapies is over the means by which an individual achieves the status "healthy." Pragmatic concerns such as cost relative to benefits and the level of intervention needed to fully affect health are the issues of empirical and rational debate.

Cognitive control is a basic method of behavioral interventions in medicine. To this end, cognitive methods of intervention with an emphasis on behavioral self-management have emerged as the treatment of choice for the variety of psycho-physiological problems encountered in medical settings. For purposes of this discussion, cognitive self-control methods provide a means for examining a number of techniques that utilize cognitive behavior modification.

Self-monitoring is a fundamental patient skill in behavioral interventions. Like the methods of biofeedback, self-monitoring is intended to bring into the patient's awareness the variety of circumstances that cue, support, and maintain behavior and/or symptoms. The purpose is to educate the patient in the broadest sense to the sequential nature of behavior and its interaction with the environment. In addition, self-monitoring sets up a reactive situation that in itself can influence behavior change. Self-monitoring alone has been shown to alter eating behavior (Romanczyk, 1974) and smoking frequency (McFall & Hammen, 1971).

The accuracy and success of self-monitoring depends on the specificity of the behavior to be monitored, the simplicity and utility of the monitoring device, good demonstration and practice with the therapist, emphasis on honesty and accuracy in recording, and rewards for the monitoring behavior as part of the treatment contract. Self-monitoring has application for symptom-related phenomena such as tension headaches, irritable bowels, insomnia, pain intensity, etc. In addition, it applies as a behavior change strategy that might be incorporated into eating and smoking-reduction programs or a program to increase exercise.

The information collected about the behavior or symptom would specify the time, place, the presence of others, thoughts or "self-talk" that occurs antecedent to the behavior, and the feelings, actions, events, thoughts, and other con-sequences of the behavior. For purposes of developing cognitive controls, the patient is encouraged to pay particular attention to the beliefs and thoughts that support the habit or accompany the symptoms. A short-term contract to collect this information can enhance the commitment to the treatment program while reducing resistance (Goldiamond, 1974).

Imagery and other forms of cognitive controls are part of the standard treatment armamentarium for the management of behavioral aspects of disease. Historically, systematic desensitization, flooding, and thought stopping were developed and successfully used for the treatment of anxiety-related symptoms such as phobias and obsessions. These are forms of imagery manipulation that modify the cognitive aspects of the anxiety with respect to the feared object or obsessional thought. These methods have direct application to the management of symptoms.

To apply these procedures, the patient is first taught relaxation. Then, in the relaxed state, a scene is described in some detail. In *systematic desensitization,* a series of scenes that increase in the intensity by which they promote anxiety are constructed into a hierarchy. These are described to the patient in increasing intensity until tension is perceived. The patient is then instructed to relax. The hierarchy is repeated until the patient can relax in the face of the most anxiety-provoking scenes.

In *flooding,* the relaxed patient is exposed to the fear-provoking scene and is encouraged to remain there in imagination or reality until the fear has completely subsided and relaxation returned. Because the patient does not physically escape from the situation and thus reduce the fear, the anxiety sensations habituate to the imagined stimuli that provoke the fear.

Thought stopping involves using imagery to substitute an alternative thought to the one that is the basis of an obsession. With the patient's cooperation, an alternative thought is developed. During relaxation, the patient is encouraged to concentrate on the unwanted thoughts until the command "stop" is given, then the alternative thought is substituted. It is the behavioral counterpart to the Rogers and Hammerstein prescription of whistling a happy tune when feeling afraid.

The value of the cognitive aspects of these imagery manipulations has not been fully explored in its application to disease. There has been a tendency to take the methods and apply them without regard to modifications that might enhance their effectiveness. Imagery manipulations do have effects on physiological processes. Schwartz, Weinberger, and Singer (1981) report a series of studies in which imagery is used to study the effects of emotional experiences on cardiovascular responses in college students. Carroll, Marzillier, and Watson (1980) have reported that relaxation imagery can be used to modify heart rate, but when compared with controls, the structured-imagery groups had higher heart rates through the testing session.

Hypnosis instructions rely heavily on the cognitive manipulations of imagery. In those conditions where hypnosis is used to modify the perception of pain, imagery instructions are directed at alterations of the pain experience (Wadden & Anderton, 1982). In the treatment of cancer, Simonton, Matthews-Simonton, and Sparks (1980) suggest that imagery and belief factors are influential in the progress of disease. Other studies of imagery manipulation via hypnosis or cognitive control of disease manifestations need to be conducted to examine systematically the impact of these cognitive methods on the progression of diseases.

Enhanced coping and stress management have become focal points of individual intervention in behavioral medicine. These methods combine techniques of relaxation and cognitive control. The patient and the behavior medicine specialist analyze the total complex within which disease occurs, with the aim of altering the patient's capacity to respond to the stress in healthful ways. The therapeutic intervention requires understanding the cognitive – behavioral perspective of the patient and retraining the patient to alter those behaviors to facilitate constructive and productive coping styles consistent with his or her life-style.

When any form of behavior change is introduced, the alteration adds stress to the person's life and there is subsequent adaptation to the change. Such an adaptation can be viewed as a response to stress requiring new coping behaviors by the patient. Diseases, surgical interventions, and rehabilitation therapies are certainly stressful and the use of stress management strategies aids in the subsequent adaptations of the individual. Excessive eating, cigarette smoking, and other maladaptive behaviors have a functional payoff (i.e., they reduce anxiety or depression, they facilitate social interaction, they are a part of the self-identity, etc.); therefore treatments designed to alter these behaviors must consider their stress-inducing aspects and make appropriate allowances for the development of new coping strategies. Similarly, stress-related symptoms have functional attributes that result in identifiable consequences that may be perceived as beneficial. They too must be responded to in a manner that facilitates coping to an altered life-style without symptoms.

Cohen and Lazarus (1979) discuss a model for coping that focuses on two distinct aspects of coping: problem solving and emotional coping. The former is an instrumental function intended to alter the threat within the environment. The latter attempts to regulate emotional – physiological responsiveness and to remove the subjective aspects of distress. When both are functioning in concert toward the aim of minimizing stress, adaptation or coping behaviors can proceed to constructive ends.

The concept of coping implies an active involvement in the process of adaptation to the consequences of change. Active coping is a positive response to environmental challenge and stress. The individual is "in control" and doing something to alter the situation. Vigilance, helplessness, and conservation – withdrawal are alternative mechanisms that reflect "passive coping" with an associated loss of control and learned helplessness. Interventions that utilize stress management procedures are designed to turn passive coping into active coping— to turn distress into eustress (Selye, 1974).

Antonovsky (1979) has emphasized the role of cognitive involvement in coping with stress in his salutogenic model of health. He stresses the need for coherence in the lives of individuals as a condition for health and suggests that stress and its associated tensions are overcome by mobilizing coping responses that modify the stress situation, control the meaning of the situation, and/or control the stress.

The four processes of coping outlined by Cohen and Lazarus (1979) provide the essential ingredients of a cognitively behavioral-oriented coping model: (1) information seeking gives the person knowledge related to the source of the distress, bringing into consciousness an understanding of the situation; (2) direct actions allow the patient to respond to the source of the distress; (3) controlled inhibition of action is also an adaptive mode of response with beneficial payoffs; and (4) intrapsychic processes such as denial, intellectualization, psychological distancing, detachment, and other defense mechanisms come into play in coping as they are used for emotional management. Cohen and Lazarus add a fifth coping mode, which is to turn to others for support and help. Effective intervention in response to stress would facilitate these adaptational behaviors. Other authors have described somewhat different coping processes with differing emphases. Moos and Tsu (1977) add goal setting, rehearsal of outcomes, and finding a purpose or meaning to the events as specific responses involving cognitive appraisal strategies. These theories and the related research give an orientation to the methods used in stress management interventions in disease.

Stress innoculation procedures have been developed and applied in a number of settings. These methods emphasize the cognitive control of emotional responsiveness and are designed to facilitate natural coping behaviors. The procedures outlined by Meichenbaum and Turk (1976) consist of three phases in training people to respond to stress: the educational phase, the rehearsal phase, and the applicational phase. The overall strategy is intended to give patients: (1) information about the sources of the stress and its effects on the body and the mind; (2) actions that the patient can engage in when the stress occurs; (3) ways to inhibit inappropriate responding that are maladaptive to the stressful situation; and (4) mechanisms of cognitively altering the perceptions and descriptions of the situation through self-talk strategies. These methods teach coping in a systematic manner that facilitates adaptation.

As a part of the education process, patients are instructed to view the sequence of events through the stressful process in terms of four phases: (1) preparing for the stressor; (2) confronting the stressor; (3) confronting the possibility of being overwhelmed by the stressor; and (4) reinforcing one's self for having coped. The use of self-talk statements in each of these four phases is developed as the plan for innoculation against the effects of stress.

The same strategies can be developed as a part of the self-management plan to deal with the stress of behavior change. In *preparation* for the stressor the patient should focus on: (1) what has to be done; (2) the plan for doing it; (3) the elimination of negative thoughts and worrys and (4) staying relaxed, calm, and in control of the situation. When *confronting* the stress, the patient should be taught to: (1) stay relaxed by taking deep breaths; (2) meet the challenge; (3) take one step at a time; (4) look for the positives in self; and (5) view tension as a positive sign for coping. The patient can be taught to *cope with the feeling* of being overwhelmed by: (1) pausing, relaxing; (2) studying the emotional state; (3) recognizing that it will pass shortly; (4) thinking about something else; and (5) doing something else. Finally, when the trial has passed, self-reward statements can be used: "It worked, the method was successful, you were successful, you were in control all along, you're making progress, you did it."

Rehearsal consists of developing and practicing these skills for the particular situation that is to be confronted and dealt with at the moment. In a behavior change program, rehearsal focuses on the practice of new behaviors that are incompatible with the old behaviors that are being changed. Rehearsal focuses on the development of alternative cognitive and behavioral response patterns that can be used to cope actively with the stress. This aspect of the procedure thus facilitates the learning of new behaviors.

The similarity between these methods and the cognitive self-control theory outlined by Meichenbaum (1977) is apparent. Meichenbaum suggests that there are three stages in self-control strategies. First, the patient becomes aware of the maladaptive behaviors by becoming an observer of thoughts, feelings, and actions. Second, by developing and emitting incompatible behaviors and thoughts, the patient develops the planned sequence needed for change. Third, the persistence and generalization of these changes lead to more effective consequences and thereby improves the incentive structure of the person's life-style and enhances self-esteem.

Self-reward is an important aspect of self-control training strategies including stress innoculation. Studies on this process are confirmatory to this idea. Bellack (1976), for example, found that subjects rewarded for adhering to a weight loss plan by giving themselves a self-rating and grade for their performance lost twice as much weight as a self-monitoring only group (see also Mahoney, 1974). Although different forms of reward have not been systematically investigated, self-praise, compliments, encouragements by others, and tangible rewards like money and gifts, vacations, and other recreational pursuits are all feasible and potentially work for most patients.

Cognitive – behavioral strategies are also used in the management of pain and other emotional states such as anxiety, anger, and depression with a great deal of success (Davidson, 1976). The applications and evaluation of these procedures to the management of emotions related to disease and illness are in the early stages of research.

A study by Kendall, Williams, Pechacek, Graham, Shisslak, and Herzoff (1979) describes a prototype for investigation of the effects of cognitive behavior treatments on stress related to surgical procedures. Using a measure of anxiety as their index of well-being, they compared a cognitive – behavioral stress-innoculation strategy with a patient education strategy in patients about to undergo cardiac cathaterization. These groups, when compared to a no-treatment control, showed anxiety reduction after the intervention. The stress-innoculation group members who had received instruction for applying coping strategies to the hospital situation were less anxious, as rated by physicians and technicians.

Social Skills Training

The objectives of social skills training are to enhance the individuals' capacity to: (1) identify personal and social needs; (2) develop strategies for having these needs met; and (3) practice behaviors that are socially appropriate for fulfilling these needs.

Assertiveness training represents a prototype for developing social process skills through behavioral intervention. The method is based on the recognition that often individuals do not have the skills to assert themselves in a manner that allows them to satisfy their needs. These skills are identifiable patterns of social behaviors that can be learned through a combination of modeling and rehearsal. Schwartz and Gottman (1976) have analyzed assertiveness into cognitive, behavioral, and physiological components. Those cognitive components include knowledge about the content of assertive behavior, self-statements made during assertive situations, and beliefs about the situation. Physiological components include increases in heart rate and other physiological signs of emotional arousal. Behavioral component, reflect the response patterns that make up assertive behaviors.

In assertiveness training a combination of skills are taught that can be used in social situations. These typically include: (1) relaxation to overcome anxieties produced in these situations; (2) self-talk to affirm the right of assertion; and (3) various behavioral skills that teach methods for physically asserting one's self, talking about feelings, disagreeing, requesting clarification, being persistent, asking for justification, speaking for one's rights, and negotiation (Bower & Bower, 1976).

A variety of methods are used in training that emphasize behavioral expression of social behaviors (e.g., structured role plays, psychodrama, relationship enhancement skills via disclosure, and confrontation). These methods expand the behavioral repetoire of the individual to allow him or her to identify and respond appropriately to the social situation. This, in turn, allows the individual to negotiate in the social world for those things that he or she needs to promote health.

These techniques, when mastered, give the individual a sense of control over the social environment. When applied in medical environments, they can provide methods for enhancing the care received (Howe, 1981) and they can also diminish social anxieties and facilitate social interactions that are often needed to implement the behaviors that result in successful behavior changes (e.g., saying no).

Interpersonal techniques have been an important area of therapeutic intervention in behavior change strategies. Though there is little systematic investigation of interpersonal processes in disease manifestation, literature on psychosocial factors in disease suggests that the social rewards that accompany disease behaviors are part of the "payoff matrix" that reinforces the behavior. From a different viewpoint, the social network of the individual seems to serve some function as a social buffer for disease. Isolated people without obvious sources of social supports seem to be a higher risk for disease than individuals with extensive, active social networks (see Chapter 1). This suggests that interpersonal interactions can be of value in the amelioration of disease symptoms. The success of Alcoholics Anonymous, Overeaters Anonymous, Weight Watchers Inc., Smokers Anonymous, among other group programs, provides testimony to the value of such involvements.

Systemic Interventions

Behavioral Management of Life-Style Changes. Behavioral and cognitive alterations function effectively when the treatment goal is to eliminate or develop a specific habit that can be identified and where behaviors can be prescribed. In a more comprehensive vein, there are many disease processes that require extensive alterations in the patterns of living. Cardiovascular disease, cancers, spinal cord injuries, extremes in obesity, alcoholism, etc. are best approached from the standpoint of altering specific behaviors within the context of altering life-style. Strategies of behavioral intervention at this level obviously require a broad range of considerations.

Such interventions demand a detailed examination of the individual's life-style from a diverse perspective. In addition to an analysis of the impact of the disease condition on living patterns, the behavioral, emotional, cognitive, familial, work, social, and environmental elements must be analyzed and addressed systematically to define the parameters of life-style change. In a general sense there are three forms of intervention that are applicable to alterations of this type: (1) environmental restructuring to make the environment compatible with enjoyable, healthy, stress-controlled living; (2) cognitive restructuring to alter perceptions, values, and belief patterns that contribute to stress reactions; (3) behavioral restructuring to modify responsiveness to arousal-producing stimuli and to increase the rewards received for behavior changes. By taking a health-oriented focus that defines the end of treatment in terms of a healthy life-style, it is possible to define these changes in living patterns in concrete terms, thus facilitating their effective implementation.

Goal-setting and *contracting* methods applied to these alterations provide a framework for designing systemic treatment interventions. Although these methods are applicable at all levels of behavioral intervention, the alteration of life-style requires extensive long-range goal planning and detailed contracting to promote compliance. The effectiveness of behavioral interventions is in large measure the result of having definable treatment goals that specify and make accountable the outcomes of the intervention. A written contract between intervention specialist and patient provides a means for negotiating specific outcomes and the time by which they are to occur. The goals define what alterations in behavior are desired and the dates by which they will be achieved. The contract sets the social expectations that these goals are to be achieved and outlines the responsibilities of both the patient and the therapist in achieving them.

The essence of goal-setting procedures is to project the particular dimension of living for the individual in all spheres of his or her life, including biological, psychological, and social. This approach involves: (1) defining the goals for the long run in concrete, pragmatic terms that include all aspects of the patient's life; (2) setting dates against which these goals are to be achieved; (3) working out specific steps that will lead to the goal; and (4) specifying responsibilities for these steps that define roles for the patient, therapist, families, friends, employees, etc.

The steps required to achieve the long-range goals are then reduced to smaller elements and put into the patient's life space in a pragmatic way. These become the short-range goals or performance changes to be implemented within a more immediate time frame. This practical distinction between long-range and short-range goals has been examined systematically by Mahoney (1974). In a study of weight loss when the treatment goals were defined in terms of daily eating habits (performance changes), weight loss occurred more rapidly and endured longer than when the goal was defined in terms of weight changes. Mahoney and Arnkoff (1979) suggest that this has three effects: (1) it makes the goals more salient to the behavior change; (2) it gives immediate increments to performance within the life situation that result in weight loss; and (3) it promotes attainable changes within a reasonable time period that remove the restrictions that are imposed by having to achieve immediate perfection. Short-term performance goals reflect a way of coping and changing behavior on an immediate basis.

Goal-setting and implementation procedures such as those just outlined are mechanisms by which individuals acquire skills in self-control while effecting modifications in life-style. In studies of planning and self-control, Kirschenbaum and his collaborators have examined the importance of the specificity of the plan in achieving the behavioral objectives (improved study habits and better grades). They found that highly specific plans done on a daily basis were conducive to self-regulatory failure leading to abandonment of the plan (Kirschenbaum & Karoly, 1977). When plans were moderately specific and meaningful choices were developed on a monthly basis, grades improved and self-monitoring of study habits was continued during the follow-up period of the study (Kirschenbaum, Tomarken, & Ordman, 1982). By implication, the implementation of planned behavior is enhanced if the plans are flexible within limits, providing choices that are consistent with the goals to be achieved.

The particular behavior changes to be implemented will necessarily vary for any individual and/or any disease. In an applied situation, treatment might include increasing exercise levels, decreasing smoking, improving family communication, etc. The armamentarium of behavioral technology used to achieve these ends might involve charting exercise on a daily basis, relaxation training, "nonsmoking imagery," and assertiveness training classes. The product of this intervention would be improved health through an altered life-style. The incorporation of these techniques into programmed treatment has been outlined elsewhere (Tapp & Garnier, 1982).

The concepts of planned change to attain identifiable, achievable goals have theoretical support from the control theory detailed in articles by Carver and Scheier (1983) and Glasser (1981). These theories speculate on the manner in which cognitive factors influence behavior through perceptual controls. The specification of goals defines the systemic endpoints that become the references values against which behaviors and their consequences are "tested." The planned activities leading to the goals become the program and event sequences that lead to the fulfillment of the system requirements. The rewards for these behaviors, via mastery, competence, and self-control, reinforce the definition of the healthy system.

By redefining the system in terms of health, alternative feedback loops are created that provide positive correction mechanisms to those resulting from the disease alternatives. It is in the context of these "positive control systems" that alterations in life-style are effected. In this model, the ultimate measure of the success of intervention is the healthy, happy individual.

A variety of behavioral and cognitive methods can be developed and incorporated into this change process. These can include exercise, relaxation, social assertiveness, imagery manipulations, cognitive restructuring, and so on. All these methods are brought to the therapeutic arena to assist patients in redefining and reprogramming their lives to achieve a healthy life (Tapp & Garnier, 1982). These concepts of therapeutic intervention reflect a theory of multilevel control systems that integrate cognitive coping skills into social – behavioral – physiological changes.

Social Systems Interventions. The role of social-stress factors as antecedents and consequences to disease manifestations has been repeatedly demonstrated. The probability of coronary heart disease increases with changes in occupation (Kaplan, Cassell, Tyroler, Cornoni, Kleinbaum, & Hames, 1971), place of residence (Syme, Borhani, & Buechley, 1965), or loss of a loved one (Engel, 1971). Individuals with fewer friends and contacts with others have higher mortality rates (Berkman & Syme, 1979).

The value of social supports in recovery from disease has not been systematically examined. Limited evidence exists suggesting that group therapies may be beneficial in aiding in recovery from coronary heart disease. Short-term involvement with a group decreased depression and hypochondriasis following a myocardial infarction (Mone, 1970). Compliance with medication, smoking decreases, decreased incidence of angina, and more effective use of nitroglycerine were reported for group participants after a myocardial infarction by Rahe, Rufflic, Suchor, and Arthur (1973).

In a systematic study of post-MI patients, those who were assigned to a group reported less social alienation, fewer exaggerated feelings of responsibility, and less competition than controls (Ibrahim, Feldman, Sultz, Staiman, Young, & Dean, 1974). These effects were not enduring, and 6-month follow-up indicated that behavior changes had not lasted. These were not therapeutic groups, however, but rather served as a focal point for supportive discussions. Wise, Cooper, and Ahmed (1982) evaluated the efficacy of short-term interventions with a group of patients with irritable bowel syndrome. They combined relaxation, stress management, and didactic training over a series of sessions. Diet changes were observed in 50% of the group and symptoms were reduced in 30%.

The value of social supportive activities such as information and support groups has been demonstrated for alcoholism, diabetes, and other diseases. It should be emphasized that, in spite of what might be apparent value in generating group supports and therapies for rehabilitation to diseases, the evaluation of the efficacy of these methods is still in its development stages.

Families and Disease. The impact of diseases on families has been well documented (Burr, Good, & Good, 1978; Findlay, Smith, Graves, & Linton, 1969; Glasser, Harrison, & Lynn, 1964; Parkes, 1975). Until recently, however, there had been no attempt to intervene systematically into family functioning to alter disease manifestations and process. The most notable recent effort is to be found in the work of Minuchin, Rosman, and Baker (1978). This is extremely important research from the standpoint of intervention because it approaches the family from a systems perspective. Recognizing that the family system is hierarchically powerful in the control of disease processes, these authors proceeded to outline the methods used to modify family functioning in disease processes. Specifically, they initiated the intervention process for families of asthmatics, juvenile diabetics, and anorexic children where disease was a part of the dynamics of the family system.

Minuchin et al. (1978) identified three factors that interact in the development of a disease: (1) the vulnerability of the child who presents the symptoms; (2) characteristics of the family transactional system that are maladaptive; and (3) the importance of the illness for the avoidance of conflict in the family. In the majority of the children of the families studied, there was a disease that had been diagnosed and identified as having a physiological basis. Asthma and diabetes, for example, were shown to be focal points for the conflicts within the family that were exacerbated by stresses. The ill child became a means for avoiding conflicts by any of three mechanisms that altered family interactions: triangulation, parent-child coalitions, or detouring.

When spouses are split in their communication patterns, the child is forced to ally with one parent or the other. In *triangulation*, the parents can express their hostility to one another by criticizing the way the other parent responds to the ill child. A hostile message is sent to the other spouse via the child's illness. *Coalitions* occur when the child sides with one parent against the other. The ill child becomes, for example, a protector of the weaker parent against the demands of the stronger. *Detouring* occurs when the disease is introduced as a means of avoiding other issues that arise within the marriage or the family functioning. The parents collude in submerging their conflicts in this manner.

The family transactional system in such families is dysfunctional in either of four characteristic ways:

Enmeshment characteristics are reflected in a high degree of responsiveness and involvement among family members. Relationships are highly interdependent, with weak personal boundaries and a poorly differentiated percept of the self, independent of the family. In addition, the normal boundaries between the adult and peer subsystems are weak, and often the executive functions of parents are confused.

Overprotectiveness is reflected in an excessively high degree of concern for the other's welfare within the family. Nurturing responses are constantly elicited by and supplied for the sick child. There is a great emphasis on what is pleasing and displeasing about behaviors that are directed toward family members, especially the sick member.

Rigidity in maintaining the status quo is reflected in strict adherence to rules and transaction patterns. Any change is perceived as a potential threat and thus there is constant stress on the family system. Typically the family has a strong commitment to denial as a defense against change and the disease of the child is seen as the only "problem" in the family.

Conflict resolution is lacking. The combination of rigidity, overprotection, and pathological enmeshment produces constant stress and sensitivity to conflict. There is an accompanying moral code that restricts conflict. As a consequence there is no clear negotiation of differences among family members and the problems that occur with stress remain unresolved. Consequently they occur repeatedly, only to be avoided. As a result, illness becomes a means of communication.

The intervention outlined by Minuchin is directed at these systemic problems. The therapeutic unit of intervention is the family. To oversimplify the process of therapy, the child must be freed from the enmeshed pattern and given individuality by support from the therapist. The parental conflict begins to emerge and becomes clarified. Overprotectiveness is addressed directly and redirected to reinforce individuality. Through relearning, the process of conflict resolution reduces the need for rigidity, and the family system is restored to a new and healthier functional equilibrium. By working with the total system, the family manifestations of the disease process are eliminated and the behavior of the family unit is modified to aid and support the diseased member to achieve a healthy functional state.

From a different perspective, Fordyce (1976) has outlined the importance of the role of the family in managing chronic pain patients. The family frequently functions as a reward system for the patient's pain behaviors, giving sympathy and attention for manifestations of pain. These rewards must be shifted in the course of treatment to reinforce those behaviors that reflect improvements.

Family interventions are clearly important from the standpoint of multisystems intervention. Research evaluating the effects of these social interventions on disease manifestations and recovery is in its development phases. Clearly the potential value of such methods should be systematically examined in terms of its relative costs and benefits.

Interventions and Compliance

Interventions in disease consist of altering the functioning of physiological systems by: (1) Changing behaviors that influence physiological reactions; (2) controlling the chemical environment of the body via drugs and/or; (3) structurally changing organ functioning via surgery. Each of these methods has its strengths and weaknesses, but ultimately their success depends on patient adherence to the treatment regimen. The patient's behavior directly influences the outcome of treatment.

Research studies of particular relevance to the success of behavioral and chemical interventions have focused on the class of behaviors that have been described as compliance or adherence behaviors. These behaviors are a major health-care problem (Masur, 1981). No matter how effective an intervention might be, if the patient does not conform to adhere to the conditions of the regimen, the treatment cannot be successful. On the other hand, when compliance occurs there is considerable potential for altering the course of disease.

Numerous problems confound compliance studies. The measurement of compliance varies from study to study and there is questionable validity in most measures. Verbal reports and counts of the number of pills taken, the most frequently used measures, are both subject to considerable error. In spite of these limitations, investigations of compliance have yielded some findings that are suggestive of relationships among patient characteristics, treatment phenomena, and compliance.

Demographic variables, in general, show little relationship to adherence to a medical regime. Haynes (1976) reviewed more than 150 studies of compliance and found no consistent relationships among age or sex and compliance. On the other hand, education, income, and occupational status have been reported to be related to preventive visits to a dentist (Kreisberg & Treiman, 1960). Conversely, lower-income children from fatherless families and with poor communication skills showed lower adherence to a regimen of treatment with immunosuppressants following a kidney transplant (Korsch, Fine, & Negrete, 1978). As Masur (1981) has noted, findings such as these may be related to access and cost considerations in the use of medical facilities. Individuals and families of limited means would have less easy access to medical services and would therefore find compliance relatively more costly than those with more available means.

The complexity of the treatment regimen lowers the adherence rates (Haynes, 1976). From another perspective, compliance rates vary with the degree of behavior changes implicit within the regimen (Scott, 1981). The development of new habits, such as taking a pill, shows more adherence than regimens that require changes in old habits or breaking previously existing habits. This hierarchy is suggestive of strategies for modifying behavior to enhance compliance (viz., the substitution of new incompatible habits may prove more effective than eliminating or modifying the old).

Side effects of medication have also been suggested as a critical variable in compliance. Those treatment regimens that produce disagreeable side effects are not adhered to and, as a result, the patient's condition does not improve. Conversely, some diseases have no notable symptoms and in the absence of symptoms there is a lack of compliance. Research on these issues does not afford any simple solutions to the problems they suggest (Masur, 1981). The use of behavioral strategies can improve compliance when the treatment is noxious. Hypnosis, relaxation, and imagery have been used to regulate the symptoms associated with immunosuppressants in the treatment of cancer (Burish, 1981). Contracting methods enhance compliance with hypertension medications.

The doctor—patient relationship has been presumed also to influence adherence. As a result there are numerous studies examining these interactive effects from a variety of perspectives (see Warner, Chapter 3, this volume). Conclusions are limited, though some of the problems inherent in the relationship between doctors and patients emerge from these investigations.

Communication gaps abound between patients and physicians. When asked to recall the doctor's instructions, patients can only recall about 40% of what they are told (Ley & Spelman, 1965), and 60% of the patients misunderstand their physician's directions (Boyd, Covington, Stanaszek, & Cousons, 1974). No doubt these phenomena reflect laws of learning for complex information. Clear, simple, step-by-step language, repeated by the patient with written instructions, would enhance the thoroughness of communication. Adherence is enhanced when patients can recall what they are told to do (Svarstad, 1976).

Social—emotional aspects of the relationship with the patient are also important for adherence. For example, McKenny and his collaborators reported 78% compliance with hypertensive medication when there was an ongoing counseling relationship during the 5 months of treatment. This compared with 15% compliance in noncounseled controls. Unfortunately, compliance stopped when counseling stopped (McKenney, Slining, Henderson, Devins, & Berr, 1973).

Patient satisfaction has been suggested as an important determinant of compliance. This hypothesis has empirical support from at least two studies. Davis (1968) reported that patients were less likely to comply when their interaction with the doctor reflected a negative social—emotional tone as assessed by an analysis of the interaction. Francis, Korsch, and Morris (1969) found a significant positive correlation between compliance as measured by verbal report and satisfaction with the physician.

Information about the disease does not appear to effect adherence to a treatment regimen, at least as an experimental variable (Masur, 1981). However, other aspects of information may be important as they relate to adherence. The health belief model as outlined in Chapter 1 postulates that certain aspects of the patient's belief about the disease (e.g., susceptibility and seriousness) influence the patient's action. The model suggests that information about the benefits and costs of compliance will be weighed to influence the behavior of the patient. Information is specifically related to the patient's perceptions of the value of the information with respect to the disease. This is a multiple-causation model, and research supporting its predictive validity has shown significant multiple correlations between components of the model and adherence (Becker, Maiman, Kirscht, Haefner, & Drachman, 1977).

Masur (1981) has extended the model to include consideration of the immediate and long-term consequences of compliance as reinforcers of behavior and has thus expanded the health beliefs model into a more comprehensive and testable theory. He suggests that the effective use of behavioral techniques to reinforce compliance would offer support to this extension. By tailoring the treatment to be compatible with the patient's life-style, using cuing stimuli such as charts and calendars to remind and record medication use, developing self-monitoring, and contracting techniques for compliance, the adherence to treatment regimens would be enhanced.

In this model, maximal information would be given to the patient about the disease, its causes, the prognosis if left untreated. Furthermore, information on the treatment would be given, including the precise nature of the treatment, its physiological effects, the specific behavioral steps to be implemented on a daily basis, the positive benefits to be accrued from these behavior changes, ways to monitor and reward the behaviors, reminders for behavior change, the involvements of significant others, and long-range benefits. A comprehensive plan, developed with patient involvement, and with follow-up dates projected over time, could be expressed in the form of a written contract for self-care and signed with appropriate social formalities and ceremonies to enhance behavioral involvement.

The involvement of significant others in compliance has been shown to be an important determinant of adherence. Heinzlmann and Bagley (1974) evaluated a program of exercise designed to prevent heart disease and improve health in men. Eighty percent of the participants whose wives had favorable attitudes toward the program had good or excellent patterns of compliance, whereas only 40% of those whose wives were neutral or negative complied. They conclude: "the husband's pattern of adherence was directly related to his wife's attitudes toward the program."

Stuart and Davis (1972) evaluated factors influencing adherence to a weight-control program. Those participants who reported receiving positive reinforcement from another family member showed 20% or more weight loss that was maintained for 12 months. Similar relationships between family support and adherence to a treatment program involving the use of antibuse have been demonstrated for alcoholism (Hunt & Azrin, 1973).

Becker and Green (1975) reviewed literature on the role of the family in compliance behaviors. Patient cooperation with the medical regimen was positively influenced by numerous factors within the family structure. These included: sympathy, support, and encouragement by family members; the compatibility of the normal roles and patterns with the patient's regimen; interspouse communication and attitudes; willingness to alter the environment to accommodate to the patient's needs for control; health beliefs; and the assumption of responsibility for the sick member's care.

Behavioral, psychological, and social factors have a strong and pronounced influence on adherence to treatment regimens. The factors listed in the preceding paragraph argue for holistic forms of intervention as appropriate mechanisms for influencing patient adherence to treatment regimens.

Behavioral Interventions in Disease

Research on the effects of behavioral interventions on specific disease processes is in a relatively early stage of development. It is possible to identify stages of research development that apply to investigations in this area, that are similar to the evaluation of drugs and other physiological treatment methods.

Stage 1 consists of case reports where documentation of the application of a particular method is limited to a few cases. The review of the clinical applications of biofeedback to skeletomuscular reeducation is an example of this state of research. In Stage 1 studies, data from single cases are reported in both quantitative and qualitative form. Pain ratings, symptom frequencies, etc. are charted over the course of the treatment as reflections of the change process. This form of clinical research has merit in suggesting directions for more systematic investigations. It is important that these case reports include examples of both successes and failures in the application of the method to present the broadest view possible.

Stage 2 studies consist of controlled research on clinical populations where care is given to the assignment of subjects to groups, the adherence to a treatment protocol, the use of "blind" evaluators, and so forth. The sample sizes of the groups are relatively small, and typically multiple measures of outcome are assessed. Stage 2 studies are the most characteristic of contemporary evaluation research in behavioral medicine.

Stage 3 research consists of clinical trials in the application of behavioral methods of intervention. The methods are applied and evaluated on large segments of the population who have the disease or are at risk for the disease. The most significant studies at this stage are the MRFIT studies. These are reviewed elsewhere in this volume (See Chapters 2, 3, and 17). Such studies give evaluations of intervention methods in considerable detail. More systematic research of this type needs to be done to evaluate behavioral intervention methods on both their preventive, treatment, and rehabilitation effects.

In the application of behavioral methods to the treatment of disease, it is presumed that the intervention addresses the needs of the patient, that an analysis of the behavior patterns involved has been conducted, and that the treatment program addresses the physiological status of the patient. In the development and application of these methods, it is imperative that sufficient documentation and appropriate accountability be incorporated into the treatment activities to allow them to be evaluated.

Cardiovascular Diseases.   Diseases of the heart and circulatory system have been subject to extensive behavioral interventions. The formation of the Behavioral Medicine branch of the National Heart, Lung, and Blood Institute has focused extensive research on the behavioral factors in cardiovascular disease and its treatment. Studies of the Stage 2 type are suggestive of successful models of intervention. Hypertension, for example, can be controlled by relaxation procedures. With repeated practice these techniques produce short-term diastolic decrease of about 5 to 12 mm of mercury (Surwit, Williams, & Shapiro, 1982). Hypnosis is also effective in blood pressure reduction, particularly in hypnotically susceptible patients (Friedman & Taub, 1978; Wadden & de la Torre, 1980).

Arrhythmias are a potentially serious cardiovascular condition because they frequently precede cardiac arrest. It is possible to regulate heart rate via biofeedback and relaxation in some patients, though studies of heart rate regulation in patients with arrhythmias is limited. Case studies by Weiss and Engel (1971) demonstrate the capacity of some patients to control heart rate, with some decreases in premature ventricular contractions. On the other hand, patients with third-degree heart block, where neural control of heart rate is not possible, cannot modify ventricular rates of activity.

This is an area that needs further investigation via systematic behavioral intervention. Stress is strongly implicated in the induction of sudden death (Engel, 1971). Antiarrhythmic agents are available and effective in control of heart rate. Pacemaker insertions also regulate the heart's response rate. Nevertheless, these measures are superimposed on the patient's life-style, with their subsequent side effects. Behavioral intervention methods in the treatment of arrhythmias may represent a judicious adjunct to drugs and surgical interventions.

Raynaud's disease and migraine headaches have been successfully treated with temperature biofeedback (Keefe, Surwit, & Pilon, 1979; Mitchell & White, 1977). Research suggests that relaxation procedures are equally effective (Mitchell & White, 1977). Surwit et al. (1982) conclude: "it would appear that the elevated skin temperature found to accompany relaxation or skin temperature feedback training in the treatment of migraine syndrome represents a decrease in general sympathetic outflow, which produces a reduction in migraine symptoms by minimizing cerebral vascular instability [p. 191]."

Gastrointestinal Disorders.   The GI tract is subject to a variety of disorders that are related to stress. Duodenal ulcers and ulcerative colitis are classically regarded as prototypes of psychosomatic diseases (Alexander, 1950). Nausea, vomiting, dyspepsia, diarrhea, constipation, and spastic colon can all be the result of psychophysiological reactions to stress. To the extent that this is true, they can probably be controlled by relaxation and stress management procedures (Latimer,

1981b). These conditions are often indicative of other major disorders that require extensive medical management. In these instances, the detailed examination of the biological basis of the persisting symptoms is mandatory.

Irritable bowel syndrome is characterized by a change in bowel habits and abdominal pain without detectable abnormalities. Medical treatments are aimed at removing bowel motility by high-fiber diets or the use of anticholinergic drugs. Behavioral treatments have varied. Furman (1973) reported that patients could learn to control their bowel sounds when these were amplified through an electronic stethoscope and that this resulted in improvements in symptoms. This result has not been replicated by others (O'Connell & Russ, 1978; Weinstock, 1976).

Latimer (1981b) has questioned the hypothesis that gastrointestinal motility may be the cause of irritable bowel syndrome. Though patients with this syndrome had more and longer colonic contractions than normals, they did not differ from neurotic patients who did not have reported irritable bowel syndrome. He suggests a multisystem intervention with cognitive therapy to correct maladaptive verbal behaviors, operant training to extinguish maladaptive behavior patterns and inappropriate reinforcement for symptoms by friends and relatives, and biofeedback or relaxation to alter physiological reactivity. Relaxation has been shown by several studies to be effective with irritable bowel syndrome (O'Connell & Russ, 1978; Weinstock, 1976; Youell & McCullough, 1975). Wise et al. (1982) have demonstrated the value of group methods in treatment also.

Fecal incontinence was treated successfully by Engel et al. (1974) in a classic paper on biofeedback application. They taught patients to recognize the stimuli associated with colon extension and to relax the external sphincter as a response to this stimulus. The treatment was effective in four of six patients, and the other two showed improvements. Cerulli, Nikoomanesch, and Schuster (1979) report success in 45 or 50 patients treated in a similar way. This method of treatment is the only nonsurgical intervention for this condition. Its application reflects a behavioral intervention that is very effective where there is no other noninvasive mode of treatment.

A variety of motility disorders such as esophageal motility, swallowing difficulties, and reflux esophagitis might be amenable to behavioral interventions. The few studies that have addressed these problems via biofeedback or relaxation techniques have shown promise in that patients can gain some control over motility (see Latimer, 1981a, for a review).

Vomiting is another disorder of considerable consequence that is resistant to standard medical intervention. To date, studies of intervention have been limited to case studies. The patterns of vomiting may differ depending on whether vomiting is an operant or a respondent behavior. Treatment interventions would be designed accordingly. For operant vomiting, the reward contingencies would be rearranged and alternative nonvomiting behaviors would be taught. For respondent vomiting, relaxation, stimulus removal, and stress management procedures would be most appropriate. Chronic vomiting has been eliminated by electric shock (Toister, Colin, Worley, & Arthur, 1975) or a squirt of lemon juice (Sajwaj, Libet, & Agras, 1974) to interrupt the muscle contraction pattern. These techniques in infants and retarded adults have a proven clinical effectiveness. Relaxation methods have been applied to nausea and vomiting resulting from cancer chemotherapy with success (see Chapter 19).

Bulimic vomiting has been successfully treated by a combination of methods. In a recent case study, Long and Cordle (1982) report the successful elimination of vomiting by a combination of self-monitoring, stimulus control manipulations of eating ·behavior patterns, and cognitive restructuring using rational – emotive therapeutic techniques. Systematic desensitization has also been used with success (Lang, 1965).

Pulmonary Disorders.   Asthma is a potentially life-threatening disease characterized by obstruction to the air passage to the lungs. An estimated 8.6 million people in the United States suffer from the disorder (Davis, 1972). The attack can be induced by allergens such as pollens, feathers, and dust or by other irritants to the air passages to the lungs (e.g., cold air, viral infections, aerosols). Exercise can also induce bronchospasms. Szentivanyi (1968) has suggested that asthmatics have a reduced number of beta-adrenergic receptors in the lungs, leaving them vulnerable to the constrictive effects of vagal activation. It is a frightening experience to suddenly feel that one has lost one's breath and that within any moment no air will be available to sustain life. As a result, the anxiety components of the disease are noteworthy. For the asthmatic, the disease takes on a controlling quality, restricting activity and requiring constant vigilance and preparation for the potential onset of an attack.

Relaxation techniques have been used with asthmatic children with somewhat mixed results. Increases in pulmonary volume and expiratory flow rate have been observed in asthmatic children following relaxation (Alexander, 1972; Scherr, Crawford, Sergent, & Scherr, 1975). However, the long-term effects of this form of intervention seem to be related to the attention – placebo effects implicit in these studies. When these effects were controlled, Erskine and Schonell (1979) found no effects due to relaxation on pulmonary measures. However, these studies do report reductions in medication use, number of attacks, and number of visits to the infirmary. Though there may be no change in physiological effects, there may be reductions in the anxiety that accompanies the disease.

Ikemi, Nagata, Ago, & Ikemi (1982) have followed a group of asthmatics closely through a psychosomatic, self-control treatment paradigm that included somatic treatment, stress management techniques, awareness training, cognitive restructuring, and assertiveness training. The groups that completed all five training stages showed 93% remission of symptoms at 3-year follow-up. Only 12% of the group that had somatic treatment only were improved.

Behavioral methods used as adjunctive to the treatment of asthma do not afford a cure. However, they do afford a treatment for consequences of living with the disease and they offer methods that are beneficial to the habilitation of the asthmatic. After reviewing work on the interventions into asthma treatment, Alexander (1981) concludes: "On the one hand, we are now in a position to state with considerable confidence that continued attempts to significantly alter lung function through psychological means will result in little success. On the other hand, the contributions of behaviorists to the overall treatment efforts with asthmatics should continue to be developed with all vigor [p. 392]."

Behavioral techniques have not been employed systematically in other pulmonary diseases, though there is certainly a place for their application. Chronic bronchitis, emphysema, and tension pneumothorax could be treated with relaxation and deep-breathing interventions. Certainly smoking as a major contributor to lung diseases can be treated by behavioral methods.

Urogenital Disorders.   A variety of disorders of the urogenital system have been treated by behavioral methods. Enuresis in children is a classic syndrome for behavioral interventions. The treatments for this condition involve a behavioral restructuring intended to rearrange contingencies such that: (1) the stimuli for bladder distention are made more salient; (2) alternative behavioral responses are introduced and; (3) reinforcements are given for "dry" behaviors. These methods have a great deal of clinical utility.

The control of the external urethral sphincter is an important aspect of bladder control. Excessive urinary retention or "dribbling" can result when urethral control is inadequate. EMG biofeedback has been used to teach children relaxation of the sphincter during voiding (Allen, 1977; Maizels, King, & Firlit, 1979). The method employed by Allen included parental involvement to reinforce the child's behavior.

In adults, Wear, Wear, and Cleeland (1979) report the successful use of biofeedback in training reduced incontinence, reduction in residual urine in the bladder, and control. Half the patients were successfully treated in a very few sessions.

The use of biofeedback has been extended to the treatment of neurogenic bladder syndromes in patients with a loss of neural control of the bladder resulting from spinal chord injury. In an 8-week training period, Nergardh, von Hedenberg, Hellstrom, and Ericssen (1974) reported that all patients improved and 18 of the 30 showed appropriate social continence.

Psychogenic urinary retention and psychogenic anuria are two other presenting conditions that require behavioral intervention. Doleys and Meredith (1982) report success with the former in the use of anxiety-reduction techniques. Studies of the latter syndrome are limited to date.

Sexual Dysfunctions.   The treatment of sexual – genital dysfunctions by behavioral methods has received extensive analysis and research. Intervention strategies have focused on the use of relaxation procedures in conjunction with cognitive restructuring techniques to eliminate the tensions and anxieties that disrupt sexual pleasures and performance. Mutual pleasuring and genital stimulation are common steps in all forms of behavioral treatment for sexual disorders. This serves to: (1) relax the partners; and (2) enhance the experience of sexual enjoyment by focusing the attention on the pleasures of the sexual stimulation.

In female sexual dysfunctions these methods are followed by interventions relevant to the specific dysfunction. For female unresponsiveness—frigidity—the treatment involves teaching alternative "responsive" behaviors. For orgastic dysfunctions, the treatment focuses on the use of clitoral stimulation to achieve orgasm, first by masturbation, then by intercourse. For vaginismus, the treatment involves training the muscles of the vagina to relax while inserting an object. Ultimately the penis is inserted during intercourse. In effect all of these are desensitization procedures requiring relaxation and approximation training.

For male sexual dysfunctions, the treatment strategies are similar. Erectile dysfunction—impotence—involves gradual approximations during a relaxed state to the achievement of coitus. Inadequate ejaculatory control—premature ejaculation—is treated by start – stop procedures. These involve focusing the male on the sensations that precede ejaculation. When these occur, stimulation is stopped temporarily until the ejaculatory urge goes away. Stimulation is then resumed. This process is repeated several times. The intent is to train the patient to control ejaculation by responding in a manner that prolongs the ejaculatory reflex.

The "squeeze" technique is also used as a method to disrupt the stimulus – response chain leading to premature ejaculation. When the urge to ejaculate is felt, the penis is squeezed at the base with enough pressure to: (1) retard ejaculation; and (2) distract the male from the ejaculatory sequence.

The pioneering work on treating sexual dysfunctions has been instructive in the development of treatment strategies for other physiologically based conditions. More specifically the analysis of the interrelationships between thought patterns and physiological-behavioral events has provided a prototype for the refined analysis of other interventions that utilize physiological – behavioral – cognitive – social treatment.

Central Nervous System.   *Epilepsy* is a biologically based disorder characterized by seizures of central nervous system origin. These produce temporary disruptions in consciousness accompanied by motor, sensory, or behavioral activity. They are believed to be the result of repetitive firing of groups of cells. As these continue to discharge, the adjacent neurons are involved, resulting in a spread of discharge. There are a variety of seizure types.

Patients can frequently report the events that produce seizures if they are taught to focus on the aura, the nature of stress responses, and other antecedent stimuli that precipitate the seizure. In conjunction with medication, relaxation, and desensitization the symptoms can be behaviorally controlled (Ince, 1976; Mostofsky & Balaschak, 1977). Sterman and MacDonald (1978) have reported that patients are able to use biofeedback from cortical electrical activity to reduce the incidence of seizure. This method, however, was considerably more expensive and required a greater expenditure of time than those that focus on relaxation procedures with cognitive restructuring techniques.

SUMMARY AND CONCLUSIONS

The material overviewed in this chapter indicates a role for the application of behavioral techniques to a variety of medical problems. There is a need to conduct systematic evaluative studies of the effects of these treatment interventions on disease. Beginning research is very promising, but the proof of the value of these methods on a larger scale and for a longer time period has yet to be clearly established.

The holistic perspective affords a model for the intervention into health disorders that gives systematic consideration to the biopsychosocial complex within which the individual functions and the forum within which disease is manifested. The use of multiple levels of intervention provides a comprehensive strategy for addressing and treating patient health problems. Along with the physiological consequences of the disease, the individual functions as a cognitive, emotional, behaving organism within a social network reflecting degrees of intimacy and psychological support.

The state of health is a balance among these multiple levels of functioning. Disruption of this balance at any level can throw the system into disequilibrium and disease. To paraphrase Claude Bernard: Maintaining the constancy of the holistic balance of life is the necessary condition for the free and independent life.

REFERENCES

Alexander, A. B. Systematic relaxation and flow rates in asthmatic children: Relationships to emotional precipitants and anxiety. *Journal of Psychosomatic Medicine*, 1972, *16*, 405 – 410.

Alexander, B. A. Behavioral approaches in the treatment of bronchial asthma. In C. K. Prokop & L. A. Bradley (Eds.), *Medical psychology: Contributions to behavioral medicine*. New York: Academic Press, 1981.

Alexander, F. *Psychosomatic medicine*. New York: Norton Press, 1950.

Allen, R. B. Bladder capacity and awakening behavior in the treatment of enuresis. University of Vermont unpublished doctoral dissertation, 1977. Cited by Doleys, D. M., & Meredith, R. L., Urological disorders. In D. M. Doleys, R. L. Meredith, & A. R. Ciminero (Eds.), *Behavior medicine: Assessment and treatment strategies*. New York: Plenum Press, 1982.

Andreychuk, T., & Schriver, C. Hypnosis and biofeedback in the treatment of migraine headache. *International Journal of Clinical and Experimental Hypnosis*, 1975, *23*, 172 – 183.

Antonovsky, A. *Health, stress and coping*. San Francisco: Jossey-Bass, 1979.

Becker, M. H., & Green, L. W. A family approach to compliance with medical treatment. *International Journal of Health Education*, 1975, *18*, 2 – 11.

Becker, M. H., Maiman, L. A., Kirscht, J. P., Haefner, D. P., & Drachman, R. H. The health belief model and the prediction of dietary compliance. *Journal of Health and Social Behavior*, 1977, *18*, 348 – 366.

Beiman, I., Israel, E., & Johnson, S. A. During training and posttraining effects of live and taped extended progressive relaxation, self-relaxation, and electromyogram biofeedback. *Journal of Consulting and Clinical Psychology*, 1978, *46*, 314 – 321.

Bellack, A. S. A comparison of self-reinforcement and self-monitoring in weight reduction program. *Behavior Therapy*, 1976, *7*, 68 – 75.

Benson, H. *The relaxation response*. Seminars in medicine of the Beth Israel Hospital, Boston, Mass., 1975.

Berkman, L. F., & Syme, S. L. Social networks, lost resistance and mortality: A nine-year follow-up study of Alameda County residents. *American Journal of Epidemiology*. 1979, *109*, 186 – 204.

Blanchard, E. B., & Young, L. D. Clinical applications of biofeedback training: A review of evidence. *Archives of General Psychiatry*, 1974, *30*, 573 – 589.

Bower, S. A., & Bower, G. H. *Asserting yourself: A practical guide for positive change*. Reading, Mass.: Addison-Wesley, 1976.

Boyd, J. R., Covington, T. R., Stanaszek, W., & Cousons, R. T. Drug-defaulting, III. Analysis of uncompliance patterns. *American Journal of Hospital Pharmacy*, 1974, *31*, 485 – 491.

Budman, S. H., & Wertlieb, D. Psychologists in health care settings. *Professional Psychology*, 1979, *10*, 297 – 643.

Bujatti, M., & Riederer, P. Serotonin, noradrenalin, dopamine, metabolites in transcendental meditation technique. *Journal of Psychosomatic Research*. 1976, *39*, 257.

Burish, T. G. EMG biofeedback in the treatment of stressrelated disorders. In C. K. Prokop & L. A. Bradley (Eds.), *Medical psychology: Contributions to behavioral medicine*. New York: Academic Press, 1981.

Burr, B. D., Good, B. J., & Good, M. D. The impact of illness in the family. In R. Taylor (Ed.), *Family medicine: Principles and practice*. New York: Springer-Verlag, 1978.

Caplan, G. *Principles of preventive psychiatry*. New York: Basic Books, Inc., 1964.

Carroll, D., Marzillier, J. S., & Watson, F. Heart rate and self-report changes accompanying different types of relaxing imagery. *Behavior Research and Therapy*, 1980, *18*, 273 – 280.

Carver, C. S., & Scheier, M. F. A control theory approach to human behavior and implications for problems in self-management. In P. C. Kendall (Ed.), *Advances in cognitive – behavioral research and therapy*. New York: Academic Press, 1983.

Cerulli, M. A., Nikoomanesch, P., & Schuster, M. M. Progress in biofeedback conditioning for fecal incontinence. *Gastroenterology*, 1979, *76*, 742 – 746.

Choquette, G., & Ferguson, R. J. Blood pressure reduction in "borderline" hypertensives following physical training. *Canadian Medical Association Journal*, 1973, *108*, 699 – 705.

Cohen, F., & Lazarus, R. S. Coping with the stresses of illness. In G. C. Stone, F. Cohen, & N. E. Adler & associates (Eds.), *Health psychology—A handbook*. San Francisco: Jossey-Bass, 1979.

Crasilneck, H. B., & Hall, J. A. *Clinical hypnosis: Principles and applications*. New York: Grune & Stratton, 1975.

Davidson, P. O. (Ed.). *The behavioral management of anxiety, depression and pain*. New York: Brunner/Mazel, 1976.

Davis, D. J. NIAID initiatives in allergy research. *Journal of Allergy and Clinical Immunology*, 1972, *49*, 323 – 328.

Davis, M. S. Variations in patients' compliance with doctor's advice: An empirical analysis of patterns of communication. *American Journal of Public Health*, 1968, *58*, 274 – 288.

Edelstein, P., Ross, W. D., & Schultz, J. R. The biopsychosocial approach: Clinical examples from a consultation – liaison service, Part I. *Psychosomatics*, 1982, *23*, 15 – 19; 141 – 151; 233 – 242.

Engel, B. T., Nikoomanesch, P., & Schuster, M. M. Operant conditioning of recto-sphincteric responses in the treatment of fecal incontinence. *New England Journal of Medicine*, 1974, *290*, 646 – 649.

Engel, G. L. Clinical applications of the biopsychosocial model. *American Journal of Psychiatry*, 1980, *137*, 535 – 543.

Engel, G. Sudden and rapid death during psychological stress. *Annals of Internal Medicine*, 1971, *74*, 771.

Erskine, J., & Schonell, M. Relaxation therapy in bronchial asthma. *Journal of Psychosomatic Research*, 1979, *23*, 131 – 139.

Findlay, I., Smith, P., Graves, P. J., & Linton, M. L. Chronic diseases in childhood: A study of family reactions. *British Journal of Medical Education*, 1969, 66 – 69.

Fordyce, W. F. *Behavioral methods for chronic pain and illness*. St. Louis: C. V. Mosby Co., 1976.

Francis, V., Korsch, B. M., & Morris, M. J. Gaps in doctor – patient communications. *New England Journal of Medicine*, 1969, *280*, 535 – 540.

Friedman, H., & Taub, H. A. A six month follow-up of the use of hypnosis and biofeedback procedures in essential hypertension. *American Journal of Clinical Hypnosis*, 1978, *20*, 184 – 188.

Furman, S. Internal biofeedback in functional diarrhea: A preliminary report. *Journal of Behavior Therapy and Experimental Psychiatry*, 1973, *4*, 317 – 321.

Gaarder, K. R., & Montgomery, P. S. *Clinical biofeedback: A procedural manual*. Baltimore, Md.: Williams & Wilkins Company, 1977.

Glasser, H. H., Harrison, G. S., & Lynn, D. B. Emotional implications of congenital heart disease in children. *Pediatrics*, 1964, *33*, 367 – 372.

Glasser, W. *Stations of the mind*. New York: Alfred A. Knopf, 1981.

Goldiamond, I. Ethical and constitutional issues raised by applied behavior analysis. *Toward a Constitutional Approach to Social Problems*, 1974, *2*, 1 – 83.

Greist, J. H., Klein, M. H., Eischeus, R. R., & Faris, J. Antidepressant running. *Behavioral Medicine*, 1978, *2*, 19 – 24.

Haynes, R. B. A critical review of the "determinants" of patient compliance with therapeutic regimens. In D. L. Sachet & R. B. Haynes (Eds.), *Compliance with therapeutic regimens*. Baltimore, Md.: Johns Hopkins University Press, 1976.

Heinzelmann, F., & Bagley, R. W. Response to physical exercise programs and their effects on health behavior. *Public Health Reports*, 1974, *2*, 129 – 177.

Hilgard, E. R. The alleviation of pain by hypnosis. *Pain*, 1975, *1*, 213 – 231.

Hoff, L. A. *People in crisis: Understanding and helping*. Reading, Mass.: Addison-Wesley, 1978.

Holmes, D. The use of biofeedback for treating patients with migraine headaches, Raynaud's disease and hypertension: A critical evaluation. In C. K. Prokop & L. A. Bradley (Eds.), *Medical psychology: Contributions to behavior medicine*. New York: Academic Press, 1981.

Howe, G. *Evaluating a medical consumer assertion training program: Effects on patient – physician interaction and compliance with therapeutic regimen*. Unpublished doctoral dissertation, 1981, University of Connecticut, Storrs, Connecticut.

Hunt, G. M., & Azrin, N. H. A community-reinforcement approach to alcoholism. *Behavior Research and Therapy*, 1973, *11*, 91 – 104.

Ibrahim, M. A., Feldman, J. G., Sultz, H. A., Staiman, M. G., Young, L. J., & Dean, D. Management after myocardial infarction: A controlled trial of the effect of group psychotherapy. *International Journal of Psychiatric Medicine*, 1974, *5*, 253 – 264.

Ikemi, Y., Nagata, S., Ago, Y., & Ikemi, A. Self control over stress. *Journal of Psychosomatic Research*, 1982, *26*, 51 – 56.

Ince, L. P. The use of relaxation training and a conditioned stimulus in the elimination of epileptic seizures in children: A case study. *Journal of Behavior Therapy and Experimental Psychiatry*, 1976, *7*, 39 – 42.

Jacobson, E. *Progressive relaxation*. Chicago: University of Chicago, 1938.

Kaplan, B. H., Cassell, J. C., Tyroler, J. A., Cornoni, J. C., Kleinbaum, D. G., & Hames, C. G. Occupational mobility and coronary heart disease. *Archives of Internal Medicine*, 1971, *128*, 938 – 942.

Katkin, E. S., & Goldband, S. The placebo effect and biofeedback. In R. J. Gatchel & K. P. Price (Ed.), *Clinical applications of biofeedback: Appraisal and status*. New York: Pergamon, 1979.

Katkin, E. S., & Murray, E. N. Instrumental conditioning of autonomically mediated behavior: Theoretical and methodological issues. *Psychological Bulletin*, 1968, *70*, 52 – 68.

Keefe, F. J., Surwit, R. S., & Pilon, R. N. A one-year follow-up of Raynaud's patients treated with behavioral therapy techniques. *Journal of Behavioral Medicine*, 1979, *2*, 385 – 391.

Kendall, P. C., Williams, L., Pechacek, T. F., Graham, L. E., Shisslak, C., & Herzoff, N. Cognitive behavioral and patient education interventions in cardiac catherization procedures: The Palo Alto Medical Psychology project. *Journal of Consulting and Clinical Psychology,* 1979, *47,* 49 – 58.

Kirschenbaum, D. S., & Karoly, P. When self-regulation fails: Tests of some preliminary hypotheses. *Journal of Consulting and Clinical Psychology,* 1977, *45,* 1116 – 1125.

Kirschenbaum, D. S., Tomarken, A. J., & Ordman, A. M. Specific planning and choice applied to adult self-control. *Journal of Personality and Social Psychology,* 1982, *42,* 576 – 585.

Korsch, B. M., Fine, R. N., & Negrete, V. F. Non-compliance in children with renal transplants. *Pediatrics,* 1978, *61,* 872 – 876.

Kreisberg, L., & Treiman, B. R. Socioeconomic status and utilization of dentist services. *Journal of the American College of Dentists,* 1960, *27,* 147 – 165.

Lang, R., Dehof, K., Meuver, J. A., & Jaufman, W. Sympathetic activity and transcendental meditation. *Journal of Psychosomatic Research,* 1979, *44,* 117 – 123.

Lang, P. J. Behavior therapy with a case of nervosa anorexia. In L. P. Ullman & L. Krasner (Eds.), *Case studies in behavior modification.* New York: Holt, Rinehart, & Winston, 1965.

Latimer, P. R. Biofeedback and behavioral approaches to disorders of the gastrointestinal tract. *Psychotherapy Psychosomatic,* 1981, *36,* 200 – 212. (a)

Latimer, P. R. Irritable bowel syndrome: A behavioral model. *Behavior Research and Therapy,* 1981, *19,* 475 – 483. (b)

Lavallee, Y. J., Lamontague, Y., Pinard, G., Anable, L., & Tetreault, L. Effects of EMG feedback, diazepam and their combination of chronic anxiety. *Journal of Psychosomatic Research,* 1977, *21,* 65 – 71.

Ley, P., & Spelman, M. S. Communications in an outpatient setting. *British Journal of Social and Clinical Psychology,* 1965, *4,* 114 – 116.

Lindemann, E. Symptomatology and management of acute grief. *American Journal of Psychiatry,* 1944, *101,* 141 – 148.

Long, C. G., & Cordle, C. J. Psychological treatment of binge eating and self-induced vomiting. *British Journal of Medical Psychology,* 1982, *55,* 139 – 145.

Mahoney, M. J. Self-reward and self-monitoring techniques for weight control. *Behavior Therapy,* 1974, *5,* 48 – 57.

Mahoney, M. J., & Arnkoff, D. B. Self-management. In O. F. Pomerleu & J. P. Brady (Eds.), *Behavioral medicine: Theory and practice.* Baltimore, Md.: William & Wilkins, Co., 1979.

Maizels, M., King, L. R., & Firlit, C. F. Urodynamic biofeedback: A new approach to treat vesical sphincter dyssynergia. *Journal of Urology,* 1979, *122,* 205 – 209.

Masur, F. T. Adherence to health care regimens. In C. K. Prokop & L. A. Bradley (Eds.), *Contributions to behavioral medicine.* New York: Academic Press, 1981.

Mathew, R. J., Ho, B. T., Taylor, D. L., & Semchuk, K. M. Catecholamine and dopamine-beta-hydroxylase in anxiety. *Journal of Psychosomatic Research,* 1981, *25,* 499 – 504.

McFall, R. M., & Hammen, C. L. Motivation, structure and self-monitoring: The role of non-specific factors in smoking behavior. *Journal of Consulting and Clinical Psychology,* 1971, *37,* 80 – 86.

McKenney, J. M., Slining, J. M., Henderson, H. R., Devins, D., & Berr, M. The effect of chemical pharmacy services on patients with essential hypertension. *Circulation,,* 1973, *48,* 1104 – 1111.

Meichenbaum, D. *Cognitive behavior modification: An integrative approach.* New York: Plenum, 1977.

Meichenbaum, D., & Turk, D. The cognitive – behavioral management of anxiety, anger and pain. In P. O. Davidson (Ed.), *Behavioral management of anxiety, depression, and pain.* New York: Bruner-Mazel, 1976.

Minuchin, S., Rosman, B. L., & Baker, L. *Psychosomatic families.* Cambridge, Mass.: Harvard University Press, 1978.

Mitchell, K. R., & White, R. G. Behavioral self-management: An application to the problem of migraine headaches. *Behavior Therapy,* 1977, *8,* 213 – 221.

Mone, L. Short-term group psychotherapy in post-cardiac disorders. *International Journal of Group Psychotherapy*, 1970, *20*, 99 – 121.

Moos, R. H., & Tsu, V. The crisis of physical illness: An overview. In R. H. Moos (Ed.), *Coping with physical illness*. New York: Plenum Press, 1977.

Morgan, W. P., & Horstman, D. H. Anxiety reduction following acute physical activity. *Medicine and Science in Sports*, 1976, *8*, 62.

Mostofsky, D. I., & Balaschak, B.A. Psychobiological control of seizures. *Psychological Bulletin*, 1977, *84*, 723 – 750.

Nergardh, A., von Hedenberg, C., Hellstrom, B., & Ericssen, N. Continence training of children with neurogenic bladder dysfunction. *Developmental Medicine and Child Neurology*, 1974, *16*, 47 – 52.

O'Connell, M. F., & Russ, K. L. *A case report comparing two types of biofeedback in the treatment of irritable bowel syndrome*. Ninth Annual Meeting of the Biofeedback Society of America, Alberquerque, New Mexico, 1978.

Parkes, C. M. The emotional impact of cancer on patients and their families. *Journal of Laryngology and Otolaryngology*, 1975, *89*, 1271 – 1279.

Pollock, M. How much exercise is enough? *The Physician and Sports Medicine*, 1978, 49 – 64.

Pollock, M., Wilmore, J. H., & Fox, S. M. *Health and fitness through physical activity*. New York: Wiley, 1978.

Qualls, P. J., & Sheehan, P. W. Electromyographic biofeedback as a relaxation technique: A critical appraisal and reassessment. *Psychological Bulletin*, 1981, *90*, 21 – 42.

Rahe, R. Subjects' recent life changes and their near future illness reports: A review. *Annals of Clinical Research*, 1972, *4*, 250 – 265.

Rahe, R. H., Mahan, J., L., & Arthur, R. J. Prediction of near future health change from subject's preceding life changes. *Journal of Psychosomatic Research*, 1970, *14*, 401 – 406.

Rahe, R. H., Rufflic, C. F., Suchor, R. J., & Arthur, R. J. Group therapy in the outpatient management of post-myocardial infarction patients. *International Journal of Psychiatric Medicine*, 1973, *4*, 77 – 92.

Reinking, R. H., & Hutchings, D. *Follow-up and extension of "Tension headaches—what method is most effective?"* Paper presented at meetings of the biofeedback society, Colorado Springs, Colorado, 1976. Cited by Burish, T. G. EMG biofeedback in the treatment of stress-related disorders.

Romanczyk, K. Self-monitoring in the treatment of obesity parameters of reactivity. *Behavior Therapy*, 1974, *5*, 531 – 540.

Sajwaj, T., Libet, J., & Agras, S. Lemon juice therapy: The control of life threatening rumination in a six-month old infant. *Journal of Applied Behavioral Analysis*, 1974, *7*, 557 – 563.

Scherr, M. S., Crawford, P. L., Sergent, C. B., & Scherr, C. A. Effect of biofeedback techniques on chronic asthma in summer camp environment. *Annals of Allergy*, 1975, *35*, 289 – 295.

Schwartz, G. Testing the biopsychosocial model: The ultimate challenge facing behavioral medicine. *Journal of Consulting Psychology*, 1982, *50*,, 1040 – 1053.

Schwartz, G. E., Weinberger, D. A., & Singer, J. A. Cardiovascular differentiation of happiness, sadness, anger, and fear following imagery and exercise. *Psychosomatic Medicine*, 1981, *43*, 343 – 364.

Schwartz, G. E., & Weiss, S. M. Yale conference on behavioral medicine: A proposed definition and statement of goals. *Journal of Behavioral Medicine*, 1978, *1*, 3 – 12.

Schwartz, R. M., & Gottman, J. M. Toward a task analysis of assertive behavior. *Journal of Consulting and Clinical Psychology*, 1976, *44*, 910 – 920.

Scott, C. S. Patient compliance. In J. J. Braunstein & R. P. Toister (Eds.), *Medical applications of the behavioral sciences*. Chicago: Yearbook Medical Publishers, 1981.

Selye, H. *Stress without distress*. New York: Lippincott, 1974.

Sheppard, R. J., & Sidney, K. H. Effect of physical exercise on plasma growth hormone and cortisol levels in human subjects. *Exercise and Sports Science Review*, 1973, *3*, 1 – 12.

Simkins, L. Biofeedback: Clinically valid or oversold? *The Psychological Record*, 1982, *32*, 3 – 17.

Simonelli, C., & Eaton, R. P. Cardiovascular and metabolic effects of exercise. *Postgraduate Medicine*, 1978, *63*, 71 – 77.

Simonton, O., Mathews-Simonton, S., & Sparks, T. F. Psychological intervention in the treatment of cancer. *Psychosomatics*, 1980, *21*, 226 – 233.

Skyler, J. F. Diabetes and exercise: Clinical implications. *Diabetes Care*, 1979, *2*(3), 307 – 311.

Sterman, M. B., & MacDonald, L. R. The effects of central cortical EEG feedback training in poorly controlled seizures. *Epilepsia*, 1978, *19*, 207 – 222.

Stuart, R. B., & Davis, B. *Slim chance in a fat world*. Chicago: Research Press, 1972.

Surwit, R. S., Shapiro, D., & Good, M. I. A comparison of cardiovascular biofeedback, neuromuscular biofeedback and meditation in the treatment of borderline essential hypertension. *Journal of Consulting and Clinical Psychology*, 1978, *46*, 252 – 263.

Surwit, R. S., Williams, R. B., & Shapiro, D. *Behavioral approaches to cardiovascular disease*. New York: Academic Press, 1982.

Svarstad, B. Physician – patient communication and patient conformity with medical advice. In D. Mechanic (Ed.), *The growth of bureaucratic medicine*. New York: Wiley, 1976.

Syme, S. L., Borhani, N. D., & Buechley, R. W. Cultural mobility and coronary heart disease in an urban area. *American Journal of Epidemiology*, 1965, *82*, 334 – 346.

Szentivanyi, A. The beta-adrenergic theory of the atopic abnormality in bronchial asthma. *Journal of Allergy*, 1968, *42*, 203 – 244.

Tapp, J. T., & Garnier, J. G. *The happy life workbook*. Psychological Health Services, Miami, Florida, 1982.

Thomson, J. K., Jarvie, G. J., Lahey, B. B., & Cureton, K. J. Exercise and obesity: Etiology, physiology and intervention. *Psychological Bulletin*, 1982, *91*, 55 – 79.

Throll, D. A. Transcendental meditation and progressive relaxation: Their psychological effects. *Journal of Clinical Psychology*, 1981, *37*, 776 – 781.

Toister, R. P., Colin, J., Worley, L. M., & Arthur, D. Faradic therapy of chronic vomiting in infancy: A case study. *Journal of Behavioral Therapy and Experimental Psychiatry*, 1975, *6*, 55 – 59.

Wadden, T. A., & Anderton, C. H. The clinical use of hypnosis. *Psychological Bulletin*, 1982, *9*, 215 – 243.

Wadden, T. A., & de la Torre, C. Relaxation therapy as an adjunct treatment for essential hypertension. *Journal of Family Practice*, 1980, *11*, 901 – 908.

Wear, J. B., Wear, R. B., & Cleeland, C. Biofeedback in urology using urodynamics: Preliminary observations. *Journal of Urology*, 1979, *19*, 464 – 468.

Weinstock, S. A. The reestablishment of intestinal control in functional colitis. *Biofeedback and self-regulation*, 1976, *1*, 324.

Weiss, T., & Engel, B. T. Operant conditioning of heart rate in patients with premature ventricular contractions. *Psychosomatic Medicine*, 1971, *33*, 301 – 321.

Wise, T. N., Cooper, J. N., & Ahmed, S. The efficacy of group therapy for patients with irritable bowel syndrome. *Psychosomatics*, 1982, *23*, 465 – 474.

Wolpe, J. The practice of behavior therapy. *The Current Status of Systematic Densitization*, 1969, 961 – 965.

Wood, P. D., & Haskell, W. L. Interrelation of physical activity and nutrition on lipid metabolism. In P. L. White, & T. Mondeika, *Diet and exercise: Synergism in health maintenance*. American Medical Association, Chicago, 1982.

Youell, K. J., & McCullough, J. P. Behavioral treatment of mucous colitis. *Journal of Consulting and Clinical Psychology*, 1975, *43*, 740 – 745.

Zimmerman, R. S. *Health: Attainment, maintenance, and optimization—the psychologist as behavioral coach*. Paper read at the Max Planck Institute for Psychiatry, Munich, West Germany, 1981.

10   Behavioral Pediatrics

Annette M. La Greca
Wendy L. Stone
University of Miami

INTRODUCTION

The term "child health care psychology" has been used to refer to the behavioral aspects of medical treatment that apply uniquely to children and adolescents. As Wright (1979) has recently noted, two major components are subsumed under child health care psychology. One component involves child mental health problems that are identified in medical settings. Pediatricians and family practitioners have been found to encounter a substantial proportion of mental health problems in the course of their medical practice (Salk, 1978). One set of investigators (McClelland, Staples, Weisberg, & Berger, 1973) noted that pediatricians provided support and counseling on child-rearing and behavior management issues for 37% of their "well-child" visits. Moreover, studies examining referral patterns in pediatric medical practice suggest that the frequency of mental health problems observed by pediatricians is about five times greater than the referral rate to psychiatric outpatient and inpatient services (Goldberg, Regier, McAnarny, Pless, & Roghmann, 1979). Clearly, many child mental health problems are initially surfacing in medical settings.

The second major component of child health care psychology involves the contribution of psychological factors to physical disease. In the case of children and adolescents, this latter area has been frequently termed "behavioral pediatrics." Behavioral pediatrics focuses particularly on issues such as psychological factors contributing to the etiology of various childhood diseases (e.g., asthma), the psychological sequelae of various medical problems (e.g., cardiac surgery, leukemia), and psychological factors that contribute to the maintenance of adequate medical care (e.g., compliance in children with juvenile diabetes). This interplay of emotional and physical factors in children's medical problems has received increasing attention from the medical community, due to the recognition that emotional and physical problems often occur concurrently (Salk, 1978; Shore & Goldston, 1978). An investigation of the types of problems encountered in outpatient pediatric practice disclosed that only 12% of the child patients presented purely physical problems, but some 52% evidenced a combination of medical and psychological concerns (Duff, Rowe, & Anderson, 1972).

The present chapter focuses on the behavioral pediatrics component of child health care psychology. There is a substantial body of literature in behavioral pediatrics; the present chapter attempts to provide an overview of several major topics of interest. First, as an orientation to this extensive area, a brief discussion of major developmental concerns and issues that affect the study of behavioral pediatrics is presented.

ISSUES RELEVANT TO BEHAVIORAL PEDIATRICS

When dealing with medical problems in children and adolescents, a number of concerns arise that are unique to this population and that have a major impact on our understanding of the interplay of physical and psychological factors. Perhaps of most importance is the recognition that children undergo rapid and uneven *developmental change* (see Mash & Terdal, 1981). As a result, the impact of the disease process is likely to differ considerably for children of varying ages. The developmental status of the child will differentially affect both the short-term and long-range consequences of physical illness. This can best be illustrated by considering the effects of chronic illness on children. The nature of the initial impact may be very different for a preschooler as compared with an adolescent, due to the differential levels of cognitive, emotional, and social maturity. A major life adjustment to chronic disease may be more readily accomplished for the younger child, but may represent an unwelcome intrusion on the already established life routine of an adolescent. On the other hand, the nature of the disease may play a larger role in shaping the subsequent social and emotional development of a young child but have a less formative influence on the adolescent.

A second issue of concern in behavioral pediatrics is the role of the *family* in the etiology, management, and course of the disease. Children are primarily under the social control of significant others in their environment (Evans & Nelson, 1977). How these significant others respond to the child will have important implications for the health status and psychological adjustment of the child (Magrab & Calcagno, 1978; Pless, Roghmann, & Haggerty, 1972; Talbot & Howell, 1971).

Finally the issue of *individual differences* in emotional functioning or behavioral style is an important one for behavioral pediatrics. According to Steinhauer, Mushin, and Rae-Grant (1974):

The child who has difficulty separating from parents may have problems coping with hospitalization. The previous phobic child is likely to develop inordinate fears of minor procedures, while the hyperactive child will have difficulty tolerating forced immobilizations. The child who already fears and resents authority figures can be expected to rebel against doctors and nurses, whereas a previously shy and withdrawn child whose illness involves some deformity is prone to extreme self-consciousness which may seriously interfere with his (her) relationships. (p. 827).

Although the importance of individual differences in children's responses to illness has been widely recognized (Petrillo & Sanger, 1980; Steinhauer et al., 1974; Travis, 1976), it is a seriously understudied area.

The remainder of this section is devoted to a closer examination of these three critical issues for behavioral pediatrics—the child's developmental status, the role of the family, and individual differences in emotional functioning and behavioral style.

Developmental Status

Achenbach (1978) aptly notes that: "even small differences in developmental level can have a large impact on (children's) capabilities, the ways in which they construe situations, the kinds of experiences they have, and the behavior they elicit from others (p. 761)." Thus, the child's developmental status is an important variable to consider in the understanding of health and physical illness in children. Most notably, developmental status includes the child's levels of cognitive and social/emotional functioning. These specific aspects of development may significantly affect the etiology, course, and management of disease.

Assuming that cognitive functioning is within normal limits, the child's level of cognitive maturity will, in part, determine how health and illness are viewed and thus may mediate the psychological impact of disease onset and treatment management. Recent investigations (Campbell, 1975; Cook, 1975; Perrin & Gerrity, 1981; Simeonsson, Buckley, & Monson, 1979) have demonstrated that children's conceptions of health and illness follow a developmental progression that closely parallels changes in cognitive abilities. In this framework, preschoolers typically regard illness causation as something magical or as a consequence of "bad" behavior. Children in the early elementary school years generally view illness as a result of specific external agents (e.g., germs) or their failure to adhere to health rules; children at this age also believe that recovery results from strict adherence to rigid health rules (a delightfully compliant period from a medical standpoint!). A major cognitive shift is observed as the child enters adolescence; the individual typically becomes more aware of the complexities of illness and health and is able to view illness and recovery as a sophisticated interaction of both internal and external factors. However, appreciation of the hypothetical long-range consequences of illness may not be apparent until later adolescence or early adulthood.

Similar developmental trends in children's understanding of death have been documented (Koocher, 1973).

Clearly, these developmental differences will be important for the child's medical treatment. For instance, preschoolers may be especially vulnerable to the belief that hospitalization is a punishment for bad behavior or some transgression (Prugh et al., 1953). Consequently, preparatory procedures prior to and during hospitalization may need to carefully address and clarify this issue in order to minimize undue anxiety and stress in the child and prevent emotional problems from surfacing once the child returns home.

The individual's level of social maturity is another important developmental factor to consider in understanding the impact of disease on children. The preschool years are generally marked by close ties between the child and parents. Separation from parents, as when a child is hospitalized for extended time periods, may be an extreme source of stress for children in this age range, affecting both the child and family. The difficulties associated with hospitalizing preschool-aged children have been well documented (Aisenberg, Wolff, Rosenthal, & Nadas, 1973; Kenney, 1975; Prugh et al., 1953; Robertson, 1970; Visintainer & Wolfer, 1975). During the early elementary school years, peer contacts begin to increase in importance as regular friendship patterns are established (Hetherington & Parke, 1979). The child whose illness results in many school absences or involves an obvious physical handicap may be particularly at risk for difficulties in establishing successful peer relationships (Korsch, Negrete, Gardner, Weinstock, Mercer, Grushkin, & Fine, 1973; Magrab & Calcagno, 1978; O'Malley, Koocher, Foster, & Slavin, 1979; Travis, 1976). In adolescence, the extreme importance of peer group activities, and the need to feel accepted by peers (Hetherington & Parke, 1979) can present other complications. Adolescents have been found to deny or neglect their medical care so as not to appear "different" from others (Heisler & Friedman, 1981; Kagen, 1976; Simonds, 1979). This especially has been noted in teenagers with chronic conditions such as diabetes (Greydanus & Hoffman, 1979; Simonds, 1979). On the other hand, peer pressures to drink or smoke may contribute to poor health practices among teens (Horan & Harrison, 1981; Levitt & Edwards, 1970). Thus, the child or adolescent's frame of social reference will be an important developmental issue to consider.

Although developmental level will be a critical variable for understanding children's health care problems, common methods of assessing developmental level have proven to be problematic. Most often, researchers have used "chronological age" as an index of developmental level. However, many studies include a very broad age range of children; it is not uncommon to find preschoolers and adolescents as subjects in the same study (e.g., Kalnins, Churchill, & Terry, 1980). Such broad age ranges do not adequately take into account marked qualitative differences among preschoolers, elementary-aged children and adolescents. Moreover, chronological age is, at best, an overall summary index for the many cognitive, social, emotional, and behavioral changes that occur throughout childhood and adolescence, and problems can arise when a child's functioning falls outside normal limits (Achenbach, 1978). This is especially true in the case of children with cognitive deficits, such as mental retardation. Here, the child's *mental age* may provide a more satisfactory measure of developmental level. The inclusion of mental age as a variable would be especially critical for researching medical conditions associated with a higher than normal prevalence of cognitive problems, as is the case with seizure disorders (Stores, 1978; Tartar, 1972; Willis & Thomas, 1978) and cerebral palsy (Wright, Schaefer, & Solomons, 1979).

In summary, some sensitive index of developmental status will be important to the study of behavioral pediatrics. Investigations that take into account both the child's developmental level and the degree to which the child falls within the normal range of functioning are needed to understand fully the complex interplay of physical and psychological factors in children.

Role of the Family

It has often been observed that children are under the social control of significant others—usually their parents (Evans & Nelson, 1977; Mash & Terdal, 1981). Consequently, the child's medical care may be fully, or at least partially the responsibility of the parents and other family members. Furthermore, the manner in which the parents cope with the child's physical problems will have implications for the child's adjustment, just as the child's reactions to illness will have an impact on family members. Researchers in behavioral pediatrics must take into account the role of the family in the etiology, sequelae, treatment, and management of physical disease.

Even within a normal functioning family, a child's illness/medical problems can have a critical impact on the entire family system. Stress, anxiety, and grief have been well documented as normal parental reactions at the time of initial diagnosis for a child's serious medical problems (Adams & Lindeman, 1974; Battle, 1975; Chodoff, Friedman, & Hamburg, 1964). Siblings of the affected child may also experience stress and other behavioral complications (Heisler & Friedman, 1981; Lavigne & Ryan, 1979). How the family eventually copes with the child's medical problem will be a determining factor in how the child adjusts as well. In the case of chronic physical conditions with a complicated treatment regimen (e.g., fibrocystic disease), family members may need to assume a large degree of responsibility in supervising and implementing daily management. In other instances, home management of chronic problems may require changes in the entire family routine, as may be the case with juvenile diabetes, where the child's dietary restrictions and complex daily regimen may precipitate major life changes for the entire family (Garner & Thompson, 1978).

Although the role of the family is always an important consideration in child health care, it is especially critical when the family situation itself is less than optimal. Problems with health care delivery and psychological functioning are almost sure to emerge when a child develops a serious or chronic illness within the context of an already problematic family situation (Bronheim, 1978; Magrab & Papadopoulou, 1978; Steinhauer et al., 1974). Moreover, the psychosocial stress resulting from problematic family interactions has been implicated in the onset and/or course of several pediatric problems, including asthma (Bronheim, 1978; Khan, Staerk, & Bonk, 1974; Purcell, 1975; Wright et al., 1979), juvenile diabetes (Baker & Barcai, 1970; Garner & Thompson, 1978; Koski & Kumento, 1975), and anorexia nervosa (Bruch, 1971), among others. The weight of the evidence suggests that understanding the role and functioning of the family is particularly important for behavioral pediatrics.

How has family functioning been assessed? Until the present, this has been a generally neglected variable. Most often, researchers have taken a limited view of the family, assessing either the child, the parents (most always the mother only), or the siblings of the affected child, without accounting for the family system as a whole. Even when family relationships have been examined, they are often characterized as simplistically unidirectional; the child's illness is thought to affect the siblings without consideration of how siblings' functioning can affect the child's adjustment. Although further discussion of methodological issues in assessing the family is beyond the scope of this chapter, it is important that the reader be sensitized to the issue of the family's role as literature in behavioral pediatrics is reviewed. (For further details on family assessment see Drotar, 1981 and Melamed & Johnson, 1981.)

Individual Differences in Emotional Functioning/ Behavioral Style

Although certain behavioral characteristics may predispose a child to a given illness, the vast majority of child health problems affect children from a very varied population with no particular premorbid behavioral characteristics, and with varying degrees of emotional adjustment. Consequently, although certain behavioral trends have emerged, one can expect a tremendous degree of variability in children's responses to a particular illness. One can also expect that efforts to find a typical "personality style" or common behavioral characteristics associated with a given illness are likely to prove problematic. Despite this, early investigators invested tremendous energy looking for personality characteristics associated with a wide array of children's health problems (Loughlin & Mosenthal, 1944; McGavin, Schultz, Peden, & Bowen, 1940; Swift, Seidman, & Stein, 1967). By and large, more sophisticated conceptualizations of child health and improved methodology recently have led to the formulation of more complicated research questions.

Major questions of interest include: "What factors (demographic, physical, and psychosocial) are predictive of positive and negative health outcomes for children afflicted with a particular illness?" and "In what manner do the personality characteristics or behavioral style of the individual interact with the demands of the particular illness?" Concerted efforts to answer questions such as these are very much needed.

Regarding the methodology available for studying individual differences, empirically based efforts to classify children's behavior disorders have produced several checklists with excellent psychometric properties that may be of use to researchers in behavioral pediatrics. One example is the Behavior Problem Checklist (Quay, 1977), which assesses four factor-analytically derived problem behavior traits that occur in children and adolescents. This instrument can be suitably employed with psychologically deviant and clinically normal populations; developmental norms are provided (Quay & Peterson, 1975/1979). Considerable support for the validity and reliability of this behavioral checklist has been reviewed (Quay, 1977, 1979).

SELECTED TOPICS OF INTEREST IN BEHAVIORAL PEDIATRICS

Several major topics of interest within behavioral pediatrics have emerged, each with its own particular set of concerns and issues. These topics include: chronic illness in children; the impact of hospitalization and surgery; life-threatening illness; and interdisciplinary problems (e.g., hyperactivity), among others. This chapter section provides a brief overview for several areas, highlighting major issues and suggestions for future investigations.

Chronic Illness in Children

The increasing ability of modern medical treatment to save and extend lives has been a major contributing factor to the growing importance of chronic pediatric conditions. Some estimates suggest that as much as 50% of pediatric practice is now concerned with the chronically disabled child (Magrab & Calcagno, 1978). Epidemiological surveys indicate that at least one in ten children will develop a chronic illness prior to age 15 (Pless & Roghmann, 1971), and this may represent an underestimate of the problem. Table 10.1 lists some of the more common chronic medical conditions found in children and adolescents.

Congenital heart defects and juvenile diabetes provide illustrations of life-saving medical practices. Rowland (1979) estimates that approximately 30,000 children each year are diagnosed as having congenital heart disease. Increasingly sophisticated diagnostic and surgical techniques have led to a much more optimistic outlook for such problems. With current medical care, a child with congenital heart disease who survives the first year of life has much improved chances for continued growth and positive prognosis.

TABLE 10.1
Sampling of Medical Conditions in Children and Adolescents

Problem	Typical Age of Onset/Detection
I. *Chronic conditions*	
Asthma	first 10 years of life
Blindness/visual impairment	at birth/early infancy
Cérebral Palsy	early infancy
Cystic Fibrosis	infancy
Deafness/hearing impairment	infancy
Epilepsy	early childhood
Heart Disease (acquired)	5 to 15 years of age
Heart Disease (congenital)	at birth
Hemophilia	at birth
Hypoglycemia	neonatal period
Juvenile Diabetes	early to middle childhood
Juvenile Rheumatoid Arthritis	prepubertal years
Peptic Ulcers	5 to 12 years of age
Sickle Cell Anemia	at birth
Spinal Bifida	at birth
Turner's Syndrome	at birth
Ulcerative Colitis	10 to 14 years of age
II. *Life-threatening conditions*	
Anorexia Nervosa	adolescence
Leukemia	3 to 5 years of age and older
Muscular Dystrophy	throughout childhood
Renal Disease (Dialysis and kidney transplants)	throughout childhood
Sudden Infant Death	6 months of age or less
Tuberculosis	even across prepubertal years; increased incidence in adolescence
III. *Developmental disorders*	
Acne	adolescence
Articulation disorders	preschool and early elementary school years
Encopresis	preschool through middle elementary school years
Enuresis	preschool through middle elementary school years
Hyperactivity	preschool through middle elementary school years
Infantile Colic	early infancy
Sleep disturbances	preschool years through early elementary years
Stuttering	3 to 5 years
Thumbsucking	preschool years
Tics	8 to 12 years of age

Based on statistics provided by Wright, Schaefer, and Solomons, 1979.

Such has been the case with juvenile diabetes as well. Prior to the discovery of insulin, a diagnosis of juvenile diabetes meant certain death. Now, some 60 years later, increasing emphasis on methods to carefully control the course of this disease has led to increased life expectancy and a more positive health outlook for some 150,000 children (Danowski, 1970; Drash, 1971).

The area of chronic illness provides rich examples of several aspects of behavioral pediatrics. Psychological and emotional factors may contribute to the etiology of certain chronic physical conditions that develop during middle childhood—most notably asthma, peptic ulcers, and ulcerative colitis. Age of onset of chronic diseases may contribute to differential sequelae. For instance, in the case of juvenile diabetes, diagnosis at a very early age may facilitate the child's adjustment to this complex disease, but may have a disruptive influence on the family system, as parents and significant others must assume a large role in the daily management of this disease. By contrast, diagnosis of juvenile diabetes in an adolescent may have less impact on the family routine, but may be a source of extreme emotional distress for the more cognitively aware adolescent, who may be intensively concerned about the implications of the disease for social interactions and future life plans.

With most chronic conditions, perhaps the largest area of interplay between medical and psychological factors can be seen in the difficulties of daily management of the disease. This interplay is most apparent in those diseases requiring complicated treatment regimens. Several of these major issues within chronic illness are considered in the following sections.

A. Psychosocial Correlates of Chronic Illness. Considerable energy has been directed toward investigating personality correlates of various chronic diseases. Research on children with cystic fibrosis, for instance, suggested that anxiety and depression were common psychological concomitants of this disease (Cytryn, Vanmoore, & Robinson, 1973; Lawler, Nakielny, & Wright, 1966; Tropauer, Franz, & Dilgard, 1970). Similar investigations of children with asthma (Leigh & Marley, 1967; Meijer, 1976; Purcell & Weiss, 1970), juvenile diabetes (Baker & Barcai, 1970; Sullivan, 1978), cerebral palsy (Freeman, 1970), and juvenile arthritis (McAnarney, Pless, Satterwhite, & Friedman, 1974) can be found, among others. More recently, the findings of this research have been questioned and underlying assumptions reexamined.

The two key assumptions behind much of the work on psychosocial correlates of chronic illness are: (1) that psychological factors play a major role in the etiology of the disease; and/or (2) that the disease has a major formative influence on the developing child to the extent that a common personality type or typical behavioral pattern might be expected among children sharing a particular chronic disease. As a consequence, researchers developed a common strategy of comparing groups of chronically ill children with physically healthy controls, in an effort to isolate the personality correlates of the particular disease. This research strategy and the underlying assumptions have proved to be very problematic.

In terms of disease etiology, advances in medical research have given greater emphasis to the role of genetic and biological factors in the etiology of many chronic illnesses that were previously thought to have a large psychogenic component. Improved methodology in psychological investigations has also led researchers to conclude that the importance of psychological factors had been overstated. Asthma provides perhaps the best illustration of this medical/psychological trend.

Asthma is predominantly a childhood disorder, affecting up to 4% of the child population (Graham, Rutter, Yule, & Pless, 1967; Wright et al., 1979). It is characterized by: "severe difficulties breathing, manifested in coughing, sneezing, and shortness of breath, which results from a narrowing of the air passages, usually due to increased mucus secretion or excessive swelling of the trachea and bronchi (Schwartz & Johnson, 1981, p. 237)." This disease has a long history of debate over psychological versus physiological factors responsible for its etiology (Mattsson, 1975). Both medical and psychological researchers have been at fault for identifying causative factors from studies that are correlational in nature (Bronheim, 1978).

During the 50s and 60s, a psychogenic view predominated (see Bronheim, 1978 and Wright et al., 1979 for reviews). "Overprotective mothering" was thought to be a prime etiological factor by some (Long, Lamont, Whipple, Bandler, Blom, Burgin, & Jessner, 1958; Pinkerton, 1967, 1970; Rees, 1963); others implicated an overly demanding but nonsupportive maternal style (Little & Cohen, 1951) and other maternal factors (Block, 1969; Garner & Wenar, 1959). A recent medical text (Jolly, 1976) highlights psychological factors by describing children with bronchial asthma and their parents in the following manner:

> (they) are commonly nervous, disturbed children, often described by their parents as being unduly sensitive. They are often introspective, this state usually having been brought on by the parents, one or both of whom are likely to be overanxious. It is because of this relationship that many children with asthma are free of their attacks when away from home and why many improve in boarding school (p. 356).

Fortunately, further efforts to identify physiological factors contributing to asthma coupled with more carefully controlled systematic investigations of the role of psychological factors (e.g., see Purcell, Brady, Chai, Muser, Molk, Gordon, & Means, 1969) have led to a different perspective. It is thought that at least two subgroups of asthmatics can be identified; one in which the disease is precipitated by infection and allergens, and one in which psychological stress may play a role, though even in this case a genetic or biological predisposition to the disease has been posited (Purcell, Weiss, & Hahn, 1972; Schwartz & Johnson,

1981). The view that psychological factors play a major role in the etiology of asthma has not been supported. According to Werry (1979): "There is no evidence that all asthmatic children have significant psychopathology or abnormal parenting. Indeed, . . . when all asthmatic children in the population are studied, differences from normal children become almost imperceptible (p. 146)."

Research efforts have now become attuned to identifying asthmatic subgroups, as well as focusing more directly on the coping strategies that may improve disease management. This trend toward identifying and studying subgroups within the clinical population, and emphasizing factors involved in disease management has been advocated for the study of other chronic illnesses as well (Drotar, 1981; Drotar et al., 1981; Johnson, 1980).

Aside from etiological concerns, studies examining the psychological sequelae of various chronic illnesses also have come into question. Studies in this area have been plagued by a number of very serious methodological flaws, including: (1) small sample size; (2) inclusion of children spanning a very broad age range, without investigating developmental trends in the data; (3) use of instruments with questionable psychometric properties; (4) inappropriate control and comparison groups; (5) neglecting to include age of disease onset as a variable; and (6) disregard for the premorbid functioning of the child and family. (See Drotar, 1981; Gayton & Friedman, 1973; Melamed & Johnson, 1981 for more detailed discussions of these issues.) A number of studies have drawn questionable conclusions from their findings. For instance, Panides and Ziller (1981) recently examined the degree to which the severity of disease (asthma in this case) was related to behavior problems. Mild asthmatics were found to display more acting-out behavior problems than those with more severe forms of the illness, and these results were interpreted to suggest that mild asthmatics were psychologically "healthier" as they were less compliant and more aggressive than the more seriously affected group!

Given these methodological problems, cautious interpretations of research findings are needed. Drotar (1981) summarizes the state of the art nicely:

> . . . recent research employing objective measures and controlled designs suggests that (a) no one personality pattern is associated with a given illness . . . (b) the personality strengths of chronically ill children outweigh their deficits, . . . and (c) chronic illness is a life stressor which, in interaction with other variables, may contribute to increased risk but is *not* the sole cause of adjustment problems (p. 218).

More productive directions for the future research on children's chronic illnesses will involve understanding the factors that differentiate those with positive and negative adjustments to their illnesses, so that those at risk for problems can be identified and aided sooner. Those with effective coping strategies may serve as models for developing appropriate interventions.

B. Psychological Factors in the Management of Chronic Illness. An important and growing area is the study of factors that enable children and adolescents to cope more effectively with chronic illness. Successful management of chronic illness includes the satisfactory implementation of a daily or regular treatment regimen as well as effectively handling the unique limitations and restrictions presented by the illness in various life contexts (e.g., school, family, peer group).

As far as medical management is concerned, compliance with prescribed treatment recommendations has proven to be a problem of critical concern. Rates of noncompliance have been found to be alarmingly high across all chronic medical populations (Rosenstock, 1975). Noncompliance among children with chronic illness and their families is especially serious given the deleterious long-range health consequences that can result from poor disease control (Bronheim, 1978; Garner & Thompson, 1978).

Special problems can arise in obtaining medical compliance from children with chronic illness, as they are largely dependent on other family members (usually the parents) for their medical care. Often, the responsibility for care is diffused among several family members, further complicating disease management. Moreover, at some point, children must be taught and encouraged to assume greater responsibility for self-care, so they can eventually manage their treatment in an effective and independent manner. Yet, the road to independence is often fraught with difficulties, as when a child uses his or her illness in a manipulative manner. One researcher reported that a significant minority of children with diabetes admitted to falsifying routine urine tests in order to receive extra attention from parents, to obtain extra sweets, or to avoid punishment for poor test results (Simonds, 1975).

Although research in this area has just recently begun to receive the detailed attention it merits, several general trends are apparent. Factors that have been found to be related to medical compliance for children and adolescents with chronic illness include: (1) lack of adequate knowledge of the disease and its treatment (Delbridge, 1975; Fireman, Friday, Gira, Vierthaler, & Michaels, 1981); (2) complexity and inconvenience of treatment (Simonds, 1979); (3) quality of patient – physician relationship (Francis, Korsch, & Morris, 1969; Korsch, Gozzi, & Francis, 1968); (4) presence of other life stressors (Bradley, 1979); (5) beliefs in the effectiveness of medical care and other health beliefs and attitudes (Becker & Maiman, 1975; Becker, Radius, Rosenstock, Drachman, Shuberth, & Teets, 1978); and (6) presence of other emotional difficulties or behavioral problems (Knowles, Guest, Lampe, Kessler, & Sillman, 1965; Simonds, 1979).

Illnesses differ in the demands placed on the child and family for medical care. Further analyses of treatment compliance for various diseases should more closely examine the subcomponents of the treatment program. Critical variables to consider in future investigations of medical compliance include the children's developmental level, the role of the family in disease management, and individual differences in children's behavioral styles. Of particular interest are identifying those factors that place a child or family "at risk" for noncompliance and designing intervention strategies that will enable children and families to manage treatment more effectively.

It is important to note that coping with chronic illness extends beyond handling the routine aspects of medical care. Children with chronic conditions often face major life adjustments that do not arise for the physically healthy child. Children who must forgo certain peer activities due to activity limitations, for example, will need to develop alternate strategies for initiating and maintaining friendships. For children with chronic illnesses, Drotar (1981) advocates a closer developmental examination of children's adjustment within various life contexts, including the family, school, peer group, and hospital or medical setting. In this manner, we may better understand the particular stressors associated with a given illness across the life-span, as well as learn effective methods for coping with these life demands.

Hospitalization and Surgery

The importance of considering children's psychological reactions to hospitalization and surgery was not recognized until the mid 1950s. Shore and Goldston (1978) describe the emerging concern with psychological aspects of medical care at that time as stemming from three historic forces: the humanist tradition, which recognized childhood as a discrete phase of development; the increase in knowledge about the interrelationships between psychological and physiological processes; and the growing interest in preventive approaches to adult psychological dysfunctions. Landmark events in the development of interest in children's hospitalization experiences were Bowlby's classic studies of long-term effects of a child's early separation from parents (1952, 1975), and Robertson's (1952) production of the British film, "A Two-Year Old Goes to the Hospital," which vividly portrayed a child's emotional reactions to separation and hospitalization.

Research in the 50s and early 60s focused on the negative effects of hospitalization on the child. The problematic responses described as accompanying and following hospitalization included: severe stress reactions as well as behavior problems such as aggression, eating and sleep disturbances, phobias, regression, enuresis, and encopresis (for reviews see Johnson, 1979; Peterson & Ridley-Johnson, 1980; Shore & Goldston, 1978; Siegel, 1976). Maladaptive responses such as these have been conceptualized as resulting from a combination of factors upsetting the child's psychological equilibrium. For example, Visintainer and Wolfer (1975) describe five categories of threats to the child faced with hospitalization and surgery: physical harm; separation from parents; the unknown, uncertainty of appropriate behavior; and loss of control or autonomy.

From the mid-60s to the present, literature in the field has assumed a more positive focus, that of suggesting methods of alleviating the traumatic aspects of the child's hospital experience. Two distinct types of articles addressing this issue can be delineated: those describing and validating techniques of psychological preparation for the child and/or the parents, and those advocating the availability of specific resources or provisions within the hospital environment. Both approaches reflect the growing emphasis on viewing a child's reactions within a developmental framework.

   A. *Developmental Considerations in Children's Reactions to Hospitalization.*   The influence of a child's developmental level on hospitalization experience has been recently receiving more attention. Not only do children have different anxieties and fears at different ages, but similar concerns are often manifested in different forms according to maturational stage. Prugh and Eckhardt (1980) describe the following age-specific fears related to hospitalization: separation anxiety in the older infant and younger preschool child; fear of body mutilation in the older preschool child; fear of loss of control of feelings or impulses in the school-aged child; and fear of loss of independence or identity in the adolescent.

   Furthermore, the degree and nature of anxiety reactions to hospitalization and medical procedures have been found to follow developmental trends. Katz, Kellerman, and Siegel (1980) describe behavioral indications of anxiety during an uncomfortable medical procedure as following a developmental progression from diffuse vocal protest and skeletal activity in younger children toward greater verbal expression and increased muscle tension in older children. The authors found younger children to display more overall behavioral anxiety, involving a greater variety of anxious behaviors lasting for a longer period of time. Similar developmental differences were found by Powazek, Goff, Schyving, and Paulson (1978) in a study of children in isolation rooms; younger children displayed more anxious behaviors, whereas older children reported a greater degree of anxiety.

   Although a developmental framework is essential for understanding children's reactions to hospitalization and surgery, other issues also merit careful consideration. Much of the early research in this area predates the routine inclusion of procedures (both formal and informal) to prepare children for hospitalization and surgery. Given that children today are better prepared for their hospital stay, further efforts should focus on isolating the various aspects of the hospital experience that are most stressful for the child (e.g., ICU, receiving injections). In this manner, suitable restructuring of hospital environments and health care routines could be accomplished. Information on the strategies employed by children and families to cope with stressful hospital experiences could stimulate the development of intervention approaches to better aid children and families experiencing hospital-related stress. Further, the impact of the *quality* of the hospital experience on future health care behaviors needs to be evaluated.

   It is very possible that the case of the "traumatic" effects of hospitalization and surgery has been overstated. A recent follow-up report on children of preschool age who underwent heart surgery disclosed no major psychological effects (La Greca & Diamond, 1982). Many of the early reports on hospital-related trauma relied heavily on case studies and anecdotal reports of children's postoperative behaviors (Danilowicz & Gabriel, 1971; Jackson, Winkley, Faust, Cermak, &

Burtt, 1953), subjective reports from potentially stressed parents (Jackson et al., 1953; Linde, Rasof, Dunn, & Rabb, 1966), or projective tests (Aisenberg et al., 1973), which tend to overestimate pathology in normal samples (Cox & Sargent, 1950). Postoperative follow-up of children's behavior was rarely conducted, and in the few cases where such information was available, the weight of the evidence suggests that children who came from dysfunctional family situations or who experienced behavioral/emotional problems prior to admission were most likely to display long-term effects (Vernon, Schulman, & Foley, 1966). For the majority of children with positive health outcomes, the stress of hospitalization and surgery appears to be a temporary one. Further research in this area must account for the presurgical functioning of the child and family, the nature of the health outcome postsurgery (positive or negative), as well as the long-range impact of hospital-related stress.

B. *Psychological Preparation for Hospitalization and Surgery.*   The literature on hospitalization reflects a general consensus that all children can benefit from preparatory procedures of one type or another. In fact, Azarnoff and Woody (1981) report that psychological preparation of children for admission and for medical and surgical procedures is now recommended by the American Academy of Pediatrics. Preparation methods may vary according to the range of applicability to different hospital situations, the time at which they are presented or introduced, and their degree of formality and integration into hospital procedures. In addition, preparation may directly address the child, the parents, or both. For example, Kenny (1975) suggests that the physician's role includes preparing the child for the hospital experience, preparing the parents to cope with the reaction of the child to the experience, and preparing parents to cope with their own concerns about the hospitalization.

Despite the importance of hospital preparation programs, it appears that many children and families do not receive such services. Two recent studies have surveyed hospitals regarding their use of preparatory procedures. Peterson and Ridley-Johnson (1980) found 74% of the 62 nonchronic care pediatric hospitals surveyed to employ some type of formal prehospital preparation procedures. However, the average percentage of children in the hospitals typically receiving prehospital preparation was only 42%. The hospitals reported using a variety of preoperative techniques, the most frequent being narrative explanations, printed material such as coloring books, and play therapy.

In a more recent and wider range study, Azarnoff and Woody (1981) sent questionnaires to 2911 children's hospitals and general acute hospitals accepting pediatric patients. Of the 1427 responders, they found only 33% to provide regular, planned preparation services. Hospitals offering preparation procedures typically had more beds for children and accepted children within a wider age range. Those without preparation services often cited low pediatric census and not enough staff as explanations. The most common preparation methods prior to admission were tours and group discussion. During hospitalization, the most common procedures reported were coloring books and informal conversations as events occurred.

Currently, a wide variety of materials are available for use in hospital preparation programs, and many are commercially distributed. These include storybooks, coloring books, filmstrips, and movies (see Altshuler, 1974 and Wolinsky, 1971 for lists and reviews). The purpose of these materials may be to prepare the child for hospitalization and/or for a particular medical procedure. Aside from commercial availability, some hospitals subscribe to commercial preparations and place their hospital stamp on it. As Roberts (1979) describes, serious questions have been raised regarding the adequacy of commercial preparations. Descriptions of procedures in some materials may contain misinformation in their misrepresentation or disregard of the child's feelings and their discrepancy from the actual procedures employed. Most importantly, these products lack validation that they are indeed assuaging a child's fears. In fact, Roberts (1979) points to the potential detrimental effect on a child of preparation materials that lead to unrealistic expectancies of painless and reassuring circumstances.

Individual hospitals may also develop their own materials and procedures for preparing children; in addition to books, filmstrips, and movies, they may include preadmission tours of pediatric wards, group discussions, puppet shows, and play sessions. Once again, these techniques more often than not lack empirical validation and in some cases may not fulfill their purported function (Roberts, Wertele, Boone, Ginther, & Elkins, 1981).

Although systematic investigations of the effectiveness of various methods of psychological preparation on reducing a hospitalized child's stress have been increasing in frequency within the past decade, the literature remains limited. Most notably, studies have focused predominantly on children preparing for routine elective surgery (e.g., tonsillectomy, tooth extractions), with relatively little attention directed toward those awaiting high-risk surgical procedures. Furthermore, numerous methodological difficulties have been noted (see Siegel, 1976, for a critical review). As the research methodology becomes more refined, the interactions of developmental level, time of preparation, type of medical problem, and previous hospital experience with the efficacy of different techniques are being investigated.

To date, the most systematic research has been on the use of modeling techniques in preparation for hospitalization and surgery. The modeling procedure typically involves having the child view a film of another child coping with various medical procedures without experiencing adverse consequences. Relatively consistent support has been found for the effectiveness of modeling techniques in reducing anxiety in hospitalized children (Melamed, Meyer, Gee, & Soule, 1976; Melamed & Siegel, 1975; Melamed, Yurchesen, Fleece, Hutchenson, & Hawks, 1978).

In addition to supporting the efficacy of filmed modeling on reducing children's hospital-related anxiety, Melamed and her associates found interactions between a child's age, previous hospitalization experience, and the timing of the film presentation. Specifically, younger children were found to profit more from immediate preparation (the day of the hospitalization), whereas older children benefited more from viewing the film 1 week prior to hospitalization (Melamed et al., 1976). Additionally in comparing modeling films with demonstration films of varying lengths, children with no prior hospitalization experience were actually sensitized by the short demonstration film (i.e., their anxiety levels rose, Melamed et al., 1978).

Although great strides have been made in the past 20 years, the studies described point to the need for much more work in this area. A dual approach is needed: from the service point of view, more systematic implementation and wider accessibility of preparation procedures are necessary. From the research point of view, a wider range of controlled studies of different preparation techniques is needed, with particular emphasis on the effects of variables such as developmental level, time of preparation, previous hospital experience, severity of illness, and number of exposures to the preparation material. Finally, systematic evaluations of parent-preparation procedures, a largely neglected area, are in need of further exploration.

Life-Threatening Illness

Medical technological advances within the past 10 years have led to dramatic changes in the course of life-threatening illnesses. Diseases that once were acutely fatal have now become chronically life threatening. Concomitant with increased life expectancy and survival rates have appeared a constellation of unique psychological and emotional stresses for the patient, the family, and the health care professionals providing treatment. This section reviews the recent trends in the literature concerning the psychological aspects of life-threatening illness from the aforementioned three perspectives. The predominant trend in the literature to present cancer as a prototype of the study of life-threatening illness will be reflected. (See Table 10.1 for a listing of several life-threatening pediatric illnesses.)

A. The Child's Perspective

The literature in this field can be classified into three principal areas: the child's understanding of death, psychological sequelae of treatment, and overall psychosocial adjustment. The overall focus has been shifting from an emphasis on death to an increased interest in the child's subjective experiences and quality of life.

1. Understanding of Death. The issue of how much a fatally ill child with a life-threatening illness should be told about the illness has been closely intertwined with questions regarding the extent of the child's ability to comprehend the concept of death. The focus of much of the literature in this area consequently has been on developmental issues. The major assumptions of earlier research recently have been challenged: (1) that a child's lack of intellectual ability to comprehend the concept of death implies unawareness of impending death; and (2) that expression of death anxiety is necessarily overt. Consistent with the second assumption, earlier studies on the fatally ill child's concept of death have relied exclusively on parental or staff observations of a child's overt expressions of anxieties and fears. In contrast, recent approaches have been more child centered in their use of projective techniques to assess a child's covert fears. The weight of evidence at this point suggests the following developmental sequence. The primary concerns of the fatally ill child under 5 are loneliness and fear of separation and abandonment; at 6 years of age, the child can have an awareness of the seriousness of the illness and experience anxiety about future body integrity even though the child's concept of death may not be fully formed and concerns may not be expressed overtly; and at 10 years of age, the child begins to display more overt awareness of and anxiety about impending death (Gogan, O'Malley, & Foster, 1977; Kalnins, 1977; Spinetta, 1974; Spinetta, Rigler, & Karon, 1973; Waechter, 1971).

A related issue is how much a child should be told about fatal illness. Gogan et al. (1977) trace the transition from a "protective" approach in the 50s and 60s to a more currently accepted "open" approach. The "protective" approach has been challenged on the basis of eroding a child's trust in caregivers, as children seem to discover for themselves the seriousness of their condition (Binger, Albin, Feuerstein, Kushner, Zoger, & Mikkelsen, 1969; Bluebond-Langner, 1974; Vernick & Karon, 1965). Proponents of the "open" approach advocate evaluating the child's own understanding of his or her condition (Kalnins, 1977) and informing the child—at his or her own level of understanding—of the name, nature, and seriousness of the illness (Koocher & Sallan, 1978). Recent studies have generally provided support for the "open" approach. For instance, one study found that disease-related communication with children is not necessarily accompanied by depression, as was previously thought (Kellerman, Rigler, Siegel, & Katz, 1977). Furthermore, open communication between a fatally ill child and his or her family has been found to be associated with the child's nondefensiveness and basic satisfaction with himself or herself (Spinetta & Maloney, 1978), as well as with the parents' adjustment after the child's death (Spinetta, Swarner, & Sheposh, 1981).

2. *Psychological Sequelae and Treatment.*   Dangerous illnesses often require aggressive treatments that have serious side effects. The use of drugs, radiation, and/or surgery in treating a cancer patient is accompanied by uncomfortable symptoms and changes in physical appearance that can have a profound effect on a child. Changes in physical appearance may include alopecia (hair loss), skin discoloration, dramatic weight changes, and scars or amputations resulting from surgery. It has been well documented that children with visible defects, regardless of the extent of the handicap, tend to have social adjustment problems (Goldberg, 1974). However, little systematic study of the effects of specific body changes resulting from cancer treatment has been conducted. Alopecia has received the most attention. Hair loss has been found to be extremely anxiety provoking for

both children and their parents, children's reactions ranging from defensive flippant joking to social withdrawal to manipulative behavior with parents, siblings, and teachers (Heffron, Bommelare, & Masters, 1973). Adolescents have been described as experiencing the highest level of anxiety, presumably due to the increased importance of personal appearance and peer group acceptance (Moore, Holton, & Marten, 1969). Parental reactions to hair loss are described as contributing strongly to the child's self-perception (Katz, Kellerman, Rigler, Williams, & Siegel, 1977).

3. Psychosocial Adjustment. Although many descriptive accounts of the stigmatized effect of a child's cancer have been published, few investigators have attempted systematic study of the long-term adjustment of cancer survivors. The stigma that such a child may experience has been explained in terms of fear of contagion, discomfort with the child's physical appearance or uncertain future, and reminding us of our own tenuous mortality (Gogan et al., 1977).

A child who has experienced frequent or lengthy hospitalizations may have a difficult time returning to school. Aside from peer rejection, the child often faces differential treatment by teachers as well as intense pressure to "catch up" with missed work. The child's responses to these stresses may be decreased school participation, separation anxiety, and/or school phobia (Katz et al., 1977; Lansky, Lowman, Vats, & Gyulay, 1975).

Two recent studies have investigated the long-term psychological adjustment of 115 survivors of childhood cancer, aged 5 to 36, returning for their annual follow-up examinations. The first study found 23% of the individuals to exhibit moderate or severe psychological impairments, with an additional 36% demonstrating mild impairments (O'Malley et al., 1979). However, interpretation of these findings is limited by the absence of a control group. In the second paper, an association was found between better adjustment (as rated from interviews) and younger age at diagnosis, higher intelligence, less self-reported depression or anxiety, and a smaller self-ideal discrepancy (Koocher, O'Malley, Gogan, & Foster, 1980). Although these studies suggest that adjustment problems are commonly experienced by adult survivors of childhood cancer, it is also apparent that the majority coped extremely well with many complicated and challenging life demands (Drotar, 1981). Clearly, the need for more systematic and controlled longitudinal studies of adjustment and coping cannot be overstated.

B. The Family's Perspective

The omnipresent prospect of a child's death forces family members to face daily uncertainty as well as maintain the difficult stance of guarded optimism and cautious hope. Family role, rules, and routines often shift to accommodate this situation. As the thrust of research on life-threatening illness moves in the direction of considering the whole child, family research has expanded to a more comprehensive "systems" approach that includes assessments of the child's siblings as well as the parents.

Early family studies concentrated almost exclusively on the mothers of fatally ill children. These mothers have been found to follow somewhat predictable patterns of coping. Disbelief and denial of the diagnosis is followed sequentially by anxiety and sadness, guilt, and finally calm acceptance (Natterson & Knudson, 1960). The coping process by which the family prepares for the child's death before it occurs is referred to as "anticipatory grief" (Lindemann, 1944). During this process family members gradually separate themselves from the patient, mourning the illness as well as the impending death. Although this may be an effective coping mechanism for the family, the effects on the child of the parents' increased emotional distance is unclear. Some authors have hypothesized that the child's perception of this parental detachment leads to an increasing sense of isolation (Spinetta, 1974, 1977; Spinetta & Maloney, 1975; Spinetta, Rigler, & Karon, 1974; Waechter, 1971).

More recently, efforts have been made to include both parents in family research. Parenting roles have been cited as particularly subject to disruption when a child develops a life-threatening illness (Koocher & Sallan, 1978). Feelings of guilt often accompany the discipline process and the child may learn to be quite manipulative (Heffron et al., 1973). Levels of marital stress have been found to be significantly higher in parents of fatally ill children as compared with parents of hemophilic or "control" children (Lansky, Cairns, Hassanein, Wehr, & Lowman, 1978). Furthermore, families of leukemic children usually are forced to face one or more serious stresses that affect their coping abilities, such as illness or death of other family members, while caring for their leukemic child (Kalnins et al., 1980). However, despite the high level of marital tension and family stress, the incidence of separation or divorce remains low, no higher than population divorce statistics (Kalnins et al., 1980; Lansky et al., 1978). Following the death of the child, parental adjustment has been found to be positively related to a consistent philosophy of life, an ongoing source of emotional support, and prior open communication with the child about the illness (Spinetta et al., 1981).

Siblings of seriously ill children often demonstrate a range of behavioral problems including enuresis, encopresis, poor school performance, school refusal, depression, and "separation anxiety" (Binger et al., 1969). Heffron et al. (1973) describe a cycle of jealousy, teasing, and guilt found in siblings. Gogan et al. (1977) describe the persistence of sibling problems—including sibling rivalry and feelings of guilt and exclusion from family crises—5 or more years after the diagnosis of cancer. More recently, investigators have found siblings of children with cancer to experience feelings similar to those of the sick child: anxiety, fear for their own health, and social isolation (Cairns, Clark, Smith, & Lansky, 1979).

An important direction for the future is a more comprehensive examination of the family unit as a whole. The advent of specific methodologies to assess various aspects of family functioning (Lewis, Beavers, Gosett, & Phillips, 1976; Moos &

Moos, 1976; Olson, Sprenkle, & Russell, 1979; Straus & Tallman, 1971) should further our understanding of the challenges and problems faced by families of fatally ill children.

C. Health Care Professionals

Providing treatment for sick or dying children is a complex and painful task from the perspective of all caregivers. From a medical stance, the advent of new treatment methods has caused a shift in the physician's priorities from alleviation of pain and discomfort to pursuing treatment protocols that often involve traumatic and painful procedures and side effects. Furthermore, counseling a patient or the parents on the life-threatening aspects of the illness, and trying to convey a sense of guarded optimism, may be difficult for a physician whose self-esteem is dependent on medical successes (Gogan et al., 1977; Koocher & Sallan, 1978).

Caregivers frequently experience extreme reactions to seriously ill or dying children, ranging from overinvolvement to avoidance to ambivalent approach-avoidance (Gogan et al., 1977). Furthermore, Frader (1979) describes residents' reactions to working on a pediatric intensive care unit as involving depression and an increased need for extra emotional support.

The psychological aspects of health care delivery encompass several areas. They include providing appropriate outlets for caregivers to discharge their emotions; focusing on the quality of a child's experiences by humanizing and personalizing hospital environments, involving family members in the child's care, and considering the "whole child" in planning treatment regimens; and providing the family with ongoing access to psychological consultation services within the hospital (Gogan et al., 1977).

D. Conclusion

This section has reviewed psychological aspects of life-threatening illnesses from different perspectives. Advocacy of open communication with the child, increased interest in the child's subjective experience and quality of life, and greater consideration of long-term adjustment difficulties have been described as recent trends in the literature. However, a strong need for more systematic investigations continues to exist. Increased life expectancy has created a crucial need for longitudinal studies of adjustment problems so that difficulties can be anticipated and preventive measures instituted. Control groups consisting of chronically ill children are necessary in order to identify psychological issues specific to dying children. A further suggestion for future research is the more systematic investigation of developmental issues as they interact with adjustment. For instance, an understanding of the relationships between age of diagnosis and the child's coping style, treatment by friends and family, and later psychosocial adjustment would be helpful in designing appropriate psychological interventions.

Interdisciplinary Problems

Although behavioral pediatrics, by nature, is likely to involve the collaborative efforts of professionals in medicine, psychology, nursing, and sociology, among other areas, a coordinated interdisciplinary approach to treatment and research has been slow to develop. However, the diagnosis, treatment, and understanding of certain developmental — pediatric problems have gradually demanded the involvement of several disciplines. Hyperactivity, or Attention Deficit Disorder with Hyperactivity in current nomenclature, serves as an excellent prototype of this recent biopsychosocial approach to pediatric problems and, as such, is discussed in the following section. Originally approached independently by the domains of medicine, education, and psychology, the current view of the diagnosis, etiology, and treatment of hyperactivity in children reflects a multidisciplinary and developmental perspective.

A. Attention Deficit Disorder with Hyperactivity (ADDH)—Descriptive and Etiology

ADDH is a frequently diagnosed childhood behavior disorder that is defined as a child's frequent failure to comply in age-appropriate fashion with situational demands for restrained activity, sustained attention, resistance to distracting influences, and inhibition of impulsive responding (Routh, 1978). Although estimates of the prevalence rates for hyperactivity have varied widely, recent epidemiological studies employing careful diagnostic criteria show the incidence to be between 1 and 2% of the school-aged population (Lambert, Sandoval, & Sassone, 1978; Schachar, Rutter, & Smith, 1981).

The past 15 years have seen a shift away from defining hyperactivity in terms of motor activity level to an emphasis on problems with organizing and sustaining attention and inhibiting impulsive responding. Recent conceptualizations of ADDH support a constitutional predisposition to attentional problems; other behavioral difficulties, such as excessive motor activity, are seen as secondary to and resulting from primary attentional deficits (Douglas & Peters, 1980).

Another recent trend in this area is that ADDH is now viewed as a lifelong disorder, rather than a transient behavior problem, with different symptoms or problematic behaviors becoming salient during different developmental periods (Barkley, 1978; O'Leary, 1980). Although problems of motor overactivity seem to decline with age, difficulties with impulsive responding and sustained attention may persist through adolescence and adulthood. In addition, effective social functioning appears to become more problematic with increased age for those who display aggressive behaviors concomitant with attentional deficits (Loney, Kramer, & Milich, 1979).

There is a considerable lack of consensus in the literature regarding the etiology of ADDH. Its origins have been attributed to neurological abnormalities, low CNS arousal state, genetic factors, social influences, and reactions to noxious physical and chemical agents, such as lead poisoning, maternal smoking, fluorescent lighting, and allergy to food additives (see Barkley, 1981; Routh, 1978; and Varga, 1979 for reviews). In addition, sugar consumption has recently been associated with increased destructive and aggressive behavior in hyperactive children (Prinz, Roberts, & Hartman, 1980). Lack of solid empirical support for any one theory has led to the suggestion that hyperactivity is a "common clinical expression for a variety of etiological processes [Varga, 1979, p. 415]."

B. Assessment and Diagnosis

An important issue pervading the literature is the accurate diagnosis of ADDH. Until recently, differential diagnosis between hyperactivity and aggressive conduct disorders was a very difficult task. The overlap between the behaviors thought to be representative of each disorder was so great that there existed legitimate concern as to whether the two could be reliably distinguished (Lahey, Green, & Forehand, 1980; O'Leary, 1980; Quay, 1979; Sandberg, Wieselberg, & Shaffer, 1980). However, the current emphasis on attentional deficits versus motor activity in ADDH should help to clarify this diagnostic confusion.

Current DSM III criteria required for the diagnosis of Attention Deficit Disorder with Hyperactivity include the following: (1) *inattention* (e.g., difficulty concentrating on school work, easily distracted); (2) *impulsivity* (e.g., acts before thinking, difficulty awaiting turn in games or group situations); (3) *hyperactivity* (e.g., excessive running or climbing, difficulty sitting still); (4) *onset* of problems *prior to age 7;* (5) difficulties not due to schizophrenia, affective disorder, or severe or profound mental retardation (American Psychiatric Association, 1980). A diagnosis of Attention Deficit Disorder without Hyperactivity can be made if activity level behaviors are not problematic.

In order to facilitate the reliable diagnosis of ADDH, several authors have advocated a multidisciplinary approach to assessment (Silber, 1981; Varga, 1979; Weiss & Hechtman, 1979). The following types of evaluations are recommended for a comprehensive assessment:

1. A *physical examination* to rule out the possibility of competing medical or neurological factors contributing to hyperactive behaviors is a necessary first step. In addition, physicians' clinical impressions can aid in identifying ADDH (Lambert et al., 1978). However, Sleator and Ullman (1981) caution that physicians cannot necessarily diagnosis ADDH accurately from standard office visits; other sources of input are needed as well. These authors found that only 20% of a group of hyperactive children were diagnosed as such during routine physical examinations.

2. A careful *social* and *environmental history* should be obtained from the parents. Specific behavioral problems of the past and present should be described in terms of their frequency, severity, duration, and relationship to situational factors. Parent behavioral checklists may supplement this information. An accu-

rate diagnosis requires evidence that problems with attention and impulsive responding have persisted over time.

3. *Psychoeducational assessment* should be conducted to determine the presence of learning disorders that frequently occur with hyperactivity. In addition, information can be gained about a child's ability to concentrate and sustain attention in a one-to-one situation. The presence of emotional factors that might contribute to attentional problems (such as preoccupation with a family crisis) should also be determined for differential diagnosis.

4. Although attentional problems and hyperactive behaviors have been found to occur with considerable day-to-day variability and situational specificity, they are most apparent in classroom situations that require self-application (Abikoff, Gittelman, & Klein, 1980; Routh, 1980; Varga, 1979; Weiss & Hechtman, 1979; Whalen, Collins, Henker, Alkus, Adams, & Stapp, 1978; Zentall, 1980). Thus, *direct observation of classroom behavior* is an invaluable tool in gaining the information necessary to make an accurate diagnosis. Moreover, *teachers' reports* of the child's behavior, obtained from interviews and behavioral checklists, should always be included in the assessment process.

C. Treatment

The two most common treatment approaches to ADDH are the use of psychostimulant medications and the use of psychological techniques involving cognitive and behavioral principles. Each is discussed in terms of its efficacy in improving social behaviors as well as academic performance.

1. Psychostimulant Treatment. The use of stimulant medications such as methylphenidate (Ritalin) and dextroamphetamine (Dexedrine) is currently the most common treatment for hyperactivity. Reviews have found drug therapy to result consistently in short-term improvements in social, but not academic behaviors (Barkley, 1981). Teacher rating scales reflect improved attention, cooperation, and compliance, and behavioral observation methods generally find decreased movement and fidgeting with drug treatment. However, no consistent achievement gains, either short-term or long-term, have been associated with drug therapy (Barkley, 1981; O'Leary, 1980; Routh, 1978), nor should they be expected from this treatment alone as it cannot remediate the accumulated cognitive effects of the child's attentional deficits (see Douglas & Peters, 1980; Weingarten, Rapoport, Buchsbaum, Bunney, Ebert, Mikkelsen, & Caine, 1980).

Drug treatment may have other liabilities as well. Short-term physical side effects such as increased heart and blood pressure rates (O'Leary, 1980), insomnia, decreased appetite, and irritability (Barkley, 1981), and temporary growth suppression (Roche, Lipman, Overall, & Hung, 1979) have been reported. Moreover, the potential detrimental effects of long-term drug use have not been well studied (Barkley, 1981). The psychosocial impact of chronic drug use also has been largely neglected; possible disadvantages are undesirable causal attributions, which may interfere with children learning more adaptive social behavior and parents learning more appropriate parenting and child management skills (Silber, 1981; Wright et al., 1979). Further evaluation of the physical and psychological concomitants of stimulant drug therapy will require concerted interdisciplinary efforts.

2. *Psychological Treatment: Cognitive and Behavioral Interventions.* There are two broad categories of psychological interventions: operant conditioning and self-control techniques. Self-control methods include problem solving, self-instruction, and cognitive modeling. All involve teaching the child to use cognitive strategies to mediate behavioral responses. For example, the child may be taught to improve academic performance by slowly going through the steps necessary for solving a math problem, or to decrease aggression by examining alternative responses to a frustrating situation. Currently, there is suggestive evidence that self-control methods may lead to improvements in academic, though not social situations (O'Leary, 1980; Routh, 1978). However, in their review of research in this area, Hobbs, Moguin, Tyroler, and Lahey (1980) describe a number of methodological improvements that are necessary before the clinical utility of these techniques can be fully documented, such as the inclusion of appropriate treatment control groups and measures to assess the durability and generalizability of responses from laboratory to natural settings. These authors also highlight the need for researchers to specifically delineate the problem behaviors in the natural environment that are affected by intervention rather than focusing solely on changes in general psychiatric labels or psychoeducational tests.

Operant conditioning techniques involve provision of rewards for good classroom behavior. Rewards may be social, as in positive teacher attention, or concrete, as utilized in token reinforcement procedures. In home-contingency programs, children are rewarded at home for their behavior in school. These programs typically involve establishment of specific behavioral contracts that are evaluated daily. In addition, educationally oriented groups for parent training in child management have been used to teach parents operant conditioning principles.

Research reviews generally indicate that operant techniques emphasizing reinforcement of classroom behavior, teacher consultation, and home-based reinforcement lead to improved social behavior on observation as well as teacher rating scales (Barkley, 1981; O'Leary, 1980). In addition, academic production rates have been found to increase in home or classroom-based reinforcement programs, when academic behaviors are targeted (O'Leary, 1980).

Although cognitive and behavioral interventions hold much promise for aiding parents, teachers, and children to cope more effectively with attention-deficit and hyperactive behaviors, a combination of psychological and psychopharmacological treatments may be desirable in some cases (Barkley, 1981). It is just recently that researchers have begun to explore combinations and comparisons of different treatment methods for ADDH; this is an important avenue for interdisciplinary research.

3. Combination of Drug and Psychological Treatments.   Recently studies have begun to compare the major treatment approaches to ADDH (Gittelman-Klein, Klein, Abikoff, Katz, Gloisten, & Kates, 1976). For example, Pelham and associates (Pelham, Schnedler, Bologna, & Contreras, 1980) assessed the individual and combined efforts of Ritalin and behavioral intervention focusing on teacher and parent training. Although both treatments were independently effective in improving behavior, only the combination of Ritalin and behavioral intervention resulted in classroom behavior that resembled that of the nonhyperactive controls. Just as diagnosis has been recently conceptualized as a multidisciplinary process, the most effective treatment for hyperactive children may involve combinations that capitalize on the strengths of several different methods. For example, the effects of drug treatment and behavioral contracting may complement each other and lead to improvement in both social and academic functioning. Pelham et al.'s (1980) results clearly demonstrate the need for further research involving multidisciplinary approaches to treatment.

4. Other Approaches.   Many other treatment approaches for ADDH have been advocated though less systematically evaluated. The implementation of dietary regimens, particularly the Feingold diet, has received much public attention (Connors, 1980; Connors, Goyette, Southwick, Lees, & Andrulonis, 1976). Recent interest stems from Feingold's (1975) hypothesis that hyperactivity results from an intolerance to salicylates and food additives. Although evidence has been presented both for and against this treatment, the more carefully controlled studies provide very limited support for its clinical utility (Barkley, 1981; Connors, 1980). Fewer than 10% of the children with ADDH are believed to be sensitive to the presence of food additives in their diet (Barkley, 1981). Moreover, the long term nutritional effects of this diet are unknown.

Studies of vitamin deficiencies or excessive sugar content in the diets of children with hyperactivity have not yielded any clinically impressive findings and have been fraught with methodological problems (Barkley, 1981). At the present time, there is very limited empirical support for interventions based on these findings.

Environmental manipulation, or restructuring the environment to enable the child to cope successfully with increasing stimuli, is an approach that can be implemented along with other treatment procedures. Wright et al. (1979) reviews recommendations that have been proposed in the literature. These include keeping activities brief and within a child's capability for sustained attention, making sure the child is attending before giving instructions, and keeping directions as brief and specific as possible. However, Barkley (1981) cautions that such approaches are unlikely to facilitate academic performance, unless accompanied by other operant behavioral strategies.

5. Conclusions Regarding Treatment.   Although positive results have been obtained for both drug and psychological interventions, there is a general consensus that these effects are short-term and do not significantly alter a prognosis for a child with ADDH (Barkley, 1978, 1981; O'Leary, 1980). Accordingly, Barkley (1978) has recommended that treatment emphasis be shifted away from providing expectations of a cure, and toward providing strategies for coping with attentional deficits and their effects. In this light, intervention may be best conceptualized as an ongoing process that involves physicians, psychologists, teachers, and parents, as well as the child.

D. Summary and Conclusions

ADDH is currently conceptualized as a lifelong disorder involving situation-specific behaviors that vary somewhat with age. The heterogeneity of children diagnosed as hyperactive will require careful investigation of etiological factors that may have implications for clinical treatment. A multidisciplinary approach to diagnosis, consisting of input from parents, educators, physicians, and psychologists, has been advocated. Both psychostimulant medication and psychological interventions have been associated with short-term behavioral improvements, though long-term effects have yet to be documented. The potential potency of combinations of treatments has received some support and warrants further investigation. The lack of a long-term "cure" for hyperactivity suggests that treatment be conceptualized as an ongoing process with an emphasis on teaching coping strategies to parents, teachers, and the child. Along these lines, assessment of the efficacy of parent training, environmental manipulation, and social skills training for hyperactive children is recommended, and interdisciplinary research efforts in these areas are advocated.

SUMMARY AND CONCLUSIONS

The research summarized in the present chapter represents a brief overview of several major areas of interest within behavioral pediatrics. Investigation of the behavioral aspects of neonatology (Quinn, Sostek, & Davitt, 1978), teenage pregnancy (Scott, Field, & Robertson, 1981), developmental problems (Coates & Thorenson, 1981; Doleys, Schwartz, & Ciminero, 1981), accident prevention (Kanther, 1976; Lieberman, Emmet, & Carlson, 1976), mental retardation and sensory impairments (Cox & Edelin, 1978; Leland, 1978), as well as health-risk factors for children and adolescents (Coates & Thorenson, 1980; Horan & Harrison, 1981) additionally fall within the realm of behavioral pediatrics and are important areas of study in their own right. However, regardless of the specialized medical area of interest, several methodological concerns arise that have broad implications for the entire field.

For one, the advancement of research in behavioral pediatrics will be largely dependent on the type of measures that are employed to document psychosocial variables. Too often, researchers have relied on measures with questionable reliability and validity for child and family populations. Measures designed for use with psychiatric populations, such as projective tests, may be very inappropriate and misleading when used with essentially "normal" populations of children with a particular medical problem and their families. Other difficulties, such as over-reliance on subjective reports rather than objective assessment and the absence of information on developmental norms for many measures, present distinct handicaps for researchers interested in the medical problems of children and adolescents. Furthermore, a number of investigators have employed "scaled-down" versions of psychosocial measures designed for use with adults; the validity of such an approach to child assessment has been seriously questioned (Achenbach, 1978). The assessment process differs considerably for children and adults; recognition of and attention to these differences will be critical for behavioral pediatrics. (See Evans & Nelson, 1977; Hetherington & Martin, 1979; La Greca, 1983 for detailed descriptions of the child and family assessment process.) At the present time, there is an urgent need for the development of psychometrically sound methods to assess psychologically important variables in children and families within a medical setting. (The reader is referred to several sources for detailed information on the assessment of children's medical problems: Balaschak & Mostofsky, 1981; Foreyt & Goodrick, 1981; Melamed & Johnson, 1981.)

A second area of concern is that of the types of research designs commonly employed in medical – psychosocial pediatric research. The vast majority of studies have been correlational and/or cross-sectional in nature. Although this has provided an excellent starting point for generating meaningful hypotheses, many interesting questions regarding the etiology, course, and long-range consequences of medical problems can be answered only through more painstaking experimental and longitudinal research efforts. A related issue is the need for more careful attention to the parameters of control populations. The limitations of studies that have neglected to include a control group or have employed physically healthy controls have already been noted (Drotar, 1981; Melamed & Johnson, 1981). In addition, studies examining the impact of various psychoeducational interventions on medical status (e.g., Fireman et al., 1981) or medical interventions on psychosocial status (e.g., allergies in hyperactive children) often have failed to include appropriate attention and/or placebo controls where ethically possible.

As has been mentioned throughout this chapter, there is a critical need for investigators to evaluate the premorbid functioning and/or behavioral characteristics of the child and family in order to examine more closely how these variables interact with the course and management of treatment. Most populations in behavioral pediatrics include heterogeneous groups of children and families. With the growing emphasis on developing positive strategies for improving disease management and strengthening personal coping skills, knowledge of how these individual differences interact with the onset and course of disease will be invaluable for improving the quality of health care and generating more positive health outcomes for children and adolescents.

Finally, the nature of research in behavioral pediatrics mandates a greater emphasis on interdisciplinary research efforts. To fully appreciate the interplay of medical and psychosocial variables, collaborative efforts among investigators with expertise in medical and psychosocial areas are very much needed.

REFERENCES

Abikoff, H., Gittelman, R., & Klein, D. F. Classroom observation code for hyperactive children: A replication of validity. *Journal of Consulting and Clinical Psychology,* 1980, *48*(5), 555 – 565.

Achenbach, T. M. Psychopathology of childhood: Research problems and issues. *Journal of Consulting and Clinical Psychology,* 1978, *46,* 759 – 776.

Adams, J., & Lindemann, E. Coping with long-term disability. In G. V. Coelho, D. A. Hamburg, & J. E. Adams (Eds.), *Coping and adaptation.* New York: Basic Books, 1974.

Aisenberg, R. B., Wolff, P. H., Rosenthal, A., & Nadas, A. S. Psychological impact of cardiac catherization. *Pediatrics,* 1973, *51,* 1051 – 1059.

Altshuler, A. *Books that help children deal with a hospital experience.* Washington, D.C.: U.S. Government Printing Office, 1974. DHEW Publication No. (HSA) 74 – 5402.

American Psychiatric Association. *Diagnostic and statistical manual of mental disorders (DSM III).* Washington, D.C.: 1980.

Azarnoff, P., & Woody, P. D. Preparation of children for hospitalization in acute care hospitals in the U.S. *Pediatrics,* 1981, *68*(3), 361 – 368.

Baker, L., & Barcai, A. Psychosomatic aspects of diabetes mellitus. *Modern Trends in Psychosomatic Medicine,* 1970, *2,* 105 – 123.

Balaschak, B. A., & Mostofsky, D. I. Seizure disorders. In E. J. Mash & L. G. Terdal (Eds.), *Behavioral assessment of childhood disorders.* New York: Guilford Press, 1981.

Barkley, R. A. Recent developments in research on hyperactive children. *Journal of Pediatric Psychology,* 1978, *3*(4), 158 – 163.

Barkley, R. A. *Hyperactive children: A handbook for diagnosis and treatment.* New York: Guilford, 1981.

Battle, C. U. Chronic physical disease: Behavioral aspects. *Pediatric Clinics of North America,* 1975, *22*(3), 525 – 531.

Becker, M. H., & Maiman, L. A. Sociobehavioral determinants of compliance with health and medical care recommendations. *Medical Care,* 1975, *8,* 10 – 24.

Becker, M. H., Radius, S. M., Rosenstock, I. M., Drachman, R. H., Shuberth, K. C., & Teets, K. C. Compliance with a medical regimen for asthma: A test of the Health Belief Model. *Public Health Records,* 1978, *93,* 268 – 277.

Binger, C. M., Albin, A. R., Feuerstein, R. C., Kushner, J. H., Zoger, S., & Mikkelson, C. Childhood leukemia: Emotional impact on patient and family. *New England Journal of Medicine,* 1969, *280,* 414 – 418.

Block, J. Parents of schizophrenic, neurotic, asthmatic, and congenitally ill children: A comparative study. *Archives of General Psychiatry,* 1969, *20,* 659 – 674.

Bluebond-Langner, M. I know, do you? A study of awareness communication, coping in terminally ill children. In B. Schoenberg, A. C. Carr, A. Kutscher, D. Peretz, & I. Goldberg (Eds.), *Anticipatory grief.* New York: Columbia University Press, 1974.

Bowlby, J. Maternal care and mental health 1952 (2nd ed.). *World Health Monograph #2.* Geneva, Switzerland.

Bowlby, J. Attachment theory: Separation, anxiety, and mourning. In S. Arieti (Ed.), *American Handbook of Psychiatry* (2nd ed., Vol. 2). New York: Basic Books, 1975.

Bradley, C. Life events and the control of diabetes mellitus. *Journal of Psychosomatic Research,* 1979, *23,* 159 – 162.

Bronheim, S. P. Pulmonary disorders: Asthma and cystic fibrosis. In P. R. Magrab (Ed.), *Psychological management of pediatric problems,* Vol. I., Sec. III. Baltimore, Md.: University Park Press, 1978.

Bruch, H. Changing approaches to anorexia nervosa. *International Psychiatry Clinics,* 1971, *45,* 3–24.

Cairns, N. U., Clark, G. M., Smith, S. P., & Lansky, S. B. Adaptation of siblings to childhood malignancy. *Journal of Pediatrics,* 1979, *95,* 484–487.

Campbell, J. D. Illness is a point of view: The development of children's concept of illness. *Child Development,* 1975, *46,* 92–100.

Chodoff, P., Friedman, S. B., & Hamburg, D. Stress, defenses and coping behavior: Observations in parents and children with malignant disease. *American Journal of Psychiatry,* 1964, *120,* 743–749.

Coates, T. J., & Thorenson, C. E. Obesity among children and adolescents: The problem belongs to everyone. In B. B. Lahey & A. F. Kazdin (Eds.), *Advances in clinical child psychology* (Vol. 3). New York: Plenum Press, 1980.

Coates, T. J., & Thorenson, C. E. Sleep disturbance in children and adolescents. In E. J. Mash & L. G. Terdal (Eds.), *Behavioral assessment of childhood disorders.* New York: Guilford Press, 1981.

Connors, C. K. A teacher rating scale for use in drug studies with children. *American Journal of Psychiatry,* 1969, *126,* 884–888.

Connors, C. K. *Food additives and hyperactive children.* New York: Plenum Press, 1980.

Connors, C. K., Goyette, C. H., Southwick, D. A., Lees, J. M., & Andrulonis, P. A. Food additives and hyperkinesis: A controlled double-bind experiment. *Pediatrics,* 1976, *58,* 154–166.

Cook, S. *The development of causal thinking with regard to physical illness among French children.* Master's thesis, University of Kansas, Kansas City, 1975.

Cox, B. P., & Edelin, P. Hearing deficits. In P. R. Magrab (Ed.), *Psychological management of pediatric problems.* Baltimore: University Park Press, 1978.

Cox, B., & Sargent, H. TAT responses of emotionally disturbed and emotionally stable children: Clinical judgment versus normative data. *Journal of Projective Techniques,* 1950, *14,* 61–74.

Cytryn, L., Vanmoore, P. V. P., & Robinson, H. E. Psychological adjustment of children with cystic fibrosis. In E. J. Anthony & C. Koupernik (Eds.), *The child and his family* (Vol. 2). New York: John Wiley and Sons, 1973.

Danilowicz, D. A., & Gabriel, H. P. Postoperative reactions in children: "Normal" and abnormal responses after cardiac surgery. *American Journal of Psychiatry,* 1971, *120,* 185–188.

Danowski, T. S. Diabetes in children. In T. S. Danowski (Ed.), *Diabetes as a way of life.* New York: Coward-McCann, Inc., 1970.

Delbridge, L. Educational and psychological factors in the management of diabetes in childhood. *Medical Journal of Australia,* 1975, *2,* 737–739.

Doleys, D. M., Schwartz, M. S., & Ciminero, A. R. Elimination problems: Enuresis and encopresis. In E. J. Mash & L. G. Terdal (Eds.), *Behavioral assessment of childhood disorders.* New York: Guilford Press, 1981.

Douglas, V. I., & Peters, K. G. Toward a clearer definition of the attentional deficit of hyperactive children. In G. A. Hale & M. Lewis (Eds.), *Attention and cognitive development.* New York: Plenum Publishing Corp., 1980.

Drash, A. Obesity and diabetes in childhood. *Journal of the Florida Medical Association,* 1971, *58,* 38–40.

Drotar, D. Psychological perspectives in chronic childhood illness. *Journal of Pediatric Psychology,* 1981, *6,* 211–228.

Drotar, D., Doershuk, C. F., Boat, T. F., Stern, R. C., Matthews, L., & Boyer, W. Psychosocial functioning of children with cystic fibrosis. *Pediatrics,* 1981, *67,* 338–343.

Duff, R. S., Rowe, D. S., & Anderson, F. P. Patient care and student learning in a pediatric clinic. *Pediatrics,* 1972, *50,* 839–846.

Evans, I., & Nelson, R. O. Child assessment. In A. R. Ciminero, D. S. Calhoun, & H. E. Adams (Eds.), *Handbook of behavioral assessment.* New York: Wiley, 1977.

Feingold, B. *Why your child is hyperactive.* New York: Random House, 1975.

Fireman, P., Friday, G. A., Gira, C., Vierthaler, W. A., & Michaels, L. Teaching self-management skills to asthmatic children and their parents in an ambulatory care setting. *Pediatrics*, 1981, *68*, 341–348.

Foreyt, J. P., & Goodrick, G. K. Childhood obesity. In E. J. Mash & L. G. Terdal (Eds.), *Behavioral assessment of childhood disorders*. New York: Guilford Press, 1981.

Frader, J. E. Difficulties in providing intensive care. *Pediatrics*, 1979, *64*(1), 10–16.

Francis, V., Korsch, B. M., & Morris, M. J. Gaps in doctor–patient communication: Patients' response to medical advice. *New England Journal of Medicine*, 1969, *280*, 235–240.

Freeman, R. D. Psychiatric problems in adolescents with cerebral palsy. *Developmental Medicine and Child Neurology*, 1970, *12*, 64–70.

Garner, A. M., & Thompson, C. W. Juvenile diabetes. In P. R. Magrab (Ed.), *Psychological management of pediatric problems*. I. Baltimore, Md.: University Park Press, 1978.

Garner, A., & Wenar, C. *The mother–child interaction in psychosomatic disorders*. Champaign, Ill.: University of Illinois Press, 1959.

Gayton, W. F., & Friedman, S. B. Psychosocial aspects of cystic fibrosis: A review of the literature. *American Journal of Diseases of Children*, 1973, *126*, 856–859.

Gittelman-Klein, R., Klein, D. F., Abikoff, H., Katz, S., Gloisten, A. C., & Kates, W. Relative efficacy of methylphenidate and behavior modification in hyperkinetic children: An interim report. *Journal of Abnormal Child Psychology*, 1976, *4*, 361.

Gogan, J. L., O'Malley, J. E., & Foster, D. J. Treating the pediatric cancer patient: A review. *Journal of Pediatric Psychology*, 1977, *2*(2), 42–48.

Goldberg, I. D., Regier, D. A., McAnarny, T. K., Pless, I. B., & Roghmann, K. J. The role of the pediatrician in the delivery of mental health services to children. *Pediatrics*, 1979, *63*(6), 898–909.

Goldberg, R. T. Adjustment of children with invisible and visible handicaps: Congenital heart disease and facial burns. *Journal of Counseling Psychology*, 1974, *21*(5), 428–432.

Graham, P., Rutter, M., Yule, W., & Pless, I. B. Childhood asthma: A psychosomatic disorder? Some epidemiological considerations. *British Journal of Preventive and Social Medicine*, 1967, *21*, 78–85.

Greydanus, D. E., & Hoffman, A. D. Psychological factors in diabetes mellitus: A review of the literature with emphasis on adolescence. *American Journal of Diseases of Children*, 1979, *133*, 1061–1066.

Heffron, W. A., Bommelare, K., & Masters, R. Group discussion with the parents of leukemic children. *Pediatrics*, 1973, *52*, 831–837.

Heisler, A. B., & Friedman, S. B. Social and psychological considerations in chronic disease: With particular reference to the management of seizure disorders. *Journal of Pediatric Psychology*, 1981, *6*, 239–250.

Hetherington, E. M., & Martin, B. M. Family interaction. In H. C. Quay & J. S. Werry (Eds.), *Psychopathological disorders of childhood* (2nd ed.). New York: Wiley, 1979.

Hetherington, E. M., & Parke, R. D. *Child psychology: A contemporary viewpoint* (2nd ed.). New York: McGraw-Hill, 1979.

Hobbs, S. A., Moguin, L. E., Tyroler, M., & Lahey, B. B. Cognitive behavioral therapy with children: Has clinical utility been demonstrated? *Psychological Bulletin*, 1980, *87*(1), 147–165.

Horan, J. J., & Harrison, R. P. Drug abuse by children and adolescents: Perspectives on incidence, etiology, assessment, and prevention programming. In B. B. Lahey & A. E. Kazdin, *Advances in clinical child psychology* (Vol. 4). New York: Plenum Press, 1981.

Jackson, K., Winkley, R., Faust, D. A., Cermak, E. G., & Burtt, M. M. Behavior changes indicating emotional trauma in tonsillectomized children. *Pediatrics*, 1953, *12*, 23–27.

Johnson, M. R. Mental health interventions with medically ill children: A review of the literature 1970–1977. *Journal of Pediatric Psychology*, 1979, *4*, 147–164.

Johnson, S. B. Psychosocial factors in juvenile diabetes: A review. *Journal of Behavioral Medicine*, 1980, *3*, 95 – 116.

Jolly, H. *Diseases of children* (3rd ed.). Oxford: Blackwell Scientific Publications, 1976.

Kagen, L. B. Use of denial in adolescents with bone cancer. *Health and Social Work*, 1976, *1*, 71 – 87.

Kalnins, I. V. The dying child: A new perspective. *Journal of Pediatric Psychology*, 1977, *2*(2), 39 – 41.

Kalnins, I. V., Churchill, M. P., & Terry, G. E. Concurrent stresses in families with a leukemic child. *Journal of Pediatric Psychology*, 1980, *5*, 81 – 92.

Kanthor, H. A. Car safety for infants: Effectiveness of prenatal counseling. *Pediatrics*, 1976, *58*, 320 – 322.

Katz, E. R., Kellerman, J., Rigler, D., Williams, K. O., & Siegel, S. E. School intervention with pediatric cancer patients. *Journal of Pediatric Psychology*, 1977, *2*(2), 72 – 76.

Katz, E. R., Kellerman, J., & Siegel, S. E. Behavioral distress in children with cancer undergoing medical procedures: Developmental considerations. *Journal of Consulting and Clinical Psychology*, 1980, *48*(3), 356 – 365.

Kellerman, J., Rigler, D., Siegel, S. E., & Katz, E. R. Disease-related communication and depression in pediatric cancer patients. *Journal of Pediatric Psychology*, 1977, *2*(2), 52 – 53.

Kenny, T. J. The hospitalized child. *Pediatric Clinics of North America*, 1975, *22*(3), 583 – 593.

Khan, A. U., Staerk, M., & Bonk, C. Hypnotic suggestibility compared with other methods of isolating emotionally prone asthmatic children. *The American Journal of Clinical Hypnosis*, 1974, *17*, 50 – 53.

Knowles, H. C., Guest, G. M., Lampe, R. N., Kessler, M., & Sillman, T. G. The course of juvenile diabetes treated with unmeasured diet. *Diabetes*, 1965, *14*, 239 – 273.

Koocher, G. P. Childhood, death, and cognitive development. *Developmental Psychology*, 1973, *9*, 369 – 375.

Koocher, G. P., O'Malley, J. E., Gogan, J. L., & Foster, D. J. Psychological adjustment among pediatric cancer survivors. *Journal of Child Psychology and Psychiatry*, 1980, *21*, 163 – 173.

Koocher, G. P., & Sallan, S. E. Pediatric oncology. In P. R. Magrab (Ed.), *Psychological management of pediatric problems* (Vol. 1). Baltimore, Md.: University Park Press, 1978.

Korsch, B., Gozzi, E., & Francis, V. Gaps in doctor – patient interaction and patient satisfaction. *Pediatrics*, 1968, *42*, 855.

Korsch, B. M., Negrete, V. F., Gardner, J. E., Weinstock, C. L., Mercer, A. S., Grushkin, C. M., & Fine, R. N. Kidney transplantation in children: Psychosocial follow up studies on child and family. *Journal of Pediatrics*, 1973, *83*, 339 – 408.

Koski, M., & Kumento, A. Adolescent development and behavior: A psychosomatic follow-up study of childhood diabetes. In Z. Laron (Ed.), *Diabetes in juveniles: Medical and rehabilitation aspects. Modern problems in pediatrics*. New York: Karger, 1975.

La Greca, A. M., & Diamond, E. L. *Cardiac surgery with preschool-aged children: The aftermath for children and parents*. Unpublished manuscript, University of Miami, 1982.

La Greca, A. M. Interviewing and behavioral observations. In C. E. Walker & M. C. Roberts (Eds.), *Handbook of clinical child psychology*. New York: John Wiley and Sons, 1983.

Lahey, B. I., Green, K. D., & Forehand, R. On the independence of ratings of hyperactivity, conduct problems, and attention deficits in children: A multiple regression analysis. *Journal of Consulting and Clinical Psychology*, 1980, *48*(5), 566 – 574.

Lambert, N. M., Sandoval, J., & Sassone, D. Prevalence of hyperactivity in elementary school children as a function of social system definers. *American Journal of Orthopsychiatry*, 1978, *48*(3), 446 – 463.

Lansky, S. B., Cairns, N. U., Hassanein, R., Wehr, B. M., & Lowman, J. T. Childhood cancer: Parental discord and divorce. *Pediatrics*, 1978, *62*, 184 – 188.

Lansky, S. B., Lowman, J. T., Vats, T., & Gyulay, J. School phobia in children with malignant neoplasms. *American Journal of Diseases in Children*, 1975, *129*, 42 – 46.

Lavigne, J. V., & Ryan, M. Psychologic adjustment of siblings of children with chronic illness. *Pediatrics*, 1979, *63*, 616 – 627.

Lawler, R. H., Nakielny, W., & Wright, N. A. Suicidal attempts in children. *Canadian Medical Association Journal*, 1963, *89*, 751 – 754.

Lawler, R. H., Nakielny, W., & Wright, N. A. Psychological implications of cystic fibrosis. *Canadian Medical Association Journal*, 1966, *94*, 1043 – 1046.

Leigh, D., & Marley, D. *Bronchial asthma*. Oxford, England: Pergammon Press, 1967.

Leland, H. Mental retardation. In P. R. Magrab (Ed.), *Psychological management of pediatric problems* (Vol. 2). Baltimore, Md.: University Park Press, 1978.

Levitt, E. E., & Edwards, J. A. A multivariate study of correlative factors in youthful cigarette smoking. *Developmental Psychology*, 1970, *2*, 5 – 11.

Lewis, J. M., Beavers, W. R., Gosett, J. T., & Phillips, V. A. *No single thread: Psychological health in family systems*. New York: Brunner/Mazel, 1976.

Lieberman, H. M., Emmet, W. L., & Carlson, A. H. Pediatric automotive restraints, pediatricians, and the Academy. *Pediatrics*, 1976, *58*, 316 – 319.

Linde, L., Rasof, B., Dunn, O., & Rabb, E. Attitudinal factors in congenital heart disease. *Pediatrics*, 1966, *38*, 92 – 101.

Lindemann, E. Symptomatology and management of acute grief. *American Journal of Psychiatry*, 1944, *101*, 141 – 148.

Little, S., & Cohen, L. Goal setting behavior of asthmatic children and their mothers for them. *Journal of Personality*, 1951, *19*, 376 – 389.

Loney, J., Kramer, J., & Milich, R. The hyperkinetic child grows up: Predictors of symptoms, delinquency, and achievement at follow-up. Presented as part of symposium, K. D. Gadow, Chairman, *Psychosocial aspects of drug treatment for hyperactivity*. Annual meeting of the American Association for the Advancement of Science, Houston, Texas, 1979.

Long, R. T., Lamont, J. H., Whipple, B., Bandler, L., Blom, G. E., Burgin, L., & Jessner, L. A psychosomatic study of allergic and emotional factors in children with asthma. *American Journal of Psychiatry*, 1958, *114*, 890 – 899.

Loughlin, W. C., & Mosenthal, H. O. Study of the personalities of children with diabetes. *American Journal of Diseases of Children*, 1944, *29*, 555 – 571.

Magrab, P. R., & Calcagno, P. L. Psychological impact of chronic pediatric conditions. In P. R. Magrab (Ed.), *Psychological management of pediatric problems* (Vol. 1). Baltimore, Md.: University Park Press, 1978.

Magrab, P. R., & Papadopoulou, Z. L. Renal disease. In P. R. Magrab (Ed.), *Psychological management of pediatric problems* (Vol. 1). Baltimore, Md.: University Park Press, 1978.

Mash, E. J., & Terdal, L. G. Behavioral assessment of childhood disturbances. In E. J. Mash & L. G. Terdal (Eds.), *Behavioral assessment of childhood disorders*. New York: Guilford Press, 1981.

Mattsson, A. Psychologic aspects of childhood asthma. *Pediatric Clinics of North America*, 1975, *22*, 77 – 88.

McAnarney, E. R., Pless, I. B., Satterwhite, B., & Friedman, S. B. Psychological problems of children with chronic juvenile arthritis. *Pediatrics*, 1974, *53*, 523.

McClelland, C. Q., Staples, W. P., Weisberg, I., & Berger, M. E. The practitioners' role in behavioral pediatrics. *Journal of Pediatrics*, 1973, *82*, 325 – 331.

McGavin, A. P., Schultz, E., Peden, G. W., & Bowen, B. D. The physical growth, the degree of intelligence and the personality adjustment of a group of diabetic children. *The New England Journal of Medicine*, 1940, *223*, 119 – 127.

Meijer, A. Generation chain relationships in families of asthmatic children. *Psychosomatics*, 1976, *17*, 213.

Melamed, B. G., & Johnson, S. B. Chronic illness: Asthma and juvenile diabetes. In E. J. Mash & L. G. Terdal (Eds.), *Behavioral assessment of childhood disorders*. New York: Guilford, 1981.

Melamed, B. G., Meyer, R., Gee, C., & Soule, L. The influence of time and type of preparation on children's adjustment to hospitalization. *Journal of Pediatric Psychology*, 1976, *1*, 31 – 37.

Melamed, B. G., & Siegel, L. J. Reduction of anxiety in children facing hospitalization and surgery by use of filmed modeling. *Journal of Consulting and Clinical Psychology,* 1975, *43,* 511 – 521.

Melamed, B. G., Yurchesen, R., Fleece, L., Hutchenson, S., & Hawks, R. Effects of film modeling in the reduction of anxiety-related behaviors in individuals varying in level of previous experience in the stress situation. *Journal of Consulting and Clinical Psychology,* 1978, *46*(6), 1357 – 1367.

Moore, D. C., Holton, C. P., & Marten, G. W. Psychologic problems in the management of adolescents with malignancy. *Clinical Pediatrics,* 1969, *8,* 464 – 473.

Moos, R., & Moos, B. A typology of family social environments. *Family Process,* 1976, *15,* 357 – 371

Natterson, J. M., & Knudson, A. G. Observations concerning fear of death in fatally ill children and their mothers. *Psychosomatic Medicine,* 1960, *22,* 456 – 465.

O'Leary, K. D. Pills or skills for hyperactive children. *Journal of Applied Behavior Analysis,* 1980, *13*(1), 191 – 204.

Olson, D. H., Sprenkle, D., & Russell, C. A circumplex model of marital and family systems. I: Cohesion and adaptability dimensions, family types, and clinical applications. *Family Process,* 1979, *14,* 1 – 35.

O'Malley, J. E., Koocher, G., Foster, D., & Slavin, L. Psychiatric sequelae of surviving childhood cancer. *American Journal of Orthopsychiatry,* 1979, *49,* 608 – 616.

Panides, W. C., & Ziller, R. C. The self-perceptions of children with asthma and asthma/enuresis. *Journal of Psychosomatic Research,* 1981, *25,* 51 – 56.

Pelham, W. E., Schnedler, R. W., Bologna, N. C., & Contreras, J. A. Behavioral and stimulant treatment of hyperactive children: A therapy study with methylphenidate probes in a within-subject design. *Journal of Applied Behavioral Analysis,* 1980, *13*(2), 221 – 236.

Perrin, E. C., & Gerrity, P. S. There's a demon in your belly: Children's understanding of illness. *Pediatrics,* 1981, *67,* 841 – 849.

Peterson, L., & Ridley-Johnson, R. Pediatric hospital response to survey on pre-hospital preparation. *Journal of Pediatric Psychology,* 1980, *5,* 1 – 7.

Petrillo, M., & Sanger, S. *Emotional care of hospitalized children* (2nd ed.). Philadelphia: Lippincott, 1980.

Pinkerton, P. Correlating physiologic and psychodynamic data in the study and management of childhood asthma. *Journal of Psychosomatic Research,* 1967, *11,* 11 – 25.

Pinkerton, P. Parental acceptance of the handicapped child. *Developmental Medicine and Child Neurology,* 1970, *12,* 207 – 212.

Pless, I. B., & Roghmann, K. J. Chronic illness and its consequences: Observations based on three epidemiological surveys. *Journal of Pediatrics,* 1971, *79,* 351 – 359.

Pless, I. B., Roghmann, K. J., & Haggerty, R. J. Chronic illness, family functioning, and psychological adjustment: A model for the allocation of preventive mental health services. *International Journal of Epidemiology,* 1972, *1,* 271.

Powazek, M., Goff, J. R., Schyving, J., & Paulson, M. A. Emotional reactions of children to isolation in a cancer hospital. *Journal of Pediatrics,* 1978, *92*(5), 834 – 837.

Prinz, R. J., Roberts, W. A., & Hartman, E. Dietary correlates of hyperactive behavior in children. *Journal of Consulting and Clinical Psychology,* 1980, *48*(6), 760 – 769.

Prugh, D. G., & Eckhardt, L. O. Stages and phases in the reactions of children and adolescents to illness or injury. *Advances in Behavioral Pediatrics* (Vol. 1). Greenwich, Conn.: JAI Press, 1980.

Prugh, D. E., Staub, E. M., Sands, H. H., Kirschbaum, R., & Lenihan, E. A. A study of the emotional reactions of children and families to hospitalization. *American Journal of Orthopsychiatry,* 1953, *23,* 70 – 106.

Purcell, K. Childhood asthma: The role of family relationships, personality, and emotions. In A. Davids (Ed.), *Child personality and psychopathology* (Vol. 2). New York: Wiley, 1975.

Purcell, K., Brady, L., Chai, H., Muser, J., Molk, L., Gordon, N., & Means, J. The effect of asthma in children on experimental separation from the family. *Psychosomatic Medicine,* 1969, *6,* 251 – 258.

Purcell, K., & Weiss, H. H. Asthma. In C. G. Costello (Ed.), *Symptoms of psychopathology: A handbook.* New York: Wiley, 1970.

Purcell, K., Weiss, J., & Hahn, W. Certain psychosomatic disorders. In P. Wolman (Ed.), *Manual of child psychopathology*. New York: McGraw-Hill, 1972.

Quay, H. C. Measuring dimensions of deviant behavior: The Behavior Problem Checklist. *Journal of Abnormal Child Psychology*, 1977, 5, 277 – 287.

Quay, H. C. Classification. In H. C. Quay & J. S. Werry (Eds.), *Psychopathological disorders of childhood* (2nd ed.). New York: Wiley, 1979.

Quay, H. C., & Peterson, D. R. *Manual for the Behavior Problem Checklist*. Unpublished manuscript, 1975, 1979. (Available from D. R. Peterson, School of Professional Psychology, Busch Campus, Rutgers State University, New Brunswick, N.J., 08903.)

Quinn, P. O., Sostek, A. M., & Davitt, M. K. The high-risk infant and his family. In P. R. Magrab (Ed.), *Psychological management of pediatric problems* (Vol. 2). Baltimore: University Park Press, 1978.

Rees, L. The significance of parental attitudes in childhood asthma. *Journal of Psychosomatic Research*, 1963, 7, 181 – 190.

Roberts, M. C. *Psychological preparation for pediatric hospitalization and surgery*. Paper presented at the Midwestern Psychological Association, Chicago, 1979.

Roberts, M. C., Wertele, S. K., Boone, R. K., Ginther, L. J., & Elkins, P. D. Reduction of medical fears by use of modeling: A preventive application in a general population of children. *Journal of Pediatric Psychology*, 1981, 6(3), 293 – 300.

Robertson, J. *A two-year old goes to hospital* (film). New York: University Film Library, 1952.

Robertson, J. *Young children in hospitals* (2nd ed.). London: Tavistock Publications Ltd., 1970.

Roche, A. F., Lipman, R. S., Overall, J. E., & Hung, W. The effects of stimulant medication on the growth of hyperkinetic children. *Pediatrics*, 1979, 63(6), 847 – 850.

Rosenstock, I. M. Patients' compliance with health regimens. *Journal of the American Medical Association*, 1975, 234, 402.

Routh, D. K. Hyperactivity. In P. R. Magrab (Ed.), *Psychological management of pediatric problems* (Vol. 2). Baltimore: University Park Press, 1978.

Routh, D. K. Developmental and social aspects of hyperactivity. In C. K. Whalen & B. Henker (Eds.), *Hyperactive children: The social ecology of identification and treatment*. New York: Academic Press, 1980.

Rowland, T. W. Pediatrics for the clinician: The pediatrician and congenital heart disease. *Pediatrics*, 1979, 64, 180 – 186.

Salk, L. Emotional factors in pediatric practice: An overview. In P. R. Magrab (Ed.), *Psychological management of pediatric problems* (Vol. 1). Baltimore: University Park Press, 1978.

Sandberg, S. T., Wieselberg, M., & Shaffer, D. Hyperkinetic and conduct problem children in a primary school population: Some epidemiological considerations. *Journal of Child Psychology and Psychiatry*, 1980, 21, 293 – 311.

Schachar, R., Rutter, M., & Smith, A. The characteristics of situationally and pervasively hyperactive children: Implications for syndrome definition. *Journal of Child Psychology and Psychiatry*, 1981, 22(4), 375 – 392.

Schwartz, S., & Johnson, J. H. *Psychopathology of childhood: A clinical-experimental approach*. New York: Pergamon Press, Inc., 1981.

Scott, K. G., Field, T., & Robertson, E. (Eds.), *Teenage parents and their offspring*. New York: Grune & Stratton, 1981.

Shore, M. F., & Goldston, S. E. Mental health aspects of pediatric care: Hospital review and current status. In P. R. Magrab (Ed.), *Psychological management of pediatric problems* (Vol. 1). Baltimore: University Park Press, 1978.

Siegel, L. J. Preparation of children for hospitalization: A selected review of the research literature. *Journal of Pediatric Psychology*, 1976, 1(4), 26 – 30.

Silber, L. *Behavioral alternatives to pharmacotherapy in the treatment of hyperactive children*. Paper presented to the Conference on Drug Management of Childhood Behavior Disorders, Chapel Hill, N.C., 1981.

Simeonsson, R. J., Buckley, L., & Monson, L. Conceptions of illness causality in hospitalized children. *Journal of Pediatric Psychology*, 1979, *4*, 77 – 84.

Simonds, J. F. Study of diabetic attitudes in children and parents. In *Seventh allied health postgraduate course in diabetes*. Kansas City, Mo.: American Diabetes Association, 1975.

Simonds, J. F. Emotions and compliance in diabetic children. *Psychosomatics*, 1979, *20*, 544 – 551.

Sleator, E. K., & Ullman, R. K. Can the physician diagnosis hyperactivity in the office? *Pediatrics*, 1981, *67*(1), 13 – 17.

Spinetta, J. J. The dying child's awareness of death: A review. *Psychological Bulletin*, 1974, *81*(4), 256 – 260.

Spinetta, J. J. Adjustment in children with cancer. *Journal of Pediatric Psychology*, 1977, *2*(2), 49 – 51.

Spinetta, J. J., & Maloney, L. J. Death anxiety in the outpatient leukemic child. *Pediatrics*, 1975, *65*, 1034 – 1037.

Spinetta, J. J., & Maloney, L. J. The child of cancer: Patterns of communication and denial. *Journal of Consulting and Clinical Psychology*, 1978, *46*(6), 1540 – 1541.

Spinetta, J. J., Rigler, D., & Karon, M. Anxiety in the dying child. *Pediatrics*, 1973, *52*, 841 – 845.

Spinetta, J. J., Rigler, D., & Karon, M. Personal space as a measure of a dying child's sense of isolation. *Journal of Consulting and Clinical Psychology*, 1974, *42*, 751 – 756.

Spinetta, J. J., Swarner, J. A., & Sheposh, J. P. Effective parental coping following the death of a child from cancer. *Journal of Pediatric Psychology*, 1981, *6*, 251 – 263.

Steinhauer, P. D., Mushin, D. N., & Rae-Grant, Q. Psychological aspects of chronic illness. *Pediatric Clinics of North America*, 1974, *2*(4), 825 – 840.

Stores, G. School children with epilepsy at risk for learning and behavior problems. *Developmental Medicine and Child Neurology*, 1978, *20*, 502 – 508.

Strauss, M. A., & Tallman, I. SIMFAM: A technique for observational measurement and experimental study of families. In J. Aldous (Ed.), *Family problem solving*. Hinsdale, Ill.: Dryden Press, 1971.

Sullivan, B. Self-esteem and depression in adolescent diabetic girls. *Diabetes Care*, 1978, *1*, 18 – 22.

Swift, C. R., Seidman, F., & Stein, H. Adjustment problems in juvenile diabetes. *Psychosomatic Medicine*, 1967, *29*, 555.

Talbot, N. B., & Howell, M. C. Social and behavioral causes and consequences of disease among children. In N. B. Talbot, J. Kagan, & L. Eisenberg (Eds.), *Behavioral science in pediatric medicine*. Philadelphia: W. B. Saunders, 1971.

Tartar, R. E. Intellectual and adaptive functioning in epilepsy. *Diseases in the Nervous System*, 1972, *33*, 763 – 770.

Travis, G. *Chronic illness in children: Its impact on child and family*. Stanford, Calif.: Stanford University Press, 1976.

Tropauer, A., Franz, M. N., & Dilgard, V. W. Psychological aspects of the care of children with cystic fibrosis. *American Journal of Diseases of Children*, 1970, *119*, 424.

Varga, J. The hyperactive child: Should we be paying more attention? *American Journal of Diseases of Children*, 1979, *133*, 413 – 418.

Vernick, J., & Karon, M. Who's afraid of death on a leukemia ward? *American Journal of Diseases of Children*, 1965, *109*, 393 – 397.

Vernon, D., Schulman, J., & Foley, J. Changes in children's behavior after hospitalization. *American Journal of Diseases of Children*, 1966, *3*, 581 – 593.

Visintainer, M. P., & Wolfer, J. A. Psychological preparation for surgical pediatric patients: The effective children's and parent's stress responses and adjustment. *Pediatrics*, 1975, *56*, 187 – 202.

Waechter, E. Children's awareness of fatal illness. *American Journal of Nursing*, 1971, *7*, 1168 – 1172.

Weingarten, H., Rapoport, J. L., Buschsbaum, M. S., Bunney, W. E., Jr., Ebert, M. H., Mikkelson, E. J., & Caine, E. D. Cognitive processes in normal and hyperactive children and their responses to amphetamine treatment. *Journal of Abnormal Psychology*, 1980, *89*(1), 25 – 37.

Weiss, G., & Hechtman, L. The hyperactive child syndrome. *Science*, 1979, *205*, 1348 – 1354.

Werry, J. S. Psychosomatic disorders, psychogenic symptoms and hospitalization. In H. C. Quay and J. S. Werry (Eds.), *Psychopathological disorders of childhood* (2nd ed.). New York: Wiley, 1979.

Whalen, C. K., Collins, B. E., Henker, B., Alkus, S. R., Adams, D., & Stapp, J. Behavior observations of hyperactive children and methylphenidate (Ritalin) effects in systematically structured classroom environments: Now you see them, now you don't. *Journal of Pediatric Psychology,* 1978, *3*(4), 177 – 187.

Willis, D. J., & Thomas, E. D. Seizure disorders. In P. R. Magrab (Ed.), *Psychological management of pediatric problems* (Vol. 2). Baltimore: University Park Press, 1978.

Wolinsky, G. F. Materials to prepare children for hospital experience. *Exceptional Children,* 1971, *37,* 527 – 528.

Wright, L. A comprehensive program for mental health and behavioral medicine in a large children's hospital. *Professional Psychology,* 1979, 458 – 466.

Wright, L., Schaefer, A. B., & Solomons, G. *Encyclopedia of pediatric psychology.* Baltimore: University Park Press, 1979.

Zentall, S. S. Behavioral comparisons of hyperactive and normally active children in natural settings. *Journal of Abnormal Child Psychology,* 1980, *8*(1), 93 – 109.

IV LIFE-STYLES AND HEALTH

11 Nutritional Basis of Health and Disease

Daryl Greenfield
University of Miami

INTRODUCTION

Nutrition and its effect on behavior and development have increasingly generated interest and research. In 1977 an international research symposium was held in Washington, D.C. that summarized both animal and human research on the behavioral effects of energy and protein deficits (Brozek, 1979). In 1979, *Human Nutrition, A Comprehensive Treatise,* was published with chapters dealing with malnutrition and mental development, brain neurotransmitters, mental development in children, behavior and brain biochemistry associated with iron deficiency, obesity in the young child, failure to thrive in the young child, drug – nutrient interrelationships, cardiac failure, the relationship of diet and nutritional status to cancer and megavitamins, and food fads, among others. In 1980, Conners reviewed the effects of food additives on hyperactivity in children. A current volume sponsored by the Nestle Foundation (Brozek & Schurch, 1984) is aimed exclusively at assessing the key issues in studying malnutrition and behavior. In 1982 a new journal, *Nutrition and Behavior,* became a focal point for research on the interrelationships among nutrition and behavior, neuroscience, ecology, anthropology, and zoology.

The present chapter focuses on a few key issues to acquaint the reader with the complexity of the research problems involved and how these complexities may ultimately be resolved. Specific discussions of obesity, anorexia (Chapter 12) and diabetes (Chapter 18) appear elsewhere in this volume.

Basic Fundamentals of Nutrition

"We are what we eat." Not surprisingly, food and the human body are made up of the same classes of chemicals: water, carbohydrates, fats, proteins, vitamins, and minerals. A protein-rich food such as red meat, or a carbohydrate-rich food such as a piece of fruit, or a human body all contain these six classes of chemicals; they differ only in the relative amount of each. Each of these classes of chemicals makes identifiable contributions to the metabolic processes of all cells in the body.

The carbohydrates, which are the sugars, starches, and fibers, are compounds composed of carbon, hydrogen, and oxygen arranged as monosaccharides ($C_6H_{12}O_6$), pairs of monosaccharides bonded together called disaccharides, or long chains of monosaccharides bonded together called polysaccharides. Simple carbohydrates, the monosaccharides glucose, fructose, and galactose all have the same chemical formula, $C_6H_{12}O_6$, but vary in structure and form the basis for the disaccharide sugars such as sucrose and lactose and the complex polysaccharides such as starch, glycogen, and cellulose. Sucrose, the familiar table sugar, is glucose bonded to fructose; lactose, commonly known as milk sugar, is glucose bonded to galactose.

The carbohydrates play many important roles in body metabolism. Along with fats and proteins they are the major source of energy for the body. Glucose, commonly referred to as blood sugar, ordinarily is the sole source of energy for the brain and central nervous system. Homeostatic mechanisms normally maintain a constant glucose level between 80 and 120 mg/100 ml of blood. When blood sugar levels drop too low, hunger is often experienced and a meal will raise the blood glucose level, as carbohydrates in the meal can be broken down to their simple form (monosaccharides) by the process of hydrolysis in the presence of water, which is abundant in the blood. In addition, glucose stored in the liver as the polysaccharide glycogen can be broken down to glucose and released into the blood. Thus, these homeostatic mechanisms normally avoid hypoglycemia, or an abnormally low blood sugar level.

Conversely, if blood sugar levels become too high, following a meal rich in carbohydrates, for example, the pancreas releases insulin into the blood, which results in an uptake of glucose, which is stored in muscle and liver cells as glycogen and as fat. This homeostatic mechanism thus avoids hyperglycemia, or an abnormally high blood sugar concentration. Glycogen in muscle can later be used as energy for the muscle, and glycogen stored in the liver can be returned to the blood as glucose when blood glucose levels drop too low or under conditions such as stress when the adrenal glands secrete the hormone epinephrine.

Finally, fiber has as its major components a number of polysaccharides including cellulose, hemicellulose, and pectin. Cellulose, like the polysaccharide starch, is abundant in plants and is comprised of long strings of glucose molecules. The human digestive tract has many enzymes that can hydrolyze the bonds in starch, but no enzymes that will hydrolyze the bonds in cellulose. Thus cellulose passes through the digestive tract relatively unchanged. Fiber plays an important laxative role, attracting water into the digestive tract. Recently fiber has been associated with reduced colon cancer (Burkitt, Walker, & Painter, 1974). Fiber has also been hypothesized to play a role in the development of atherosclerosis. A number of animal models have related fiber to reduced atherosclerosis: Kritchevsky and Tepper, 1968, Moore, 1967, rabbits; Kritchevsky, Davidson, Shapiro, Kim, Kitagawa, Malhotra, Nair, Clarkson, Bershon, and Winter, 1974, baboons; and Kritchevsky, Davidson, Kim, Krendel, Malhotra, Vander Watt, Du Plessis, Winter, Ipp, Mendelsohn, and Bersohn, 1977, monkeys. Also pectin has been shown to be effective in lowering serum lipid levels in humans (Kay & Truswell, 1977). The role of fiber in the development of atherosclerosis and in reducing serum lipid levels remains a tentative hypothesis requiring additional investigation.

The lipids, fats and oils, are also a source of energy for the body. The liver cells are capable of storing a limited amount of glycogen. Fat storage is unlimited and an efficient form of energy, as a pound of fat can be oxidized to supply 3500 kcal of energy for the body's needs. Fat stored in muscle, for example, provides, in conjunction with muscle glycogen, energy for the muscle cells when they are active. The heart, which requires a constant energy source, utilizes fat for energy.

The lipids are also required for a variety of metabolic processes. Linoleic acid, for example, is essential for growth and must be provided through the diet. In food, fat "carries" the fat soluble vitamins. Fat also insulates and protects the body from physical damage. The layer of fat below the skin insulates the body from extremes in temperature because it is a poor conductor of heat. Fat also protects a number of organs from damage, such as the hard pad of fat beneath each kidney.

Ninety-five percent of lipids in the diet are in the form of triglycerides, an organic compound like the carbohydrates, containing carbon, hydrogen, and oxygen arranged as a glycerol molecule with three fatty acid molecules attached to it. Some tryglycerides carry a maximum number of hydrogen molecules and are referred to as saturated fats. Carbon atoms that bond with hydrogen molecules in the saturated fats can form double bonds with each other. These molecules with fewer hydrogen atoms and double bonds between carbon atoms are referred to as unsaturated fats. Polyunsaturated fats, those with at least two carbon double bonds and four fewer hydrogen atoms than saturated fats (such as the essential nutrient, linoleic acid), have been shown to reduce serum cholesterol level (Keys, Anderson, & Grande, 1965), which rises with the ingestion of saturated fats, thus potentially playing a role in heart disease.

Other dietary lipids include phospholipids such as the choline containing lecithin and the sterols such as cholesterol. The role of choline in neurotransmitter function and cholesterol as a risk factor for heart disease are discussed later in this chapter.

Proteins, like lipids and carbohydrates, are an energy source for the body and contain carbon, hydrogen, and oxygen. In addition, proteins contain nitrogen, and this nitrogen-carrying amino group (NH_2) in combination with an acid group (COOH) bonds with a central carbon atom to form the bases of a number of common amino acids that link together to form proteins. Proteins play many crucial roles in body metabolism. At least eight of the more than 20 essential amino acids, the building blocks of the cells, cannot be synthesized by the body and must be ingested. The role of such amino acids like tryptophan in brain functioning and the effects of inadequate protein in the diet for normal development are detailed later in this chapter.

Vitamins are the fourth organic substance contained in food and in the human body. Some vitamins, like the proteins and carbohydrates, are attracted by the positive (H+) and negative (OH−) ions of water and are transported free in the blood. Excesses of these water-soluble vitamins are excreted. Other vitamins are carried by proteins along with fat in the lymphatic system. Excesses of these fat-soluble vitamins are stored in the body. Vitamins play crucial metabolic roles, aiding in the digestion, absorption, and metabolism of the carbohydrates, lipids, and proteins.

Finally, two classes of minerals, the macrominerals calcium, chloride, magnesium, phosphorus, potassium, sodium, and sulphur, and the trace element microminerals such as iron, iodine, and zinc play important roles in the body. Micronutrients are needed in small amounts, about .1 gm per day. A micronutrient such as calcium is an important component of teeth and bones, cell membrane activity, synapse activity, muscle activity including the heart, blood clotting, and as a cofactor in many enzymatic reactions. A micronutrient such as iron is required in even smaller amounts, less than .01 gm/day but again plays important roles in body and brain function, as highlighted later in this chapter.

Inadequate Energy Needs

In developing third world countries many individuals, usually children, fail to receive adequate nutrient intake to meet their daily energy requirements. *Protein-calorie malnutrition* (PCM), which was first described near the turn of this century, afflicts approximately .5% to 20% of the world's population in its most severe form and 3.5% to 46.4% to a more modest degree (Bengoa, 1974).

Inadequate energy intake combined with inadequate protein intake creates a problem for the developing organism because protein is an essential structural element in living organisms. The essential amino acids, which are indispensable for growth and development, cannot be synthesized from materials already available in the human body. Protein requirements for the human infant are actually greater per unit of body weight (Hathaway, 1957) than adult requirements.

Much research interest has focused on the potential consequences of inadequate energy intake on the developing fetus and young organism. Numerous animal models have been generated to study the effects of PCM on the development and functioning of the brain and nervous system and the behavioral consequences of undernutrition. There is also a substantial body of research using humans to investigate the relationship between nutrition and behavior.

ANIMAL STUDIES OF NUTRITIONAL DEFICIT

Effects on Growth and Neural Systems

Animal research in nutrition allows manipulation of the animal's nutritional status over extended time periods, thereby allowing researchers to make strong cause and effect statements about a nutrient's or class of nutrient's effect on growth and development. Such manipulation is clearly unethical and undesirable in human studies. In addition, one cannot easily isolate nutrition as an independent variable in a natural setting with humans. Poor nutrition is usually only one of many potentially undesirable elements in an environment of a child at risk for inadequate growth and development.

Early work with animals (Chase, Lindsley, & O'Brien, 1969; Winick & Noble, 1965) showed that inadequate food intake produced inadequate brain growth in the developing organism, with deficits in such indices as brain weight, brain cell number, and DNA. Similar results were obtained when a small number of human infants who died from malnutrition were compared to infants who died from accidental causes (Winick & Rosso, 1969).

Despite the importance of this work, researchers were concerned about the functional consequences of such findings. Would a child with a smaller head circumference or fewer brain cells learn at a slower than normal rate? Would such a child be less intelligent? Such concerns have led to a greater emphasis in current research to study systems that are likely to have a direct role in determining behavior.

One such line of work is exemplified by Wurtman and Wurtman (1977a, 1977b). They have extensively studied the role of nutrition on neurotransmitters in the brain and have shown that dietary manipulations can influence neurotransmitter activity.

PCM has a diversity of long-term effects. Research in animals has shown the long-term effect of PCM on structural changes in the brain. For example, perinatal rats fed low protein diets had significantly fewer alpha- and beta-adrenergic binding sites in their brains (Keller, Munaro, & Orsingher, 1982). Decreases in neurotransmitter levels also follow chronic PCM in the early life of the animal (Lee & Dubos, 1972; Sereni, Principi, Perletti, & Piceni Sereni, 1966; Showmaker & Wurtman, 1971; Stern, Morgane, Miller, & Resnick, 1975, for example). Cohen and Wurtman (1979), however, report similar effects following a single meal. Consumption of a meal changes not only the plasma concentration of tryptophan, choline, and tyrosine, but brain levels of neurotransmitters as well. For example, tryptophan, an essential amino acid, is the precursor of the neurotransmitter serotonin. If rats are injected with a low dose of tryptophan when blood tryptophan levels are lowest, serotonin levels rise significantly in the brain.

Acetylcholine (ACh) is also affected by a rat's diet. Rats injected with a saline solution containing choline chloride showed rises in serum and brain choline levels, followed by a significant rise in brain ACh levels (Cohen & Wurtman, 1975). Weanling rats subjected to a 5-day dietary choline deficiency showed a 30 – 35% decrease in brain ACh levels (Nagler, Dettbarn, Seifter, & Levenson, 1968). Varying the choline level in drinking water for 3 days also led to elevated levels of brain choline and ACh levels (Cohen, 1976). In studies where different brain areas were examined following choline administration (Cohen & Wurtman, 1976; Hirsch, Growdon, & Wurtman, 1977), all three areas examined, the caudate nucleus, the cortex and the hippocampus, showed significant increases in ACh levels. The increase in the caudate nucleus, an area rich in cholinergic interneurons and the increase in the hippocampus, a region rich in cholinergic nerve terminals, would likely indicate that ACh increase following choline administration occurs not only in the cell bodies but at the boutons and terminals where ACh is released.

Finally, rats who ingest a single protein-containing meal that raises tyrosine levels in the brain also show an accelerated formation of the neurotransmitter norepinephrine (Gibson & Wurtman, 1978).

If daily diet can also effect neurotransmitter levels, the potential exists for dietary treatment of diseases that may be linked to neurotransmitter levels. Nondietary administration of tyrosine, which stimulates synthesis of the neurotransmitter dopamine, has been effectively used to treat depression (Gelenber, Wojcik, Growden, et. al., 1980). Tyrosine administration has also been shown to reduce blood pressure in hypertensive rats (Sved, Fernstrom, & Wurtman, 1979).

Effects on Behavior

Research relating nutrition to brain and nervous system function is clearly important in both a theoretical and applied sense. In addition to this work, however, much effort has gone into linking inadequate nutrition to maladaptive or suboptimal behavior in both subhuman and human populations.

A large body of research has been generated relating the effects of PCM to behavior in subhuman animal populations. The majority of animal work has been conducted with rats. Although there are some inconsistencies in findings, early and chronic PCM produces diverse long-term behavioral effects despite nutritional rehabilitation. It is not clear which specific developmental processes are affected, and whether the underlying causes of the deficit are structural changes in the nervous system or functional deficits resulting from the malnourished animal interacting less with the environment.

The types of behavioral tests used to determine how malnourished rats differ from normal rats often involve some sort of learning or problem solving. Performance on these tasks is also influenced by a number of other psychological processes such as motivation, state of arousal, or level of anxiety. Such processes may underlie the obtained differences between malnourished and normal animals. This same problem makes pinpointing specific process deficits in studies with human populations difficult.

Although structural changes in the brain have been noted as a result of malnutrition, some researchers have accounted for behavioral differences in malnourished animals in terms of inadequate environmental interactions. Levitsky (1979), for example, proposed that malnutrition serves as a form of "functional isolation" in that the organism lacks the motivation or the energy to explore the environment. According to this view, malnutrition has consequences similar to exposure to an impoverished environment.

Boelkins and Hegsted (1979), working with subhuman primates, report long-term consequences of early low protein diets on visual habituation tasks. Squirrel monkeys that had experienced either 6 weeks of undernutrition or 20 weeks of partial isolation took longer to habituate to a checkerboard pattern than did well-fed monkeys raised in an enriched environment. They regard their data as being consistent with Levitsky's proposal (1979) that malnutrition serves to functionally isolate the animal from the opportunity for learning. Zimmerman (1979), on the other hand, whose lab has produced the most work on the long-term consequences of malnutrition in monkeys (see Riopelle, 1974), argues that measurable behavioral changes associated with severe nutritional deprivation are minimal and that rehabilitation quickly eliminates any deficits.

HUMAN DEVELOPMENTAL STUDIES

Effects on Growth

Waterlow and Rutishauser (1974) distinguish between two forms of severe PCM, marasmus and kwashiorkor. Marasmus has an early onset, with poor growth evident from birth. Infants typically show a growth in weight for age below 60% for their culture, within the first few months of life. The etiology of marasmus often involves an early abrupt weaning in combination with an unsanitary food source, which results in infections such as gastroenteritis. These infections are often treated by fasting the child, which exacerbates the condition.

Kwashiorkor, on the other hand, displays a later onset. The child often receives adequate nutrition at the breast for the first half year of life. Weaning at this point, however, is followed by a high carbohydrate, low protein diet that increases the child's susceptibility to infection. Illness, in combination with a low protein intake, often result, in kwashiorkor.

Distinguishing between these two forms of PCM has relevance for assessing the effects of PCM on behavior. It should be noted, however, that many factors such as geographical area, dietary practices, types and rates of infection play a role in the etiology of PCM and in reality the two forms of PCM, may show considerable overlap. Schrimshaw and Behar (1961), for example, present a model in which children can either alternate between these two forms of PCM or show symptoms of both, referred to as Marasmus – Kwashiorkor.

Effects on Behavior

Most researchers would agree that severe PCM occurring chronically throughout the first year of life (marasmus) results in severe intellectual deficits as measured by a standardized developmental test. Severe but acute PCM occurring during the second year of life has not consistently been associated with retardation in intellectual functioning. The relationship between moderate and mild forms of PCM and behavior is less clear.

A number of studies dealing with severe PCM and behavior used retrospective research designs. Data on the infant's birth weight, morbidity, achievement of developmental milestones, and general intellectual development prior to and immediately after the episode of malnutrition are lacking. These studies, which show poorer intellectual ability in infants who were malnourished, cannot distinguish whether the malnutrition caused intellectual retardation or whether intellectual retardation preceded and possibly contributed to the infant becoming malnourished. In an impoverished environment where parents have difficulty meeting the demands of an infant, a less active and demanding infant may not receive necessary care.

Attempts to overcome the problems inherent in a retrospective design by matching malnourished children with either control children or siblings for comparison purposes are also unsatisfactory. Finding matched controls on all relevant variables other than nutrition may not be possible. Using siblings as matched controls also has problems, as having a malnourished child and a well-nourished child within the same family implies differential treatment, differential response to the treatment, or both. Many of the early studies examining the relationship of PCM to intellectual functioning (see Pollitt & Thomson, 1977, for an extensive review) add little to our understanding of the role of undernutrition in intellectual development.

A second major problem with many of the early studies involves the issue of construct validity of the dependent measures used to assess intellectual development. Studies relating PCM to cognitive functioning have typically been carried out in third world countries. Intellectual development in these populations, however, has been assessed using global intelligence tests such as the Wechsler or Bayley, which have been standardized on U.S. populations. The test items, which are often culture specific may not be tapping the same underlying process in the different cultures. For example, Hertzig, Birch, Richardson, and Tizard (1972) compared malnourished children, matched controls, and siblings of the malnourished children in Jamaica, using the Wechsler Full Scale IQ as the dependent measure. Mean IQs of the three groups were 57.7, 61.8, and 66.0 respectively. These means were all significantly different at the .10 level. What is striking about these results is that the control group, the majority of whom were rated by their teachers as doing average or better in their school work, had a mean IQ below the cutoff level used in the United States to classify a child as mentally retarded.

Significantly lower than average IQ scores in a normal contrast group is consistently found in studies where IQ tests standardized in a Western culture are lifted and directly applied in a developing country. It is therefore unclear whether these tests are tapping the same functions of cognition in these populations, and thus the difficulty in interpreting the results.

Over the last several years there has been a major shift in research focus from studying severely malnourished children to studying children with moderate to mild PCM. Habicht (1979) points to a number of reasons for such a shift in emphasis. Severe forms of PCM have many known ill effects in addition to poor intellectual development and one need not show lower IQ scores as a justification for prevention and treatment. One might argue that limited resources targeted for severely malnourished infants should go directly for prevention and treatment and not for a demonstration of an IQ deficit. Much less is known about the cognitive development implications of moderate to mild PCM and the problem has greater potential significance because the number of children affected by moderate to mild PCM is 10 to 100 times greater than the number of children affected by severe PCM.

A large data base has been assembled relating moderate to mild PCM and cognitive development, including a number of prospective longitudinal intervention studies carried out in Columbia, Guatemala, and Mexico. These studies have been detailed elsewhere (Brozek, Coursin, & Read, 1977) and have produced a large number of published findings (for example, Brozek, 1979; Chavez & Martinez, 1979 [Mexico]; Freeman, Klein, Kagan, & Yarbrough, 1977 [Guatemala]; McKay, Sinistrera, McKay, Gomez, & Lloreda, 1978 [Cali, Columbia]; Mora, Clement, Christiansen, Ortiz, Vuori, & Wagner, 1979 [Bogota, Columbia]).

Several prospective longitudinal studies identified pregnant mothers at risk for a malnourished child, by choosing families where a malnourished child already existed. Nutritional supplementation was begun by the third trimester of pregnancy and often the child received a continued food supplement through the first few years of life. Some studies included behavioral stimulation as an additional variable, usually in the form of teaching the mother how to interact with her infant.

These longitudinal prospective studies avoided the problem associated with inappropriate cognitive measures by often standardizing the test on the target culture and including in the test battery as many behavioral measures as possible.

Although the various findings from these studies are too numerous to detail here, some general conclusions from this research can be drawn. Mild to moderate PCM contributes to less than optimal development in children, but the exact magnitude of the independent effects of undernutrition on behavior and the specific behavioral process impacted is unclear. Mild to moderate PCM is viewed as one of a number of social, nutritional, and psychological factors, including poor sanitation, low income, inadequate housing, low parental education, and poor child – caretaker interaction, which interact to contribute to less than optimal development.

The atheoretical nature of the test batteries used have made it difficult to isolate the specific behavior process being impacted, as tests both within and across ages are measuring multiple behavioral processes. In addition, the independent effect of undernutrition on poor behavior has been difficult to isolate because of the difficulty of finding an environment with only one risk factor present, and the nonadditive effect of multiple factors. Mild to moderate PCM by itself would be unlikely to result in measurable differences in behavior if adequate environmental stimulation were present. A number of risk factors occurring simultaneously, however, will increase the probability of a poor developmental outcome in an interactive manner. Sulzer, Wesley, and Leonig (1973), for example, in a retrospective analysis compared the effects of past nutritional status (as measured by a composite index of height for age and weight for height) and present nutritional status (presence or absence of anemia) on an IQ measure. Anemia alone produced no IQ deficit, whereas short stature alone (poor past nutrition) resulted in a 4-point IQ deficit. Short stature in combination with anemia resulted in a 10-point IQ deficit.

Finally it has proven difficult to impact nutrition as a single factor while keeping all other factors constant. For example, simply giving food to hungry people may not be a way of isolating nutrition as an independent variable. In the Bogota study (Mora, de Parades, Wagner, de Navarro, Suescun, Vuori, Christiansen, & Herrera, 1979) it was determined prior to supplementation that the diet of the pregnant women who would participate in the study was deficient in both protein and calories (average intake was 36 grams of protein and 1600 calories per day). The nutritional intervention provided 850 additional calories and 38.4 additional grams of protein to the pregnant mother's diet and an additional 600 calories and 30 grams of protein to every other member of the family. The infants born to supplemented mothers were not that much heavier than infants born to unsupplemented mothers. Dietary surveys revealed the reason for this outcome. Supplemented mothers increased their daily intake by only 130 calories and 20 grams of protein. What likely occurred was that part of the resources initially used to produce the 1600-calorie diet were diverted for other uses. The change in the family, then was not simply nutritional.

NUTRITIONAL DEFICITS

A more specific nutritional deficit than inadequate energy is a lack of sufficient amounts of a single nutrient such as a vitamin or trace element. Vitamins are catalysts in chemical reactions and like trace elements are not found in large quantities in the body. Nevertheless, an insufficient amount of an essential vitamin or trace element can have a severe effect on the organism.

It is beyond the scope of this chapter to detail the known effects associated with insufficient amounts of each vitamin and trace element. A number of sources are available (Goodhart & Shils, 1980, for example) that detail these effects. The present discussion is directed only to the effects of iron deficiency on behavior. This deficiency has been chosen because it is the most prevalent nutritional deficiency in the United States and has received considerable research attention. Iron plays important roles in oxygen transport in the blood, mitochondrial redox reactions, immunocompetence, and possibly neurotransmitter synthesis and catabolism.

Iron Deficiency

According to data from the most recent National Health and Nutrition Examination Survey II (Lane & Johnson, 1981), iron deficiency is a major problem in the U.S., with its greatest impact occurring during the first few years of life. Under a year of age, for example, estimates range from 13.3% in white females to 38.6% in black males. A number of factors interact to determine iron status, including gestational age, growth rate, breast versus bottle feeding, and the timing of the introduction of solid food (Siimes, 1981).

The normal infant passes through three hematopoietic phases during the first year of life, with the aforementioned factors determining the timing, not the ordering of the phases: (1) During the first 2 to 3 months of life, erythropoiesis is suppressed due to factors augmenting tissue oxygenation at a given hemoglobin level. Iron stores actually rise regardless of dietary iron supply, due to a shift of iron from red blood cells to storage sites. "Anemia" normally noted at 8 to 10 weeks is not associated with reduced stores or diminished tissue oxygenation and is termed "physiologic." (2) Hemoglobin concentration and transferrin saturation reaches a low around 3 to 4 months and erythropoiesis recommences. The duration of this period depends on a combination of factors including iron stores, dietary iron, and growth rate. Total hemoglobin usually rises but hemoglobin concentration remains stable due to the expanded blood volume associated with growth. (3) Without iron intake, storage sites become exhausted (termed iron deficiency) and, although total body iron remains stable, physical growth and increased blood volume result in a fall in hemoglobin concentration resulting in iron-deficiency anemia. By the end of the first year of life an increasing number of infants become iron deficient and anemic (Lane & Johnson, 1981).

A number of studies have been conducted relating iron deficiency to behavior in infants, preschool children, adolescents, and adult women, who also show higher iron-deficiency prevalence than men because of monthly blood loss. (See Leibel, Greenfield, & Pollitt, 1979, for greater detail). It is clear from published research that during infancy, iron-deficiency anemia has a negative impact on behavior. What is less clear is the specific behavioral process that is being affected by iron insufficiency. Numerous authors (Cantwell, 1974; Lozoff, Brittenham, Viteri,

Wolf, & Urrutia, 1982; Oski & Honig, 1979) have concluded that results show that iron-deficiency anemia negatively impacts cognitive development in infancy. This conclusion, however, is limited by the fact that the most widely used behavioral measure in these studies has been the Bayley Scales of Infant Development. More specifically, the Bayley Scales have a moderately low correlation of .1 to .2 with tests of intelligence obtained after the period of infancy (McCall, 1979). This low predictability is likely due to the Bayley's sampling of a large number of different behaviors, only some of which are cognitive, as they emerge during the first 2 years of life. Behaviors such as smiling in a mirror, searching for a fallen spoon, transferring toys from one hand to the other normally emerge around 5 months of age. A 5-month-old infant lacking in these and other age-appropriate skills, not all of which would be considered cognitive, would be judged developmentally delayed. Obviously, very different behaviors must be used to assess delays at other ages during infancy.

Because of the small number of subjects used and the choice of the Bayley scales as the dependent measure, no firm conclusions concerning the impact of iron deficiency on cognition are possible. It is clear that iron is having an effect on behavior, but whether that effect relates to poor attention, reduced reactivity, or deficits in cognition is presently unknown.

A study conducted with preschool children in Cambridge, Mass. (Pollitt, Leibel, & Greenfield, 1983) indicates how one could choose a test battery that would allow an assessment of which specific process is affected by iron deficiency. The behavioral test battery in this study was derived from a theoretical model developed for the study of normal – retardate difference in the specific processes involved in attention, learning, and memory (Fisher & Zeaman, 1973). Use of this model allowed these researchers to conclude that iron deficiency produces reversible deficits in attentional processes.

One interesting finding hints at an important need for further research on the biochemical link between iron deficiency and behavior. Initially it was thought that behavioral alterations associated with iron-deficiency anemia resulted from the impact on reduced circulating hemoglobin mass. Oski and Honig (1979) report reversibility of behavioral deficits 7 to 10 days following iron repletion therapy. Iron therapy over this short time span has no significant effect on circulating hemoglobin mass. These results are consistent with anecdotal reports from physicians that behavioral symptoms associated with iron deficiency are eliminated very quickly.

The results have two important implications. First, the role of iron in affecting behavior is likely related to iron's metabolic or enzymatic function. Although the specific mechanism is unknown, a number of hypotheses are tenable (Leibel, et al., 1979). One hypothesis relates to neurotransmitter activity in the brain. Iron is essential for phenylalanine hydroxylase activity, which catalyzes phenylalanine to tyrosine, which, as discussed earlier, plays a role in neurotransmitter formation. Tyrosine hydroxylase (unique to catecholamine-containing neurons) is the first and rate-limiting enzyme in catecholamine biosynthesis and requires ferrous iron as a cofactor. Tryptophan hydroxylase, which is the rate-limiting enzyme in the synthesis of serotonin, may require iron as a cofactor (Youdim, Hamon, & Bourgoin, 1975). Aldehyde oxidase functions in the catabolism of serotonin and is an iron-containing metalloflavoprotein. Monoamine oxidase (MAO) limits the duration of action of the neurotransmitters serotonin, dopamine, and norepinephrine by oxidizing them after their release or uptake into the presynaptic nerve fiber (Snyder, 1976). Sourkes (1972) has shown that both riboflavin and iron deficiency result in reduced hepatic MAO activity in rats, which is reversed following repletion of the missing vitamin or mineral.

A second series of hypotheses relates to iron's role in oxidative metabolism in the brain. The average adult male consumes 250 ml of oxygen per minute in the basal state. Some 50 ml/minute of this oxygen is accounted for by the brain. Thus an organ that constitutes roughly 2% of body weight accounts for 20% of oxygen consumption. A child's brain, on the other hand, accounts for more than 50% of the total body basal oxygen consumption. Various hemes, iron-flavoproteins and iron-dependent enzymes are components of the Krebs cycle and cytochrome pathways, both of which are essential to oxidative metabolism.

The second implication of the results of the Oski and Honig study (1979) is that if iron plays its role in an enzymatic or metabolic fashion, then behavior may be affected prior to significant decreases in hemoglobin concentration, or early on in the etiology of this deficiency. Many more children suffer from the precursor of iron-deficiency anemia (i.e., iron deficiency).

The high prevalence of iron deficiency in an otherwise well-nourished population, and its large impact in the developing human organism make the issue of its role in behavior and brain development an important one. As indicated previously, the specific behavioral process affected by iron deficiency early in life is not known. In addition, the specific enzymatic or metabolic process in which iron affects behavior is also unknown. Clearly additional research is needed.

Short-Term Fasting

In addition to the chronic effects of insufficient energy and inadequate amounts of missing nutrients, many individuals, especially school-age children, skip a meal and are subjected to a short-term fast. Despite a large body of anecdotal evidence from teachers (Pollitt, Gargiulo, Gersovitz, Greenfield, Teodori, Wetsel, & Witenberg, 1976) that the initiation of school feeding programs improves school performance, very little research has been conducted on the effects of skipping a meal on behavior in humans.

Cahil (1976) and Havel (1972) have described the events in the transition from a fed to a fasted state. Briefly, this transition involves a sequence, orchestrated largely by shifts in circulating insulin/glucagon ratios (Unger, 1971), such that different endogenous fuel sources are mobilized to provide the organism with sufficient energy. A complex series of adjustments serves the purpose of providing adequate energy substrates for brain metabolism without undue sacrifice of critical somatic tissue such as muscle. In the adult the following sequence of steps from the last meal occurs:

1. 4 – 5 hours—Hepatic glycogen begins to return to the peripheral circulation in the form of glucose.
2. 8 – 10 hours—Decreasing blood glucose and insulin levels reduces muscle and adipose glucose utilization. At this point more than 50% of muscle energy needs are met by oxidation of free fatty acids. The liver also begins to catabolize free fatty acids as an energy source.
3. 12 – 16 hours—Liver glycogen is depleted and gluconeogenesis is used to produce glucose for cerebral consumption. Hepatic keto acid (beta hydroxybutyrate, acetoacetate) production is increased and some of the ketones, along with free fatty acids, are used as a fuel source for muscle, sparing glucose for the brain.

Because glycogenolysis is the major buffer of blood glucose for the brain against a short-term fast (12 – 18 hours), and because the brain accounts for more than 50% of body oxygen consumption in children, and the child has less available energy stores due to the higher brain/liver weight ratio of a child as compared to an adult (Sokoloff, 1976), one might expect that a short-term fast has a greater impact on the child than the adult. These theoretical projections are borne out. Whereas the adult who has fasted for 24 hours does not show a plasma glucose decline below 60 mg/dl (mean plasma level = 100 mg/dl at the start of the fast) (Fajans & Floyd, 1976), the fasted child shows a significant fall in capillary blood glucose within 8 hours (Chaussain, 1973).

One recent study (Pollitt, Leibel, & Greenfield, 1981) relating short-term fasting and behavior in 9 – 11-year-old children is worth mentioning. These children were fed a prescribed meal at 5:00 p.m. and were kept overnight in a clinical research center so that their food intake could be monitored. On one occasion the children were fed a prescribed breakfast at 8:00 a.m. On a second occasion (these treatments were randomized for order) no breakfast was administered. All children received a battery of psychological tests at 11:00 a.m. prior to lunch. Thus, on the day that they skipped breakfast the children had fasted for roughly 18 hours. Blood was drawn following the administration of the behavioral tests to relate behavior to blood chemistry.

A comparison was made for analysis purposes of the children who showed large differences versus small differences in glucose concentration from the no-breakfast to breakfast conditions. The children with large glucose differences compared to children who handled the fast better in the sense that the fast did not significantly impact their glucose level, performed more poorly on a test requiring reflexive as opposed to impulsive behavior (the Matching Familiar Figures test), but better on a short-term memory task. These results (i.e., heightened arousal leading to better short-term memory, but poorer cognitive processing style) were consistent with results obtained with adults under conditions of moderate stress such as noise (Poulton, 1976).

The implication of the results of this study is intriguing. Short-term fasting may be another form of stress that needs to be added to the equation in our understanding of the role of stress in behavioral medicine. Clearly more research on this topic is needed.

Hypoglycemia

A condition related to fasting, hypoglycemia, is worth mentioning. "Reactive hypoglycemia" is the term used to describe a fall in blood glucose level below 50 mg/100 ml of blood usually 2 − 3 hours after the ingestion of a meal. The term has also been applied to the symptoms associated with this condition, including anxiety, sweating, weakness, and palpitations. These symptoms, however, are not unique to hypoglycemia. As indicated earlier in this chapter, homeostatic mechanisms exist to maintain blood glucose levels in a stable range, and when blood glucose levels drop below this range, glucose is released from the liver. Part of this mechanism involves the release of catecholamines that cause these symptoms. Catecholamine release under other conditions such as stress results in the same symptoms. These symptoms, then, are unlikely to be due to hypoglycemia unless blood sugar levels have fallen below 50 or 40 mg/100 ml of blood. In addition, hypoglycemia is promptly relieved by the ingestion of food or sugar. Consistent relationships between low blood sugar, elimination of symptoms by ingestion of food or sugar, and the presence of reported symptoms of hypoglycemia have not been found. The most common cause of hypoglycemia is the use of drugs such as insulin that lower blood sugar and thus may be a problem in diabetes. Data from the Mayo Clinic (Service, 1976) report fewer than 100 cases of hypoglycemia a year from the over a quarter of a million patients seen yearly. The symptoms commonly associated with this condition are thus likely due to catecholamine release in the absence of blood glucose levels below 40 or 50 mg/100 ml.

NUTRIENT OVERCONSUMPTION

Fats are an essential part of one's diet and play key roles in many aspects of metabolic function. According to the recent goals set by the Senate Select Committee on Nutrition and Human Needs (1980), Americans should obtain less than 30% of their total daily caloric intake from fat, a substantial reduction from present consumption levels. The recommended reduction in fat content has largely resulted from concerns about the relationship between dietary fat and atherosclerosis. Recent data show that Americans obtain 40 − 45% of their caloric intake from fat.

Atherosclerosis is a result of fat accumulation, especially in the form of cholesterol and cholesterol esters, in the cells that line the arterial walls. Recent focus has been on the role of high density lipoprotein cholesterol in the development of this condition (Gordon, Castelli, Hjortland, Kannel, & Dawber, 1977).

Both genes and the environment are thought to interact in the development of this condition. Genetic factors seem to predispose individuals to high, medium, or low values of serum cholesterol levels. With increased age, nutritional factors tend to elevate these levels (Eaton, Allen, Koopmans, Ellis, Abrams, & Schade, 1981). Dietary attempts to reduce serum cholesterol levels only seem to bring values down to levels approximating values present earlier in life or near the low, medium, or high value preset by genetic factors.

The etiology of atherosclerosis is complex and a number of factors in addition to genes and diet have been implicated. Hamilton and Whitney (1979), for example, list over 30 risk factors including smoking, high blood pressure, lack of exercise, obesity, and stress. Some of these factors, including excess caffeine consumption (Sved, 1976) and trace element deficiencies (Johnson, Peterson, & Smith, 1979), remain unproved in their relation to coronary disease.

Although it is clear that nutritional factors play an important role in the development of atherosclerosis, it has been difficult to assess diet's exact role. It is not easy to demonstrate, for example, a dose response relationship between serum cholesterol and dietary cholesterol (Quinao, Grundy, & Ahrens, 1971). Because of the relative homogeneity of cholesterol in the American diet and the large reduction in intake of fats needed to reduce serum cholesterol levels, it has been difficult to demonstrate different dietary habits in the United States as they relate to the development of atherosclerosis. In addition, although there are a large number of epidemiologic studies relating coronary risk to high cholesterol levels (Stamler, 1979), reduced coronary risk does not seem to correlate with reduction by clinical trial of serum cholesterol levels (Olson, 1979). Thus, within a culture, differences between people with and without cardiovascular disease seem to depend on factors other than diet.

The relationship between diet and the development of atherosclerosis is a complex one. Although dietary habits across cultures correlate with serum cholesterol level, lower cholesterol availability does not always lead to lower rates of heart disease. In Finland, for example, where dietary cholesterol is one-third less available than in the United States, higher rates of coronary disease occur (Connor & Connor, 1972). Nonetheless, given the repeated correlation between serum cholesterol level and the risk of coronary disease, it would be wise to err on the side of caution and follow recommendations for reduced fats in the diet.

Salt is another important nutrient in the diet. Recommended ingestion in the form of sodium chloride is approximately 100 to 500 mg/day. In many cultures the actual intake of salt far exceeds these values. Average intake in the United States has been estimated at 10 gm/day and in Japan, 14 gm/day in the south, 26 gm/day in the north (Dahl, 1972). Dahl (1958) hypothesized that the excess results from an acquired taste, beginning with the unnecessarily high levels of salt found in infant food (Dahl, 1972).

A number of studies have confirmed the correlation between salt intake and hypertension (Dahl, 1972; Isaacson, Modlin, & Jackson, 1963; Prior, Evans, Harvey, Davidson, & Lindsey, 1968). Dahl (1972), for example, shows the correlation between sodium intake and hypertension in a number of different countries. The Eskimo, for example, who have very low salt intake, show virtually no hypertension in their society. Northern Japan, on the other hand, with very high salt intake, had 38% hypertensives in the sample studied. Work with animals confirms this relationship. Dahl (Dahl, Knudsen, Meine, & Leitl, 1968) has shown that the severity of hypertension in rats is related directly to the level of salt intake. The younger the animal when fed a high-salt diet, the more rapidly hypertension develops.

Although other factors such as genetics play a role in hypertension, this risk factor for coronary disease (Cohn, 1977) has clearly been shown to be related to salt intake. Fortunately, dietary sodium restriction appears to lead to large decreases in blood pressure in about one-third of patients who restrict their diet to 1 to 2 gm of salt/day. Another one-third of patients so treated show mild decreases in blood pressure. About one-third of patients show no decrease in blood pressure (Dahl, 1972). Low levels of salt ingestion in the diet would thus seem a prudent measure.

CONCLUSION

The role of nutrition in behavior and psychological development is an expanding field only touched upon in this chapter. An attempt was made to highlight a number of key areas in order to give the reader a feel for some of the issues that are now being addressed and are likely to develop further as our knowledge base in this area expands. Because of the expanded sophistication of the methods involved in this research, increased collaboration of investigators from many different biobehavioral and psychosocial disciplines is needed for the research to develop in a meaningful way.

REFERENCES

Alfin-Slater, R., & Kritchevsky, D. *Human nutrition: A comprehensive treatise* (Vol. 3A). New York: Plenum Press, 1979.

Alfin-Slater, R., & Kritchevsky, D. *Human nutrition: A comprehensive treatise* (Vol. 3B). New York: Plenum Press, 1980.

Bengoa, J. M. The problem of malnutrition. *WHO Chronicle*, 1974, *28*, 3 – 7.

Boelkins, R. C., & Hegsted, D. M. Consequences of early protein and energy malnutrition in monkeys. In J. Brozek (Eds.), *Behavioral effects of energy and protein deficits*. Washington, D.C.: NIH Publication 79 – 1906, 55 – 67, 1979.

Brozek, J. *Behavioral effects of energy and protein deficits.* Washington, D.C.: NIH Publication 79–1906, 1979.

Brozek, J., Coursin, D. B., & Read, M. S. Longitudinal studies on the effects of malnutrition, nutritional supplementation, and behavioral stimulation. *Bulletin of the Pan American Health Organization,* 1977, 237 – 249.

Brozek, J., & Schurch, B. (Eds.). *Malnutrition and behavior: Critical assessments of key issues.* Lausanne: The Nestle Foundation, 1984.

Burkitt, D., Walker, A., & Painter, N. Dietary fiber and disease. *Journal of the American Medical Association, 229,* 1068, 1974.

Cahil, G. F., Jr. Starvation in man. *Clinical Endocrinology and Metabolism,* 1976, *5,* 397.

Cantwell, R. The long-term neurological sequelae of anemia in infancy. *Pediatric Research,* 1974, *8.*

Chase, H., Lindsley, W., & O'Brien, D. Undernutrition and cellular development. *Nature,* 1969, *221,* 554 – 555.

Chaussain, J. L. Glycemic response to 24 hour fast in normal children and children with ketotic hypoglycemia. *Journal of Pediatrics,* 1973, *82,* 438.

Chavez, A., & Martinez, C. Behavioral effects of undernutrition and food supplementation. In J. Brozek (Ed.), *Behavioral effects of energy and protein deficits.* Washington, D.C.: NIH Publication 79 – 1906, 216 – 228, 1979.

Cohen, E. L. *In vivo studies of the effect of the availability of choline on the biosynthesis and content of acetylcholine in brain.* Unpublished doctoral dissertation, Massachusetts Institute of Technology, 1976.

Cohen, E. L., & Wurtman, R. J. Brain acetylcholine: Increase after systemic choline administration. *Life Science,* 1975, *16,* 1095.

Cohen, E. L., & Wurtman, R. J. Brain acetylcholine: Control by dietary choline. *Science,* 1976, *191,* 561.

Cohen, E. L., & Wurtman, R. J. Nutrition and brain neurotransmitters. In M. Winick (Ed.), *Human nutrition: A comprehensive treatise* (Vol. 1). New York: Plenum Press, 1979.

Cohn, J. N. Heart disease in hypertensive patients. *Med. Clin. North Am.,* 1977, *61,* 581.

Conners, C. K. *Food additives and hyperactive children.* New York: Plenum Press, 1980.

Connor, W. I., & Connor, S. L. The key role of nutritional factors in the prevention of coronary heart disease. *Preventive Medicine,* 1972, *1,* 49.

Dahl, L. K. Salt intake and salt need. *New England Journal of Medicine,* 1958, *258,* 1152.

Dahl, L. K. Salt and hypertension. *American Journal of Clinical Nutrition,* 1972, *25,* 231.

Dahl, L. K., Knudsen, K. D., Meine, M. A. & Leitl, G. J. Effects of chronic excess salt ingestion. Modification of experimental hypertension in the rat by variations in the diet. *Circulation Research,* 1968, *22,* 11.

Eaton, R. P., Allen, R. C. Jr., Koopmans, H. E., Ellis, H., Abrams, J., & Schade, D. S. Overview of lipoprotein metabolism. In P. J. Garry (Ed.), *Human nutrition clinical and biochemical aspects.* Washington, D.C.: The American Association for Clinical Chemistry, 1981, 109 – 120.

Fajans, S. S., & Floyd, J. C. Fasting hypoglycemia in adults. *New England Journal of Medicine,* 1976, *294,* 766.

Fisher, M. A., & Zeaman, D. An attention – retention theory of retardate discrimination learning. In N. Ellis (Ed.), *International Review of Research in Mental Retardation, 6.* New York: Academic Press, 1973.

Freeman, H. E., Klein, R. E., Kagan, J., & Yarbrough, C. Relations between nutrition and cognition in rural Guatemala. *American Journal of Public Health,* 1977, *67,* 233 – 239.

Gelenberg, A., Wojcik, J. D., & Growdon, J. H. et. al. Tyrosine for the treatment of depression. *American Journal of Psychiatry,* 1980, *137,* 622 – 623.

Gibson, C. J., & Wurtman, R. J. Physiological control of brain norepinephrine synthesis by brain tyrosine concentration. *Life Science,* 1978, *22,* 1399 – 1406.

Goodhart, R. S., & Shils, M. E. *Modern nutrition in health and disease* (6th ed.). Philadelphia: Lea & Febiger, 1980.

Gordon, T., Castelli, W. P., Hjortland, M. C., Kannel, W. B., & Dawber, T. R. High density lipoprotein as a protective factor against heart disease. *American Journal of Medicine*, 1977, *62*, 707 – 714.

Habicht, J. P. Public health implications of present evidence for long-term behavioral consequences of energy and protein deficits. In J. Brozek (Ed.), *Behavioral effects of energy and protein deficits*. Washington, D.C.: NIH Publication 79 – 1906, 331 – 356, 1979.

Hamilton, E. M. N., & Whitney, E. N. Atherosclerosis: What causes it, and can we prevent it? In *Nutrition: Concepts and controversies*. St. Paul: West Publ. Co., 1979.

Hathaway, M. *Heights and weights of children in the United States*, US Dept. Agric. Home. Econ. Res. Rep. No. 2, 1957.

Havel, R. J. Caloric homeostasis and disorders of fuel transport. *New England Journal of Medicine*, 1972, *287*, 1186.

Hertzig, M. E., Birch, H. G., Richardson, S. A., & Tizard, J. Intellectual levels of school children severely malnourished during the first two years of life. *Pediatrics*, 1972, *49*, 814 – 823.

Hirsch, M. J., Growdon, J. H., & Wurtman, J. Increase in hippocampal acetylcholine following choline administration, *Brain Research*, 1977, *332*, 383 – 385.

Hodges, R. *Human nutrition: A comprehensive treatise* (Vol. 4). New York: Plenum Press, 1979.

Isaacson, L. C., Modlin, M., & Jackson, W. P. U. Sodium intake and hypertension. *Lancet*, 1963, *1*, 946.

Jelliffe, D., & Jelliffe, E. F. *Human nutrition: A comprehensive treatise*, (Vol. 2). New York: Plenum Press, 1979.

Johnson, C. J., Peterson, D. R., & Smith, E. R. Myocardial tissue concentrations of magnesium and potassium in men dying suddenly from ischemic heart disease. *American Journal of Clinical Nutrition*, 1979, *32*, 967.

Kay, R., & Truswell, A. Effect of citrus pectin on blood lipids and fecal steroid excretion in man. *American Journal of Clinical Nutrition*, 1977, *30*.

Keller, E., Munaro, N., & Orsingher, O. Perinatal undernutrition reduces alpha and beta adrenergic receptor binding in adult rat brain. *Science*, 1982, *215*, 1269 – 1270.

Keys, A., Anderson, J., & Grande, F. Serum cholesterol response to changes in the diet. *Clin. Exp.* 1965, *14*, 747.

Kritchevsky, D., & Tepper, S. Experimental atherosclerosis in rabbits fed cholesterol free diets: Influence of chow components. *Journal of Atherosclerosis Research*, 1968, *8:*

Kritchevsky, D., Davidson, L., Shapiro, I., Kim, H., Kitagawa, M., Malhotra, S., Nair, P., Clarkson, T., Bersohn, I., & Winter, P. Lipid metabolism and experimental atherosclerosis in baboons: Influence of cholesterol-free, semi-synthetic diets. *American Journal of Clinical Nutrition*, 1974, *27*.

Kritchevsky, D., Davidson, L., Kim, H., Krendel, D., Malhotra, S., Vander Watt, J., Du Plessis, J., Winter, P., Ipp, T., Mendelsohn, D., & Bersohn, I. Influence of semi-purified diets on atherosclerosis in African green monkeys. *Exp. Mol. Pathol.*, 1977, *26*.

Lane, J. M., & Johnson, C. J. Prevalence of iron deficiency. In F. A. Oski, & H. A. Pearson (Eds.), *Iron nutrition revisited—Infancy, childhood, adolescence*. Columbus: Ross Laboratories, 1981.

Lee, C., & Dubos, R. Lasting biological effects of early environmental influences. *Journal of Experimental Medicine*, 1972, *136*, 1031.

Leibel, R., Greenfield, D. B., & Pollitt, E. Iron deficiency: Behavior and brain biochemistry. In M. Winick (Ed.), *Human nutrition: A comprehensive treatise* (Vol.1). New York: Plenum Press, 1979.

Levitsky, D. A. Comment on rodent studies. In J. Brozek (Ed.), *Behavioral effects of energy and protein deficits*. Washington, D.C.: NIH Publication 79 – 1906, 39 – 41, 1979.

Lozoff, B., Brittenham, G., Viteri, F., Wolf, A., & Urrutia, J. The effects of short-term oral iron therapy on developmental deficits in iron-deficient anemic infants. *The Journal of Pediatrics*, 1982, *100*(3), 351 – 357.

McCall, R. B. The development of intellectual functioning in infancy and the prediction of later IQ. In J. Osofsky (Ed.), *Handbook of infant development*. New York: John Wiley & Sons, 1979.

McKay, H., Sinistrera, L., McKay, A., Gomez, H., & Lloreda, P. Improving cognitive ability of chronically deprived children. *Science*, 1978, *200*, 270 – 278.

Moore, J. The effect of the type of roughage in the diet on plasma cholesterol levels and aortic atherosis in rabbits, *British Journal of Nutrition*, 1967, *27*.

Mora, J. O., Clement, N., Christiansen, N., Ortiz, N., Vuori, L., & Wagner, M. Nutritional supplementation, early stimulation, and child development. In J. Brosek (Ed.), *Behavioral effects of energy and protein deficits*. Washington, D.C.: NIH Publication 79 – 1906, 255 – 269, 1979.

Mora, J. O., de Parades, B., Wagner, M., de Navarro, L., Suescun, J., Vuori, L., Christiansen, N., & Herrera, M. G. Nutritional supplementation and the outcome of pregnancy. I. Birth weight. *American Journal of Clinical Nutrition*, 1979, *32*, 455.

Nagler, A. L., Dettbarn, W. D., Seifter, E., & Levenson, S. M. Tissue levels of acetylcholine and acetylcholinesterase in weanling rats subjected to acute choline deficiency. *Journal of Nutrition*, 1968, *94*, 13.

Olson, R. Is there an optimum diet for the prevention of coronary heart disease? In R. I. Levy, B. M. Rifkind, B. H. Dennis, & N. Ernst (Eds.), *Nutrition, lipids and coronary heart disease: A global view of nutrition in health and disease*. New York: Raven Press, 1979.

Oski, F., & Honig, A. The effects of therapy on the developmental scores of iron deficient infants. *Journal of Pediatrics*, 1979, *92*, 21 – 25.

Pollitt, E., Gargiulo, M., Gersovitz, M., Greenfield, D., Teodori, M., Wetsel, W., & Witenberg, S. *The US school feeding program: Modes of evaluating its effects on the behavior of recipients*. New York: The Ford Foundation, 1976.

Pollitt, E., Leibel, R., & Greenfield, D. Brief fasting, stress, and cognition in children. *The American Journal of Clinical Nutrition*, 1981, *34*, 1526 – 1533.

Pollitt, E., Leibel, R., & Greenfield, D. Iron deficiency and cognitive test performance in preschool children. *Nutrition and Behavior*, 1983, *1*, 137–146.

Pollitt, E., & Thomson, C. Protein-calorie malnutrition and behavior: A view from psychology. In R. J. Wurtman, & J. J. Wurtman (Eds.), *Nutrition and the brain*. New York: Raven Press, 1977.

Poulton, E. C. Arousing environmental stress can improve performances, whatever people say. *Aviation Space Environmental Medicine*, 1976, *47*, 1193 – 1204.

Prior, I. A. M., Evans, J. G., Harvey, H. P., Davidson, F., & Lindsey, M. Sodium intake and blood pressure in two Polynesian populations. *New England Journal of Medicine*, 1968, *279*, 515.

Quinao, E., Grundy, S. M., & Ahrens, E. I. Effects of dietary cholesterol on the regulation of total body cholesterol in man. *Journal of Lipid Research*, 1971, *12*, 233.

Riopelle, A. J. Early protein deprivation and behavior deficit reconsidered. In J. Cravioto, L. Hambraeus, & B. Vahlquist (Eds.), *Early malnutrition and mental development*. Symposia of the Swedish Nutrition Foundation XII. Uppsala: Almquist and Wiksell, 1974.

Schrimshaw, N. I., & Behar, M. Protein malnutrition in young children. *Science*, 1961, *133*, 2039 – 2047.

Sereni, F., Principi, N., Perletti, L., & Piceni Sereni, L. Undernutrition and the developing rat brain. I. Influence on acetylcholinesterase and succinic acid dehydrogenase activities and on norepinephrine and 5-OH thryptamine tissue concentrations. *Biol. Neonate*, 1966, *10*, 254.e

Service, F. J. Hypoglycemias. *Comparative Therapy*, 1976, *2*, 27.

Showmaker, W. J., & Wurtman, R. J. Perinatal undernutrition: Accumulation of catecholamines in rat brain. *Science*, 1971, *171*, 1017.

Siimes, M. A. Pathogenesis of iron deficiency in infancy. In F. A. Oski, & H. A. Pearson (Eds.), *Iron nutrition revisited—Infancy, Childhood, Adolescence*. Columbus: Ross Laboratories, 1981.

Snyder, S. H. Catecholamines, serotonin and histamine. In F. J. Siegel, R. W. Albers, R. Katzman, & B. W. Agranoff (Eds.), *Basic neurochemistry*. Boston: Little, Brown, & Co., 1976.

Sokoloff, L. Circulation and energy metabolism of the brain. In G. J. Siegel, R. W. Albers, R. Katzman, & B. W. Agranoff (Eds.), *Basic neurochemistry*. Boston: Little, Brown & Co., 1976.

Sourkes, T. L. Influence of specific nutrients on catecholamine synthesis and metabolism. *Pharm. Rev.*, 1972, *24*, 349.

Stamler, J. Population studies. In R. I. Levy, B. M. Rifkind, B. H. Dennis, & N. Ernst (Eds.), *Nutrition, lipids and coronary heart disease: A global view of nutrition in health and disease.* New York: Raven Press, 1979.

Stern, W. C., Morgane, P. J., Miller, M., & Resnick, O. Protein malnutrition in rats: Response of brain amines and behavior to foot shock stress. *Experimental Neurology,* 1975, *47,* 56.

Sulzer, J. L., Wesley, H. H., & Leonig, F. Nutrition and behavior in Head Start children: Results from the Tulane study. In D. Kallen (Ed.), *Nutrition, development and social behavior.* DHEW Publ. 73 – 242, 1973.

Sved, I. B. The effects of caffeine. *Journal of the American Pharmacology Association,* 1976, *16,* 568.

Syed, A. F., Fernstrom, J. D., & Wurtman, R. J. Tyrosine administration reduces blood pressure and enhances brain norepinephrine release in spontaneously hypertensive rats. *Proceedings of the National Academy of Science, USA,* 1979, *76,* 3511 – 3514.

Unger, R. H. Glucagon and the insulin glucagon ratio in diabetes and other catabolic illnesses. *Diabetes,* 1971, *20,* 834.

U.S.D.A.—H.E.W. *Nutrition and your health: Dietary guidelines for Americans.* Washington, D.C.: US Department of Agriculture, 1980.

Waterlow, J. C., & Rutishauser, H. Malnutrition in man. In J. Cravioto, L. Hambraeus, & B. Vahlquist (Eds.), *Early malnutrition and mental development.* Uppsala, Sweden: Almqvist and Wiksell, 1974.

Winick, M. *Human nutrition: A comprehensive treatise* (Vol. *1*). New York: Plenum Press, 1979.

Winick, M., & Noble, A. Quantitative changes in DNA, RNA, and protein during prenatal and postnatal growth in the rat. *Developmental Biology,* 1965, *12,* 451.

Winick, M., & Rosso, P. The effects of severe early malnutrition on cellular growth of human brain. *Pediatric Research* 1969, *3,* 181.

Wurtman, R., & Wurtman, J. *Nutrition and the brain* (Vol. 1). New York: Raven Press, 1977. (a)

Wurtman, R., & Wurtman, J. *Nutrition and the brain* (Vol. 2). New York: Raven Press, 1977. (b)

Youdim, M. B. H., Hamon, M., & Bourgoin, S. Preparation of partially purified pig brain stem-tryptophan hydroxylase. *Journal of Neurochemistry,* 1975, *25,* 407.

Zimmermann, R. R. Nutrition and behavior: A view of the current state of research. In J. Brozek (Ed.), *Behavioral effects of energy and protein deficits.* Washington, D.C.: NIH Publication 79 – 1906, 87 – 93, 1979.

12

Eating Disorders: Obesity and Anorexia

Nancy T. Blaney
Florida International University

Eating disorders constitute behavioral syndromes that incur particularly high risks for the individual. The extremes—either undereating or overeating—respectively produce anorexia and obesity, both of which have morbid medical sequellae.

As both disorders represent disturbances in the regulation of food intake, existing theory and research on the various proposed hunger-satiety mechanisms will be briefly noted (see Garfinkel & Coscina, 1982, for a detailed discussion) before the disorders are discussed.

Animal research has shown that bilateral lesions of the ventromedial hypothalamus (VMH) produce hyperphagia, causing weight to nearly double. Lesions in the adjacent region, the lateral hypothalamus (LH) produce aphagia, and consequent severe weight loss and even death. Thus for many years the VMH has been viewed as the "satiety center" and the LH, the "feeding center." This concept has been challenged, however, with evidence that hunger regulation involves multiple neurochemical mechanisms rather than reflecting the action of any single neuroanatomical site (Leibowitz, 1976). Further, experiments involving these neurochemical mechanisms have reproduced the range of behaviors found in hypothalamically lesioned animals (Stricker & Zigmond, 1976).

Fuel availability, another proposed mechanism, has varied effects depending on whether the fuel is glucose, lipids, or proteins. Glucose has a short-term and lipids have a long-term regulatory role. Amino acid regulation of food intake is a relatively new area. However, it is clear that, (1) protein intake can be closely regulated separately from caloric intake; (2) dietary amino acids may affect brain neurotransmitters; and (3) they can in turn control subsequent protein intake.

Further, there is evidence that signals from the gastrointestinal system regulate food intake (Koopmans, 1978), giving rise to the concept of the gut – brain axis of shared hormones. The functions of these hormones are not yet completely understood, however.

Besides these physiological mechanisms, psychological processes affect the regulation of food intake and are considered in the following sections. The chapter is divided into two parts, focusing on obesity and anorexia. In each, the psychological and physiological characteristics of the condition, its etiology, treatment, and outcome are examined.

OBESITY

Obesity, or an excess of body fat, is one of the most common medical problems afflicting Americans. Bray (1976) cites statistics showing that among adults, approximately 20% or more of males are obese, and 25% to 40% of females. Diagnosis generally is by comparison of weight with standard height – weight charts, or by measures of skinfold thickness and/or body density, with 20% overweight defined as a serious problem. The label "serious" connotes more than cosmetic concerns, as obesity poses increased health risks such as cardiovascular disease, diabetes mellitus, hyperlipidemia, endometrial carcinoma (Bray, 1978), and breast cancer (Donegan, Harts, & Rimm, 1978). In the 40 – 70 age group, being 30% overweight increases mortality among men and women respectively to 42% and 36% above average (Waxler & Liska, 1975). Although obesity occurs secondary to a number of disease processes, this is not the case for most obesity. The discussion that follows focuses on situations in which the obesity is primary, having no other known cause.

Obesity is closely tied to social class, being more common in the lower socioeconomic group than in the middle or upper (Noppa & Hällström, 1981). This class difference already is apparent by age 6 for both sexes, though especially strong for girls. Because its occurrence is tied to cultural norms, it appears inappropriate to view obesity solely as an abnormal trait of the individual.

Characteristics

Body image disturbance—as reflected in overestimating body size—has been found to characterize the obese (Slade & Russell, 1973b). Among obese women, degree of obesity is associated with degree of overestimation (Pearlson, Flournoy, Simonson, & Slavney, 1981). However, overestimation has been found among normal weight controls (Garner, Garfinkel, Stancer, & Moldofsky, 1976; Slade, 1977) and has failed to be predictive of weight loss (Pearlson et al., 1981). The general conclusion is that body image disturbance is a consequence of obesity, not a cause, and characterizes primarily childhood-onset obesity (Stunkard & Mendelson, 1967).

In eating patterns, the obese have been presumed to differ from nonobese. Though research has failed to establish any single eating style characteristic of obese adults (Mahoney, 1975), obese children do eat more rapidly than nonobese children (Drabman, Hammer, & Jarvie, 1977; Waxman & Stunkard, 1980). As the assumption of an obese eating style underlies various behavioral treatments of obesity, it is important to determine if laboratory failure to find one accurately represents what occurs in natural environments as well. To this end, Stunkard and colleagues utilized a fast-food setting for observing obese and normal weight patrons eating either a high- or low-calorie meal. They found no evidence for a distinctively obese eating style. Only a small but significant difference was observed, which showed that obese did not slow their eating during the last part of a large meal as much as nonobese, suggesting differences in the satiety process (Stunkard, Coll, Lundquist, & Meyers, 1980).

Apart from its initial causes, obesity has consequences that may in themselves be of causal import. Rodin (1981) cites data documenting this as a vicious cycle wherein the fat get fatter due to a fourfold effect of weight gain: (1) fat storage capacity of adipose cells increases; (2) basal levels of insulin rise, facilitating fat storage by speeding conversion of sugar to fat; (3) feelings of hunger increase due to rapid sugar utilization; and (4) energy expenditure diminishes due to reduced activity and to lowered metabolism that results from dieting, and from fat tissue being metabolically more inert than lean tissue. The last point suggests that dieting itself perversely may contribute to maintaining overweight by each successive dieting episode further lowering the metabolic rate.

Etiological Explanations

Organic factors.   Genetics, metabolic and endocrine disorders, and adipose cell function have been suggested as organic bases for the etiology of obesity.

The difficulties of disentangling the *genetic* contribution to human obesity from that of the environment has led to a focus on animal research where the genetic component is easier to evaluate. Summarizing this literature, Foch and McClearn (1980) conclude that there is considerable evidence, for both animals and humans, of both single-gene and polygenic influence on adult body weight and obesity, though single-gene obesity in humans likely accounts for only a small proportion of cases. They emphasize that obesity can arise as a result of any one or a combination of several channels of influence. Each channel comprises an interaction of genes with environmental factors to determine individual phenotypes. In their view, one channel could be the number of fat cells, another the efficiency of metabolic processes, another the sensitivity of the hypothalamus to nutrient levels. Regarding heritability, they cite data showing that heritability estimates for humans cluster in the .60s for weight, with twin studies yielding heritability estimates for obesity of .77 to .88. These appear to be relatively stable throughout life. Foch and McClearn conclude that, although the existence of genetic influences on human obesity is clear, what is not clear is the relative importance of the effects and how they interact with environmental influences. They stress the need for developmental studies to investigate individual differences as a function of this interaction.

Rodin (1977) has summarized the data regarding whether obesity is caused by *metabolic* or *hormonal disturbances,* concluding that, although serious disturbances do exist, they are not etiological. Studies of experimentally induced obesity and weight loss show the associated changes to be a consequence, and not a cause of obesity. For example, Sims and colleagues demonstrated that, when normal-weight persons overeat and become obese, they evidence the same metabolic and endocrine abnormalities shown by the spontaneously obese, with three exceptions: (1) weight gain is accomplished only by increasing fat cell size, not number; (2) more calories are required to maintain the induced obesity; and (3) induced obesity is associated with a decrease, rather than the usual rise, in plasma-free fatty acids. This last phenomenon is thought to be due primarily to the high carbohydrate diet necessary to induce overweight. When weight and caloric intake are reduced, the metabolic and endocrine changes diminish (Sims, Danforth, Horton, Bray, Glennon, & Salans, 1973; Sims, Goldman, Gluck, Horton, Kelleher & Rowe, 1968; Sims & Horton, 1968).

As Rodin notes, such disturbances are not causal in a single way for all obese. It is now clear that individual differences in these functions are important and interact with other factors to determine whether obesity results for a given person.

Because excess fat must be stored, a key to understanding obesity may lie in understanding the development and function of *adipose* cells in which fat is stored. The prevailing view is that: (1) fat storage can be accomplished by increases in cell size, number, or both; (2) adult adipose cell number is not altered by dietary changes or weight loss; and, (3) decreases in cell size resulting from dieting are reversed when normal food intake resumes. This constancy in adipose cell function originates from early childhood experiences and is thought to constitute a lifelong propensity to manufacture fat.

Two studies have illustrated the importance of early childhood feeding experiences in determining adult adipose cell number and size. Knittle and Hirsch (1968) found that the number and size of fat cells in rats was related to food availability during a critical early development period; leaner rats had fewer and smaller cells. Once the cell number was established, further weight changes occurred only through changes in cell size, not number. This has implications for human obesity. Knittle (1975) found the critical period for human adipose tissue development occurred between birth and age 2. By that time obese children have more and larger fat cells than normals. Weight loss after age 2 did not alter the number of adipose cells among obese children. These continued to increase in number, a pattern not found in normal-weight children. Although these studies suggest that early eating experiences can permanently alter adipose tissue and predispose toward obesity, they do not clarify what causes the initial overeating that leads to adipose tissue changes.

Sjöström (1980) contends that this deterministic view of obesity is based on methodological artifact. He argues that fat cell number continues to increase past the supposed critical early development period, and that this "critical period" concept is limited. Sjöström cites data showing that for the first 12 months there was no increase in fat cell number. Only size increased, with cells reaching adult size during this time. The method used for measuring fat cell number in the Knittel and Hirsch studies may have falsely given the impression of rapid proliferation of fat cells during early development because only cells above a certain size were able to be counted. Sjöström and colleagues, on the other hand, have used biopsy specimens to microscopically count and measure fat cells. This method allows cells of all sizes to be included, and reveals the unsuspectedly high proportion of small fat cells during early development.

The finding that increases in fat cell number occur past the "critical period" suggests that weight gain at any age may irreversibly increase fat cell number, thereby predisposing toward future weight gain. This suggests that an important treatment focus for severe obesity may be to prevent future weight gain as a way to interrupt this weight escalation cycle, rather than to attempt the frustrating goal of weight reduction.

A Comprehensive Model

As noted earlier, extensive animal research has focused attention on the hypothalamus as the mechanism regulating both hunger and satiety. Whether hypothalamic dysfunction underlies human obesity has been the subject of some controversy, however.

Studies have found behaviors among obese humans that parallel those of the VMH-lesioned animal (cf. Rodin, 1977). But, as Rodin points out, these behaviors seem to exist apart from obesity. As hypothalamic dysfunction of the magnitude of the VMH animal is extremely rare in humans, it is unlikely to explain very much of human obesity. Friedman and Stricker (1976) believe that the focus on hypothalamic controls of hunger and satiety has been misplaced. They argue that hunger comes and goes according to normal fluctuations in metabolic fuel availability, with hunger stimuli arising in the liver as the organ most directly responsive to such fluctuations. Their focus, then, is on the biochemical and physiological energy metabolism processes associated with hunger and satiety rather than on central neurological control.

Stricker (1978) has synthesized findings from animal research into a model proposing two fundamentally different types of obesity, each with a distinct origin. Primary obesity is viewed as resulting from nutrients being rapidly removed from the bloodstream due to hyperlipogenesis, leading to chronic feelings of hunger (i.e., failure of satiety) and consequent overeating. In other words, metabolically induced fat accumulation actually causes the overeating. Primary hyperphagia, on the other hand, has no metabolic basis. Fat simply results from, rather than causes the overeating. Spontaneous hypophagia returns weight to normal if there is not some other stimulus keeping food intake elevated. Stricker notes that two forms of primary hyperphagia exist, each functioning to optimize general arousal level via food intake. In one, general arousal level is low and food is used as a stimulant. In the other, arousal is too high and food is used for its calming properties. These distinctions between types of obesity, derived from animal models, have important implications for behavioral treatment of human obesity, which is discussed later.

Psychological Factors

Perhaps the most visible proponent of the psychological etiology of obesity is Hilde Bruch (1973), who has proposed two types of psychogenic obesity, developmental and reactive. In her view, developmental obesity results from early learning problems in differentiating hunger from emotional tensions and nonfood discomforts and is characterized by personality disturbances. Reactive obesity, usually of adult onset, occurs in reaction to a stressful or traumatic event and serves to stabilize emotional functioning and decrease anxiety. More generally, psychological explanations for obesity focus on emotionality (both anxiety and depression), external cue responsiveness, and restraint theory.

Emotionality. The psychosomatic hypothesis that excessive eating represents a way to control emotionality has been examined experimentally. Results show that anxiety does not lead to overeating among the obese (Schachter, Goldman, & Gordon, 1968), except with very tasty food (McKenna, 1972), and that eating does not reduce anxiety (Herman & Polivy, 1975). Though overall support is not strong for the psychosomatic hypothesis, inconsistencies in results suggest that totally dismissing it would be imprudent without better experimental evidence (Leon & Roth, 1977; Rodin, 1977). In addition, there is concern regarding whether the hypothesis has been definitively tested in that: (1) anxiety manipulations may have been insufficiently threatening; and (2) taste ratings made in laboratory settings may not generalize to eating behavior in natural environments.

Epidemiological evidence also casts doubt on the psychogenic etiology of obesity (Hällström & Noppa, 1981). Obesity has been found to be associated with low, rather than high levels of both anxiety and depression among suburban and rural men and, to a lesser extent, among women (Crisp, Queenan, Sittampaln, & Harris, 1980). In the latter study, however, the few massively obese younger women were very anxious. This led the authors to suggest that these may overlap with the highly anxious and depressed obese, usually females, who seek help to reduce obesity. It may be these who account for the link between psychological disturbance and obesity in the clinical literature. On the other hand, in the first random-sample, prospective study of obesity reported, Noppa and Hällström

(1981) did find weight gain among females to be positively related to depth of depression but unrelated to most personality variables. They concluded that psychosocial variables, rather than personality, may be of causal importance in adult female weight gain.

Efforts to find an "obese personality type" have been mostly unproductive (Leon & Roth, 1977). Mendelson's (1966) classification of obesity along an emotional stability continuum illustrates the variety among the obese, from those who are emotionally stable but eat simply to reduce tension to those for whom eating is of pathologically central importance.

Given the long-standing assumption that depression leads to overeating, and thus obesity, it is surprising how seldom this proposition has been examined directly, particularly as clinical evidence suggests that depression causes decreases in eating as well. Baucom and Aiken (1981) clarified this differential response somewhat with their experimental induction of depression among both obese and nonobese subjects who were either dieting or not dieting at the time of the study. Results showed that for dieters, regardless of weight, depression led to increased eating, whereas for nondieters depression led to decreased eating. Baucom and Aiken suggest that the increased eating among dieters may be due either to a depression-induced loss of control of eating restraint, or to reinforcers for dieting losing their effectiveness during depression. As they indicate, further research is needed to determine which mechanism accounts for the results, and if the pattern holds true for more enduring and naturally occurring depression.

For the most part, studies supportive of the psychogenic origin of obesity are methodologically flawed. Psychological problems that cause obesity are not distinguished from those that result from being obese. This is particularly important for, even if psychological problems are not etiological, they may result from dieting per se or from the chronic pattern of alternating weight gain and loss. Further, samples of emotionally disturbed obese seeking help cannot be regarded as representative of the general population of overweight persons. Finally, as Rodin (1977) has noted, the failure of substitute psychological problems to emerge after sudden removal of overweight by surgery strongly challenges the assumptions underlying an exclusively psychogenic model of obesity.

External Cue Responsiveness.   According to this approach, in obese persons eating is not tied to internal states. It is influenced primarily by external environmental cues unrelated to physiological hunger or emotionality. Obesity results, then, from being overly susceptible to external cues such as time of day or availability of food. Early research suggested that the obese are not responsive to internal states such as stomach contractions (Stunkard & Koch, 1964) or actual food intake (Schachter et al., 1968). It is now clear, however, that normals do not show internal regulation either (Spiegel, 1973; Wooley, Wooley, & Dunham, 1972) and that some obese are as responsive as normals to internal caloric regulation (Wooley, 1971).

Externality among the obese has been posited as a more generalized sensitivity to external stimuli, not food specific. Rodin (1981), who earlier advocated this view, has concluded that the external – internal distinction is too simplistic an explanation for obese – normal differences. It is now apparent that neither are all overweight persons externally responsive nor all normals internally so. Further, both response modes exist at each weight level and neither is strongly related to degree of overweight. Nevertheless, externality does exist among the adult obese and seems to precede overeating and subsequent weight gain. For example, Rodin and Slochower (1976) found that girls who where hyperresponsive to external cues (measured at pretest) were the ones who gained the most weight in a summer camp abundant with easily obtainable food. The most striking aspect of the data is that the subjects were not overweight and had no history of weight problems. Further, this study suggests that external responsiveness may determine weight primarily in the short run, with long-term weight regulation influenced more by physiological (e.g., metabolic rate, adipose tissue characteristics) and phychological (e.g., body image) factors.

Because generalized, and not merely food-specific externality is suggested as a precursor of weight gain, it is important to determine when this begins. Does it exist in human infants, and if so, what relationship does it have to characteristics of parents and babies? Milstein (cited in Rodin, 1981) compared babies of overweight couples with babies of normal-weight couples, measuring visual responsiveness and sucking response to glucose versus plain water solutions as measures of external responsiveness. The predicted differences were found. Babies of overweight parents were significantly more responsive to differences in taste and visual stimuli. Heavier babies showed stronger preference for the glucose solution the sweeter it became.

Milstein's data suggest that: (1) general external responsiveness to environmental stimuli predisposes toward overeating in food abundant situations; and (2) this responsiveness appears early in development. Data from Costanzo and Woody (1979), however, challenge this assumption. Although children 7 to 12 did show evidence of external responsiveness to salient food cues, there was no evidence that this derived from a more general style of externality. They concluded that the: "causal priority of general externality in the overeating of the obese. . . does not bear up well developmentally (p. 2295)." They propose, instead, that the food-related externality stems from obesity and later generalizes to other stimuli, thereby giving rise to a more pervasive external responsiveness.

Rodin (1978, 1981) suggests that a more useful etiological framework would be to consider internal and external responsiveness not as a dichotomy, but as two variables that interact with and thus mutually influence one another. (Rodin also suggests methodological refinements to measure internal responsiveness and define external cues more accurately than was done in earlier studies.)

Such methodological and conceptual refinements may be insufficient to extend our understanding of obesity, however, in that social – psychological variables of causal import in eating behavior and obesity would still remain unaddressed. Krantz (1978) contends that strong social pressures (e.g., self-consciousness, concern for looking good to others, stigmas regarding obesity) influence experimental settings by eliciting situationally appropriate behavior that has been misinterpreted as external responsiveness. Krantz urges that these social context variables be taken seriously as determinants of behavior and be studied in their own right, along with variables from conceptual frameworks other than externality.

Restraint Theory. Restraint theory stems from Nisbett's view that there is a biologically determined "set point" for body weight that the extremely obese have reached. Less obese diet to remain below this point, leaving them chronically hungry and thus more sensitive to food cues (Nisbett, 1972). Extending this concept, Herman and Mack (1975) proposed that the restraint of eating (i.e., dieting), not degree of overweight, is the predictor of behaviors, including externality. They contend that overeating results when this self-control mechanism of restraint is disrupted by other events, such as emotional distress (Polivy & Herman, 1976a) or alcohol (Polivy & Herman, 1976b). The stress due to dieting, rather than hunger per se, is suggested as the mediator between dieting and behavior (Hibscher & Herman, 1977).

Recently, Ruderman and Wilson (1979) examined the restraint theory prediction that restraint disinhibition in the form of a food preload leads to increased eating, or counterregulation, and that this is characteristic of the obese. That is, they addressed the question of whether or not experimenter-induced violation of food intake restrictions would lead to subsequent abandonment of restraint. They also examined the assumed cognitive underpinnings of counterregulation, that believing one has already overindulged (via a food preload, for example) leads to temporary abandonment of restraint. From their own data and reanalyses of earlier data, Runderman and Wilson found that, although restraint is indeed a more powerful behavioral predictor than weight, this may be more true for normals than for the obese. Restraint predicted counterregulatory eating only for normals, not for obese. Among obese, restraint predicted the extent of regulation of food intake, with unrestrained obese better than the restrained at regulating intake. Restraint, then, appears to predict different kinds of eating behavior for normals and obese. Concerning cognitions, data supported the prediction that perceived overindulgence leads to further eating among the restrained, regardless of weight. Ruderman and Wilson concluded that, although restraint proved to be a strong predictor of eating, the failure to find counterregulation among the obese necessitates evaluation of the extent to which restraint predicts behaviors of the obese.

Treatment

It is obvious that, if diet is controlled so that fewer calories are taken in than are expended, weight loss should result. Yet dieting is singularly ineffective for long-term maintenance of weight loss, working primarily for only the moderately overweight. Eating more frequent but smaller meals has been thought to make weight loss and maintenance easier. Data cited by Leon (1976), however, suggest that when carefully investigated, such food intake patterns do not result in superior weight loss. Attention has been given to determining client characteristics predictive of outcome, but with little promise. A review by Stuart (1980) indicates that results are highly inconsistent, with even multivariate approaches yielding solutions that account for very small portions of the variance. An exception that merits further research is the Jeffery, Wing, and Stunkard (1978) report that weight loss early in treatment (first week) predicts weight loss later.

Exercise also merits particular attention, regarding potential both to prevent obesity among children (Nelson, 1978) and to facilitate long-term weight loss of fat rather than lean body mass (Brownell & Stunkard, 1980).

A neglected dimension in the treatment literature concerns food palatability, cited by Wooley, Wooley, and Dyrenforth (1979) as the only consistently emerging difference between obese and normals. Among obese, food intake is more dependent on palatability, becoming increasingly so after weight loss (Rodin, Slochower, & Fleming, 1977). Jeffery and Coates (1978) note the potential usefulness of training persons to regulate food intake in part on the basis of palatability as a way of increasing treatment efficacy. In the following sections, treatment approaches examined include organic, psychotherapeutic, and behavioral.

Surgery.   Jejunoileal bypass surgery creates a shunt to bypass a portion of the small intestine, producing a state of malabsorption that results in rapid weight loss. As a weight loss technique, it should be viewed as a last resort as it carries the risks of major surgery plus long-term negative side effects (e.g., diarrhea, electrolyte imbalance). Nonetheless, it provides the opportunity to study the psychological effects of sudden weight loss uncontaminated by the psychological effects of the weight loss procedure itself (e.g., dieting demands on self-control).

Surgically induced weight loss has been shown to be associated with improvements in mood, interpersonal and vocational effectiveness, self-esteem, and body image, and with decreases in depression; changes in the latter three were proportional to weight loss (Solow, Silberfarb, & Swift, 1974). Although accuracy of self-perception (as shown in self-sketches) adjusts to the drastically lowered weight during the first year after surgery, negative attitudes toward the body seem unaffected (Schiebel & Castelnuovo-Tedesco, 1978). These appear to be intractable and independent of perceptual accuracy. Another study suggests that bypass patients express increased satisfaction with their state of being, though symptoms of depression may remain (Kalucy & Crisp, 1974).

The effect of jejunoileal bypass on eating behavior is unclear, some studies showing that eating decreases, others that it remains the same (Leon, 1976). Taste responsiveness does appear to be altered by the surgery (Bray, Barry, Benfield, Castelnuovo-Tedesco, & Rodin, 1976), suggesting that intestinal tract changes affect perceived palatability. Specifically, responsiveness to sweet tastes changed to be like that of normal-weight persons for bypass patients but not for obese who merely lost weight (Rodin, Moskowitz, & Bray, 1976).

Fasting.   Although certainly resulting in weight loss, prolonged fasting incurs risk of serious physical complications such that it also should be used only as a last resort, and then under close medical supervision. A review of the literature (Leon, 1976) indicates that hunger sensations vanish after the first few days, unlike the chronic hunger produced on low-calorie diets. Psychological distress is varied, possibly as a function of: (1) overall adjustment prior to fasting; (2) the importance of food as a means of solving emotional problems; and (3) the length of the fast (longer duration associated with more distress). Weight loss maintenance results are equivocal.

Psychotherapeutic Approaches.   Individual psychotherapy for obesity focuses on the conflicts presumed to underlie the eating problem. Bruch's work (1973, 1977b) is typical of this approach, though her patients, who have sought psychotherapy, may not be representative of the "normal" obese. Further, evaluation of psychotherapy's effectiveness is difficult because much of the work is reported as case studies or as an adjunct to other techniques. Specific weight loss and follow-up data are not the norm. More recently, Stunkard (1980) suggests a "cautious optimism" for the efficacy of psychoanalysis, particularly with cases of body image disparagement or bulimia. It should be noted, however, that the primary presenting problem in the sample was not obesity, but rather anxiety or depression, again suggesting the unrepresentativeness of these subjects.

Leon's (1976) review of group approaches indicates that insight-oriented psychotherapy has produced negligible weight changes, whereas groups focusing on problems in diet adherence have resulted in weight loss for adult women, though not for adolescents. Even this weight loss is temporary, however, as weight progress tends to cease when the groups cease. As with individual approaches, evaluation is difficult due to the absence of specific weight loss and follow-up data.

Self-help groups, both lay and commercial, represent an increasingly frequent approach to weight loss (see Stuart & Mitchell, 1980). The general approach is to announce each member's weight status at each meeting to generate social pressure to lose weight. A study of TOPS (Take Off Pounds Sensibly) groups by Stunkard, Levine, and Fox (1970) demonstrated that this approach produces weight loss, though not as much as TOPS groups instructed in behavior modification techniques by a trained TOPS leader (Jordan & Levitz, 1973) or a behavior modification professional (Levitz & Stunkard, 1974).

Behavioral Approaches.   Since Stuart's (1967) demonstration of its effectiveness, behavioral treatment of obesity has mushroomed, until at present it is used by over 400,000 people weekly in lay group formats and is even viewed as a prototype for the development of behavioral medicine (Stunkard, 1979).

The first controlled outcome study (Harris, 1969) showed stunning promise, with behaviorally treated obese losing nearly three times as much as untreated controls gained. Subsequent research demonstrated behavioral treatment to be superior to either social pressure or psychotherapy (Wollersheim, 1970), even when professionals highly committed to psychotherapeutic approaches were utilized (Penick, Filion, Fox, & Stunkard, 1971). However, in the latter study the variability of weight loss was greater for behavioral treatment subjects, a finding since reported by others. Stunkard (1979) pointed out that behavioral treatment was not especially effective for as many as half his subjects. Perhaps a more flexible behavioral approach than is usually used would meet the individual weight loss needs of a larger proportion of patients. A 1 − year follow-up of the Penick et al. (1971) study shows that, in terms of weight-loss maintenance rather than initial loss, behavioral treatment subjects did not fare significantly better than others (Stunkard, 1977).

In other words, the early optimism regarding behavioral treatment for obesity has diminished as it has become apparent that initial weight loss is not predictive of maintenance, and that considerable variability exists regarding the efficacy of this approach for different individuals. Stunkard and Mahoney (1976) conclude that it is primarily for mild to moderate obesity that behavioral therapy is superior to other approaches.

1. Behavioral Techniques.   As outlined by Wooley et al. (1979), the assumption that faulty eating habits underlie excess food consumption and consequent overweight led to treatment strategies focusing on changing these learned habits. In general, these strategies include: (1) immediately reinforcing (via money, social approval, self-reward) appropriate or reduced eating; (2) reducing pleasurable reinforcements for eating (via aversive or covert conditioning); (3) increasing the salience during eating of long-term negative consequences of eating; (4) eliminating environmental food cues; and (5) restricting time and place of eating to reduce discriminative stimuli that elicit eating. In addition to these environmental controls of eating, nutritional planning and increased energy expenditure have been suggested as useful treatment strategies.

A summary of the effectiveness of specific techniques (Leon, 1976) suggests the following conclusions. Therapist-provided rewards and reinforcements appear to be effective, particularly in institutional settings. Results for contingency contracting (i.e., a reward—penalty system contingent on weight loss) are mixed, though positive if contracting occurs during the maintenance phase (Wing, Epstein, Marcus, & Shapira, 1981). The efficacy of self-reward and self-monitoring is unresolved, though self-reward for changing habits (rather than for weight loss) is associated with weight loss and maintenance; the amount of reduction is related to the degree of habit change. Classical conditioning procedures such as aversive training, covert sensitization (i.e., pairing of eating with noxious stimuli), and coverant control (i.e., systematically using thoughts and images to modify eating) all yield rather weak effects. Jeffrey (1976) noted that goal-setting techniques need research attention, particularly setting realistic goals on an intermediate, even weekly basis.

Additional variables have been suggested as determinants of success of behavioral treatments. These include booster sessions, therapist – client continuity, pace of treatment, cognitive factors, family support, and individualizing programs. For example, comparing individual and group behavior therapy, Kingsley and Wilson (1977) found that weight differences at 1 – year follow-up were due not to original treatment, but to participation in booster sessions. Therapist – client continuity has been shown as the variable most closely associated with weight loss (Stuart & Guire, 1978). Pace of treatment also appears to be important, with slower paced groups (i.e., meeting alternate weeks) producing a more consistent rate of weight loss than more frequent groups (Jeffery et al., 1978).

The importance of cognitive factors is illustrated by the association of weight loss maintenance with viewing self as normal weight (Fransella, 1970) or thin rather than formerly fat (Stuart & Guire, 1978). The latter study also suggested the importance of patients believing they have learned new self-management skills. Such data underscore the importance of including cognitive factors in both treatment and outcome evaluation far more extensively than is presently done.

Family support has been shown to be a critical variable in the etiology and treatment of obesity in both children and adults (cf. Stuart, 1978). For example, Matson (1977) found that positive social reinforcement by spouse was related to weight loss and maintenance. Brownell, Heckerman, Westlake, Hayes, and Monti (1978) found greater weight loss for women whose husbands were cooperative and trained with them than for women whose husbands were either cooperative but untrained or uncooperative. The magnitude of weight loss was considerably larger than usual, with nearly one-third occuring during the 6-month maintenance phase. This suggests that spouse training may facilitate both weight loss and long-term maintenance.

Regarding individualizing programs, Yates (1978) advocates having clients rate the difficulty and usefulness for them of various strategies prior to their use. Clients then can self-tailor programs to consist of strategies they perceive as beneficial and not so difficult as to discourage continued use. This would then facilitate both positive experiences and self-attributions of efficacy. The value of this is shown by the superiority of self-designed treatment over strategies to control either eating behavior or environmental food cues (Loro, Fisher, & Levenkron, 1979). Although all three approaches produced treatment weight losses, only for the individualized group did losses continue during follow-up. Treatment outcome also may be affected by individual differences on dimensions unrelated to weight, such as internal-external control, as shown by Chambliss and Murray (1979) and Kincey (1980).

Stuart (1980) suggests tailoring programs to focus on differences in the weight loss process, as a function of initial weight. Those who are relatively heavy initially have greater difficulty than less obese in maintaining weight loss, especially as it necessitates greater adjustment socially, psychologically, and physiologically. Elaborating on Stricker's (1978) view of two types of obesity that have fundamentally different origins, Wooley et al. (1979) propose a schema for tailoring treatment to type of obesity. The reader is referred to Wooley et al. for details of the schema. In general, it elaborates how responses to both dietary restriction and fasting vary as a function of type of obesity (primary obesity or primary hyperphagia) and arousal level (low or high). Discomfort from and ability to cope with treatment are predicted to differ substantially for each group.

2. Sources of Failure. It is now apparent that inducing, generalizing, and maintaining eating behavior changes are not necessarily influenced by the same variables (Kingsley & Wilson, 1977). For the most part, long-term evaluation of weight loss maintenance has been neglected in the treatment literature, leading Stunkard and Penick (1979) to target this as the next frontier in obesity treatment research. In their own 5-year follow-up, Stunkard and Penick found that, paradoxically, subjects who lost weight in treatment tended to gain during follow-up, whereas failures to lose in treatment tended to lose later. These data illustrate the importance of long-term evaluation as well as the value of reporting data on individual subjects rather than the more common reporting of group means only.

Similar results emerged in a study comparing the effectiveness of behavior therapy, pharmacotherapy (fenfluramine), and their combination (Stunkard, Craighead, & O'Brien, 1980). Although both pharmacotherapy and combined treatment produced greater weight loss during treatment than behavior therapy alone, this effect was reversed by the 1-year follow-up. By that time, behavior therapy patients regained significantly less weight than others. Despite its somewhat lower treatment weight loss, behavior therapy produced better maintenance of the loss that did occur, an effect that pharmacotherapy appeared to compromise.

Stuart (1980) sees the disappointing long-term efficacy of behavior therapy as due to six problems common in treatment programs. First, focus is often on negative change goals (e.g., suppressing problem eating, often through aversive procedures) rather than on developing constructive ways to attain pleasures in life. Second, there is incomplete planning regarding specifics of managing personal environments. Thus clients fail to learn healthful means of promoting weight loss. Instead, they are focused on the short-term goal of weight loss rather than on the long-term process of weight control. Third, interventions usually are direct (i.e., to control eating behavior) rather than indirect (i.e., to control the *urge* to eat). Consequently clients are not equipped to cope effectively with their eating urges before focusing on eating. Fourth, techniques of service delivery often overlook the distinct advantages that lay personnel and self-help groups can have over professionals (see Stuart, 1980, for details). Fifth, assessments generally are made at the end of treatment, rather than as an ongoing part of the treatment process. When the latter is done, ongoing programs can be modified to increase effectiveness for individual participants. Sixth, service delivery is incomplete in that it generally is short-lived and fails to offer services during the entire painstaking process of weight loss and adjustment. Stuart presents a convincing case that, when these six problems are remedied, behavior therapy can in fact result in long-term maintenance of weight loss.

Quite apart from weight loss maintenance, there is a growing concern that the magnitude of weight loss occurring during behavioral treatment is so modest as to be of minimal clinical significance. Wooley et al. (1979) examined the reasons for small weight losses to occur at a decelerating rate. They concluded that, rather than indicating poor treatment compliance, this reflects predictable compensatory metabolic changes that slow weight loss and promote regain. Treatment should be planned to counter these metabolic effects as much as possible (such as by increasing energy expenditure and alternating brief periods of dieting with returns to normal eating).

Two additional issues have hindered the refinement of behavioral treatments of obesity. One concerns the assumed "obese eating style" discussed earlier. This clearly is no longer a valid underpinning for behavioral treatment. The failure to find an association between changes in eating behavior and weight loss has been noted by various investigators (e.g., Brownell & Stunkard, 1978; Jeffery et al., 1978). The other issue concerns the assumption of externality among the obese, also discussed earlier. This should be abandoned as a basis for treatment presumed applicable to all obese persons (Rodin, 1981). Jeffery and Coates (1978) emphasize the need to explore other conceptual frameworks for treatment design, noting the possible importance of self-concept and body image, beliefs about ability to control eating habits, "obesogenic" life-styles and environments, and coping responses to stress.

Stunkard (1979), in reviewing the accomplishments of behavior therapy, concludes that perhaps we have reached the limits of the effectiveness of behavioral techniques alone and need to combine them with other technologies. He also suggests applying them to larger groups, focusing on life-style changes, and working through nonclinical avenues (e.g., the food industry, media, educational settings, work sites). In fact, Brownell, Stunkard, and Albaum (1980) demonstrated that a sign encouraging the use of stairs rather than escalators in a natural setting did result in significant modification of exercise patterns for both obese and nonobese. The investigators suggest that modifications of routine activities such as this may facilitate adherence to activity programs designed to promote weight loss.

Schachter (1981, 1982) contends that the relative ineffectiveness of weight treatment programs is due largely to their self-selected samples—only the most difficult cases seek help. His data show that in nontherapeutic populations people do lose weight and keep it off. Schachter concludes that the absence of such success in treatment research findings has led to an erroneous view of obesity as intractable.

3. Research Issues.   Mahoney (1976) lists common flaws in studies of the behavioral treatment of obesity: lack of no-treatment controls and attention – placebo controls; incompleteness in procedural descriptions and reporting of outcome data for all subjects; failure to explore other variables that may contribute to change; and absence of adequate follow-up. Stuart (1980) suggests that follow-up should be a minimum of 1 year, preferably 2 or 3, in order to assess the "yoyo" effect of repeated weight loss – weight gain cycles. Others (e.g., Wilson, 1978) disagree regarding the necessity of no-treatment controls. They argue that, inasmuch as data clearly show that untreated controls do not lose weight due to the mere passage of time, their use is unproductive.

Offering specific suggestions for methodological improvements, Wilson (1978) emphasizes the need to provide a more meaningful context in which to evaluate weight loss. He suggests using multiple outcome measures such as indices of social, physical, and psychological functioning, and direct measures of both cardiovascular health and eating in the natural environment. To standardize data, he suggests the following: (1) reporting individual as well as group data; (2) using two weight measures—absolute weight and a weight reduction quotient—in addition to skinfold measures; (3) completely describing clients and therapists; (4) reporting proportion of clients who improve plus attrition rates; and, (5) reporting the clinical significance of treatment effects, cost effectiveness, and emotional cost to clients. Further, Wilson notes the need to determine the effectiveness of component parts of treatment programs and to establish maintenance and follow-up as integral parts of both treatment and client expectations.

Even with standardization, however, weight loss may not be the most appropriate outcome criterion. Weight loss and behavior change fail to be correlated (Brownell & Stunkard, 1978). Wooley et al. (1979) suggest that it may be preferable to use food intake as the outcome criterion because weight loss may vary for reasons unrelated to eating. However, to accurately assess food intake, naturalistic observations must include measures of food left over as well as food chosen, as obese leave fewer leftovers than normals (Krasener, Brownell, & Stunkard, 1979). And, because amount left over varies with palatability (Ballard, Gipson, Gutenberg, & Ramsey, 1980), outcome measures should include assessments of palatability too.

ANOREXIA

Anorexia nervosa is a disorder in which the patient, usually female, relentlessly pursues thinness to the point of emaciation while simultaneously denying that she is too thin. Patients are resistant to attempts to help them and often require hospitalization and tube-feeding to prevent nutritional crisis or death. There are two syndromes of anorexia, one in which weight control is achieved by fasting or dieting, and bulimia, characterized by binge-eating with weight control by vomiting and purging. Some view anorexia as a distinct disorder (Russell, 1965), others as an extreme form of culturally encouraged dieting (Garner & Garfinkel, 1980).

Reported prevalence of anorexia is increasing, possibly due to more frequent recognition of mild forms (Crisp, Palmer, & Kalucy, 1976) and a heightened awareness of the disorder (Bemis, 1978). For females, prevalence estimates range from 1.6 per 100,000 population (Kendell, Hall, Hailey, & Babigian, 1973) to 1 of 250 high school age women (Crisp et al., 1976), with most cases occurring in the upper social classes (Garner, Garfinkel, Schwartz, & Thompson, 1980; Kalucy, Crisp, & Harding, 1977). Males account for 5 − 15% of cases (Bemis, 1978) with prognosis being poorer than for females.

Precipitating factors have been found in up to two-thirds of patients (Morgan & Russell, 1975), generally consisting of situations for which the person is unprepared (e.g., puberty, heterosexual experiences, marriage). Beumont, Abraham, and Simson (1981) report that a majority of their patients thought a "sexual challenge" had precipitated their illness. However, because psychosexual history was the focus of this study, one can question whether the result would obtain if a broader conceptual framework were utilized to study precipitating factors.

Although it is often reported that premorbid obesity leads to anorexia, Bemis (1978) notes that reviews of case reports fail to support this notion. Dieting also has been said to precede the onset of anorexia, yet its role as precipitator is unclear. The literature on precipitating factors provides little insight into the process that makes a person vulnerable to factors that might precipitate the onset of anorexia.

Characteristics

Excessive weight loss is described as the cardinal symptom of anorexia (Bemis, 1978; Feighner, Robins, Guze, Woodruff, Winokur, & Munoz, 1972). Amenorrhea and diminished sexual interest are often cited as characteristic of anorexia. This fails to be consistent with bulimia symptoms. Bulimics are more sexually active than dieters (Casper, Eckert, Halmi, Goldberg, & Davis, 1980; Garfinkel, Moldofsky, & Garner, 1980) and rarely show amenorrhea (Russell, 1979). Beumont et al. (1981) conclude that anorexia has a variable effect on heterosexual behavior, with some patients increasing, and others decreasing their sexual activity.

Hyperactivity (e.g., being perpetually active and denying fatigue) is a frequently cited symptom (Bruch, 1973; Thomä, 1977) and has been demonstrated by pedometric measurement (Stunkard, 1972). Halmi and colleagues found hyperactivity to be positively correlated with weight gain, leading them to suggest that perhaps the most active women represent a less seriously ill subgroup of anorexics (Halmi, Goldberg, Casper, Eckert, & Davis, 1979).

Though findings are not entirely consistent (cf. Casper, Halmi, Goldberg, Eckert, & Davis, 1979; Crisp & Kalucy, 1974), it appears that anorexics manifest a distorted body image and overestimate weight and size of certain body regions (cf.

Garfinkel, Moldofsky, Garner, Stancer, & Coscina, 1978). This perceptual disturbance is not general but is specific to horizontal body dimensions (Slade &
Russell, 1973a) and may be a function of low self-esteem (Wingate & Christie,
1978). Body size disturbance is relatively stable and is associated with failure to
develop satiety aversion to sucrose (Garfinkel et al., 1978), suggesting that
internal satiety cues may be altered in anorexia. The degree of overestimation is
associated with denial of illness, less weight gain, and generally poorer outcome
(Casper et al., 1979). The perceptual disturbance may underlie the self-perpetuat-
ing aspect of the disorder in that the thinner the anorexic becomes, the more she
overestimates her actual size and curtails her food intake to become slimmer.

The attitudes of anorexics toward weight differ from those of normal controls
(Fransella & Crisp, 1979) and predicted weight gain in a 5-week treatment program
(Goldberg, Halmi, Eckert, Casper, Davis, & Roper, 1980). The most extensively
validated instrument to assess anorexic attitudes is the Eating Attitudes Test (EAT;
Garner & Garfinkel, 1979), consisting of 40 items presented in a 6-point Likert
format. The EAT taps a broad range of behaviors and attitudes found frequently in
anorexic populations and has detected previously undiagnosed anorexics (Garner
& Garfinkel, 1980).

Criteria for diagnosing anorexia have been described by Feighner et al. (1972)
and include *age of onset* (between 10 and 30 years), *weight loss* (at least 25% of
premorbid weight and/or 15% below weight norms for age and height), *distorted
attitude/behavior toward food/weight, periods of overactivity, amenorrhea, no
medical illness, no major psychiatric disorder,* and at least *one* of the following—
bulimia, vomiting, hypothermia, bradycardia, or lanugo. Additionally, the *Diagnostic and Statistical Manual of Mental Disorders,* third edition (*DSM* III;
American Psychiatric Association, 1980), emphasizes the "intense fear of becoming obese" along with "refusal to maintain a minimal normal body weight."

Recently, numerous investigators have suggested that bulimia is a subgroup of
anorexia with differential etiology and symptomatology, implying both the need
for differential diagnosis and treatment, and less of a reliance on weight loss as a
primary diagnostic indicator. Beumont, George, and Smart (1976) distinguished
anorexics according to weight loss method, finding that dieters/fasters and vomi-
ters/purgers differed in terms of personality, premorbid weights, and course of
illness. Further study has shown that fasters are more introverted, deny hunger, and
evidence little psychic distress. Bulimics, however, are extroverted, admit to a
strong appetite, have more somatic complaints, are more sensitive interpersonally,
and evidence greater depression and anxiety (Casper et al., 1980). The *DSM* III
(1980) treats bulimia as totally distinct from anorexia.

Lack of self-control is viewed as the core problem of bulimia, implying: (1) that
a distinct group of women may be predisposed to have anorexia develop with
bulimia (Garfinkel et al., 1980); and (2) that vomiting and purging may be
adaptive responses to the lack of control over eating (Crisp. Hsu, & Harding,
1980). The elevated prevalence among bulimics of kleptomania (Casper et al.,

1980), hoarding of food (Crisp et al., 1980), and alcohol and street drug usage (Garfinkel et al., 1980) also are taken as evidence of impaired control.

Bulimia has been estimated to be nearly as frequent as the dieting – fasting syndrome and is characterized by older onset (Casper et al., 1980), poor prognosis in the form of greater metabolic devastation (Crisp et al., 1980), and longer duration of illness, repeated hospitalization, and poorer social adjustment (Garfinkel, Moldofsky, & Garner, 1977; Halmi, Brodland, & Loney, 1973). Russell (1979) emphasizes the habit-forming nature of the bingeing – purging pattern, which leads to serious physical complications including potassium loss, renal failure, epileptic seizures, permanent loss of bowel reactivity, and to the severe, frequently suicidal depression that makes bulimia so difficult to treat. Disagreement exists regarding whether premorbid obesity does (Beumont et al., 1976; Garfinkel et al., 1980) or does not (Casper et al., 1980) differentiate bulimia.

Etiology and Treatment

Unlike obesity, the notions of etiology and treatment are intertwined with anorexia and so will be discussed together.

Organic Approaches. The two primary organic explanations for anorexia focus on genetics and dysfunction of the hypothalmic – pituitary – gonadal axis. According to Ross (1977), evidence for genetic factors is inconclusive. He notes, for example, a study by Halmi and Brodland of monozygotic twins wherein one of each pair was anorexic, yielding a concordance rate of about 50% in the co-twin.

Concerning the hypothalamic – pituitary – gonadal axis, data are more complex. Some investigators conclude that the dysfunction is secondary to starvation (Vigersky & Loriaux, 1977; Wakeling, Souza, Gore, Sabur, Kingstone, & Boss, 1979). Gold and colleagues report that the dysfunction includes pathologic growth hormone responses to thyrotropin-releasing hormone in addition to previously known hormonal abnormalities (e.g., in luteinizing and follicle-stimulating hormone, and other growth hormone responses) (Gold, Pottash, Sweeney, Martin, & Davies, 1980). On the other hand, Walsh and associates believe the dysfunction to be out of proportion to emaciation, being due in part to psychological factors (Walsh, Katz, Levin, Kream, Fukishima, Hellman, Weiner, & Zumoff, 1978). They suggest that the independent hypothalamic disturbance proposed by Russell (1965) may cause anorexics to be less sensitive to negative feedback from plasma cortisol.

The greater than chance occurrence of anorexia in patients with gonadal dysgenesis (Turner syndrome) is another argument for a genetic basis for anorexia. According to this view, persons with abnormally low or high gonadatropin – estrogen levels may be at risk (Kron, Katz, Gorzynski, & Weiner, 1977). Contrasting views, however, hold that the occurrence of the two disorders is no greater than chance. Anorexia is proving to be more common than previously thought, and the anorexia body image disturbance suggests that psychological factors contribute to etiology (Darby, Garfinkel, Vale, Kirwan, & Brown, 1981).

At present, data do not permit definitive conclusions regarding the etiological role of hypothalamic dysfunction in anorexia. Bemis (1978) correctly concludes that etiology most likely involves an interaction of organic and psychological variables, rather than organic variables only, and that continued research on both is necessary.

Assessing the effectiveness of medical treatment alone is problematic. In one of the few controlled studies Goldberg and colleagues found cyproheptadine (a weight-inducing drug with more benign side effects than the often used chlorpromazine or amitriptyline) produced weight gain in a seriously ill subgroup of anorexics with a history of massive weight loss and previous outpatient treatment failures (Goldberg, Halmi, Eckert, Casper, & Davis, 1979). Casper et al. (1979) speculate that traditional appetite stimulants probably would not be useful because anorexics have appetites but deny feelings of hunger. If anorexia were merely starvation, tube-feeding should cure the disorder, but it does not.

Psychodynamic Approaches.   The traditional psychodynamic view is that psychosexual difficulties underlie anorexia. Factors such as fantasies of oral impregnation, sexual immaturity, rejection of femininity, fear of pregnancy have been offered as contributing to etiology. Rampling (1978) succinctly typified this approach when he wrote that anorexia represents a regression in psychosexual development as a maladaptive solution to the maturational demands of adolescence.

In one of the few systematic investigations of the psychosexual history of anorexics, Beumont et al. (1981) found there to be no common pattern in behavior, attitudes, or knowledge. They concluded that sexual factors are not etiological in anorexia, a conclusion also reached by Dally, Gomez, and Isaacs (1979). The fact that anorexia develops in persons who do not develop secondary sex characteristics, due to having gonadal dysgenesis (Turner syndrome), makes it unlikely that anorexia arises as a defense against either the heterosexual implications of puberty or fantasies of oral impregnation (Kron et al., 1977).

Finding the psychosexual approach inadequate, others (e.g., Bruch, 1973, 1977a; Sours, 1974) have turned toward disturbances in the mother – child relationship as etiological. Bruch (1973) sees the childhood pattern resulting in a severe deficiency of autonomy and effectiveness in the child, leading to herculean efforts at control in various life domains. This drive for achievement precedes the syndrome that manifests itself in maladaptive control over eating behavior.

In treatment, Thomä (1977) has argued that insight into psychodynamic processes is essential. Bruch (1973) focuses instead on perceptual body image defects and the sense of incompetence, aiming to help the patient feel responsible for therapeutic accomplishments. Effectiveness of either approach is questionable. Traditional psychoanalysis has not proven to be impressively successful, and the value of Bruch's approach is difficult to assess (Bemis, 1978).

Behavioral Approaches. Due to the emphasis on overt behavior, etiology is viewed in terms of impaired food intake as a learned behavior maintained by environmental reinforcement (Blinder, Freeman, & Stunkard, 1970). Behavioral treatment is based on social learning theory and consists of reinforcement for weight gain or constructive changes in eating behavior, with focus on specific behaviors such as number of mouthfuls, caloric intake, and time spent eating.

Inherent in many behavioral programs is an emphasis on rapid weight gain, one-half pound per day in some, which necessitates an enormous food intake. This has been criticized as inappropriate and akin to sanctioning bulimia (Bemis, 1978), possibly leading to compulsive eating and consequent obesity (Halmi et al., 1973), and producing medical complications including acute gastric dilatation (Jennings & Klidjian, 1974). Weight regulation, not gain, is suggested as the more appropriate focus. As in obesity, successful long-term treatment of anorexia hinges on establishing normal eating patterns rather than achieving immediate short-term weight changes.

Although behavioral treatments do effectively restore weight, the early optimism regarding their long-term efficacy in treating anorexia seems unjustified. In a limited follow-up study, Bhanji and Thompson (1974) concluded that behavioral treatment was inadequate for long-term maintenance of normal eating habits and weight and was best used for rapid weight gain during nutritional crises. Agras and associates found that positive reinforcement was relatively ineffective unless accompanied by informational feedback regarding weight and caloric intake and concluded that feedback may be the most important variable (Agras, Barlow, Chapin, Abel, & Leitenberg, 1974).

The contention that behavioral programs are effective in accomplishing short-term weight gain needs reevaluation. In a controlled randomized treatment study, Eckert and colleagues found the greater weight gain of behavior therapy patients not to be significantly different from that of controls (Eckert, Goldberg, Halmi, Casper, & Davis, 1979). They suggest that the behavioral program might have been more efficacious if individualized reinforcers had been utilized, and if reinforcement were immediate and daily rather than delayed.

Methodological problems plague research on the behavioral approach. Sample sizes are small, often reports of single case experiments. Failure to separately evaluate behavior therapy components and distinguish them from other concurrent treatment modalities make precise conclusions regarding efficacy impossible. Further, the general absence of follow-up data and the narrow focus on weight have hindered the application of behavior therapy to non-eating problems that either cause, maintain, or result from the disorder. Clearly, a broader conceptual framework is necessary to utilize behavioral techniques in a wider array of situations relevant to anorexia.

Familial Approaches. Despite long-standing interest in the topic, causal questions regarding the family's etiological role in anorexia remain virtually untouched. Even the best of studies are retrospective and speculative.

A recurring finding is that anorexic-like behaviors (Crisp, Hsu, Harding, & Hartshorn, 1980) and obesity (Garfinkel et al., 1980) are overrepresented in the families of anorexics. Enmeshed or overinvolved family relationships, poor parental relationships, and an emphasis on physical fitness also are typical (Crisp et al., 1980). Kalucy et al. (1977) described a "weight pathology" wherein family members viewed self and others in terms of size, weight, eating habits, and weight control, with these factors being equated with well-being and self-control. They view this weight pathology as a critical aspect of the disorder in that eating, shape, and weight become the vehicles of interaction and communication, thus forming the basis for the development of anorexia.

In contrast to the psychodynamic literature, Crisp et al. (1980) conclude that: (1) there is a wide variety of family relationships, not a specific anorexia type of family pathology; (2) disturbances involve the entire family, thus rendering inadequate those approaches that focus on the dyadic relationship between the patient and one parent or on issues of dominance/submissiveness or over/underprotectiveness; and (3) the familial incidence of anorexia is striking, even without appropriate control data.

Retrospective descriptions of anorexics as children are varied, ranging from asymptomatic (Kalucy et al., 1977) to shy, timid, well-behaved, competitive, and perfectionistic (Casper et al., 1980), with bulimics being more outgoing than others. Academic achievement (Morgan & Russell, 1975), even overachievement (Bruch, 1973), is frequently cited. Although infant or early childhood feeding difficulties are often mentioned, Bemis (1978) questions the significance of such recollections since feeding disturbances characterize normal children as well.

It has been suggested that if the problem resides in the style of family interaction (Rosman, Minuchin, Baker, & Liebman, 1977) with anorexia serving to meet pathological needs of the family (Crisp, Harding, & McGuinness, 1974), treatment must restructure family relationships. Rosman, Minuchin, & Liebman (1975) utilize a "family therapy lunch session" for both diagnosis and treatment in the highly charged mealtime environment. Their treatment program includes weight gain by hospital behavioral management or outpatient contingency contracting and individual counseling as needed, in addition to the family focus. Though the newness of the procedure precludes definitive evaluation of its effectiveness, incorporation of the family with treatment is promising and long overdue. Long-term follow-up ranging from 3 months to 4 years indicates at least an 86% success rate (Rosman et al., 1977).

Sociocultural Approaches. The cultural preoccupation with female slimness may be an important etiological factor in anorexia. During the last 10 years, the feminine ideal has shifted to a thinner size while improved nutrition has caused the average female under 30 to become heavier (Garner et al., 1980). Garner and Garfinkel (1980) suggest that anorexia may simply be an extreme form of relatively common dieting disorder and point out that, if so, this has important implications for views of etiology, diagnosis, and treatment.

Hypothesizing that subcultures emphasizing thinness would foster anorexia, Garner and Garfinkel (1980) found this to be true among dance and modeling groups. Further, this was not simply a function of competitiveness (e.g., music students in competitive environments failed to show the same high rate of anorexia). Within the subcultures emphasizing thinness, greater competitiveness was associated with higher scores on an anorexia attitudes questionnaire and with the number of anorexia cases.

Outcome

Definitive statements about the natural course of the disease and the long-term efficacy of treatment are virtually impossible to make due to the dearth of longitudinal studies of etiology or treatment effects. Spontaneous recovery may occur in as many as 40% of anorexics after 4 years or longer (Morgan & Russell, 1975). Serious relapses also can occur even after long periods of recovery (Crisp et al., 1980). Uncertainty also exists regarding the death rate, cited as below 5% in many studies (Hsu, 1980) but as high as 21% in longer follow-up studies (Halmi, Brodland, & Rigas, 1975).

Although initial response to treatment generally is encouraging, data cited by Bemis (1978) underscore the chronicity of the disorder, with fewer than half of anorexics satisfactorily recovering and up to 50% experiencing symptom recurrence. Long-term follow-up studies (from 4 to 8 years) show that, despite weight gain and return of menses, a large proportion of patients continue to experience weight phobia (Crisp et al., 1980; Morgan & Russell, 1975). Crisp et al. found that, although 80% showed weight at or near normal and 70% were menstruating, over 40% were intensely worried about weight and shape and two-thirds had highly variable dietary patterns.

Various attempts have been made to isolate factors predictive of good or poor outcome. For example, good prognosis recently has been found to be associated with no previous hospitalizations, hyperactivity prior to treatment, less denial and psychosexual immaturity, and admitting to having an appetite (Halmi et al., 1979). Poor prognosis has been associated with long duration of illness, older age at onset, severity of weight loss, and bulimia and vomiting (Hsu, 1980). The validity of such outcome predictors has yet to be substantiated, as the methodological criticisms of Hsu (1980) illustrate. Criteria for diagnosing anorexia have not been consistent, follow-up methods (e.g., questionnaires, phone calls) are subject to bias by anorexics' denial of illness, patients are not traced, follow-up durations are short, and outcome criteria and information are often incomplete at follow-up. Hsu further notes that none of the 16 follow-up studies he reviewed was properly designed to assess the effects of treatment.

Obviously, recovery from anorexia encompasses far more than weight gain and return of menses. Simply returning to normal weight can present distressing psychological problems to anorexics, and successfully adapting emotionally and perceptually to body changes can be a critical step in the recovery process. Pillay and Crisp (1977) found that anorexics with newly restored weight had very low self-esteem, were highly sensitive to social interactions, and were perfectionistic with a high need for order. They emphasized the potential value of directly treating these problems with combined behavioral – psychotherapeutic treatment to diminish the psychosocial maladjustment that typically characterizes "recovered" anorexics.

Conclusion

It is apparent that, for both anorexia and obesity, far too little is known about controlling the conditions and restoring normal functioning. Behavioral treatments have proven too simplistic and narrow to successfully accomplish long-range weight regulation. Indeed, it is now clear that this must be regarded as a process with biochemical, physiological, psychological, and social components, rather than as a one-time behavior change.

Several topics have potential for aiding understanding of this process and thus warrant further research. Techniques (e.g., exercise and meditation) that reduce the cognitive and emotional distress of weight regulation appear particularly promising (Foreyt, Goodrick, & Gotto, 1981). For obesity, recent research has suggested the utility of focusing on the "urge to eat" as the target of change (Youdin & Hemmes, 1978). Treatment of anorexia would particularly benefit from well-controlled prospective studies of high risk individuals. For both anorexia and obesity, longer follow-up studies are needed of treatment effects and the maintenance/recovery process. Factors that facilitate or hinder relapse need identification and careful study.

Overall, broader conceptual frameworks are needed that transcend traditional paradigm boundaries. Only then will we progress further in understanding the complexities of anorexia and obesity, and how relevant factors may have differing roles in etiology, maintenance, and change, and vary from individual to individual.

REFERENCES

Agras, W. S., Barlow, D. H., Chapin, H. N., Abel, G. G., & Leitenberg, H. Behavior modification of anorexia nervosa. *Archives of General Psychiatry*, 1974, *30*, 279 – 286.

American Psychiatric Association. *Diagnostic and statistical manual of mental disorders*, (3rd ed.) Washington, D.C.: APA, 1980.

Ballard, B. D., Gipson, M. T., Gutenberg, W., & Ramsey, K. Palatability of food as a factor influencing obese and normal-weight children's eating habits. *Behaviour Research and Therapy*, 1980, *18*, 598 – 600.

Baucom, D. H., & Aiken, P. A. Effect of depressed mood on eating among obese and nonobese dieting and nondieting persons. *Journal of Personality and Social Psychology*, 1981, *41*, 577–585.

Bemis, K. M. Current approaches to the etiology and treatment of anorexia nervosa. *Psychological Bulletin*, 1978, *65*, 593–617.

Beumont, P. J. V., Abraham, S. F., & Simson, K. G. The psychosexual histories of adolescent girls and young women with anorexia nervosa. *Psychological Medicine*, 1981, *11*, 131–140.

Beumont, P. J., George, G. C. & Smart, D. E. "Dieters" and "vomiters and purgers" in anorexia nervosa. *Psychological Medicine*, 1976, *6*, 617–622.

Bhanji, S., & Thompson, J. Operant conditioning in the treatment of anorexia nervosa: A review and retrospective study of 11 cases. *British Journal of Psychiatry*, 1974, *124*, 166–172.

Blinder, B. J., Freeman, D. M. A., & Stunkard, A. J. Behavior therapy of anorexia nervosa: Effectiveness of activity as a reinforcer of weight gain. *American Journal of Psychiatry*, 1970, *126*, 1093–1098.

Bray, G. A. *The obese patient*. Philadelphia: W. B. Saunders Co., 1976.

Bray, G. A. To treat or not to treat—that is the question? In G. A. Bray (Ed.), *Recent advances in obesity research: II*. London: Newman Publishing, 1978.

Bray, G. A., Barry, R. E., Benfield, J. R. Castelnuovo-Tedesco, P., & Rodin, J. Intestinal bypass surgery for obesity decreases food intake and taste preferences. *American Journal of Clinical Nutrition*, 1976, *29*, 779–783.

Brownell, K. D., Heckerman, C. L., Westlake, R. J., Hayes, S. C., & Monti, P. M. The effect of couples training and partner cooperativeness in the behavioral treatment of obesity. *Behaviour Research and Therapy*, 1978, *16*, 323–333.

Brownell, K. D., & Stunkard, A. J. Behavior therapy and weight change: Uncertainties in programs for weight control. *Behaviour Research and Therapy*, 1978, *16*, 301.

Brownell, K. D., & Stunkard, A. J. Physical activity in the development and control of obesity. In A. J. Stunkard (Ed.), *Obesity*. Philadelphia: W. B. Saunders Co., 1980.

Brownell, K. D., & Stunkard, A. J., & Albaum, J. M. Evaluation and modification of exercise patterns in the natural environment. *American Journal of Psychiatry*, 1980, *137*, 1540–1545.

Bruch, H. *Eating disorders. Obesity, anorexia nervosa, and the person within*. New York: Basic Books, 1973.

Bruch, H. Psychological antecedents of anorexia nervosa. In R. A. Vigersky (Ed.), *Anorexia nervosa*. New York: Raven press, 1977. (a)

Bruch. H. Psychotherapy in eating disorders. *Canadian Psychiatric Association Journal*, 1977, *22*, 102–108. (b)

Casper, R. C. Eckert, E. D., Halmi, K. A., Goldberg, S. C., & Davis, J. M. Bulimia. Its incidence and clinical importance in patients with anorexia nervosa. *Archives of General Psychiatry*, 1980, *37*, 1030–1035.

Casper, R. C., Halmi, K. A., Goldberg, S. C., Eckert, E. D., & Davis, J. M. Disturbances in body image estimation as related to other characteristics and outcome in anorexia nervosa. *British Journal of Psychiatry*, 1979, *134*, 60–66.

Chambliss, C. A., & Murray, E. J. Efficacy attribution, locus of control, and weight loss. *Cognitive Therapy and Research*, 1979, *3*, 349–353.

Chediak, C. The so-called anorexia nervosa. Diagnostic and treatment considerations. *Bulletin of the Menninger Clinic*, 1977, *41*, 453–474.

Costanzo, P. R., & Woody, E. Z. Externality as a function of obesity in children: Pervasive style or eating specific attribute? *Journal of Personality and Social Psychology*, 1979, *37*, 2286–2296.

Crisp, A. H., Harding, B., McGuinness, B. Anorexia nervosa. Psychoneurotic characteristics of parents: Relationship to prognosis. *Journal of Psychosomatic Research*, 1974, *18*, 167–173.

Crisp, A. H., Hsu, L. K. G., & Harding, B. The starving hoarder and voracious spender: Stealing in anorexia nervosa. *Journal of Psychosomatic Research*, 1980, *24*, 225–231.

Crisp. A. H., Hsu, L. K. G., Harding, B., & Hartshorn, J. Clinical features of anorexia nervosa. A study of a consecutive series of 102 female patients. *Journal of Psychosomatic Research*, 1980, *24*, 179–191.

Crisp, A. H., & Kalucy, R. S. Aspects of the perceptual disorder in anorexia nervosa. *British Journal of Medical Psychology,* 1974, *47,* 349 – 361.

Crisp, A. H., Palmer, R. L., & Kalucy, R. S. How common is anorexia nervosa? A prevalence study. *British Journal of Psychiatry,* 1976, *128,* 549 – 554.

Crisp, A. H., Queenan, M., Sittampaln, Y., & Harris, G. "Jolly fat" revisited. *Journal of Psychosomatic Research,* 1980, *24,* 233 – 241.

Dally, P., Gomez, J., & Isaacs, A. J., *Anorexia nervosa.* London: William Heinemann Medical Books Ltd., 1979.

Darby, P. L., Garfinkel, P. E., Vale, J. M., Kirwan, P. J., & Brown, G. M. Anorexia nervosa and "Turner Syndrome": Cause or coincidence? *Psychological Medicine,* 1981, *11,* 141 – 145.

Donegan, W., Harts, A., & Rimm, A. The association of body weight with recurrent cancer of the breast. *Cancer,* 1978, *41,* 1590 – 1594.

Drabman, R. S., Hammer, D., & Jarvie, G. J. Eating styles of obese and nonobese black and white children in a naturalistic setting. *Addictive Behaviors,* 1977, *2,* 83 – 86.

Eckert, E. D., Goldberg, S. C., Halmi, K. A., Casper, R. C., & Davis, J. M. Behavior therapy in anorexia nervosa. *British Journal of Psychiatry,* 1979, *134,* 55 – 59.

Feighner, J. P., Robins, E., Guze, S. B., Woodruff, R. A., Winokur, G., & Munoz, R. Diagnostic criteria for use in psychiatric research. *Archives of General Psychiatry,* 1972, *26,* 57 – 63.

Foch, T. T., & McClearn, G. E. Genetics, body weight, and obesity. In A. J. Stunkard (Ed.), *Obesity.* Philadelphia: W. B. Saunders Co., 1980.

Foreyt, J. P., Goodrick, G. K., & Gotto, A. M. Limitations of behavioral treatment of obesity: Review and analysis. *Journal of Behavioral Medicine,* 1981, *4,* 159 – 174.

Fransella, F. Measurement of conceptual change accompanying weight loss. *Journal of Psychosomatic Research,* 1970, *14,* 347 – 351.

Fransella, F., & Crisp, A. H. Comparisons of weight concepts in groups of neurotic, normal, and anorexic females. *British Journal of Psychiatry,* 1979, *34,* 79 – 86.

Friedman, M. I., & Stricker, E. M. The physiological psychology of hunger : A physiological perspective. *Psychological Review,* 1976, *83,* 409 – 431.

Garfinkel, P. E., & Coscina, D. V. The physiology and psychology of hunger and satiety. In M. R. Zales (Ed.), *Eating, sleeping, and sexuality.* New York: Bruner/Mazel, 1982.

Garfinkel, P. E., Moldofsky, H., Garner, D. M. Prognosis in anorexia nervosa as influenced by clinical features, treatment, and self-perception. *Canadian Medical Association Journal,* 1977, *117,* 1041 – 1045.

Garfinkel, P. E., Moldofsky, H., & Garner, D. M. The heterogeneity of anorexia nervosa. *Archives of General Psychiatry,* 1980, *37,* 1036 – 1040.

Garfinkel, P. E., Moldofsky, H., Garner, D. M., Stancer, H. C., & Coscina, D. V. Body awareness in anorexia nervosa: Disturbances in "body image" and "satiety." *Psychosomatic Medicine,* 1978, *40,* 487 – 498.

Garner, D. M., & Garfinkel, P. E. The Eating Attitudes Test: An index of the symptoms of anorexia nervosa. *Psychological Medicine,* 1979, *9,* 273 – 279.

Garner, D. M., & Garfinkel, P. E. Socio-cultural factors in the development of anorexia nervosa. *Psychological Medicine,* 1980, *10,* 647 – 656.

Garner, D. M., Garfinkel, P. E., Schwartz, D., & Thompson, M. Cultural expectations of thinness in women. *Psychological Reports,* 1980, *47,* 483 – 491.

Garner, D. M., Garfinkel, P. E., Stancer, H. C., & Moldofsky, H. Body image disturbances in anorexia nervosa and obesity. *Psychosomatic Medicine,* 1976, *38,* 327 – 336.

Gold, M. S., Pottash, A. L. C., Sweeney, D. R., Martin, D. M., & Davies, R. K. Further evidence of hypothalamic – pituitary dysfunction in anorexia nervosa. *American Journal of Psychiatry,* 1980, *137,* 101 – 102.

Goldberg, S. C., Halmi, K. A., Eckert, E. D., Casper, R. C., & Davis, J. M. Cyproheptadine in anorexia nervosa. *British Journal of Psychiatry,* 1979, *134,* 67 – 70.

Goldberg, S. C., Halmi, K. A., Eckert, E. D., Casper, R. C., Davis, J. M., & Roper, M. Attitudinal dimensions in anorexia nervosa. *Journal of Psychiatric Research*, 1980, *15*, 239 – 251.

Hällström, T., & Noppa, H. Obesity in women in relation to mental illness, social factors, and personality traits. *Journal of Psychosomatic Research*, 1981, *25*, 75 – 82.

Halmi, K., Brodland, G., & Loney, J. Prognosis in anorexia nervosa. *Annals of Internal Medicine*, 1973, *78*, 907 – 909.

Halmi, K., Brodland, G., & Rigas, C. A follow-up study of 79 patients with anorexia nervosa: An evaluation of prognostic factors and diagnostic criteria. In R. D. Wirt, G. Winokur, & M. Roff (Eds.), *Life history research in psychopathology* (Vol. 4). Minneapolis: University of Minnesota Press, 1975.

Halmi, K. A., Goldberg, S. C., Casper, R. C., Eckert, E. D., & Davis, J. M. Pretreatment predictors of outcome in anorexia nervosa. *British Journal of Psychiatry*, 1979, *134*, 71 – 78.

Harris, M. B. Self-directed program for weight control: A pilot study. *Journal of Abnormal Psychology*, 1969, *74*, 263 – 270.

Herman, C. P. & Mack, D. Restrained and unrestrained eating. *Journal of Personality*, 1975, *43*, 647 – 660.

Herman, C. P., & Polivy, J. Anxiety, restraint, and eating behavior. *Journal of Abnormal Psychology*, 1975, *84*, 666 – 672.

Hibscher, J. A., & Herman, C. P. Obesity, dieting, and the expression of "obese" characteristics. *Journal of Comparative and Physiological Psychology*, 1977, *91*, 374 – 380.

Hsu, L. K. G. Outcome of anorexia nervosa. A review of the literature (1954 to 1978). *Archives of General Psychiatry*, 1980, *37*, 1041 – 1046.

Jeffery, R. W., Wing, R. R., & Stunkard, A. J. Behavioral treatment of obesity: The state of the art 1976. *Behavior Therapy*, 1978, *9*, 189 – 199.

Jeffery, R. W., & Coates, T. J. Why aren't they losing weight? *Behavior Therapy*, 1978, *9*, 856 – 860.

Jeffrey, D. B. Behavioral management of obesity. In W. E. Craighead, A. E. Kazdin, & M. J. Mahoney (Eds.), *Behavior modification: Principles, issues, and applications*. Boston: Houghton Mifflin Co., 1976.

Jennings, K. P., & Klidjian, A. M. Acute gastric dilatation in anorexia nervosa. *British Medical Journal*, 1974, *2*, 477 – 478.

Jordan, H. A., & Levitz, L. S. Behavior modification in a self-help group. *Journal of the American Dietetic Association*, 1973, *62*, 27 – 29.

Kalucy, R. S., & Crisp, A. H. Some psychological and social implications of massive obestiy. *Journal of Psychosomatic Research*, 1974, *18*, 465 – 473.

Kalucy, R. S., Crisp, A. H., & Harding, B. A study of 56 families with anorexia nervosa. *British Journal of Medical Psychology*, 1977, *50*, 381 – 395.

Kendell, R. E., Hall, D. J., Hailey, A., & Babigian, H. M. The epidemiology of anorexia nervosa. *Psychological Medicine*, 1973, *3*, 200 – 203.

Kincey, J. Target setting, self-reinforcement pattern, and locus of control orientation as predictors of outcome in a behavioral weight-loss programme. *Behaviour Research and Therapy*, 1980, *18*, 139 – 145.

Kingsley, R. G., & Wilson, G. T. Behavior therapy for obesity: A comparative investigation of long-term efficacy. *Journal of Consulting & Clinical Psychology*, 1977, *45*, 288 – 298.

Knittle, J. Early influences on development of adipose tissue. In G. A. Bray (Ed.), *Obesity in perspective*. Washington, D.C.: US Government Printing Office, 1975.

Knittle, J. L., & Hirsch, J. Effect of early nutrition on the development of rat epididymal fat pads: Cellularity and metabolism. *Journal of Clinical Investigation*, 1968, *47*, 2091 – 2098.

Koopmans, H. S. The intestinal control of food intake. In G. A. Bray (Ed.), *Recent advances in obesity research: II*. Westport, Conn.: Technomic Publishing Co., 1978.

Krantz, D. S. The social context of obesity research: Another perspective on its place in the field of social psychology. *Personality and Social Psychology Bulletin*, 1978, *4*, 177 – 183.

Krasener, H. A., Brownell, K. D., & Stunkard, A. J. Cleaning the plate: Food left over by overweight and normal weight persons. *Behaviour Research and Therapy*, 1979, *17*, 155 – 156.

Kron, L., Katz, J. L., Gorzynski, G., & Weiner, H. Anorexia nervosa and gonadal dysgenesis. *Archives of General Psychiatry*, 1977, *34*, 332 – 335.

Leibowitz, S. F. Brain catecholaminergic mechanisms for control of hunger. In D. Novin, W. Wyrwicka, & G. A. Bray (Eds.), *Hunger: Basic mechanisms and clinical implications*. New York: Raven Press, 1976.

Leon, G. R. Curent directions in the treatment of obesity. *Psychological Bulletin*, 1976, *83*, 557 – 578.

Leon, G. R., & Roth, L. Obesity: Psychological causes, correlations, and speculations. *Psychological Bulletin*, 1977, *84*, 117 – 141.

Levitz, L. S., & Stunkard, A. J. A therapeutic coalition for obesity: Behavior modification and patient self-help. *American Journal of Psychiatry*, 1974, *131*, 423 – 427.

Loro, A. D., Fisher, E. B., & Levenkron, J. C. Comparison of established and innovative weight-reduction treatment procedures. *Journal of Applied Behavior Analysis*, 1979, *12*, 141 – 155.

Mahoney, M. J. The obese eating style: Bites, beliefs, and behavior modification. *Addictive Behaviors*, 1975, *1*, 47 – 53.

Mahoney, M. J. The behavioral treatment of obesity: A reconnaissance. *Biofeedback and Self-Regulation*, 1976, *1*, 127 – 133.

Matson, J. L. Social reinforcement by the spouse in weight control: A case study. *Journal of Behavior Therapy and Experimental Psychiatry*, 1977, *8*, 327 – 328.

McKenna, R. J. Some effects of anxiety level and food cues on the eating behavior of obese and normal subjects: A comparison of the Schachterian and psychosomatic conceptions. *Journal of Personality and Social Psychology*, 1972, *22*, 311 – 319.

Mendelson, M. Psychological aspects of obesity. *International Journal of Psychiatry*, 1966, *2*, 599 – 612.

Morgan, H. G., & Russell, G. F. M. Value of family background and clinical features as predictors of long-term outcome in anorexia nervosa: Four year follow-up study of 41 patients. *Psychological Medicine*, 1975, *5*, 355 – 371.

Nelson, R. A. Exercise in the treatment of obesity. In G. A. Bray (Ed.), *Recent advances in obesity research: II*. London: Newman Publishing, 1978.

Nisbett, R. E. Hunger, obesity, and the ventromedial hypothalamus. *Psychological Review*, 1972, *79*, 433 – 453.

Noppa, H., & Hällström, T. Weight gain in adulthood in relation to socioeconomic factors, mental illness, and personality traits: A prospective study of middle-aged women. *Journal of Psychosomatic Research*, 1981, *25*, 83 – 89.

Pearlson, G. D., Flournoy, L. H., Simonson, M., & Slavney, P. R. Body image in obese adults. *Psychological Medicine*, 1981, *11*, 147 – 154.

Penick, S. B., Filion, R., Fox, S., & Stunkard, A. J. Behavior modification in the treatment of obesity. *Psychosomatic Medicine*, 1971, *33*, 49 – 55.

Pillay, M., & Crisp. A. H. Some psychological characteristics of patients with anorexia nervosa whose weight has been newly restored. *British Journal of Medical Psychology*, 1977, *50*, 375 – 380.

Polivy, J., & Herman, C. P. Clinical depression and weight change: A complex relation. *Journal of Abnormal Psychology*, 1976, *85*, 338 – 340. (a)

Polivy, J., & Herman, C. P. Effects of alcohol on eating behavior: Influence of mood and perceived intoxication. *Journal of Abnormal Psychology*, 1976, *85*, 601 – 606. (b)

Rampling, D. Anorexia nervosa: Reflections on theory and practice. *Psychiatry*, 1978, *41*, 296 – 301.

Rodin, J. Bidirectional influences of emotionality, stimulus responsivity, and metabolic events in obesity. In J. D. Maser & M. E. P. Seligman (Eds.), *Psychopathology: Experimental models*. San Francisco: W. H. Freeman and Co., 1977.

Rodin, J. Has the distinction between internal versus external control of feeding outlived its usefulness? In G. A. Bray (Ed.), *Recent advances in obesity research: II*. London: Newman Publishing Ltd., 1978.

Rodin, J. Current status of the internal – external hypothesis for obesity. What went wrong? *American Psychologist*, 1981, *36*, 361 – 372.

Rodin, J., Moskowitz, H. R., & Bray, G. A. Relationship between obesity, weight loss, and taste responsiveness. *Physiology and Behavior*, 1976, *17*, 591 – 597.

Rodin, J., & Slochower, J. Externality in the nonobese: Effects of environmental responsiveness on weight. *Journal of Personality and Social Psychology*, 1976, *33*, 338 – 344.

Rodin, J., Slochower, J., & Fleming, B. Effects of degree of obesity, age of onset, and weight loss on responsiveness to sensory and external stimuli. *Journal of Comparative and Physiological Psychology*, 1977, *91*, 586 – 597.

Rosman, B. L., Minuchin, S., Baker, L., & Liebman, R. A family approach to anorexia nervosa: Study, treatment and outcome. In R. A. Vigersky (Ed.), *Anorexia nervosa*. New York: Raven Press, 1977.

Rosman, B. L., Minuchin, S., & Liebman, R. Family lunch session: An introduction to family therapy in anorexia nervosa. *American Journal of Orthopsychiatry*, 1975, *45*, 846 – 853.

Ross, J. L. Anorexia nervosa. An overview. *Bulletin of the Menninger Clinic*, 1977, *41*, 418 – 436.

Ruderman, A. J., & Wilson, G. T. Weight, restraint, cognitions and counter regulation. *Behaviour Research and Therapy*, 1979, *17*, 581 – 590.

Russell, G. F. M. Metabolic aspects of anorexia nervosa. *Proceedings of the Royal Society of Medicine*, 1965, *58*, 811 – 814.

Russell, G. Bulimia nervosa: An ominous variant of anorexia nervosa. *Psychological Medicine*, 1979, *9*, 429 – 448.

Schachter, S. Self-treatment of smoking and obesity. *Canadian Journal of Public Health*, 1981, *72*, 401 – 406.

Schachter, S. Recidivism and self-cure of smoking and obesity. *American Psychologist*, 1982, *37*, 436 – 444.

Schachter, S., Goldman, R., & Gordon, A. Effects of fear, food deprivation, and obesity on eating. *Journal of Personality and Social Psychology*, 1968, *10*, 91 – 97.

Schiebel, D., & Castelnuovo-Tedesco, P. Studies of superobesity: III. Body image changes after jejuno-ileal surgery. *International Journal of Psychiatry in Medicine*, 1978, *8*. 117 – 123.

Sims, E. A. H., Danforth, E., Horton, E. S., Bray, G. A., Glennon, J. A., & Salans, L. B. Endocrine and metabolic effects of experimental obesity in man. *Recent Progress in Hormone Research*, 1973, *29*, 457 – 496.

Sims, E. A. H., Goldman, R. F., Gluck, C. M., Horton, E. S., Kelleher, P. C., & Rowe, D. W. Experimental obesity in man. *Transactions of the Association of American Physicians*, 1968, *81*, 153 – 170.

Sims, E. A. H., & Horton, E. S. Endocrine and metabolic adaptation to obesity and starvation. *American Journal of Clinical Nutrition*, 1968, *21*, 1455 – 1470.

Sjöström, L. Fat cells and body weight. In A. J. Stunkard (Ed.), *Obesity*. Philadelphia: W. B. Saunders Co., 1980.

Slade, P. D. Awareness of body dimensions during pregnancy: An analogue study. *Pscyhological Medicine*, 1977, *7*, 245 – 252.

Slade, P. D., & Russell, G. F. M. Awareness of body dimension in anorexia nervosa: Cross-sectional and longitudinal studies. *Psychological Medicine*, 1973, *3*, 188 – 199. (a)

Slade, P. D., & Russell, G. F. M. Experimental investigations of bodily perception in anorexia nervosa and obesity. *Psychotherapy and Psychosomatics*, 1973, *22*, 359 – 363. (b)

Solow, C., Silberfarb, P. M., & Swift, K. Psychosocial effects of intestinal bypass surgery for severe obesity. *New England Journal of Medicine*, 1974, *290*, 300 – 304.

Sours, J. A. The anorexia nervosa syndrome. *International Journal of Psychoanalysis*, 1974, *55*, 567 – 576.

Spiegel, T. A. Caloric regulation of food intake in man. *Journal of Comparative and Physiological Psychology*, 1973, *84*, 24 – 37.

Stricker, E. M. Hyperphagia. *New England Journal of Medicine*, 1978, *298*, 1010 – 1013.

Stricker, E. M., & Zigmond, M. J. Brain catecholamines and the lateral hypothalamic syndrome. In D. Novin, W. Wyrwicka, & G. A. Bray (Eds.) *Hunger: Basic mechanisms and clinical implications.* New York: Raven Press, 1976.

Stuart, R. B. Behavioral control of overeating. *Behaviour Research and Therapy,* 1967, *5,* 357 – 365.

Stuart, R. B. *Act thin: Stay thin.* New York: W. W. Norton, 1978.

Stuart, R. B. Weight loss and beyond: Are they taking it off and keeping it off? In P. O. Davidson & S. M. Davidson (Eds.), *Behavioral medicine: Changing health lifestyles.* New York: Bruner/Mazel, 1980.

Stuart, R. B., & Guire, K. Some correlates of the maintenance of weight lost through behavior modification. *International Journal of Obesity,* 1978, *2,* 225 – 235.

Stuart, R. B., & Mitchell, C. Self-help groups in the control of body weight. In A. J. Stunkard (Ed.), *Obesity.* Philadelphia: W. B. Saunders Co., 1980.

Stunkard, A. New therapies for the eating disorders: Behavior modification of obesity and anorexia nervosa. *Archives of General Psychiatry,* 1972, *26,* 391 – 398.

Stunkard, A. J. Behavioral treatments of obesity: Failure to maintain weight loss. In R. B. Stuart (Ed.), *Behavioral self-management.* New York: Bruner/Mazel, 1977.

Stunkard, A. J. Behavioral medicine and beyond: The example of obesity. In O. F. Pomerleau (Ed.), *Behavioral medicine: Theory and practice.* Baltimore: Williams & Wilkins, 1979.

Stunkard, A. J. Psychoanalysis and psychotherapy. In A. J. Stunkard (Ed.), *Obesity.* Philadelphia: W. B. Saunders Co., 1980.

Stunkard, A., Coll, M., Lundquist, S., & Meyers, A. Obesity and eating style. *Archives of General Psychiatry,* 1980, *37,* 1127 – 1129.

Stunkard, A. J., Craighead, L. W., & O'Brien, R. Controlled trial of behavior therapy, pharmacotherapy, and their combination in the treatment of obese hypertensives. *Lancet,* 1980, *2,* 1045 – 1047.

Stunkard, A., & Koch, C. The interpretation of gastric motility: I. Apparent bias in the reports of hunger by obese persons. *Archives of General Psychiatry,* 1964, *11,* 74 – 82.

Stunkard, A., Levine, H., & Fox, S. The management of obesity. Patient self-help and medical treatment. *Archives of Internal Medicine,* 1970, *125,* 1067 – 1072.

Stunkard, A. J., & Mahoney, M. J. Behavioral treatment of the eating disorders. In H. Leitenberg (Ed.), *Handbook of behavior modification and behavior therapy.* Englewood Cliffs, N.J.: Prentice – Hall, Inc., 1976.

Stunkard, A., & Mendelson, M. Obesity and the body image: I. Characteristics of disturbances in the body image of some obese persons. *American Journal of Psychiatry,* 1967, *123,* 1296 – 1300.

Stunkard, A. J., & Penick, S. B. Behavior modification in the treatment of obesity. The problem of maintaining weight loss. *Archives of General Psychiatry,* 1979, *36,* 801 – 806.

Thomä, H. On the psychotherapy of patients with anorexia nervosa. *Bulletin of the Menninger Clinic,* 1977, *41,* 437 – 452.

Vigersky, R. A., & Loriaux, D. L. Anorexia nervosa as a model of hypothalamic dysfunction. In R. A. Vigersky (Ed.), *Anorexia nervosa.* New York: Raven Press, 1977.

Wakeling, A., Souza, V. F. A., Gore, M. B. R., Sabur, M., Kingstone, D., & Boss, A. M. B. Amenorrhea, body weight, and serum hormone concentrations, with particular reference to prolactin and thyroid hormones in anorexia nervosa. *Psychological Medicine,* 1979, *9,* 265 – 272.

Walsh, T. B., Katz, J. L., Levin, J., Kream, J., Fukishima, D. K., Hellman, L. D., Weiner, H., & Zumoff, B. Adrenal activity in anorexia nervosa. *Psychosomatic Medicine, 1978, 40,* 499 – 506.

Waxler, S. H., & Liska, E. S. Obesity and self-destructive behavior. In A. R. Roberts (Ed.) *Self-destructive behavior.* Springfield, Ill.: Charles C. Thomas, Publisher, 1975.

Waxman, M., & Stunkard, A. J. Caloric intake and expenditure of obese boys. *Journal of Pediatrics,* 1980, *96,* 187 – 193.

Wilson, G. T. Methodological considerations in treatment outcome research on obesity. *Journal of Consulting and Clinical Psychology,* 1978, *46,* 687 – 702.

Wing, R. R., Epstein, L. H., Marcus, M., & Shapira, B. Strong monetary contingencies for weight loss during treatment and maintenance. *Behavior Therapy,* 1981, *12,* 702 – 710.

Wingate, B. A., & Christie, M. J. Ego strength and body image in anorexia nervosa. *Journal of Psychosomatic Research,* 1978, *22,* 201 – 204.

Wollersheim, J. P. Effectiveness of group therapy based upon learning principles in the treatment of overweight women. *Journal of Abnormal Psychology,* 1970, *76,* 562 – 574.

Wooley, O. W. Long-term food regulation in the obese and nonobese. *Psychosomatic Medicine,* 1971, *33,* 436 – 444.

Wooley, O. W., Wooley, S. C., & Dunham, R. B. Can calories be perceived and do they affect hunger in obese and nonobese humans? *Journal of Comparative and Physiological Psychology,* 1972, *80,* 250 – 258.

Wooley, S. C., Wooley, O. W., & Dyrenforth, S. R. Theoretical, practical, and social issues in behavioral treatments of obesity. *Journal of Applied Behavior Analysis,* 1979, *12,* 3 – 25.

Yates, B. T. Improving the cost-effectiveness of obesity programs: Three basic strategies for reducing cost per pound. *International Journal of Obesity,* 1978, *2,* 249 – 266.

Youdin, R., & Hemmes, N. S. The urge to overeat—the initial link. *Journal of Behavior Therapy and Experimental Psychiatry,* 1978, *9,* 227 – 233.

13 Smoking: Psychophysiological Causes and Treatments

Nancy T. Blaney
Florida International University

Smoking is an indisputable health risk. Smokers of both sexes show higher death rates at all ages compared to nonsmokers (World Health Organization, 1979). It is estimated that smoking is responsible for up to 35% of all cancer deaths among males and 10% of those among females in the United States (Hammond & Seidman, 1980). Though the risk of lung cancer from smoking is well known, the risk of cardiovascular disease is far greater (Garfinkel, 1979). Specifically, cardiovascular disease (CVD) accounts for nearly 59% of excess deaths of male smokers (compared to nonsmokers) whereas lung cancer accounts for barely 15% of excess deaths, all cancers combined only 26%. Among women, CVD accounts for nearly two-thirds of excess deaths, with lung cancer only 7.2%, all cancers combined 13%.

Smoking rates among youth are alarmingly high, with perhaps 25 – 30% becoming occasional or regular smokers by age 15. The recent finding that multiple CVD risk factors are familial and observable early in life suggests that smoking would add to risk that children in such families already experience (Blonde, Webber, Foster, & Berenson, 1981). The trend toward increased smoking among females has led to the assessment that females starting to smoke now may be shortening their life expectancy by 6 years, comparable to that of male smokers (Peto, 1979). Notably, smoking has been shown to be a risk factor for myocardial infarction in young women who are in good health and not otherwise at risk (Slone, Shapiro, Rosenberg, Kaufman, Hartz, Rossi, Stolley, & Miettinen, 1978).

Data document the association between habitual cigarette smoking and chronic tendencies to perceive oneself as experiencing high stress (Conway, Vickers, Ward, & Rahe, 1981). Furthermore, substantial increases in smoking occur as larger numbers of crises are experienced (Lindenthal, Myers, & Pepper, 1972). Thus stress and smoking are interrelated risk factors.

Although it generally has been presumed that heavier smoking leads to greater risk, recent data suggest that some light or moderate smokers may incur a risk equivalent to that of the heavy smoker (Vogt, Selvin, Widdowson, & Hulley, 1977). Even nonsmokers may be at risk simply from absorbing the carbon monoxide (CO) in a smoke-filled room. Russell, Cole, and Brown (1973) demonstrated that such "passive smoking" for about 1 hour can lead to a CO absorption equivalent to that from actively smoking and inhaling one cigarette.

Physiological Mechanisms

Both carbon monoxide and nicotine have been implicated as the myocardial risk-causing agents in cigarette smoke (Astrup & Kjeldsen, 1979). Smoking both low- and high-nicotine cigarettes causes increases in heart rate and blood pressure (cf. Aronow, 1975). Smoking any cigarettes, even nonnicotine, results in elevated carboxyhemoglobin levels (Aronow, Dendinger, & Rokaw, 1971). The physiological mechanisms by which these risks occur are detailed by Aronow (1975). Heart rate and blood pressure increases are caused by nicotine increasing catecholamine discharge and by acting directly on arterial chemoreceptors to produce vasoconstriction. Elevated myocardial infarction risk appears due to nicotine's action in: (1) increasing the myocardial oxygen demand but not supply; (2) increasing thrombotic tendency due to enhanced platelet adhesiveness; and (3) lowering the ventricular fibrillation threshold. Carboxyhemoglobin (COHb) elevation aggravates the aforementioned reactions by: (1) displacing oxygen from hemoglobin, thereby decreasing the myocardial oxygen supply; (2) lowering the ventricular fibrillation threshold; and (3) possibly aiding in the development of atherosclerosis. Additionally, smoking may impair pulmonary function, decreasing oxygen supply still further. The rise in COHb after smoking is greater for women than for men (Russell, Wilson, Cole, Idle, & Feyerabend, 1973). This is particularly disturbing given the increase in smoking among women in recent years and the fact that it is harder for women than men to quit smoking (Dicken, 1978).

Prevalence

In 1978 some 54 million Americans smoked 615 billion cigarettes (Krasnegor, 1979). Contrary to fears that increases in smoking continue unabated, recent data offer room for cautious optimism. Warner (1977) shows that the per capita projected increases in cigarette consumption would have been as much as one-third larger in the absence of the years of antismoking campaigns. Trends in teenage smoking between 1968 and 1979 (Scarpetti & Datesman, 1980) indicate that teenagers are no longer starting to smoke at earlier ages and that there is an overall decrease in the proportion of teenagers who smoke. This is particulary true for boys, though not for older teenage girls. Smoking rates for girls now exceed those for boys (Bachman, Johnston, & O'Malley, 1981; Scarpetti & Datesman, 1980), and the median age for both sexes for beginning to smoke is 12 years. Nonetheless, over 20% of teenage smokers have begun by age 10 or younger, and nearly half express a desire to quit (Williams, Carter, & Wynder, 1981).

From this brief review it is obvious that smoking behavior represents a considerable risk to health. Though most studies have been done on cigarette smoking, there is also risk associated with pipe and cigar smoking (World Health Organization, 1975). The ingestion of smoke from tobacco into the lungs is a well-known hazard. Yet the behavior persists.

This chapter reviews some of the theories of smoking and the effects of interventions designed to change smoking behavior. With rare exceptions, the studies have focused on the smoking of cigarettes.

THEORIES OF SMOKING

Even if the utopian aim of preventing smoking onset entirely can someday be achieved, the present task must focus upon those who already are smokers. Both to motivate them to cease and to aid them in the process, knowledge of *why* people smoke is essential—hence the concern with theories of smoking. The predominant theories are either psychological in nature, focusing upon affective, personality, and social variables, or physiological, and are examined in the following section.

Psychological Theories

The point of departure for psychological theorizing is Tomkins' (1966, 1968) fourfold typology of the uses of smoking for managing affect. Tomkins viewed smoking as either for pleasure (positive affect), for sedation and tension reduction (negative affect), for both inducing pleasure and reducing anxiety (addictive), or autonomous (habitual). Three additional smoking motives—stimulation, sensorimotor manipulation, and social reward—have been suggested from factor analyses of the Reasons for Smoking scale (RFS) developed from Tomkins' model (Ikard, Green, & Horn, 1969). Subsequent experimental research has supported the validity of the RFS model by demonstrating the following: (1) negative affect smokers smoke more under distress (Ikard & Tomkins, 1973); (2) taste adulterations reduce smoking more for high- than low-pleasure smokers, whereas increased awareness of smoking leads to reductions for habit but not for pleasure smokers (Leventhal & Avis, 1976); and (3) for addictive smokers, deprivation results in greater distress (Costa, McCrae, & Bosse, 1980; Leventhal & Avis, 1976).

Others disagree, however, that the motives proposed by Tomkins relate to actual smoking behavior. Adesso and Glad (1978) report that, although subjects could be categorized into the categories proposed by Tomkins, these did not relate to actual smoking in either positive or negative affect conditions in which others present either were or were not smoking. An earlier study (Glad & Adesso, 1976) suggested that, even during distress, only the presence of others smoking led to increased smoking by subjects and only then among light smokers. A nonexperimental study (Joffe, Lowe, & Fischer, 1981) also failed to support the predictive validity of the RFS motives. In this study, smokers categorized according to the RFS self-monitored naturally occurring smoking using the RFS motives. Only the self-monitoring report of sensorimotor manipulation predicted smoking status 3 months later. Clearly, additional research is needed to fully establish the RFS predictive validity for naturally occurring smoking and should utilize both the RFS and self-monitoring approaches.

Various attempts have been made to relate smoking to personality characteristics, though most such studies have utilized smoker/nonsmoker designs and so are subject to severe limitations regarding inferences about causality (Dunn, 1973). Few firm conclusions can be drawn about the relationship between personality variables and smoking (Simon & Primavera, 1976; Smith, 1970). In this regard, a longitudinal study by Cherry & Kiernan (1976) is useful in that it relates personality characteristics to changes in smoking between the ages of 16 and 25. Specifically, they found that neurotics and extroverts who had not begun smoking by age 16 were more likely than the stable and introverts to take up the habit later.

Regarding smoking onset among youth, personality traits have not proven particularly useful in understanding adolescent smoking (Blaney, 1981), though risk taking has yet to be systematically examined. Although some investigators have concluded that the personality of adolescent smokers parallels that of deviant misbehavers (Powell, Steward, & Grylls, 1979), the more general conclusion is that a multidimensional deviance theory is not sufficient to portray the complexity of substance usage, including cigarettes (Huba, Wingard, & Bentler, 1980). In their study of personality and sexual behavior of the adolescent smoker, Malcolm and Shephard (1978) conclude that smoking onset is related more to parental and peer influence than to an inherent personality structure. A more promising use of personality characteristics in delineating smoking would be to focus on their interaction with pharmacological factors (cf. O'Connor, 1980), as the influence of personality variables may be a function in part of nicotine level and/or pharmacological dependence.

Other researchers have focused on the social environment as important in understanding smoking (Mausner & Platt, 1971), particularly that of females, whose smoking has been found to be more socially influenced than has that of men (Silverstein, Feld, & Kozlowski, 1980; Tryon, Vaughter, & Ginorio, 1977), though this difference disappears when pharmacological motivation (i.e., heavy smoking) develops (Russell, Wilson, Taylor, & Baker, 1980). Russell and his colleagues (Russell, Peto, & Patel, 1974) view the psychosocial and sensory aspects of smoking, seen as principal motives in other models, as being only inducements and/or peripheral benefits to the more central pharmacological and addictive aspects of smoking. Recent research (Bosse, Garvey, & Glynn, 1980) has found addiction to be both pharmacological and psychological, suggesting the utility of theories recognizing both.

Pharmacological Theories

Such theories of smoking assume that pharmacological addiction is the major component maintaining smoking behavior. Russell et al. (1974) conclude that classifying smokers along this dimension is more useful than utilizing their profiles on the types of smoking derived from Tomkins. Indeed, subsequent research (Russell, 1980) has demonstrated two pharmacologically distinct types of smokers in terms of their use of nicotine. The "peak-seekers" show a blood nicotine profile of repeated high peaks, suggesting that the reaction derived from the nicotine peaks is the basis for smoking. "Trough-maintainers" are heavier smokers who show smaller peaks relative to the absolute level of blood nicotine, suggesting that they smoke to maintain a high blood nicotine level and avoid withdrawal effects. This parallels the Leventhal and Cleary (1980) classification of pharmacological models as being either fixed-effect (i.e., rewarding) or nicotine regulation (i.e., avoidance of withdrawal) models.

However, because the effects of nicotine are short-lived and so cannot fully explain either the persistence of smoking or the high recidivism rate among former smokers (Russell, 1971a, 1971b), Leventhal and Cleary (1980) conclude that the fixed-effects (rewarding) model is insufficient to explain all smoking behavior.

Regarding the nicotine regulation model, the data are more impressive. Numerous studies have demonstrated that smokers compensate for varying nicotine levels in cigarettes by modifying their smoking patterns so that their blood nicotine levels remain the same (Russell, 1980; Russell, Jarvis, Iyer, & Feyerabend, 1980). This compensation appears to occur largely by increases in number of puffs and depth of inhalation. Accordingly, there is increased concern that the presumed health advantages of low-nicotine cigarettes may be offset by the health risks posed by greater CO exposure (Russell, 1980; Russell et al., 1980). Russell (1980) suggests that developing a low-CO, low-tar but medium- rather than low-nicotine cigarette would be a more logical way to minimize health risk from smoking.

The studies of Schachter (1977) and his colleagues are also an experimental demonstration of nicotine regulation. Experimentally altering blood nicotine level by varying urinary pH should presumably lead to increased smoking to replace lost nicotine, as low pH is acidic, causing alkaloid nicotine to be excreted. Results were as expected: Subjects with acidified urine (due to taking vitamin C or Acidulin) showed an increase in smoking from base levels (Schachter, Kozlowski, & Silverstein, 1977). Lowered urinary pH, due to the effects of stress, is also the reason suggested by Schachter for why people seem to smoke to reduce negative affect. If the stress-induced drop in urinary pH is blocked, hence preventing nicotine excretion, then high stress should not lead to increased smoking, an effect experimentally demonstrated by Schachter, Silverstein, and Perlick (1977).

Despite these data, however, the nicotine regulation model has been criticized. Regarding research with low-nicotine cigarettes, showing that compensatory smoking patterns develop as a way to maintain nicotine intake, Stepney (1980) points out that the compensatory smoking patterns associated with low-nicotine cigarettes may be due to such cigarettes differing in other ways that could significantly alter the process of smoking. Thus, such experiments cannot be taken as having conclusively established the importance of nicotine relative to other smoke constituents. Further, the amount of compensation is not sufficient to maintain previous nicotine levels. Also, the pattern of withdrawal effects argues against a primarily addictive view of smoking. Heavy and light smokers do not seem to differ in severity of withdrawal, with withdrawal effects being worse for those who reduce but do not cease than for those who cease completely (Shiffman & Jarvik, 1976). Leventhal and Cleary (1980) further discuss the inadequacies of a solely pharmacologic addiction model, emphasizing that smoking has a long developmental history in which smokers differ concerning reasons for starting and continuing to smoke, as well as in rates of developing dependency on cigarettes. Leventhal and Cleary argue that individual differences, as suggested by Schachter (1977), cannot account for these phenomena, and that there is no convincing evidence showing that different underlying mechanisms are associated with differences in smoking levels.

Combined Models

Both Stepney (1980) and Leventhal and Cleary (1980) propose alternative models with an entirely different focus in which nicotine is a psychological tool, used to control emotional arousal. In support of his view, Stepney (1980) reviews studies showing how smoking paradoxically both increases and reduces stress, depending on the context in which smoking occurs. A stimulant effect is obtained under conditions of low arousal but a depressant effect under conditions of high (auditory) stress. Further, Stepney notes the dual manner in which smoking-induced changes in arousal appear to improve performance—either by increasing arousal and thus behavioral alertness, or by reducing arousal and thereby reducing the behavioral disruption caused by stress. He concludes that smoking is rewarding and continues not as a means of avoiding nicotine withdrawal, as other pharmacological models suggest, but solely as a means of controlling arousal.

Leventhal and Cleary (1980) propose a multiple regulation model in which emotions, not nicotine, are being regulated. In their view, the illusion that it is nicotine that is being regulated arises because various emotional states have become conditioned to nicotine level as the smoking habit has developed. The craving resulting from a change in homeostasis can come from two sources: (1)

nicotine itself via the dysphoria resulting from declines in plasma nicotine; and (2) external stimulation in the form of negative situations that become conditioned to drops in plasma nicotine levels. Leventhal and Cleary made several assumptions in their model: (1) several emotional processes can operate simultaneously; (2) they can combine algebraically to intensify one another and the nicotine-based response; (3) nicotine level changes generate physiological sensations that can be conditioned to the emotional states and that constitute the basis of the craving response; and, (4) nicotine facilitates reactions that help the smoker adapt to situational stress by increasing or decreasing arousal as the situation requires.

Leventhal and Cleary posit that such smoking-induced behavioral adaptation leads to the development of schematic memories of motoric and physiological reactions that they label "emotional memory." This emotional memory integrates external situational cues with the internal nicotine state and various associated emotional and motoric experiences, and maintains the homeostatic combination of these. In their view, eliciting any component of this schematic memory can arouse any of the other components. Thus the schema is the source of craving experienced by smokers when they see someone else smoke. The oft cited individual differences among smokers, they contend, are due to the different elements incorporated into individuals' schemas. Leventhal and Cleary conclude that the smoker ultimately attempts to "protect" his nicotine level because its link, via the emotional memory, is such that declines in plasma nicotine elicit negative emotional experiences. In explaining the development of the smoking habit, their model suggests that smoking: (1) initially regulates emotional responses to situational stress; (2) then regulates the craving that has become conditioned to these external situational cues; and (3) then regulates the craving and distress resulting from changes in plasma nicotine levels. They emphasize that it is regulation of emotions, not nicotine, that is the core of the dependence process, and that smoking does not maintain plasma nicotine levels but supresses emotional distress that drops in plasma nicotine levels would induce. The model points clearly to the interactions among emotional and biological systems in the development and maintenance of smoking behavior.

As Stepney (1980) has noted, the question of how to get people to stop smoking will not be answered so long as the psychological components of the pharmacological effects of smoking are ignored. Psychological involvement with smoking increases with age (Bosse et al., 1980), a fact that underscores the importance of disembedding from the smoker's life-style the use of smoking as a psychological tool. Leventhal and Cleary (1980) address the same issue, utilizing the Robins, Davis, and Goodwin (1974) data showing that the more drug use was integrated into a person's everyday life prior to military service, the greater the likelihood of postservice addiction. Extending this to smoking, Leventhal and Cleary suggest that using nicotine across numerous life situations allows the development of a broad-based emotional smoking schema that could make cessation particularly difficult.

INTERVENTION

Intervention efforts can be categorized as either indirect or direct. Indirect efforts consist of community and school programs, which may seek either to prevent onset or modify ongoing smoking behavior. Direct interventions consist of cessation efforts aimed at changing behavior in the established smoker. Until recently, research on both types of intervention efforts failed to include adequate evaluation and follow-up components and tended to ignore theoretically based knowledge of human behavior. As a result, relatively few intervention studies have provided systematic evaluations of theoretically derived strategies that improve our understanding of the processes underlying the initiation, maintenance, cessation, or recidivism of smoking behavior. The following paragraphs present an assessment of the state of intervention efforts, both indirect and direct, with prevention being discussed first. No attempt is made to provide an exhaustive review.

Prevention

The topic of prevention has many facets, from a focus on the very young to the need to establish a preventive nonsmoking attitude in public media and entertainment. It is increasingly recognized that smoking is a pediatric concern (Williams & Wynder, 1976) and that young children are perhaps the most appropriate intervention targets. Tennant (1979) found that a high level of awareness of health-abusing behaviors already exists among preschoolers, though some studies suggest that children may be unaware of just how personal the health risk can be for them (Rawbone, Keeling, Jenkins, & Guz, 1978).

Preventing the well-documented fetal risk from maternal smoking is an important though perverse form of prevention in that its success requires maternal smoking cessation. Results are mixed and range from effects of antismoking efforts during pregnancy being negligible (Donovan, 1977) to somewhat more positive outcomes (Baric, MacArthur, & Sherwood, 1976; Danaher, Shisslak, Thompson, & Ford, 1978). Overall, the success rates for interventions are modest, and methodological problems preclude optimism at this point.

Clearly the ultimate key to reducing fetal risk is prevention of smoking onset. The recognition that smoking is a cultural phenomenon, fostered by the social environment, has directed attention to efforts to modify the larger social environment to make it more conducive to nonsmoking and less reinforcing to smoking. Nostbakken (1979) has urged the establishment of a nonsmoking norm by ensuring that media programming reflect nonsmoking beliefs and attitudes. Efforts to modify community knowledge and behaviors by using mass media campaigns, however, have shown limited usefulness for media alone in reducing smoking (Meyer, Nash, McAlister, Maccoby, & Farquhar, 1980). Survey data from Champion and Bell (1980) show that although health education has discouraged the moderate user of tobacco, the heavy user has remained uninfluenced. The more appropriate goal at present for mass media would appear to be that of disseminating information and creating a normative nonsmoking environment rather than attempting to accomplish substantial behavior change directly, a task for which they clearly are not suited. Leventhal (1973) argues that preventive measures will be unsuccessful to the extent that their behavioral and habit aspects are ignored, aspects not well addressed by mass media. Media efforts, then, are best thought of as adjuncts to more direct intervention strategies based on psychological and pharmacological theories of smoking.

Indirect Interventions

Community studies.   Numerous reviewers have documented the shortcomings of community studies, and the reader is referred to those for further detail (Bradshaw, 1973; Evans, Henderson, Hill, & Raines, 1979; Leventhal & Cleary, 1980). The need for more systematically developed and pretested communications is a frequently cited problem, as is the lack of evidence of overall effectiveness. A study that rises above much of the criticism leveled at community programs is the Stanford Heart Prevention Program (Meyer et al., 1980; Stern, Farquhar, Maccoby, & Russell, 1976), which utilized three communities to compare the effectiveness of a mass media campaign on changes in heart disease risk factors with that of a media campaign supplemented with face-to-face instruction for high risk individuals. The third community served as a control group. The media-plus-instruction community was significantly different from the control, whereas the media-only community was not. Though it has been noted that the smoking reductions are neither particularly large nor dramatically different from those obtained with therapy studies (Leventhal, Safer, Cleary, & Gutman, 1980), the Stanford study nonetheless demonstrates a potentially useful combination of cost-efficient, large-scale approaches to stimulating behavior change.

As Leventhal and Cleary (1980) point out, however, there is a dearth of research showing how community norms and values interact with intervention efforts to either facilitate or hinder behavior change. Knowledge of such effects is particularly crucial for community studies in that the effectiveness of media campaigns may be quite different in contexts that are supportive versus those that are antagonistic or neutral. The more positive antismoking climate noted earlier may have set the stage for a new level of success with media campaigns, providing they are tailored to the psychological and pharmacological experiences of smokers at all stages of the dependence process. To the extent that future media campaigns contain components that systematically address psychopharmacological factors differentiating types of smokers and degrees of addiction, and to the extent that they are cognizant of community values, media campaigns may become appropriate and effective vehicles for inducing greater changes in smoking behavior.

School studies.   Interventions aimed at children and adolescents are based on the premise that preventing smoking from starting in the first place is far more productive than getting people to stop once they have become regular smokers (see

Blaney, 1981, for a critical review of this topic). Even if youngsters have begun smoking, many dislike aspects of smoking, and few smoke heavily enough to be addicted, suggesting that they are important targets for intervention (Nye, Haye, McKenzie-Pollock, Caughley, & Housham, 1980).

Just how early interventions need to occur in order to be effective has become disturbingly apparent. Hansen (1978) found distant past behavior was related to current smoking habits even as early as the sixth grade, suggesting that behavioral patterns underlying or leading to smoking have already been established by that age. Developmental changes in attitudes, showing a decrease in antismoking sentiments, have been reported for grade school children (Pederson, Stennett, & Lefcoe, 1981) and young adolescents (Schneider & Vanmastrigt, 1974). All this suggests the appropriateness of the developmental focus urged by Blaney (1981) and Leventhal and Cleary (1980). Nonetheless, there has been a particular lack of data explaining why children start to smoke or what means are most effective in preventing or reducing their smoking.

Recent longitudinal data (Murray & Cracknell, 1980) suggest that adolescents' smoking behavior and attitudes simply cannot be attributed to smokers having more siblings, friends, and parents who smoke. These investigators suggest that to understand the decision to smoke we must also examine: (1) whether these social influencers actively encourage smoking; and (2) the strength of the counterarguments available to nonsmokers. Their data show that, as nonsmokers grow older, they begin to see smoking in a positive light and acquire an image of smoking as being relaxing without actually ever having smoked. Murray and Cracknell conclude that when smoking is actively encouraged and counterarguments are few or weak, prosmoking views are likely to develop that in turn facilitate smoking onset. They note the need to examine strategies used by nonsmokers who have successfully resisted the temptation to become smokers as larger numbers of their friends start to smoke.

One such strategy may center on the smoking status label a person assigns himself. Hunter, Webber, and Berenson (1980) suggest that much could be learned regarding the transition from nonsmoker to adopter by studying "experimental nonadopters." These are individuals who try smoking but neither adopt it nor label themselves as smokers. Because they often are incorporated into the category of exsmoker in surveys, much information regarding them is lost. Further, Hunter et al. (1980) argue that because most children try smoking at some time or other, it is the experimental nonadopters who are the most appropriate target of intervention programs that should be designed specifically to reinforce their nonadopting behavior.

Sex differences in the process of becoming a smoker particularly need systematic examination. Limited available data suggest the process may be somewhat different for each sex regarding social, psychological, and physiological dimensions. For example, at the age when girls are finally becoming regular smokers boys are starting to quit and become exsmokers (Hunter et al., 1980). And though in general the perceived pleasures of smoking increase with age among adolescents, this occurs earlier for boys than for girls, who show greater concerns for health than do boys (Murray & Cracknell, 1980). Girls seem to experience greater social pressures to smoke but also greater physiological sensitivity to nicotine, a conflict apparently resolved by their becoming lighter smokers and smoking more low-nicotine brands than males (Silverstein et al., 1980).

Only recently have interventions begun focusing on grade school and early adolescent years. Interventions prior to the late 1970s focused on older adolescents and were mostly unsuccessful in modifying smoking habits. This is not surprising given that the greatest risk for smoking onset appears to be around age 12, not older adolescence.

The earlier research warrants other criticisms too. Interventions were often nonsystematic, focused only on imparting knowledge of health risks, and failed to include adequate evaluation or follow-up. Even the methodologically rigorous investigations of teaching methods and message themes (Creswell, Huffman, Stone, Merki, & Newman, 1969; Creswell, Stone, Huffman, & Newman, 1971) suffer from a failure to objectively validate smoking self-reports and from a focus that is too narrow to answer broader questions concerning the process of becoming a smoker and what kinds of communications are most effective at different points in that process. This latter criticism also pertains to evaluations of the School Health Curriculum Project (SHCP) (Bureau of Health Education, 1977), the widely used elementary school curriculum emphasizing physiology, health maintenance, and the effects of environmental and individual abuse (e.g., by smoking). Unfortunately, SHCP evaluations do not answer questions regarding the interactive effects of the curriculum and variables relevant to the process of becoming— or refraining from becoming—a smoker. Green (1979) concluded her review of this area with the disappointing observation that, despite the proliferation of prevention programs, we still do not know what types of interventions effectively keep youth from becoming smokers.

More recent studies, however, provide the basis for some optimism, as the focus has shifted toward one of teaching coping skills that enable students to resist peer and other pressures to smoke. Evans and his colleagues report success in reducing smoking onset with their program to "inoculate" students to resist peer, parent, and media pressure to smoke (Evans, Rozelle, Mittelmark, Hansen, Bane, & Havis, 1978). Their intervention utilizes specially created videotapes and written responses to questions based on them, small group discussions, classroom posters, and posttest feedback to students regarding their smoking behavior and future intentions about smoking.

Believing effectiveness would be enhanced by the addition of roleplaying, and peer rather than adult presentation of material, McAlister and his colleagues conducted an inoculation intervention incorporating these variables (McAlister, Perry, Killen, Slinkard, & Maccoby, 1980; McAlister, Perry, & Maccoby, 1979). They utilized peer leaders to implement an intervention aimed at sixth- and seventh-graders to teach them appropriate responses to social pressures to smoke. Results showed that: (1) the smoking rate increased less at the experimental than at the control school; (2) a schoolwide antismoking climate may have been established at the experimental school (McAlister et al., 1979); and (3) at both 1 year (McAlister et al., 1980) and at 33 months (Telch, Killen, McAlister, Perry, & Maccoby, 1982) the smoking onset rate was significantly lower at the experimental school.

Similar success is reported in a more detailed study of curriculum components conducted by Hurd and his colleagues (Hurd, Johnson, Pechacek, Bast, Jacobs, & Luepker, 1980). The most successful aspects of their broad-spectrum approach were the combination of the social pressures curriculum (including roleplaying), presentation by respected peer opinion leaders, and public commitment from students regarding their reasons for not smoking. By making it clear to students that a majority of their peers do not yet smoke, the commitment procedure may alter the schoolwide climate regarding smoking. This may have an effect similar to the peer leader procedure employed by McAlister et al. (1979).

A more generalized approach to teaching coping skills to resist pressure to smoke is represented by the Life Skills Training (LST) program (Botvin, Eng, & Williams, 1980; Williams, 1980). The purpose of the program is to help students develop basic life skills relevant to adolescent problems, including smoking. An outside specialist conducted 10 weekly classroom sessions for eighth- through tenth-graders, utilizing group discussion techniques, role modeling, and behavior rehearsal. Topics covered included myths and realities of smoking, awareness of advertising techniques, self-image, decision making, coping with anxiety, communication skills, social skills, and assertiveness. Analysis of smoking onset rates at the end of the program indicated that significantly fewer of the experimental than control group students began smoking, and that this was inversely related to grade level, with the greatest prevention occurring for eighth-graders.

In addition to teaching students to resist social pressures to smoke, recent interventions have shifted the message content from the long-term health risks to the more immediate physiological effects of smoking. This has been found to be effective in reducing smoking rates among both older adolescents (Perry, Killen, Telch, Slinkard, & Danaher, 1980) and sixth-grade children (Hansen, 1978). However, a direct comparison of the two types of messages failed to yield the predicted differences among ninth-graders (Hill, 1980), though this may not be an appropriate evaluation of differential effectiveness, as even the immediate effects message may need the context of a multicomponent, peer-based intervention to be maximally effective.

Despite the encouraging results cited in the preceding paragraphs, there remain concerns regarding the optimal timing and packaging of antismoking interventions. At least two studies suggest that interventions may have some kind of enabling effect on smoking, quite contrary to that intended. Pederson et al. (1981) report that their smoking awareness curriculum appeared to result in less negative attitudes toward smoking among the elementary school children exposed to it, raising the question of possibly increased vulnerability to smoking onset. Jason and Mollica (1979) found that decreases in smoking occurred only among those experimenting with smoking in their junior high sample, with regular smokers actually increasing in smoking. This raises the question of differential effects of smoking interventions, and the implied need to tailor programs to subgroups who differ on dimensions relevant to smoking rate or onset. Duncan (1977) proposes a stress-reduction model for the development of drug dependence that views drug usage in part as due to individuals with poor coping skills being confronted with stressful, unsupportive environments. Such a model well might be extended to smoking intervention research to determine what levels and kinds of stress might facilitate succumbing to peer pressures or lead to solitary experimentation, with interventions ultimately being tailored to those at greatest risk.

Overall, one can conclude that advances are being made in indirect interventions aimed at modifying smoking behavior (though methodologically rigorous designs are not yet the norm), the role of teachers and parents has been insufficiently explored in school-based interventions, and controlled studies are needed to determine the differential effectiveness of components of the more successful broad-spectrum programs. This latter point is acknowledged by various investigators (Hurd et al., 1980; Perry et al., 1980; Spitzzeri & Jason, 1979).

Direct Interventions

For many years the smoking cessation clinic has been a widely used means for smokers to attempt to modify their smoking behavior. Despite its popularity, however, this approach has shown disappointing effectiveness with smoking reductions due primarily to nonspecific treatment factors and tending to be neither permanent nor superior to unaided efforts. Clearly there is great need for carefully designed, systematically evaluated interventions that significantly improve on the clinic success rate. Recent reviews (Bernstein & Glasgow, 1979; Frederiksen & Simon, 1979) form the basis for much of the following assessment of current efforts. The framework utilized is that suggested by Frederiksen and Simon (1979), with programs grouped according to whether they address the antecedents of smoking, the smoking event itself, or the consequences of smoking.

Antecedents

Programs addressing antecedents evidence a wide range of goals, seeking to alter or control smoking-eliciting cues that are both external (social, environmental) and internal (physiological, emotional, cognitive). In this category are approaches that utilize drugs, stimulus control, covert sensitization, systematic desensitization and relaxation, and hypnosis.

1. Drug approaches. Here the focus has been twofold—on psychoactive drugs and on nicotine. For the most part, psychoactive drugs have proved ineffective in modifying smoking. This is true for both antianxiety drugs and stimulants, with methodological problems plaguing the few positive results for the latter (Frederiksen & Simon, 1979). The principal focus has been on nicotine, either in the form of a nicotine substitute or on nonsmoking modes of administering nicotine directly. On the whole, lobeline sulfate, the most widely studied nicotine substitute, has been shown to be relatively ineffective.

The most promising of the drug approaches concerns the direct administration of nicotine, either orally or intravenously, which has been shown to reduce smoking. The advantage of such direct administration is that it bypasses the smoke-based inhalation of tar and CO, now considered more harmful than nicotine. Nicotine chewing gum is the most easily administered and widely used mode of direct nicotine administration. It is superior to psychological treatment (Raw, Jarvis, Feyerabend, & Russell, 1980) and produces blood nicotine concentrations similar to those from smoking (Russell, Raw, & Jarvis, 1980). Both of these studies yielded abstinence rates near 40%. Though Raw et al. (1980) suggest that nicotine gum is probably safe even for those with cardiovascular disease, more research is needed to establish its safety and effectiveness with long-term usage. Bernstein and Glasgow (1979) suggest that attention to maximizing nicotine's metabolism and blocking its reinforcement may lead to pharmacological treatment techniques that may become vital adjuncts of nonpharmacological approaches.

2. Stimulus Control.   Smoking is associated with a wide range of environmental cues, presumably differing among individuals. Stimulus control treatment seeks gradually to narrow the range of cues that elicit smoking. Stimulus control variations have included: (1) "situational hierarchies," in which less stressful situations are the first cessation target; (2) transferring stimulus control of smoking to one cue, such as an auditory timing device; and (3) "behavioral engineering," using an automatically locking cigarette case that opens at predetermined intervals. Although case studies have demonstrated success, Bernstein and Glasgow (1979) conclude that no stimulus control studies have shown effectiveness superior to unaided efforts, other treatments, or placebo effects. Used alone, stimulus control treatments have been characterized by high attrition and relapse, and by an inability of subjects to reduce below a threshold of about 12 cigarettes daily (Levinson, Shapiro, Schwartz, & Tursky, 1971; Shapiro, Tursky, Schwartz, & Schnidman, 1971). Nicotine withdrawal has been offered as the explanation for this effect (Levinson et al., 1971), though others have suggested that the gradual reduction increases the reinforcing power of each remaining cigarette, making them increasingly harder to give up and thus perversely strengthening the habit (Flaxman, 1978; Shiffman & Jarvik, 1976).

3. Covert Sensitization.   Covert sensitization seeks to control internal cues, primarily cognitive, that elicit smoking. Representative techniques include teaching smokers to use aversive antismoking self-statements, pro-nonsmoking statements, and pairing noxious imagery (e.g., extreme nausea) with visualizations of smoking. However, none of these has demonstrated long-term effectiveness or superiority over other approaches. Aversive conditioning has been added to covert sensitization by pairing electric shock with verbalizations about and visualizations of smoking. Pairing shock with subjects' imagining the *urge* to smoke has proven the most promising approach (Berecz, 1976), although this was not effective for females. Frederksen and Simon (1979) conclude that, though additional validation and refinement are necessary, aversive conditioning of antecedent cognitions has merit in smoking cessation research. In particular, the Berecz (1976) data point to the value of punishing smoking urges, an early antecedent of smoking behavior.

4. Systematic Desensitization and Relaxation. These approaches focus on reducing the stress that leads to smoking as well as that that accompanies cessation efforts. However, systematic desensitization has not been found to be superior to aversive conditioning and counseling groups, electric shock or self-monitoring, or relaxation and covert sensitization both alone and with desensitization. In fact, both relaxation and desensitization have been found to be the least effective of various approaches.

5. Hypnosis. Although proponents have claimed success for hypnosis in smoking cessation, critical reviews of the literature have consistently concluded that its effectiveness in smoking cessation has yet to be conclusively demonstrated (Bernstein & Glasgow, 1979; Bernstein & McAlister, 1976; Frederiksen & Simon, 1979). As noted by Bernstein and Glasgow (1979), hypnosis has most frequently been used in two ways. One is to establish negative associations with cigarettes and smoking behavior. A more positive approach is to build reinforcing associations for nonsmoking or to increase motivation to follow varied nonhypnotic treatment approaches.

Smoking Behavior

A quite different approach to modifying smoking behavior is represented by programs that focus directly on the act of smoking itself, through self-monitoring or through changing either the substance smoked or the topographical characteristics of smoking.

1. Self-Monitoring. Effectiveness of this as a smoking cessation technique varies as a function of other factors, such as the specific behavior being monitored, whether monitoring occurs pre- or postbehavior, and how frequently. For example, McFall (1970) found greater smoking decreases with monitoring of resisting urges to smoke rather than of cigarettes smoked, but failed to confirm this in a subsequent study (McFall & Hammen, 1971) in which all forms of monitoring produced reductions. Larger reductions have been associated with monitoring that is pre- rather than postsmoking (Rozensky, 1974) and continuous rather than intermittent (Frederiksen, Epstein, & Kosevsky, 1975). However, continuous monitoring was found to be more aversive and led to greater attrition. Despite its usefulness for measuring smoking rate, self-monitoring has been questioned regarding reactive effects that might necessitate independent assessment of smoking rates (Frederiksen & Simon, 1979; see also Leventhal & Avis, 1976).

2. Smoking Topography. This approach seeks to change smoking characteristics such as frequency and depth of inhalation and has given rise to the concept of "controlled smoking" (Frederiksen & Simon, 1978a, 1978b) as an alternative to abstinence. This approach has been both supported (Vogt, Selvin, & Billings, 1979) and criticized (Paxton, 1980). The two treatment objectives of abstinence and controlled smoking imply different methods for measuring smoking behavior. Abstinence requires only consideration of smoking rate. Controlled smoking additionally requires measures of the way a person smokes and what is smoked, as the objective is "safer smoking" rather than cessation. Research has shown that components of smoking behavior (e.g., puff frequency and duration, interpuff interval, cigarette duration, and amount consumed) can be isolated, measured, and modified (Frederiksen, Miller, & Peterson, 1977). Changes in one component lead to compensating changes in others, presumably as a way to maintain nicotine levels. Case study research, however, has demonstrated the feasibility of structured modifications in successive components, resulting in positive changes in smoking behavior that avoid the compensation effect and generalize to the natural environment with long-term maintenance (Frederiksen & Simon, 1978a, 1978b).

Safer smoking also has been promoted by development of cigarettes containing less tar and nicotine. Unfortunately, the compensation effect noted previously may result in smokers being exposed to greater amounts of cigarette smoke as they attempt to maintain nicotine levels, thereby increasing the health risks from CO, thought by some to be even greater than those posed by nicotine. Clearly, unless smoking topography can be altered, lower-nicotine cigarettes do not represent a safe substitute for substantial reduction or cessation.

Consequences

In addition to focusing on antecedents to and characteristics of smoking, interventions may attempt to change its consequences. These consequences can be social (e.g., support, reward of nonsmoking), nonsocial (e.g., contracts, deposits), or aversive (e.g., taste, electric shock, rapid smoking, or satiation). The most usual approach has been aversive conditioning. More recently, though, attention has turned to both social and nonsocial reward of nonsmoking.

1. Aversive Conditioning. Taste aversion has been the least researched of the aversive procedures, perhaps because resulting decrements in smoking have been temporary, with long-term successes (Seltzer, 1975) not yet experimentally evaluated (Bernstein & Glasgow, 1979). Contingent electric shock, despite its early promise, has not been found in well-controlled studies to be more effective than other approaches (Russell, Armstong, & Patel, 1976) or even control conditions (Conway, 1977). Combining shock with self-management training has been suggested as a way to enhance effectiveness (Frederiksen & Simon, 1979). Data from Conway (1977) indicate that this is not the case regarding long-term maintenance. The greatest potential for shock aversion appears to be its use in altering cognitions preceding smoking (Berecz, 1976), thereby altering antecedents as discussed earlier.

More widely used is aversive conditioning via satiation smoking or cigarette smoke. Because satiation smoking (i.e., tripling daily smoking rate) has failed to be generally effective, research has focused on cigarette smoke. Early research established that rapid smoking alone was as effective as the combined procedure of blowing warm, smoky air into the smoker's face during rapid smoking (Lichtenstein, Harris, Birchler, Wahl, & Schmahl, 1973), with abstinence figures comparable to other treatments. Despite claims for the efficacy of the procedure, a recent controlled study comparing three treatment conditions found rapid smoking to be no more effective than cue exposure or simple support (Raw & Russell, 1980). Even proponents of the procedure (e.g., Glasgow, Lichtenstein, Beaver, & O'Neill, 1981) report that normally paced smoking to the point of aversion can be as effective as rapid smoking, leading them to support development of less physiologically stressful alternatives.

Rapid smoking has been criticized regarding possible health risks (e.g., nicotine poisoning and cardiovascular stress). Studying the subjective reactions to rapid smoking, Glasgow et al. (1981) failed to find evidence that rapid smoking causes nicotine poisoning as suggested by Horan, Linberg, & Hackett (1977). Regarding cardiovascular stress, although healthy persons do not seem to be at risk, those with cardiovascular problems are (Hall, Sachs, & Hall, 1979; Poole, Sanson-Fisher, German, & Harker, 1980). This is due primarily to heart muscle damage from lowered blood oxygen and cardiac arrhythmias from lowered serum potassium levels (Hall et al., 1979). Although rapid smoking is seen by some as one of the most powerful smoking cessation treatments available, it is clear that more parametric research is needed to determine the conditions that establish optimal effectiveness, and that alternative procedures are necessary for those with health risks.

2. *Social Consequences.* Establishing an environment supportive of non-smoking has long been emphasized as important in smoking treatment programs (Bernstein, 1969; Schmahl, Lichtenstein, & Harris, 1972) but its effectiveness has been unclear. Buddy systems and/or social approval (contingent on nonsmoking) from significant others have been found to be both effective and ineffective. However, strong treatment effects and 50% abstinence at 6 months have been found with a variation of social consequences utilizing reciprocal aversion (requiring one spouse to smoke whenever the other did) to stop smoking within a couple

(Lichstein & Stalgaitis, 1980). It is unclear though, whether these latter results are due to positive social influence (i.e., joint commitment), negative social influence (i.e., spouse criticism), or aversion.

3. *Nonsocial Consequences.* Typical nonsocial consequences include self-reward for abstinence, self-punishment for smoking, and contracted return of monetary deposit contingent on nonsmoking. Self-reward has been found to be less effective than either self-punishment (Murray & Hobbs, 1981) or control conditions (Conway, 1977; Murray & Hobbs, 1981). Contingency contracted return of monetary deposit has produced abstinence on both a short- and long-term basis, though recently Paxton (1980) found the effects disappeared by 2 months. This suggests the importance of an extended deposit duration to assist in early abstinence, a possibly critical period after which maintenance may be less problematic.

Multicomponent Programs

Due to the multifaceted nature of smoking behavior and the impressive but temporary effects of many behavioral interventions, reviewers have long emphasized the need for cessation programs to be multicomponent ones, focusing on maintaining as well as obtaining abstinence (Bernstein, 1969; Hunt & Matarazzo, 1970). As noted by Frederiksen and Simon (1979), such programs generally can be categorized as involving either therapist control or self-control. Examples of therapist-control approaches include rapid smoking combined with covert-conditioning and behavioral group therapy (Tongas, Patterson, & Goodkind, 1976), or combined relaxation and satiation (Sutherland, Amit, Golden, & Roseberger, 1975). Both studies have demonstrated smoking reductions and maintenance, though the latter was not notably long-term.

Self-control programs involve the subject being the primary administrator of treatment via such techniques as self-monitoring, self-reward, self-punishment, and stimulus control. Although self-control programs offer the advantages of economy and ease of administration, they also embody the assessment disadvantage that evaluation must include a measure of how completely the procedures have been followed by participants. A recent review (Frederiksen & Simon, 1979) finds self-control programs not to be superior to other approaches in either treatment effects or maintenance, though data from Flaxman (1978) show mixed results, with setting a target date for cessation enhancing self-control effects.

Glasgow, Schafer, and O'Neill (1981) examined both self-control and therapist-control approaches using either a minimal treatment program or one of two self-help behavior therapy books, finding only modest change and equal relapse rates among conditions. They did, however, find evidence suggesting that the more complex the self-help behavior therapy program, the more important therapist assistance became. Glasgow et al. (1981) also suggest that the degree of structure imposed on self-help programs may affect how well tailored to individual needs the intervention becomes and should be systematically varied and evaluated.

Several multicomponent programs (Delahunt & Curran, 1976; Lando, 1977; Tongas et al., 1976) have yielded superior 6-month abstinence rates (56 – 77%), with Powell and McCann (1981) showing 66% abstinent at 1 year. Clearly such programs merit further evaluation and implementation.

CONCEPTUAL AND METHODOLOGICAL ISSUES

A number of conceptual and methodological problems have limited the effectiveness of interventions aimed at both prevention and cessation. Thus it is disappointing, though not surprising, that long-term (5-year) follow-up figures of smoking cessation programs show only 17 – 25% abstinence rates (Evans & Lane, 1980; West, Graham, Swanson, & Wilkinson, 1977), consistent with earlier estimates (Hunt & Bespalec, 1974) of 75% relapse the first 6 months. Leventhal and Cleary (1980) attribute this to the failure to base interventions on theories of smoking, thereby providing overly simplistic motivation and skill training that pays scant attention to individual differences in the complex psychological and physiological processes underlying smoking. The present section addresses conceptual problems regarding prevention and cessation, and methodological problems in designs and measures regarding both.

Conceptual Issues

Prevention. Several seldom researched but important issues are relevant to preventing smoking onset. These include the process of becoming a smoker or remaining a nonsmoker, the consequences of starting to smoke, precocity of smoking, tailoring programs to high risk groups and the focus of studies (Blaney, 1981).

Regarding the process of becoming a smoker, it is essential that research questions address the process across time. This implies the use of longitudinal frameworks rather than the more common smoker/nonsmoker design, which limits inferences about causation (see critique in Dunn, 1973). Research on adolescent drug usage provides heuristic examples of how longitudinal data can answer process-oriented questions regarding developmental changes in variables relevant to usage, and the subsequent impact on usage rates (Jessor & Jessor, 1978; Smith & Fogg, 1978). Similar examination is needed of the process of *remaining* a nonsmoker. For example, although smoking is thought to result in part from peer pressure, is resisting smoking due to the same process, or do peers play any significant role at all in remaining a nonsmoker? Only recently have interventions addressed peer influence directly (Evans et al., 1978; McAlister et al., 1979), but still data do not address these process questions.

Nor do data clearly show how consequences of becoming a smoker might differ for students of different ages, and how these might impact self-esteem, academic achievement, and perceptions by peers. A related issue concerns precocity, or the deviance of smoking, at each age level. Beginning to smoke later, when it is an accepted part of the adolescent life-style, is quite different from early onset during childhood, yet we are unable to specify how precocious smokers differ on relevant variables.

Correspondingly, the absence of data on precocity and other variables pinpointing those at risk for early onset precludes the tailoring of interventions for such high risk groups, particularly disturbing because early onset is associated with heavy smoking later. Data from Powell et al. (1979) illustrate the importance of such tailoring in that their childhood smokers evidenced characteristics that might cause traditional antismoking interventions to actually increase rather than decrease the attractiveness of smoking.

Overall, studies on prevention and intervention have focused too narrowly on outcome criteria, with insufficient attention to process variables. A conceptual expansion utilizing psychophysiological concepts (Leventhal & Cleary, 1980), life stress (Duncan, 1977), moral development (Schneider & Vanmastrigt, 1974), and the Health Belief Model and perceived vulnerability (Stone, 1978), to name a few, would be beneficial. Theoretical frameworks have seldom been utilized in studies of smoking onset and prevention and are much needed to increase our understanding of both the behavior and the theory.

Cessation.   Although knowing the health hazards of smoking is sometimes associated with cessation, especially if the risk is personally salient (Gritz, 1977; Schwartz, 1979; Warnecke, Graham, Rosenthal, & Manfredi, 1978), more often it is not. In fact, those who most need to stop (the heavy smokers) are least likely to do so (Vogt et al., 1979), and some treatments involving smoking may actually strengthen craving if offered when plasma nicotine levels are low (Leventhal & Cleary, 1980), thus perversely reinforcing smoking. Aside from treatment considerations, issues relevant to cessation that merit further attention include motivation, self-efficacy, activity needs, and stresses.

Regarding motivation, Russell (1979) proposes a two-dimensional model for smoking cessation that addresses low and high levels of both motivation to quit and dependency (either pharmacological or nonpharmacological). This yields four motivation – dependency combinations, each requiring a different focus to maximize cessation success. For example, emphasizing treatment to break dependency is most appropriate for smokers high in both dependency and motivation. Increasing motivation is more appropriate for smokers low in both, whereas emphasis on both motivation and treatment is required for high dependency – low motivation smokers. Russell's model underscores the importance of matching the intervention to the smoker, and as 75% of his subjects fell into high dependency groups, shows why primarily motivational approaches so consistently fail.

Self-efficacy is another potentially important variable in cessation and maintenance of abstinence. Marlatt's (1978) theory of relapse predicts that former addicts who perceive themselves as in control (high self-efficacy), but who violate abstinence, are at great risk for relapse. This is due to the resulting cognitive dissonance and internal attributions for failure that create an expectancy for continued failure. In the first empirical test of these predictions (Condiotte & Lichtenstein, 1981), self-efficacy did emerge as important, with higher levels of self-efficacy associated with a higher probability of abstinence during both treatment and the 3-month follow-up period. Futher, there was high correspondence between smoking situations in which self-efficacy was low and those situations actually leading to relapse. However, unlike Marlatt's (1978) prediction that high self-efficacy would predispose toward total relapse if abstinence violation occurred, the present data showed just the reverse: High self-efficacy appeared to insulate subjects from complete relapse as a consequence of smoking. Other research has shown that a related control variable, nonfatalistic outlook on life, is associated with quitting smoking (Straits, 1967) and that smokers and exsmokers show differences in attributions for causes of smoking and reasons for failure to give it up (Wright, 1980). Certainly attributions regarding control and self-efficacy merit further investigation to determine their relationship to pharmacological, psychosocial, and motivational variables and to different modes of intervention.

Activity and arousal needs of smokers represent another underresearched aspect of smoking cessation efforts. It has been suggested that smoking may be a manifestation of an underlying need for activity for which interventions should provide alternative outlets (Blair, Blair, Howe, Pate, Rosenberg, Parker, & Pickle, 1980). Similarly, Noppa and Bengtsson (1980) conclude that increased physical activity is an important intervention component, particularly among those who smoke heavily. Activity and arousal needs imply a focus on physiological aspects of smoking and unfortunately have seldom been considered in intervention research (Flaxman, 1976).

Another untapped but relevant variable in cessation efforts is life stress. This is a central feature of the stress – psychosocial assets model of smoking cessation proposed by Ockene and her colleagues (Ockene, Nutall, Benfari, Hurwitz, & Ockene, 1981). Their model crosses two dimensions, stress and psychosocial assets, to predict the following cessation outcome categories: successful stoppers (low stress, high assets); two groups of recidivists (low stress, low assets; high stress, high assets) and nonstoppers (high stress, low assets). A hard-to-predict borderline group near the intersection of the stress and assets dimensions may contain both recidivists and stoppers.

Obviously maintenance of treatment-induced abstinence is the ultimate test of an intervention's effectiveness, yet it is here that smoking cessation research is most disappointing and least enlightening. Although good, long-term maintenance procedures are seen as pivotal in cessation success, inclusion of a systematic maintenance component in intervention studies is the exception rather than the rule. Clearly this must be remedied. Aspects of maintenance considered important include social reinforcement on both a short-term (Baric, 1979) and long-term (Gritz, 1977) basis, and self-control strategies that give exsmokers nonaddictive alternatives for handling feelings and situations that typically elicit smoking

(Adesso, 1979; Harrup, 1978; Tongas, 1977). Further, there is pressing need for research on the relapse process.

Methodological Issues

Though substantial progress has occurred in smoking research methodology since early reviews, important deficiencies remain. The following paragraphs highlight the major advances as well as the topics requiring continued research attention.

Validity of Measures. Various investigators have questioned whether self-report measures accurately reflect smoking behavior, either for smoking onset (Evans, Hansen, & Mittlemark, 1977; McKennell, 1980) or for cessation (Bernstein & McAlister, 1976). This concern has led to the development of objective measures of smoking. These utilize samples of: (1) carbon monoxide (CO) from blood or expired air; (2) nicotine from saliva, urine, and blood; (3) a nicotine metabolite, from blood; and (4) cotinine and thiocyanate from saliva or blood. The measures are differentially effective. Expired CO shows considerable overlap for smokers and nonsmokers but is nonetheless widely used because of its convenience. Blood samples, on the other hand, are less easily obtained but offer greater accuracy. Due to a longer half-life, cotinine has proved a more sensitive measure than plasma nicotine (Williams, Eng, Botvin, Hill, & Wynder, 1979), with serum thiocyanate being the most appropriate measure for assessing long-term abstinence and detecting very occasional smoking (Paxton & Bernacca, 1979). Various studies utilizing objective measures of smoking have established the validity of self-report data (Hurd et al., 1980; Perry et al., 1980; Williams et al., 1979) though it may be that the accuracy of self-reporting is enhanced by the inclusion of such an objective measure.

Multiple Measures. Another methodological advance concerns the use of multiple measures to assess intervention outcome, and a corresponding broadening of the kind of measures utilized. The importance of using multiple measures has been stressed repeatedly of late (Adesso & Glad, 1978; Glasgow et al., 1981), particularly measures of physiological and subjective effects of interventions in addition to their effects on behavior (Glasgow et al., 1981). The risk of assessing only behavioral change is illustrated by the Vogt et al. (1979) data showing that reductions in smoking rate did not lead to corresponding reductions in health risk, as CO and nicotine levels remained high. The importance of going beyond smoking rate to include a focus on smoking topography and substance smoked has been stressed (Frederiksen, Martin, & Webster, 1979).

Additional Issues. McFall (1978) has presented a cogent critique of smoking research that focuses on issues regarding subjects, methodology, and treatments. Subject problems seriously limiting generalizability of results include: (1) widespread use of volunteer subjects who are nonrepresentative of smokers in general, particularly in motivation to quit; and (2) failure to discuss attrition in terms of rates and characteristics of persons who leave treatment.

Measurement issues affect reliability and validity of data in various ways. Definitions and measurements of smoking have been imprecise, with measurement approaches (e.g., laboratory, self-report, naturalistic) varying across studies. Assessing change has been problematic, particularly establishing a stable estimate of base-line smoking against which to measure intervention outcome. The singular focus on outcome has meant that measurement of the process of smoking change, on both a short- and long-term basis, generally has been overlooked. There also has been a failure to use the same measures both pre- and postintervention. Treatment issues concern problems of relevance and replicability. These are due largely to the absence of theory and the resulting nonsystematic building or dismantling of interventions to isolate components or combinations of them which are effective.

Omission of unaided quitting and attention placebo control groups is a frequent failing in smoking research (Bernstein & Glasgow, 1979), as is the failure to collect long-term follow-up data regarding maintenance of cessation.

In McFall's view a possibly more productive approach would be to study the "folk methods" that have successfully aided smokers to quit on their own, without elaborate interventions. Indeed, data from Schachter (1981, 1982) suggest that smokers who attempt to quit on their own are considerably more successful than those who seek treatment. The latter are a hard-core self-selected group that is more likely to fail, particularly with a single attempt. This, then, has led to the erroneous conclusion that smoking is an intractable addiction.

The lack of an expanded time perspective for data gathering is also a common problem in research regarding smoking onset and prevention (Blaney, 1981). Other methodological problems hindering smoking onset prevention research include the following: (1) a failure until quite recently to focus on young subjects (i.e., grade school age); (2) inconsistent definitions of categories of smoker (particularly the minimal or occasional smoker), thereby obscuring an understanding of the process of movement between categories; and, (3) absence of multivariate data analyses to address longitudinal questions regarding antecedents and correlates of smoking onset as a process across time. Intervention studies too often fail to include appropriate control groups, long-term follow-up evaluation, replication, and detailed description of methodology and procedures, though recent studies are beginning to rectify these omissions.

CONCLUSION

Though problems remain, considerable progress has occurred during the past decade in interventions and research on smoking. Most notable is the increased recognition of the complexity of the problem, as shown in multicomponent interventions with multiple measures and models of smoking that emphasize the interaction of pharmacology with psychological and social factors. Recently proposed models of cessation suggesting the importance of self-efficacy, and the differential impact of various combinations of motivation − dependency or stress − assets represent an untapped potential, as do efforts to utilize nicotine gum and changes in smoking topography. Regarding adolescent smoking, the recent focus on teaching coping skills and the acknowledgment of the value of studying strategies for remaining a nonsmoker represent important advances.

Still needed is a conceptual refocusing to define smoking in terms of the process underlying onset, cessation, or maintenance of abstinence, and the expanded time perspective this implies. Such a focus is necessary before intervention programs can be tailored to maximize effectiveness for persons at different stages of the process. For example, virtually nothing is known about relapse process, yet such knowledge is essential in helping former smokers maintain long-term abstinence—currently the least impressive domain of smoking research. Attention to this and other problems cited in the previous sections should, given the increasing sophistication of measures of smoking behavior, result in significant advances in smoking interventions and research during the decade to come.

REFERENCES

Adesso, V. J. Some correlates between cigarette smoking and alcohol use. *Addictive Behaviors*, 1979, *4*, 269 − 273.

Adesso, V. J., & Glad, W. R. A behavioral test of a smoking typology. *Addictive Behaviors*, 1978, *3*, 35 − 38.

Aronow, W. S. Cigarette smoking, carbon monoxide, nicotine, and coronary disease. *Preventive Medicine*, 1975, *4*, 95 − 99.

Aronow, W. S., Dendinger, J., & Rokaw, S. N. Heart rate and carbon monoxide level after smoking high-, or low-, and non-nicotine cigarettes. A study in male patients with angina pectoris. *Annals of Internal Medicine*, 1971, *74*, 697 − 702.

Astrup, P., & Kjeldsen, K. Model studies linking carbon monoxide and/or nicotine to arteriosclerosis and cardiovascular disease. *Preventive Medicine*, 1979, *8*, 295 − 302.

Bachman, J. G., Johnston, L. D., & O'Malley, P. M. Smoking, drinking, and drug use among American high school students: Correlates and trends, 1975 − 1979. *American Journal of Public Health*, 1981, *71*, 59 − 69.

Baric, L. Preventing relapses after smoking cessation. In L. M. Ramstrom (Ed.), *The smoking epidemic, a matter of worldwide concern*. Stockholm: Almqvist & Wiksell International, 1979.

Baric, L., MacArthur, C., & Sherwood, M. A study of health education aspects of smoking in pregnancy. *International Journal of Health Education*, 1976, *19*, 1 − 16.

Berecz, J. Treatment of smoking with cognitive conditioning therapy: A self-administered aversion technique. *Behavior Therapy*, 1976, *7*, 641 − 648.

Bernstein, D. A. The modification of smoking behavior: An evaluative review. *Psychological Bulletin*, 1969, *71*, 418 − 440.

Bernstein, D. A., & Glasgow, R. E. Smoking. The modification of smoking behavior. In O. F. Pomerleau, (Ed.) *Behavioral medicine: Theory and practice*. Baltimore: Williams & Wilkins, 1979.

Bernstein, D. A., & McAlister, A. The modification of smoking behavior: Progress and problems. *Addictive Behaviors*, 1976, *1*, 89 – 102.

Blair, A., Blair, S. N., Howe, H. G., Pate, R. R., Rosenberg, M., Parker, G. M., & Pickle, L. W. Physical, psychological, and sociodemographic differences among smokers, exsmokers, and nonsmokers in a working population. *Preventive Medicine*, 1980, *9*, 747 – 759.

Blaney, N. T. Cigarette smoking in children and young adolescents: Causes and prevention. In B. Camp (Ed.), *Advances in Behavioral Pediatrics* (Vol. 2). Greenwich, Conn.: JAI Press Inc., 1981.

Blonde, C. V., Webber, L. S., Foster, T. A., & Berenson, G. S. Parental history and cardiovascular disease risk factor variables in children. *Preventive Medicine*, 1981, *10*, 25 – 37.

Bosse, R., Garvey, A. J., & Glynn, R. J. Age and addiction to smoking. *Addictive Behaviors*, 1980, *5*, 341 – 351.

Botvin, G. J., Eng, A., & Williams, C. L. Preventing the onset of cigarette smoking through life skills training. *Preventive Medicine*, 1980, *9*, 135 – 143.

Bradshaw, P. W. The problem of cigarette smoking and its control. *International Journal of the Addictions*, 1973, *8*, 353 – 371.

Bureau of Health Education. *The school health curriculum project*. Washington, D.C.: US Department of Health, Education, and Welfare, Public Health Service, Center for Disease Control, Bureau of Health Education. DHEW Publication No. (CDC) 78 – 8359, 1977.

Champion, R. A., & Bell, D. S. Attitudes toward drug use: Trends and correlations with actual use. *International Journal of the Addictions*, 1980, *15*, 551 – 567.

Cherry, N., & Kiernan, K. Personality scores and smoking behavior. *British Journal of Preventive and Social Medicine*, 1976, *30*, 123 – 131.

Condiotte, M. M., & Lichtenstein, E. Self-efficacy and relapse in smoking cessation programs. *Journal of Consulting and Clinical Psychology*, 1981, *49*, 648 – 658.

Conway, J. B. Behavioral self-control of smoking through aversive conditioning and self-management. *Journal of Consulting and Clinical Psychology*, 1977, *45*, 348 – 357.

Conway, T. L., Vickers, R. R., Ward, H. W., & Rahe, R. H. Occupational stress and variation in cigarette, coffee, and alcohol consumption. *Journal of Health and Social Behavior*, 1981, *22*, 155 – 165.

Costa, P. T., McCrae, R. R., & Bosse, R. Smoking motive factors: A review and replication. *International Journal of the Addictions*, 1980, *15*, 537 – 549.

Creswell, W. H., Huffman, W. J., Stone, D. B., Merki, D. J., & Newman, I. M. University of Illinois antismoking education study. *Illinois Journal of Education*, 1969, *60*, 27 – 37.

Creswell, W. H., Stone, D. B., Huffman, W. F., & Newman, I. M. Antismoking education study at the University of Illinois. Health Service and Mental Health Administration, *Health Reports*, 1971, *86*, 565 – 576.

Danaher, B. G., Shisslak, C. M., Thompson, C. B., & Ford, J. D. A smoking cessation program for pregnant women: An exploratory study. *American Journal of Public Health*, 1978, *68*, 896 – 898.

Delahunt, J., & Curran, J. P. The effectiveness of negative practice and self-control techniques in the reduction of smoking behavior. *Journal of Consulting and Clinical Psychology*, 1976, *44*, 1002 – 1007.

Dicken, C. Sex roles, smoking, and smoking cessation. *Journal of Health and Social Behavior*, 1978, *19*, 324 – 334.

Donovan, J. W. Randomized controlled trial of anti-smoking advice in pregnancy. *British Journal of Preventive and Social Medicine*, 1977, *31*, 6 – 12.

Duncan, D. F. Life stress as a precursor to adolescent drug dependence. *International Journal of the Addictions*, 1977, *12*, 1047 – 1056.

Dunn, W. L. Experimental methods and conceptual models as applied to the study of motivation in cigarette smoking. In W. L. Dunn (Ed.), *Smoking behavior: Motives and incentives*. Washington, D.C.: V. H. Winston & Sons, 1973.

Evans, D., & Lane, D. S. Long-term outcome of smoking cessation workshops. *American Journal of Public Health*, 1980, *70*, 725 – 727.

Evans, R. I., Hansen, W. B., & Mittelmark, M. B. Increasing the validity of self-reports of smoking behavior in children. *Journal of Applied Psychology,* 1977, *62,* 521 – 523.

Evans, R. I., Henderson, A. H., Hill, P. C., & Raines, B. E. Current psychological, social, and educational programs in control and prevention of smoking: A critical methodological review. In A. M. Gotto & R. Paoletti (Eds.), *Atherosclerosis reviews* (Vol. 6). New York: Raven Press, 1979.

Evans, R. I., Rozelle, R. M., Mittelmark, M. B., Hansen, W. B., Bane, A. L., & Havis, J. Deterring the onset of smoking in children: Knowledge of immediate physiological effects and coping with peer pressure, media pressure, and parent modeling. *Journal of Applied Social Psychology,* 1978, *8,* 126 – 135.

Flaxman, J. Quitting smoking. In W. E. Craighead, A. E. Kazdin, & M. J. Mahoney (Eds.), *Behavior modification: Principles, issues, and application.* Boston: Houghton Mifflin Co., 1976.

Flaxman, J. Quitting smoking now or later: Gradual, abrupt, immediate, and delayed quitting. *Behavior Therapy,* 1978, *9,* 260 – 270.

Frederiksen, L. W., Epstein, L. H., & Kosevsky, B. P. Reliability and controlling effects of three procedures for self-monitoring smoking. *Psychological Record,* 1975, *25,* 255 – 264.

Frederiksen, L. W., Martin, J. E., & Webster, J. S. Assessment of smoking behavior. *Journal of Applied Behavior Analysis,* 1979, *12,* 653 – 664.

Frederiksen, L. W., Miller, P. M., & Peterson, G. L. Topographical components of smoking behavior. *Addictive Behaviors,* 1977, *2,* 55 – 61.

Frederiksen, L. W., & Simon, S. J. Modification of smoking topography: A preliminary analysis. *Behavior therapy,* 1978, *9,* 946 – 949. (a)

Frederiksen, L. W., & Simon, S. J. Modifying how people smoke: Instructional control and generalization. *Journal of Applied Behavior Analysis,* 1978, *11,* 431 – 432. (b)

Frederiksen, L. W., & Simon, S. J. Clinical modification of smoking behavior. In R. S. Davidson (Ed.), *Modification of pathological behavior: Experimental analyses of etiology and behavior therapy.* New York: Gardner Press, 1979.

Garfinkel, L. Cardiovascular mortality and cigarette smoking. In L. M. Ramstrom (Ed.), *The smoking epidemic, a matter of worldwide concern.* Stockholm: Almqvist & Wiksell International, 1979.

Glad, W., & Adesso, V. J. The relative importance of socially induced tension and behavioral contagion for smoking behavior. *Journal of Abnormal Psychology,* 1976, *85,* 119 – 121.

Glasgow, R. E., Lichtenstein, E., Beaver, C., & O'Neill, K. Subjective reactions to rapid and normal paced aversive smoking. *Addictive Behaviors,* 1981, *6,* 53 – 59.

Glasgow, R. E., Schafer, L., & O'Neill, H. K. Self-help books and amount of therapist contact in smoking cessation programs. *Journal of Consulting and Clinical Psychology,* 1981, *49,* 659 – 667.

Green, D. E. Youth education. In *Smoking and health: A report of the Surgeon General.* Washington, D.C: US Department of Health, Education, and Welfare, Public Health Service, Office on Smoking and Health, DHEW Publication No. (PHS) 79 – 50066, 1979.

Gritz, E. R. Smoking: The prevention of onset. In M. E. Jarvik, J. W. Cullen, E. R. Gritz, T. M. Vogt, & L. J. West (Eds.), *Research on smoking behavior.* NIDA Research Monograph 17. Washington D.C.: US Department of Health, Education, and Welfare, 1977.

Hall, R. G., Sachs, D. P. L., & Hall, S. M. Medical risk and therapeutic effectiveness of rapid smoking. *Behavior Therapy,* 1979, *10,* 249 – 259.

Hammond, E. C., & Seidman, H. Smoking and cancer in the United States, *Preventive Medicine,* 1980, *9,* 169 – 173.

Hansen, W. B. Monitoring carbon monoxide in conjunction with immediate, delayed, withheld, and vicarious feedback as a means of deterring smoking in children. *Dissertation Abstracts International,* 1978, *39* (Part B – 4), 2009 – 2010.

Harrup, T. Addictive processes in tobacco use. In J. L. Schwartz (Ed.), *Progress in smoking cessation.* Proceedings of the International Conference on Smoking Cessation, June 1978. New York: American Cancer Society, 1978.

Hill, P. C. The impact of immediate physiological consequences versus long-term health consequences on the smoking beliefs, intentions, and behavior of adolescents. *Dissertation Abstracts International,* 1980, *40* (Part B – 8), 4027 – 4028.

Horan, J. J., Linberg, S. E., and Hackett, G. Nicotine poisoning and rapid smoking. *Journal of Consulting and Clinical Psychology*, 1977, *45*, 344 – 347.

Huba, G. J., Wingard, J. A., & Bentler, P. M. Longitudinal analysis of the role of peer support, adult models, and peer subcultures in beginning adolescent substance use: An application of setwise canonical correlation methods. *Multivariate Behavioral Research*, 1980, *15*, 259 – 280.

Hunt, W. A., & Bespalec, D. A. An evaluation of current methods of modifying smoking behavior. *Journal of Clinical Psychology*, 1974, *30*, 431 – 438.

Hunt, W. A., & Matarazzo, J. D. Habit mechanisms in smoking. In W. A. Hunt (Ed.), *Learning mechanisms in smoking*. Chicago: Aldine, 1970.

Hunter, S. M., Webber, L. S., & Berenson, G. S. Cigarette smoking and tobacco usage behavior in children and adolescents: Bogalusa heart study. *Preventive Medicine*, 1980, *9*, 701 – 712.

Hurd, P. D., Johnson, C. A., Pechacek, T., Bast, L. P., Jacobs, D. R., & Luepker, R. V. Prevention of cigarette smoking in seventh-grade students. *Journal of Behavioral Medicine*, 1980, *3*, 15 – 28.

Ikard, F. F., Green, D., & Horn, D. A scale to differentiate between types of smoking as related to the management of affect. *International Journal of the Addictions*, 1969, *4*, 649 – 659.

Ikard, F. F., & Tomkins, S. The experience of affect as a determinant of smoking behavior: A series of validity studies. *Journal of Abnormal Psychology*, 1973, *81*, 172 – 181.

Jason, L. A., & Mollica, M. *Comparative effectiveness of smoking prevention programs*. Paper presented at the meeting of the American Psychological Association, New York, September 1979.

Jessor, R., & Jessor, S. L. Theory testing in longitudinal research on marijuana use. In D. B. Kandel (Ed.), *Longitudinal research on drug use: Empirical findings and methodological issues*. Washington: Hemisphere, 1978.

Joffe, R., Lowe, M. R., & Fisher, E. B. A validity test of the Reasons for Smoking Scale. *Addictive Behaviors*, 1981, *6*, 41 – 45.

Krasnegor, N. A. Introduction. In N. A. Krasnegor (Ed.), *The behavioral aspects of smoking*. NIDA Research Monograph 26. Washington, D.C.: US Department of Health, Education, and Welfare, 1979.

Lando, H. A. Successful treatment of smokers with a broad-spectrum behavioral approach. *Journal of Clinical Psychology*, 1977, *45*, 361 – 366.

Leventhal, H. Changing attitudes and habits to reduce risk factors in chronic disease. *American Journal of Cardiology*, 1973, *31*, 571 – 580.

Leventhal, H., & Avis, N. Pleasure, addiction, and habit: Factors in verbal report or factors in smoking behavior? *Journal of Abnormal Psychology*, 1976, *85*, 478 – 488.

Leventhal H., & Cleary, P. D. The smoking problem: A review of the research and theory in behavioral risk modification. *Psychological Bulletin*, 1980, *88*, 370 – 405.

Leventhal, H., Safer, M. A., Cleary, P. D., & Gutmann, M. Cardiovascular risk modification by community-based programs for life-style change: Comments on the Stanford study. *Journal of Consulting and Clinical Psychology*, 1980, *48*, 150 – 158.

Levinson, B. L., Shapiro, D., Schwartz, G. E., & Tursky, B. Smoking elimination by gradual reduction. *Behavior Therapy*, 1971, *2*, 477 – 487.

Lichstein, K. L., & Stalgaitis, S. J. Treatment of cigarette smoking in couples by reciprocal aversion. *Behavior Therapy*, 1980, *11*, 104 – 118.

Lichtenstein, E., Harris, D. E., Birchler, G. R., Wahl, J. M., & Schmahl, D. P. Comparison of rapid smoking, warm smoky air, and attention placebo in the modification of smoking behavior. *Journal of Consulting and Clinical Psychology*, 1973, *40*, 92 – 98.

Lindenthal, J. L., Myers, J. K., & Pepper, M. P. Smoking, psychological status and stress. *Social Science and Medicine*, 1972, *6*, 583 – 591.

Malcolm, S., & Shephard, R. J. Personality and sexual behavior of the adolescent smoker. *American Journal of Drug Abuse*, 1978, *5*, 87 – 96.

Marlatt, G. A. Craving for alcohol, loss of control, and relapse: A cognitive – behavioral analysis. In P. E. Nathan, G. A. Marlatt, & T. Loberg (Eds.), *Alcoholism: New directions in behavioral research and treatment*. New York: Plenum Press, 1978.

Mausner, B., & Platt, E. S. *Smoking: a behavioral analysis*. New York: Pergamon Press, 1971.

McAlister, A., Perry, C., Killen, J., Slinkard, L. A., & Maccoby, N. Pilot study of smoking, alcohol, and drug abuse prevention. *American Journal of Public Health,* 1980, *70,* 719 – 721.

McAlister, A. L., Perry, C., & Maccoby, N. Adolescent smoking: Onset and prevention. *Pediatrics,* 1979, *63,* 650 – 658.

McFall, R. M. Effects of self-monitoring on normal smoking behavior. *Journal of Consulting and Clinical Psychology,* 1970, *35,* 135 – 142.

McFall, R. M. Smoking-cessation research. *Journal of Consulting and Clinical Psychology,* 1978, *46,* 703 – 712.

McFall, R. M., & Hammen, C. L. Motivation, structure, and self-monitoring: Role of nonspecific factors in smoking reduction. *Journal of Consulting and Clinical Psychology,* 1971, *37,* 80 – 86.

McKennell, A. C. Bias in the reported incidence of smoking in children. *International Journal of Epidemiology,* 1980, *9,* 167 – 177.

Meyer, A. J., Nash, J. D., McAlister, A. L., Maccoby, N., & Farquhar, J. W. Skills training in a cardiovascular health education campaign. *Journal of Consulting and Clinical Psychology,* 1980, *48,* 129 – 142.

Murray, M., & Cracknell, A. Adolescents' views on smoking. *Journal of Psychosomatic Research,* 1980, *24,* 243 – 251.

Murray, R. G., & Hobbs, S. A. Effects of self-reinforcement and self-punishment in smoking reduction: Implications for broad-spectrum behavioral approaches. *Addictive Behaviors,* 1981, *6,* 63 – 67.

Noppa, H., & Bengtsson, C. Obesity in relation to smoking: A population study of women in Goteborg, Sweden. *Preventive Medicine,* 1980, *9,* 534 – 543.

Nostbakken, D. Power of mass media in smoking cessation. In L. M. Ramstrom (Ed.), *The smoking epidemic, a matter of worldwide concern.* Stockholm: Almqvist & Wiksell International, 1979.

Nye, P. A., Haye, K. L., McKenzie-Pollock, D. J. B., Caughley, B. L., & Housham, R. W. What encourages and discourages children to smoke? Knowledge about health hazards and recommendations for health education. *New Zealand Medical Journal,* 1980, *91,* 432 – 435.

Ockene, J. K., Nutall, R., Benfari, R. C., Hurwitz, I., & Ockene, I. S. A psychosocial model of smoking cessation and maintenance of cessation. *Preventive Medicine,* 1981, *10,* 623 – 638.

O'Connor, K. The contingent negative variation and individual differences in smoking behavior. *Personality and Individual Differences,* 1980, *1,* 57 – 72.

Paxton, R. The effects of a deposit contract as a component in a behavioural programme for stopping smoking. *Behaviour Research & Therapy,* 1980, *18,* 45 – 50.

Paxton, R., & Bernacca, G. Urinary nicotine concentration as a function of time since last cigarette: Implications for detecting faking in smoking clinics. *Behavior Therapy,* 1979, *10,* 523 – 528.

Pederson, L. L., Stennett, R. G., & Lefcoe, N. M. The effects of a smoking education program on the behavior, knowledge and attitudes of children in grades 4 and 6. *Journal of Drug Education,* 1981, *11,* 141 – 149.

Perry, C., Killen, J., Telch, M., Slinkard, L. A., & Danaher, B. G. Modifying smoking behavior of teenagers: A school-based intervention. *American Journal of Public Health,* 1980, *70,* 722 – 725.

Peto, J. The health effects of smoking in women. In L. M. Ramstrom (Ed.), *The smoking epidemic, a matter of worldwide concern.* Stockholm: Almqvist & Wiksell International, 1979.

Poole, A. D., Sanson-Fisher, R. W., German, G. A., & Harker, J. The rapid-smoking technique: Some physiological effects. *Behaviour Research & Therapy,* 1980, *18,* 581 – 586.

Powell, D. R., & McCann, B. S. The effects of a multiple treatment program and maintenance procedures on smoking cessation. *Preventive Medicine,* 1981, *10,* 94 – 104.

Powell, G. E., Steward, R. A., & Grylls, D. G. The personality of young smokers. *British Journal of Addiction,* 1979, *74,* 311 – 315.

Raw, M., Jarvis, M. J., Feyerabend, C., & Russell, M. A. H. Comparisons of nicotine chewing gum and psychological treatments for dependent smokers. *British Medical Journal,* 1980, *281,* 481 – 482.

Raw, M., & Russell, M. A. H. Rapid smoking, cue exposure and support in the modification of smoking. *Behaviour Research & Therapy*, 1980, *18*, 363 – 372.

Rawbone, R. G., Keeling, C. A., Jenkins, A., & Guz, A. Cigarette smoking among secondary school children in 1975. *Journal of Epidemiology and Community Health*, 1978, *32*, 53 – 58.

Robins, L. N., Davis, D. H., & Goodwin, D. W. Drug use by US Army enlisted men in Vietnam: A follow-up on their return home. *American Journal of Epidemiology*, 1974, *99*, 235 – 249.

Rozensky, R. H. The effect of timing of self-monitoring on reducing cigarette consumption. *Journal of Behavior Therapy and Experimental Psychiatry*, 1974, *5*, 301 – 303.

Russell, M. A. H. Cigarette dependence: I. Nature and classification. *British Medical Journal*, 1971, *2*, 330 – 331. (a)

Russell, M. A. H. Cigarette smoking: Natural history of a dependence disorder. *British Journal of Medical Psychology*, 1971, *44*, 1 – 16. (b)

Russell, M. A. H. Smoking as a dependence disorder. In L. M. Ramstrom (Ed.), *The smoking epidemic, a matter of worldwide concern*. Stockholm: Almqvist & Wiksell International, 1979.

Russell, M. A. H. Nicotine intake and its regulation. *Journal of Psychosomatic Research*, 1980, *24*, 253 – 264.

Russell, M. A. H., Armstrong, E., & Patel, U. A. The role of temporal contiguity in electric aversion therapy for cigarette smoking: Analysis of behavior changes. *Behaviour Research and Therapy*, 1976, *14*, 103 – 123.

Russell, M. A. H., Cole, P. V., & Brown, E. Passive smoking: Absorption by nonsmokers of carbon monoxide from room air polluted by tobacco smoke. *Postgraduate Medical Journal*, 1973, *49*, Part 2, 688 – 692.

Russell, M. A. H., Jarvis, M., Iyer, R., & Feyerabend, C. Relation of nicotine yield of cigarettes to blood nicotine concentrations in smokers. *British Medical Journal*, 1980, *280*, 972 – 976.

Russell, M. A. H., Peto, J., & Patel, U. A. The classification of smoking by factorial structure of motives. *Journal of the Royal Statistical Society*, 1974, *137* (Part 3), 313 – 333.

Russell, M. A. H., Raw, M., & Jarvis, M. J. Clinical use of nicotine chewing gum. *British Medical Journal*, 1980, *280*, 1599 – 1602.

kussell, M. A. H., Wilson, C., Cole, P. V., Idle, M., & Feyerabend, C. Comparison of increases in carboxyhaemoglobin after smoking "extra-mild" and "non-mild" cigarettes. *Lancet*, 1973, *2*, 687 – 690.

Russell, M. A. H., Wilson, C., Taylor, C., & Baker, C. D. Smoking habits of men and women. *British Medical Journal*, 1980, *281*, 17 – 20.

Scarpetti, F. R., & Datesman, S. K. (Eds.) *Drugs and the youth culture. Sage annual reviews of drug and alcohol abuse* (Vol. 4) Beverly Hills: Sage Publications, 1980.

Schachter, S. Nicotine regulation in heavy and light smokers. *Journal of Experimental Psychology: General*, 1977, *106*, 5 – 12.

Schachter, S. Self-treatment of smoking and obesity. *Canadian Journal of Public Health*, 1981, *72*, 401 – 406.

Schachter, S. Recidivism and self-cure of smoking and obesity. *American Psychologist*, 1982, *37*, 436 – 444.

Schachter, S., Kozlowski, L. T., & Silverstein, B. Effects of urinary pH on smoking. *Journal of Experimental Psychology: General*, 1977, *106*, 13 – 19.

Schachter, S., Silverstein, B., & Perlick, D. Psychological and pharmacological explanations of smoking under stress. *Journal of Experimental Psychology: General*, 1977, *106*, 31 – 40.

Schmal, D. P., Lichtenstein, E., & Harris, D. E. Successful treatment of habitual smokers with warm, smoky air, and rapid smoking. *Journal of Consulting and Clinical Psychology*, 1972, *38*, 105 – 111.

Schneider, F. W., & Vanmastrigt, L. A. Adolescent – preadolescent differences in beliefs and attitudes about cigarette smoking. *Journal of Psychology*, 1974, *87*, 71 – 81.

Schwartz, J. L. Review and evaluation of methods of smoking cessation, 1969 – 77. *Public Health Reports*, 1979, *94*, 558 – 563.

Seltzer, A. P. Anti-smoking lozenge. *Journal of the National Medical Association,* 1975, *67,* 311 – 313.

Shapiro, D., Tursky, B., Schwartz, G. E., & Schnidman, S. R. Smoking on cue: A behavioral approach to smoking reduction. *Journal of Health and Social Behavior,* 1971, *12,* 108 – 113.

Shiffman, S. M., & Jarvik, M. E. Smoking withdrawal symptoms in two weeks of abstinence. *Psychopharmacology,* 1976, *50,* 35 – 39.

Silverstein, B., Feld, S., & Kozlowski, L. T. The availability of low-nicotine cigarettes as a cause of cigarette smoking among teenage females. *Journal of Health and Social Behavior,* 1980, *21,* 383 – 388.

Simon, W. E., & Primavera, L. H. The personality of the cigarette smoker: Some empirical data. *International Journal of the Addictions,* 1976, *11,* 81 – 94.

Slone, D., Shapiro, S., Rosenberg, L., Kaufman, D. W., Hartz, S. C., Rossi, A. C., Stolley, P. D., & Miettinen, O. S. Relation of cigarette smoking to myocardial infarction in young women. *New England Journal of Medicine,* 1978, *298,* 1273 – 1276.

Smith, G. M. Personality and smoking: A review of empirical literature. In W. A. Hunt (Ed.), *Learning mechanisms in smoking.* Chicago: Aldine, 1970.

Smith, G. M., & Fogg, C. P. Psychological predictors of early use, late use, and nonuse of marijuana among teenage students. In D. B. Kandel (Ed.), *Longitudinal research on drug use: Empirical findings and methodological issues.* Washington, D.C.: Hemisphere, 1978.

Spitzzeri, A., & Jason, L. A. Prevention and treatment of smoking in school age children. *Journal of Drug Education,* 1979, *9,* 315 – 326.

Stepney, R. Smoking behaviour: A psychology of the cigarette habit. *British Journal of Diseases of the Chest,* 1980, *74,* 325 – 344.

Stern, M. P., Farquhar, J. W., Maccoby, N., & Russell, S. H. Results of a two-year health education campaign on dietary behavior: The Stanford Three Community Study. *Circulation,* 1976, *54,* 826 – 833.

Stone, J. The effects of a fifth-grade health education curriculum model on perceived vulnerability and smoking attitudes. *Journal of School Health,* 1978, *48,* 667 – 671.

Straits, B. C. The discontinuation of cigarette smoking: a multiple discriminant analysis. In S. V. Zagona (Ed.), *Studies and issues in smoking behavior.* Tucson: University of Arizona Press, 1967.

Sutherland, A., Amit, Z., Golden, M., & Roseberger, Z. Comparison of three behavioral techniques in the modification of smoking behavior. *Journal of Consulting and Clinical Psychology,* 1975, *43,* 443 – 447.

Telch, M. J., Killen, J. D., McAlister, A. L., Perry, C. L., & Maccoby, N. Long-term follow-up of a pilot project on smoking prevention with adolescents. *Journal of Behavioral Medicine,* 1982, *5,* 1 – 8.

Tennant, F. S. Awareness of substance abuse and other health-related behaviors among preschool children. *Journal of Drug Education,* 1979, *9,* 119 – 128.

Tomkins, S. Psychological model for smoking behavior. *American Journal of Public Health,* 1966, *56,* 17 – 27.

Tomkins, S. A modified model of smoking behavior. In E. F. Borgatta & R. R. Evans (Eds.), *Smoking health and behavior.* Chicago: Aldine, 1968.

Tongas, P. N. The long-term maintenance of nonsmoking behavior. In M. E. Jarvik, J. W. Cullen, E. R. Gritz, T. M. Vogt, & L. J. West (Eds.), *Research on smoking behavior.* NIDA Research Monograph 17. Washington, D.C.: US Department of Health, Education, and Welfare, 1977.

Tongas, P. N., Patterson, J., & Goodkind, S. *Cessation of smoking through behavior modification.* Paper presented at the meeting of the Association for the Advancement of Behavior Therapy, New York, December 1976.

Tryon, W. W., Vaughter, R. M., & Ginorio, A. B. Smoking behavior as a function of social cues and sex: A naturalistic study. *Sex Roles,* 1977, *3,* 337 – 344.

Vogt, T. M., Selvin, S., & Billings, J. H. Smoking cessation program: Baseline carbon monoxide and serum thiocyanate levels as predictors of outcome. *American Journal of Public Health,* 1979, *69,* 1156 – 1159.

Vogt, T. M., Selvin, S., Widdowson, G., & Hulley, S. B. Expired air carbon monoxide and serum thiocyanate as objective measures of cigarette exposure. *American Journal of Public Health*, 1977, *67*, 545 – 549.

Warnecke, R. B., Graham, S., Rosenthal, S., & Manfredi, C. Social and psychological correlates of smoking behavior among black women. *Journal of Health & Social Behaior*, 1978, *19*, 397 – 410.

Warner, K. E. The effects of the anti-smoking campaign on cigarette consumption. *American Journal of Public Health*, 1977, *67*, 645 – 650.

West, D. W., Graham, S., Swanson, M., & Wilkinson, G. Five-year follow-up of a smoking withdrawal clinic population. *American Journal of Public Health*, 1977, *67*, 536 – 544.

Williams, C. L. Primary prevention of cancer beginning in childhood. *Preventive Medicine*, 1980, *9*, 275 – 280.

Williams, C. L., Carter, B. J., & Wynder, E. Prevalence of selected cardiovascular and cancer risk factors in a pediatric population: The "Know Your Body" project, New York. *Preventive Medicine*, 1981, *10*, 235 – 250.

Williams, C. L., Eng, A., Botvin, G. J., Hill, P., & Wynder, E. L. Validation of students' self-reported cigarette smoking status with plasma cotinine levels. *American Journal of Public Health*, 1979, *69*, 1272 – 1274.

Williams, C. L., & Wynder, E. A blind spot in preventive medicine. *Journal of the American Medical Association*, 1976, *236*, 2196 – 2197.

World Health Organization. *Smoking and its effect on health.* Technical Report Series 568. Geneva: WHO, 1975.

World Health Organization. *Controlling the smoking epidemic.* Technical Report Series 636. Geneva: WHO, 1979.

Wright, S. J. Actor – observer differences in attributions for smoking: Introducing ex-actors and attributions for failure to give up. *British Journal of Social and Clinical Psychology*, 1980, *19*, 49 – 50.

14　Behavioral Medicine and Alcoholism

Robert S. Davidson
Miami VA Medical Center

INTRODUCTION

In the Middle Ages, when distilling techniques were first used to produce alcohol for consumption, there was a common belief that a remedy for all disease had been discovered. In contemporary society, alcoholism is one of the nation's most serious health problems, probably claiming more lives through direct and indirect causes than all other health problems with the exceptions of cancer and cardiovascular disease (NIAAA, 1974). The use of alcohol in excessive amounts directly affects 10 to 12 million people in the United States. The total number of alcoholics in this country is estimated to be more than 5% of the population (NIAAA, 1974; Wilkinson, 1970). This rate places the United States among the nations with the highest rates of alcoholism in the world.

The cultural stereotype of the alcoholic as a skid row bum represents only about 5% of all alcoholics. Ten percent of the nation's work force are thought to be alcoholic or to have serious alcoholic problems (Chafetz, 1976; Wilkinson, 1970). Alcoholism costs the country an estimated $26 billion each year; most of these losses are through absenteeism and substandard work performance (Chafetz, 1976; NIAAA, 1974).

Alcoholism is among the major risk factors for death from cirrhosis of the liver, heart disease, and suicide (Wallgren & Barry, 1970). Alcoholics are involved in over half of all traffic accidents and resultant deaths, and perpetrators and victims of homicides have been found with significant levels of blood alcohol more often than not (NIAAA, 1974; Wilkinson, 1970). Alcoholism not only results in a variety of other medical and psychological diseases and disorders, but reduces life expectancy by 10-12 years (Chafetz, 1976; Davidson, 1979).

379

Drinking alcohol in excessive amounts is clearly a behavioral problem of major proportions. This chapter reviews the effects of alcohol, determinants of alcoholism, and systematic attempts to intervene in the behavior of the alcoholic.

DEFINITION AND DIAGNOSIS OF ALCOHOLISM

There is no uniform description of the primary components of alcoholism. For the diagnostician, this is the problem of labeling. The variety of definitions of this disease range from the conservative medical perspective of Jellinek (1960) and the pharmacological classification systems (Mello, 1979) to a holistic diagnosis involving adaptation and function in most important life areas, such as psychological, social, sexual, occupational, and family adjustment, as well as specific drinking behaviors and medical symptoms (Davidson, 1979).

The best known and most widely applied definition of alcoholism was proposed by the committee of experts brought together by the World Health Organization (WHO). According to WHO (1952): "Alcoholics are those excessive drinkers whose dependence upon alcohol has attained such a degree that it shows a noticeable mental disturbance or an interference with their bodily and mental health, their interpersonal relations, and their smooth social and economic functioning, or who show the prodromal signs of such developments [p. 16]." A simpler (although perhaps oversimplified) and more objective definition of alcoholism is a pharmacological one, which focuses upon the criteria of physical dependence and tolerance. This definition is tantamount to defining alcoholism as an addiction, with similarities to addiction to narcotic and barbiturate drugs (Mello, 1979). As a refinement, Mello further elucidates the varieties of tolerance (i.e., metabolic, behavioral, or cross-tolerance), each of which can be tested objectively.

Early behavioral studies of alcoholism focused on drinking behavior and associated topography. From this point of view, pathological behavior of any kind could be defined as any behavior not supported by the reinforcing community (Davidson, 1979). Pathological behavior defined in this way consists of behavioral excesses or deficits; behavior lacking stimulus control or under inappropriate stimulus control (such as solitary drinking).

In an effort to produce diagnostic uniformity and standardization, 65 experienced medical scholars contributed criteria for the diagnosis of alcoholism to the National Council on Alcoholism (1972). These criteria were weighted for diagnostic significance and assembled according to whether they were physiological, clinical, behavioral, psychological, and/or attitudinal. Criteria such as those proposed by this committee not only help to objectify and standardize the major dimensions involved in diagnosis, but also help to clarify the elements of a holistic definition. Such a broad-based definition appears to be useful for those who assess and treat alcoholics within a behavioral medicine framework. These are summarized in outline form in Table 14.1. Unfortunately they have not been widely adopted and used in diagnosing alcoholism.

EFFECTS OF ALCOHOL

By their own drinking behavior, alcoholics and heavy drinkers produce physical and medical symptoms that are roughly correlated with the pattern of alcohol consumption (Mello, 1979). The effects may include the immediate symptoms of intoxication and/or hangover, and the long-term consequences of physical dependence, withdrawal symptoms, or the abstinence syndrome.

Signs and symptoms of inebriation or intoxication are dose dependent and resemble the four stages of anesthesia as summarized in Table 14.2. The initial effect of small doses appears to be stimulating. Excited or uninhibited behavior may occur. Tension may be reduced, and the individual may experience an expansive feeling of sociability and well-being (Docter & Perkins, 1971; Steffen, Nathan, & Taylor, 1974). This is usually due to depression of inhibitory areas of the brain.

As larger doses depress the brain, interference with complex thought processes occurs, followed by impairment of motor coordination, balance, speech, and vision. In very large doses, blunting of pain, increases in anxiety, loss of consciousness, sedation, and sleep may be observed. Before the days of modern anesthesia, alcohol was sometimes used to prepare patients for surgery (Wallgren & Barry, 1970).

Physical dependence is one of the hallmarks of alcoholism. The pathognomonic indicator of dependence is the appearance of withdrawal symptoms (the abstinence syndrome) after alcohol ingestion is terminated. Recent research has demonstrated that exposure to low concentrations of alcohol vapor for perhaps as short a time as 1 or 2 weeks may induce physical dependence on alcohol in rats (French & Morris, 1972). Consumption of as little as 8 oz of whiskey per day or maintenance of blood alcohol levels as low as 50 mg percent may be sufficient to produce physical dependence in humans (Mello, 1979).

The abstinence syndrome includes withdrawal symptoms such as nausea, vomiting, hyperthermia, gastrointestinal irritation, convulsions, delirium tremens, and death. Long-term, steady diets of alcohol may lead to blackouts, loss of memory, pancreatitis, stomach ulceration, peripheral neuropathy, cirrhosis of the liver, cardiovascular disease, brain damage, and cancer (especially in smokers). Toxic effects of long-term consumption of large volumes of alcohol have been observed in every major organ and system in the body, including the heart, liver, intestines, brain, throat, and muscles (Mello, 1979). Diseases that may result from long-term alcohol consumption, associated symptoms and known or suspected etiological mechanisms are listed in Table 14.3.

TABLE 14.1
Physiological, Clinical, Behavioral, Psychological, and Social Diagnostic Criteria for Alcoholism
(After the National Council on Alcoholism, 1972)

Physiological
1. Dependence as evidenced by withdrawal syndrome
   Tremors
   Hallucinosis
   Withdrawal seizures
   Delirium tremens
2. Tolerance as evidenced by amount drunk
   Blood alcohol greater than 150 mg/without gross intoxication
   One fifth gal. per day of whiskey or equivalent
3. "Blackouts" from excessive drinking

Clinical
Signs of illness associated with alcohol consumption

Alcohol hepatitis	Peripheral neuropathy
Laennec's cirrhosis	Alcohol myopathy
Pancreatitis	Alcohol cardiomyopathy
Chronic gastritis	Beriberi Pellagra
Wernicke-Korsakoff syndrome	

Alcohol cerebellar degeneration in the absence of arteriosclerosis

Behavioral (Signs depend on stage of development)
   Drinking in gulps
   Surreptitious drinking
   Morning drinking
   Drinking despite medical contraindications

Psychological
   Several conscious attempts to stop
   Drinking to relieve emotional upset, e.g., anger, anxiety, jealousy, resentment
   Subjective feeling of loss of control
   Denial of obvious drinking problems
   Organization of life-style relevant to drinking, e.g., job, friends, hang-outs
   Rage and/or suicidal gestures while drinking

Familial-Social
   Complaints by spouse and family members
   Family disruptions related to alcohol
   Changes in family status, social and business relations
   Preference for bars and drinking companions
   Medical excuses from work, job loss or changes
   Frequent accidents
   Loss of interest in activities not related to drinking

TABLE 14.2
Effects of Alcohol
Immediate Effects of Alcohol (Signs and Symptoms of Intoxication)

Dose (In a 150 lb. person)	BAC (Blood alcohol concentration)	Signs	Symptoms
1 oz.	.03	Feelings of well-being, warmth	Stimulation, disinhibition
2 oz.	.05	Nystagmus, tremor driving, rational thought affected	Impaired muscular control, judgment
4 oz.	.10	Driving usually affected, unsteady gait	Slowed reaction time, ataxia
6 oz.	.15	Vomiting, blurring of vision, loss of balance, falling	Impaired balance, loss of muscular control
12 oz.	.30	Sedated	Stuporous
20 oz.	.50	Loss of consciousness	Coma
22 oz.	.55	Respiratory collapse, cardiac failure	Death

Note: Partially derived from M. Grant & P. Gwinner (Eds.), *Alcoholism in perspective*. Baltimore, Md.: University Park Press, 1979, p. 18.

TABLE 14.3
Medical Sequellae to Long-Term Alcohol Use

Disease	Symptoms	Etiology or Mechanism
Cirrhosis	Fever, loss of appetite, pain, nausea, jaundice	Unknown, fatty infiltration of cells, scarring and malnutrition suspected
Pancreatitis	Epigastric pain, jaundice, fever	Unknown, toxic effects plus malnutrition suspected
Acute gastritis	Nausea, pain, vomiting	Unknown, toxic inflammatory process suspected
Cardiomyopathy	Dyspnea, palpitations, enlargement	Fatty infiltration of muscle cells
Anemia	Weakness, irritability, GI symptoms	Folic acid, B12 deficiency
Wernicke-Korsakoff syndrome	Confabulation, perseveration, short term memory problems, dementia	Destruction of brain cells
Neuropathy	Paresthesias, lack of sensation	Damaged peripheral nerves

From Mello (1979).

Physiological Effects of Alcohol

Alcohol is rapidly absorbed into the blood from the stomach, small intestine, and colon. It is uniformly distributed throughout the body in plasma. In moderate doses it produces vasodilation which facilitates its circulation.

The major effect of alcohol is in the central nervous system, where it acts as a general anesthetic, depressing activity in higher neural centers. This effect frees the brain from inhibitory influences, resulting in an apparent stimulating effect. The integrating functions of the cortex and the reticular system are also disrupted. There is an associated depression of respiratory rate, an increase in pain threshold, an increase in catecholamine levels due to blockage of reuptake, and an increase in diuresis due to decreased tubular reabsorption of water.

Approximately 90% of the alcohol in the body is oxidized at a relatively constant rate of 10 ml/hour. This occurs primarily in the liver via alcohol dehydrogenase to produce acetylaldehyde. This is degredated to acetic acid via the action of aldehyde dehydrogenase. The byproducts of this process are used in the synthesis of cholesterol and fatty acids. The carbohydrates in alcohol are a source of energy but alcohol has no vitamins to support other nutritional needs. Because of the oxidation of alcohol, very little is excreted from the body via urine.

Excessive alcohol use puts a number of demands on the physiological and biochemical system of the body. Ethanol oxidation uses from 75 to 100% of the oxygen that is normally available for other oxidative reactions. The overproduction of acetic acid disrupts the Krebs cycle production of energy and the oxidation of free fatty acids. Concentrations of high-density lipoproteins in blood increase while low-density lipoproteins decrease. Gastric acid secretions in the stomach increase.

Over an extended period of time, these effects are disruptive to a great number of physiological functions, producing the variety of diseases that are presented by the alcohol abuser. For example, the altered oxidation of fatty acids and their release into the blood produces an accumulation of fat in the space of Disse in the liver, obstructing normal biochemical exchanges and leading ultimately to cirrhosis. Gastritis resulting from the excessive release of stomach acid is another common condition accompanying excessive alcohol consumption.

The effects of alcohol on the cardiovascular system are dependent on dosage and duration of use. Chronic excessive use produces lesions in the cells of the myocardium, producing dilated cardiomyopathy with associated congestive heart failure. On the other hand, alcohol in moderate dosages may be protective of coronary heart disease via the decrease in low-density lipoproteins that is associated with atherosclerosis (see Hammer & Schneiderman, Chapter 17).

Chronic ingestion of alcohol also produces neurological damage to cells within the central nervous system. Wernicke's encephalopathy and Korsakoff's psychosis are common syndromes among long-term alcohol users. There is some debate as to whether these effects are due to alcohol ingestion or to nutritional and vitamin deficiencies occurring secondary to poor food intake and abnormal metabolic functions. Recent studies suggest that alcohol produces neurological damage even when diet is relatively normal.

EPIDEMIOLOGY AND INCIDENCE

Epidemiological studies have brought together a great deal of information of potential relevance to the understanding of alcoholism and its amelioration. Traditional epidemiological studies have focused on the incidence and prevalence of alcoholism in large cultural or subcultural samples from the population. Such studies reveal patterns in the development of alcoholism such as age relationships, the identification of subcultural groups that show more than the expected rates of alcoholism, and other predictors of the onset and risk.

The first survey of American drinking practices reported that about 68% of the adult population drink at least once per year, while 22% reported that they had never consumed alcoholic beverages (Cahalan, 1970). In this large sample 12% were described as heavy drinkers. This included 21% of the men and 5% of the women. Later population studies have shown that the highest incidence of reported drinking problems occurs among men in their early 20s, with the average institutionalized alcoholic being in his 40s (Cahalan & Cisin, 1976). However, people do not show uniform patterns of development of drinking problems. Plateaus of severity may develop and remain constant and many people move in and out of problem or symptomatic drinking. Thus, any attempts to develop models of the time course or natural history of alcoholism represent statistical artifacts, which may not fit many individual cases.

Development of Alcoholism

There are ample data to suggest that drinking increases during teen years when individuals may be influenced heavily by peer models, by conflicts over identity, and by problems of transition to adulthood. Although an increasing number of cases of teen alcoholism have been reported, the modal peak of problems due to alcoholism is during the 20s (Cahalan & Cisin, 1976).

Studies with animals have indicated that alcohol dependence can be produced in as little as 3 days in mice (Freund, 1969) and 10 – 14 days in primates (Ellis & Pick, 1970). However, in the natural human environment, alcoholic patients have reported wide variability in the time taken to develop physical dependence. This has been supported by observation and reports of withdrawal symptoms following the removal of alcohol from the diet in patients undergoing treatment for alcoholism. In one such study, the range reported for the development of physical dependence was 1 – 32 years (Mendelson & Mello, 1979). Over half the patients in this study reported the appearance of withdrawal symptoms between the fifth and fifteenth years of heavy drinking.

Jellinek (1952) suggested that there was a common pattern of development of alcoholism distinguished by four primary phases: (1) *prealcoholic*, a time when drinking increases for relief of distress, and tolerance for increased amounts of alcohol occurs; (2) *prodromal*, when drinking increases further, the drinker becomes preoccupied with alcohol, and blackouts begin to occur; (3) *the crucial phase*, when loss of tolerance, development of guilt about drinking, fear of discovery, and social isolation occur. Morning drinking, deterioration of health, and the first hospitalization may occur in this phase; (4) *the chronic final phase*, when social and physical deterioration are present with withdrawal symptoms each time the person stops drinking. A loss of tolerance for alcohol and prolonged drinking bouts and binges are also characteristic.

Several studies have lent empirical support to Jellinek's proposed model of alcoholic development. Some investigators have found that many alcoholics reported the development of clusters of symptoms although not always in a consistent, predictable sequence (Trice & Wahl, 1958). For example, morning or daytime drinking was usually but not always reported to precede long drinking bouts or "benders."

Contradictory data has shown that the course of alcoholism varies more among individuals than Jellinek's model suggests. Park (1973), for example, used newer statistical techniques to analyze Jellinek's data, with the result that the original data did not support any overall chronological order and sequence of development of symptom patterns. Similarly, Orford (1974) examined the developmental sequence in a large sample of alcoholics in England, reporting great variation in the sequence, with no identifiable shared pattern or stages of development.

We have already reviewed data that suggest a great amount of turnover, including movements into and out of problem drinker populations (Clark & Cahalan, 1976). Some long-term follow-up studies have reported decreases, rather than increases in the number of problem drinkers first identified in college and then interviewed again 20 years later (Fillmore, 1974). Similarly, a group of Army servicemen who suffered drinking problems in Vietnam reported no further problems with drinking after returning home.

Patterns of "reactive" drinking, or drinking in the presence of situational stress, have been reported with increasing frequency. The reactive drinking pattern may develop in mid-life following acute life changes or stress beyond the person's ability to cope (Blum & Levine, 1975). Aged or recently retired persons may develop the first serious drinking problems of their lives because of inability to cope with retirement or to find constructive activities to fill the void of leisure time (Gaitz & Baer, 1971; Schuckit, 1977).

Reports such as those already reviewed, which found decreases in drinking problems after age 29 in large populations (Cahalan & Cisin, 1976), decreases in problem drinkers interviewed 20 years after problems in college (Fillmore, 1974), and decreases in problem drinking following return home from Vietnam (Goodwin, David, & Robins, 1975), suggest that alcoholism may not be an irreversible disease process that cannot be treated, but only arrested, as Jellinek originally proposed (1952).

Comparisons of plots of incidence and prevalence in large groups have been used to analyze the time course of alcoholism. Drew (1968) found that the curves of predicted prevalence (cumulative new cases reported each year) and actual prevalence (total cases each year) among three million patients treated by the Mental Health Department in Victoria, Australia in 1963 approximated each other only until age 40. By contrast, similar curves plotting predicted prevalence and actual prevalence of a chronic, incurable condition (chronic alcoholic psychosis) in New York state mental hospitals were almost identical up to age 85. The plots were smooth ogives or "S" curves. The observed decrease in incidence of alcoholism after age 40 may have been due to many factors, including mortality, spontaneous recovery, and treatment. It suggests a time-limited course of alcoholism and a definite relationship with age.

THEORIES OF ALCOHOLIC ETIOLOGY

Although there has been a great proliferation of information regarding alcoholism, especially in the last 15 years, the lack of critical information of a heuristic nature is nowhere more evident than in the relationship between theoretical models of the etiology of alcoholism and supporting data. It would seem that there are as many models as theoretical orientations, or almost as many as individual authors. Some of these models seem to wax and wane in popularity, without predictable relationship to empirical support (Conger, 1956; Franks, 1958; Jellinek, 1960; Mello, 1979; Wikler & Pescor, 1961).

Biological Models

Among the biological models, theories of genetic transmission have received the most support. Jellinek, for example, found that an overall average of 52% of all the alcoholics he studied had at least one alcoholic parent (1960). Although the expectancy rate of alcoholism in the general population is about $5-10\%$, he estimated it at $20-30\%$ in families where at least one parent is alcoholic. Although these findings are not inconsistent with genetic transmission, they could also be the result of psychosocial influences.

Goodwin (1971, 1976) recently found that 55 adult males separated in infancy from their biological parents showed increased probability of becoming alcoholic over matched adopted controls. In another study children of alcoholic biological parents raised by nonalcoholic parents showed greater probability of becoming alcoholic than did children of nonalcoholic parents adopted by alcoholic parents (Schuckit, Goodwin, & Winokur, 1972). These studies suggest the genetic transmission of alcoholism, although they lack the control implicit in twin studies.

Several twin studies, however, also support the genetic transmission model. Kaij (1960) studied 174 male twin pairs in Sweden. At least one of each twin pair was alcoholic. The rate of concordance for alcoholism was 54% for monozygotic and 28% for dizygotic twins. In addition, he found that the degree of concordance increased with the degree of alcohol abuse. In a study of 902 male Finnish twins, Partanen, Bruun, and Markkanen (1966) reported an influence of heredity on amount of drinking and "lack of control" in a young group, but no differences between monozygotic and dizygotic twins regarding "social complication" of drinking. Both studies support the proposition that there is a high probability of the transmission of alcoholism through a genetic mechanism.

Behavioral Models

Perhaps the most popular psychological model of the etiology of alcoholism is the tension-reduction hypothesis. Beginning with the study of Masserman and Yum (1946), who found that alcohol resolved an "experimental neurosis" formed by delivering electric shock to cats as they ate, most of the etiological studies of the 1950s and 1960s were designed to test this model. Essentially, the model involves two hypotheses: that alcohol reduces tension, and that tension reduction motivates alcoholics to continue drinking in order to produce tension reduction. The hypothesis and its corollaries have been reinterpreted in many ways (e.g., stress reduction—a currently popular terminology, conflict resolution, pain reduction, or negative reinforcement including avoidance of withdrawal symptoms) (Brown & Crowell, 1974; Cappell & Herman, 1972; Doleys, Groves, & Davidson, 1979).

There is some evidence to suggest that a limited dose of alcohol may reduce tension and elevate mood (Docter & Perkins, 1971). Steffen et al. (1974) found levels of muscle tension were negatively correlated with blood alcohol levels. When sober, alcoholics may state that they expect alcohol to decrease their tension, help them to "relax" and to lift their spirits. After significant amounts of maintained drinking, however, they rate their mood as actually being more anxious and depressed (McNamee, Mello, & Mendelson, 1968; Mendelson, LaDou, & Solomon, 1964; Nathan & O'Brien, 1971; Steffen et al. 1974). The study by Steffen et al. found measures of subjective distress correlated positively with blood alcohol level over a 12-day drinking period. Further reviews of the tension-reduction model of alcoholism may be found in Brown and Crowell (1974), Cappell and Herman (1972), and Franks (1970).

Social drinkers as well as alcoholics often talk as if drinking will help them to relax and reduce tension. Drinkers may therefore share a common history of cultural or verbal conditioning that may motivate drinking (McGuire, Stein, & Mendelson, 1966; Tamerin & Mendelson, 1969; Tamerin, Weiner, & Mendelson, 1970). Several other conditioning factors also appear to be important determinants of rates and patterns of alcohol consumption. In animals it has been found that monkeys will press a lever to produce an injection of alcohol into their veins

(Mello, 1979). Like their human counterparts, the monkeys continued to respond at a rate that was sufficient to keep their blood alcohol above a minimal level. Also similar to patterns observed for human alcoholics, these animals were observed to occasionally take in enough alcohol to kill themselves; and when they stopped, they quit abruptly or "cold turkey."

Several positive reinforcement functions have been observed in alcoholic patients in experimental wards that supplied alcohol to the patients as a consequence of pushing a button or performing in a mock automobile driving situation. In such situations, alcoholics chose to produce alcohol in preference to money or social companionship.

Although not as well documented, alcoholics and social drinkers have reported that they drink alcohol because it tastes good or makes them feel better. Speculation also suggests that these individuals might drink alcohol because it is expected in the social context of cocktail lounges and parties; because it makes business deals easier or sexual partners more desirable or attainable. Social reinforcement of drinking may include motivation to drink to become part of "the crowd"; to attain access to a more permissive social atmosphere; to make one the "life of the party"; to assure belonging to a social group with the companionship and fellowship involved.

Negative reinforcement functions may be even more complex and less well explored experimentally. Some of these functions may include drinking to avoid anxiety and tension (e.g., drinking to combat fear of flying or fear of public speaking); or drinking to escape or avoid pain (e.g., following surgery or a headache).

At the end of a long career of heavy drinking, the situational factors, conditioned stimuli, and conditioned reinforcers may become all-pervasive. Such phenomena are consistent with therapists' reports that alcoholics can always find an excuse to drink. Behavioral analyses suggest that under these conditions it would be difficult for anyone to resist drinking.

Risk Factor Analysis

Just as epidemiological investigations have revealed that heavy drinking increases the risks of morbidity or mortality through its medical sequelae, so risk factors that predict an increased probability to become an alcoholic have been studied. The National Council on Alcoholism (1972) reported that epidemiological and sociological studies found that the following are risk factors for the development of alcoholism: a family history of alcoholism; a history of teetotalism in the family; a history of alcoholism or teetotalism in the spouse or spouse's family; having come from a broken home; being the last child or in the last half of the birth order in a large family; coming from Irish or Scandinavian descent; having female relatives of more than one generation who have had a high incidence of recurrent depression; and heavy smoking.

In the George Washington University national survey, which was conducted in 1964 – 1965, the following were found to be at high risk to develop alcoholism: men under age 45 – 49; men of lower social status; operatives and service workers; men who completed high school but did not complete a college education; single or divorced or separated men and women; residents of large cities; those whose fathers were Latin American or Caribbean, Italian, British, or Irish; Protestants of no specific denomination; and Catholics or those without religious affiliation (Cahalan, Cisin, & Crossley, 1969). These data and others reviewed in this section suggest that the risk of alcoholism is multiply determined.

ASSESSMENT OF ALCOHOLISM

Consistent with the assumption of multiple determination of alcoholism, it would be expected that a wide range of individual differences exists among persons with alcoholic problems. This section focuses on the methods that might be used to assess alcoholism and related problems.

Before the ground rules for any assessment program can be determined, the objectives of the overall treatment should be established. For example, if the goals of a particular program are limited to reducing or eliminating drinking behavior, assessment may be restricted to the drinking problem and little else. On the other hand, if the goal of treatment is to produce improvement in many areas, which might include psychological, social, marital, and vocational functioning, a more broad-ranging assessment might be necessary in order to evaluate subsequent treatment effectiveness.

Multidimensional Assessment

Behavioral problems concerned with problems other than alcoholism have often found that assessment in areas other than the specific presenting problem may increase the possibility of successful treatment outcome. For example, in treating phobic behaviors, it was found that assessment of physiological and cognitive responses produced more accurate prediction of treatment outcome than did assessment of phobic behavior alone (Mash & Terdal, 1975). Similarly, in alcoholism, traditional treatment led to overall improvement in psychological, social, and vocational adjustment more frequently than it did to abstinence. After reviewing 384 studies of treatment of alcoholics, Emrick (1975) concluded that general improvement in many areas of life occurred in addition to reduction in drinking and associated problems.

It would thus seem important to develop tools and techniques of assessment in several areas of importance. Two helpful approaches have been: (1) the rational design of tests or measures to elicit pertinent information; and (2) the empirical analysis of differences between treated and untreated alcoholics or between alcoholics and nonalcoholics in their responses to tests.

The empirical approach to assessment has focused on the differences between alcoholics, social drinkers, and teetotalers and/or between treated and untreated alcoholics. Recent studies have begun to suggest that treatment characteristics are of less importance in predicting outcome than are patient characteristics (Kissin, Platz, & Su, 1971; Ruggels, Armor, Polich, Mothershead, & Stephen, 1975; Smart, 1978; Sobell, Sobell, & Ward, 1979).

Among the patient characteristics found predictive of treatment outcome are: age, education, marital status and stability, family discord, job stability, alcohol-related symptoms, and number of previous hospitalizations or treatments (Davidson, 1981; Smart, 1978; Sobell et al., 1979). Each of these factors should be assessed in programs aimed toward prediction of treatment outcome.

Psychological Tests

The rational design of psychological tests has led to a proliferation of questionnaires, only a few of which have been subjected to standard test construction procedures. For example, tests designed to measure directly alcoholic histories, patterns, and associated symptoms include the Manson Evaluation Test (Manson, 1948), the Alcadd (Manson, 1949), the Volume – Variability Index (Cahalan & Cisin, 1968), the Drinking Behavior Interview (Shelton, Hollister, & Gocka, 1969), the Michigan Alcoholism Screening Test (Selzer, 1971), the Alcohol Use Questionnaire (Horn, Wanberg, Adams, Wright, & Foster, 1973), the Drinking Profile Questionnaire (Marlatt, 1975), and the AlcEval (Davidson, 1974, 1980, 1981). A great deal of research has been done on this group of tests and many have been validated for the purposes for which they were developed. However, tests of this variety are often criticized for being susceptible to falsification because of their face validity. In addition, several of these tests have been validated for the discrimination of alcoholic from normal persons. The most frequent clinical need is for an instrument that will discriminate between the alcoholic and other persons with general psychiatric problems.

Several tests or instruments were originally designed to measure general psychopathology or personality and were then validated empirically using samples of clinical subpopulations. The Minnesota Multiphasic Personality Inventory (MMPI) was designed in this way. Containing 10 clinical and three validity scales, the MMPI has been the most popularly used of the personality inventories. Because it does not contain a scale developed specifically for use with alcoholic patients, three special research scales have been developed that are effective in discriminating the alcoholic from normal populations (Miller, 1976; Neuringer & Clopton, 1976).

Another test of general psychopathology, the Millon Clinical Multiaxial Inventory (MCMI), has 20 clinical and two validity scales, as well as separate scales standardized on alcoholic and drug-abusing patients. Studies with the MCMI have demonstrated its validity in discriminating alcoholic from: (1) other drug-abusing patients; and (2) general psychiatric populations. In addition, the test identifies several subtypes of alcoholics, with the suggestion that different forms of treatment might be appropriately directed to the different types of patients (Millon, 1977).

Behavioral Assessment

Several behavioral investigations have determined that alcoholics differ from normals in a number of behavioral domains. These include: muscle tension, social and behavioral skills, lack of control over drinking, and drinking topography. Measurement of frontalis EMG has frequently been used to assess general muscular tension in stress-related disorders (Steffen, 1975; Strickler, Bigelow, Wells, & Liebson, 1977). Alcoholics have been found higher than normals in resting EMG and abnormally high under abstinence (alcohol-related stress). Verbally the subjects of these studies report that they drink to reduce stress and tension (Doleys et al. 1979; Steffen, 1975). This finding supports the tension-reduction hypothesis of alcoholism etiology.

Several studies have found alcoholics to be lacking in social and behavioral skills (Doleys et al. 1979; Miller & Eisler, 1976). Although alcoholics frequently express positive assertions and feelings as well as normals, they often lack proper expression of negative assertions, such as expressions of hostile feelings or saying "no" to a proffered drink. Lack of such skills may frequently lead to drinking, whereas social and behavioral skill training may lead to increased control or avoidance of drinking (Doleys et al., 1979; Foy, Miller, Eisler, & O'Toole, 1976). Further studies are needed to standardize skills training programs and to compare their effectiveness with other types of treatment.

A long series of studies has suggested that alcoholics lose control over their drinking and that they perceive themselves as lacking in control generally, as well as in specific relation to drinking (Ludwig, Benefeldt, Wikler, & Cain, 1977; Ludwig & Wikler, 1974). This has been measured by the Locus of Control Scale, as well as several behavioral or role play situations designed to assess self-control.

Recent years have seen an increase in the experimental analysis of alcoholic drinking behavior per se. One of the repeated findings of such investigations is that alcoholics' consummatory behaviors differ from those of normal or social drinkers. For example, Schaefer, Sobell, and Mills (1971) found that alcoholics allowed to order drinks in a mock bar situation more often ordered straight (undiluted or unmixed) liquor than did social drinkers, who most frequently ordered beer, wine, or mixed drinks. The alcoholics also consumed their drinks in large gulps, while the social drinkers usually took more frequent, small sips of their drinks.

Physical fitness has also been measured in alcoholics (Frankel & Murphy, 1974; Gary & Guthrie, 1972). Alcoholic patients have been found to show improvement from low levels of physical fitness on these scales after a physical fitness training program (Frankel & Murphy, 1974; Gary & Guthrie, 1972). The relationship of physical fitness to controlled drinking or abstinence and to other characteristics of the alcoholic patient await further exploration.

The developments in assessment of alcoholism reviewed here have suggested that it is important to assess broad dimensions of personal, physical, social, and vocational areas as well as specific drinking behaviors. It has been found that patient characteristics ranging from demographic information to previous treatment and motivation for current treatment are often more predictive of treatment outcome than is the specific type of treatment. It is important to assess these factors as well as other areas in which alcoholics may show improvement as a result of successful treatment.

INTERVENTIONS

A number of treatment techniques have been applied to alcoholics. Each of the techniques tried appears to have had some success. Recent reviews suggest that no one treatment technique is a panacea in terms of treatment outcome. Clusters of patient characteristics may predict treatment outcome better than can any type of treatment (Kissin et al., 1971; Ruggels et al., 1975; Smart, 1978).

Methodological Problems in Evaluating Treatment

There has been difficulty in estimating the base rate of spontaneous change or improvement in alcoholism against which treatment effects might be judged. For example, the prevalence of alcoholism is age-related. The highest frequency of high volume drinking in this country occurs in the decade of the 20s; the highest frequency of alcohol-related problems occurs in persons aged 25 − 45 (Cahalan et al., 1969). From ages 45 − 60, the frequency of alcoholism in the general population decreases. This has been called the "maturing-out" phenomenon. Because of this age relation, it is to be expected that any reports of spontaneous change or treatment success will be smaller at younger ages (e.g., in the 20s and 30s) and greater in the 50s and 60s. This age relationship may occur independently of the effectiveness of treatment. It is probable that more alcoholics quit drinking without treatment than do with formal treatment. Other reasons for decreasing incidence of alcoholism with increasing age are death, incarceration, hospitalization, and medical complications.

Base rates of spontaneous change have been estimated in several ways. First, there have been a few studies of the fate of untreated alcoholics. The earlier studies of this type estimated that rates of change in untreated alcoholics were very low (e.g., 1 − 10%, see Kendell & Staton, 1965; Lemere, 1953). These estimates were based only on alcoholics who became totally abstinent. Of course, when overall improvement and moderate drinking are assessed as measures of change, the base rates of improvement are much higher (Emrick, 1975). In Emrick's review of 384 studies of alcoholic treatment, seven studies were found that followed alcoholics who received no formal treatment. The average rate of change for untreated patients was 13% who became abstinent and 43% who appeared somewhat improved. For 17 studies that used minimal treatment groups with less than five outpatient sessions or 2 weeks inpatient treatment as controls, 21% of the patients became abstinent over time and 43% improved. No statistical or practical differences were found between no-treatment and minimal-treatment rates of change. Emrick (1975) concluded that most treatments do not significantly increase abstinence rates, but do contribute significantly to decreasing rates of alcohol intake and overall improvement beyond the rate of change without treatment. In summary, very little difference in treatment outcome between treatments has been found in large-scale studies or reviews. The main effect that treatment may offer is an increased probability of reduction of alcohol drinking and related problems, as well as reduced risk of more serious disorders.

Historical and Traditional Forms of Treatment

The most frequent forms of treatment of alcoholism until the last decade were verbal psychotherapy, antabuse, and Alcoholics Anonymous (AA). Antabuse (disulafram) produces a chemically based hypersensitivity to ethanol. By itself it is a nontoxic substance with minimal effects. When pretreated with disulfram, the ingestion of ethanol causes the concentrations of blood aldehyde to rise in the body. Vasodilation results in flushing, pulsing headaches, and sweating. This is followed by vomiting, weakness, vertigo, blurred vision, and mental confusion. The effect serves as a punishment for alcohol ingestion and is effective if antabuse is taken on a daily basis. Unfortunately, noncompliance renders the treatment ineffective.

Alcoholics Anonymous is a social treatment. The individual is provided with social supports from concerned others who are alcoholic but who have chosen this means of changing their life-style. Treatment involves confronting the reality of alcoholism as a disease and implementing alternative cognitive and behavioral strategies to reinforce abstinence.

None of these forms of treatment by themselves has been found significantly more effective than the rates of change without treatment quoted previously (Emrick, 1975; Fox, 1967; Hill & Blane, 1967; Wallerstein, 1957). More sophisticated measurement of outcome might show greater frequency of success with these treatments, but the problems of compliance with antabuse regimens and long-term versus short-term attendance at AA complicate these analyses.

The most current psychiatric treatment for alcoholism is a broad spectrum combination of group and individual psychotherapy, auxiliary therapies (occupational, recreational, and physical), AA meetings, and antabuse. Treatment at Veterans Administration health-care facilities is probably representative of such programs. A large-scale study has been completed by the Veterans Administration (1979) of inpatient treatment at 17 health-care facilities of 849 patients with primary alcohol problems. The median duration of treatment was 45 days. Treatment consisted of various combinations of group and individual counseling, AA meetings, antabuse, and goal setting. The eight goals of the program were: to decrease drug and alcohol problems, medical problems, and illegal behaviors, and to increase self-support, self-esteem, social interaction, management of personal affairs, and work. Follow-up data on 495 patients (58% of original sample) indicated that 41.8% were rated as having no more than minimal problems in each of the eight treatment goal areas. Most improvement was in areas of alcohol abuse, psychological problems, social interaction, and obtaining satisfaction from socially acceptable sources. Reported days of alcohol use during the prior month decreased from 17.29 at admission to 6.63 at 24-month follow-up. Reported days intoxicated decreased from 13.44 to 1.69 (53% reported abstinence). Least improvement was in medical problems and failure to become economically self-supporting (56% were employed at follow-up compared to 37% at admission). Patient characteristics at intake were better predictors of outcome than was treatment type. Fifty-two percent of the sample were readmitted for a median length of 21 days of additional treatment.

Most of the 384 studies reviewed by Emrick (1975) also involved broad-spectrum combinations of treatment. His conclusion was that these programs contributed to overall improvement, but not significantly to rates of abstinence when compared to no treatment. This finding was replicated by the RAND study conducted under the direction of Stanford Research Institute using a sample of eight of 44 NIAAA-funded alcoholic treatment centers (Ruggels et al., 1975). This large-scale study found a significantly greater rate of overall improvement, including moderate drinking, following complete treatment, than following minimal or no treatment in over 2000 cases. Of even greater interest was the general finding that alcoholics who continued to drink moderately after treatment, even though they may have been severely "physically addicted" before treatment, were at no greater risk for relapse than were abstinent patients (Ruggels et al., 1975). This clearly indicates that programs that aim at reducing (but not necessarily eliminating) rates of alcohol consumption should have a place in the array of possible treatment modalities.

Controlled Drinking Strategies

As reported earlier, several studies have found that improvement in areas not related to drinking (e.g., in personal, social, occupational, and marital adjustment) have been observed in nonabstinent graduates of treatment programs (Ruggels et al., 1975). In addition, many alcoholics have chosen to control, rather than to abstain completely from drinking when the choice was made available (Ewing & Rouse, 1973; Lloyd & Salzberg, 1975; Miller & Munoz, 1976).

Teaching a controlled drinking strategy might be the treatment of choice for those who will opt for nothing else, and also for those on whom all other efforts have been ineffective. A review of treatment outcome studies has indicated that only a minority of alcoholics achieve and maintain total abstinence (Emrick, 1974,

1975). In particular, young patients have done poorly in abstinence-oriented programs (Voegtlin & Broz, 1949). Moreover, following controlled drinking intervention programs, at least some clients have chosen and maintained total abstinence (Ewing & Rouse, 1973; Miller, 1976; Vogler, Compton, & Weissbach, 1975).

By far the largest number of former alcoholic patients who have become controlled drinkers as a function of treatment have done so following specific therapies with controlled drinking as an explicit goal. These therapies have included aversive conditioning (Mills, Sobell, & Schaefer, 1971; Sobell & Sobell, 1973; Wilson, Leaf, & Nathan, 1975), biofeedback of blood alcohol levels (Huber, Karlin, & Nathan, 1976; Lovibond & Caddy, 1970; Vogler, et al., 1975), and training in ordering mixed rather than straight, undiluted drinks and to sip, rather than to gulp, drinks (Mills, Sobell et al., 1971). A broad-spectrum behavior therapy including ward therapy, avoidance conditioning with shock, videotaped feedback, behavioral rehearsal, stimulus control training and a list of personal do's and don'ts (Sobell & Sobell, 1973, 1974; Vogler et al., 1975) have also been reported effective. Davidson and Bremser (1977) have also developed a program for teaching alcoholics to control their consumption by pausing an increasing length of time between sips of very small alcoholic drinks. Because of the success noted in controlled drinking treatment programs, further research is indicated. It might be especially productive to investigate which type of patient is most successful at learning controlled drinking.

Multiple Risk Factor Reduction

Current emphases in preventive medicine focus on secondary, as well as on primary prevention (Saward & Sorensen, 1978). Secondary prevention attempts to stabilize or improve health in patients who may have already developed pathology or who are at high risk to develop pathology. Approaches such as this may be termed risk factor intervention programs (Breslow, 1972). Personal habits such as smoking, diet, lack of exercise, alcohol drinking, and bodily processes such as hypertension and high cholesterol levels may be modified to achieve better health.

One potential means of producing controlled drinking is through a program similarly aimed at secondary prevention or multiple risk factor reduction. As indicated earlier, alcoholics are at increased risk of a multitude of physical, physiological, and psychological disorders because of their high rate of alcohol ingestion. Multiple risk factor reduction might be constructively programmed through an educational approach to self-control.

It should be possible to deliver information regarding risk factors in alcoholism to alcoholic patients in the context of teaching them self-control. For example, communication of the fact that heavy drinking shortens the lives of alcoholics by 10 – 12 years might reduce drinking in alcoholics. Each one of the major risk factors could perhaps be presented in this manner, combined with a specific program for prevention or elimination of further risk.

Self-Control Procedures

Educational programs of the past (Cameron, Campbell, & Cipywnyk, 1977; Cappiello, 1977) have suggested the possibility of secondary prevention by teaching patients about etiology, symptomatology, and therapy. Although many critics have suggested that informational training alone may not be maximally effective, no systematic programs of this sort have yet been designed and applied to alcoholic patients.

Self-help manuals and self-control programs developed for public consumption are frequently on current booklists and in bookstores (Alberti & Emmons, 1974; Carnegie, 1936; Fensterheim & Baer, 1975; Mahoney & Thoresen, 1974; Miller & Munoz, 1976; Rosen, 1976). Several manuals have been written for patients to learn the techniques of relaxation and/or systematic desensitization (Baker, Cohen, & Saunders, 1973; Clark, 1973; Morris & Thomas, 1973; Phillips, Johnson, & Geyer, 1972; Rosen, 1976). Only a few of these programs have attempted experimental analysis and evaluation of these self-administered techniques or programs to particular target populations.

Some manuals and programs have been developed for use of therapists with alcoholics, or for the use of alcoholics who did not have access to a therapist (Mertens & Fuller, 1963, 1964; Miller & Munoz, 1976). It is not known at this point whether these manuals or programs have enjoyed success with alcoholic patients, as there are no known reports of their controlled or experimental use.

Relaxation Training

To the extent that alcoholic patients drink alcohol in response to stressful or tension-producing situations, more constructive means of tension reduction should serve as effective therapy. Relaxation is a response that can be learned or conditioned to occur in response to formerly tension-producing cues or stimuli. To the extent that a patient can be trained to respond with relaxation to formerly tension-producing stimuli, alcohol should become a less preferred means of tension reduction.

Relaxation has actually been incorporated into treatment programs with alcoholic patients. Alcoholic treatment programs of many orientations have incorporated relaxation training (Doleys et al., 1979; Lazarus, 1965; Pomerleau, Pertschuk, Adkins, & Brady, 1980). In most of these programs, it has been claimed that relaxation provided an important coping and stress-reduction strategy following treatment. Separate analyses of the contribution of relaxation alone have not been reported.

Blake (1965, 1967) studied the effects of aversive conditioning alone compared with aversion combined with relaxation training. He found that 59% of the group receiving combined treatment improved or remained abstinent after one year, compared to 50% for the aversion-only group. Other groups have reported similar advantage for a combination of relaxation and aversion (Lanyon, Primo, Terrell, & Wener, 1972).

In a more recent experimental demonstration, 14 male alcoholics who had been maintained on antabuse for 6 months were divided into control and experimental groups (Strickler et al., 1977). Each then had base line measurement of frontalis muscle tension (by electromyogram or EMG), relaxation instructions (for experimental subjects), a tape recording describing life on an island in Chesapeake Bay (control), and a final tape of drink-related stimuli (an alcoholic verbalizing approach – avoidance conflicts and deciding to drink again following treatment, with street and bar sounds in the background). Relaxation training reduced levels of EMG in the presence of drink-related stimuli. Control subjects increased in EMG levels (up to 17 – 23 microvolts, unusually high levels). This study demonstrated that relaxation training, even of very brief duration, may reduce levels of muscle tension of alcoholics in the presence of drinking-related stress stimuli.

These studies have demonstrated that relaxation training can be helpful to alcoholic patients, alone and in combination with other treatments. Although the mechanism of action is unknown, relaxation may be helpful because of broad-ranging effects including reduction in muscle tension, reduction in general sympathetic arousal, increase in stress management, and resultant feelings of increased self-control.

Exercise

A sedentary life-style is a serious risk factor that increases the probability of coronary heart disease (Frank, Weinblatt, Shapiro, & Sager, 1966; Morris, Heady, Raffle, Roberts, & Parks, 1953; Paffenbarger & Hale, 1975). It has been suggested that most alcoholics lead sedentary lives and are physically unfit (Frankel & Murphy, 1974; Gary & Guthrie, 1972).

Exercise programs have been studied in alcoholic patients. For example, Frankel and Murphy (1974) trained 20 hospitalized male alcoholic patients to jog 5 days per week for 4 weeks or to a 20-mile distance. Jogging led to a marked increase in physical fitness and psychological improvement in self-esteem and reduction of sleep disturbance, as compared to controls with normal activity. However, no change in number of drinking episodes was reported following this program.

In another program, 214 alcoholics aged 28 – 56 were trained 1 hour per day for 84 days (Gary & Guthrie, 1972). This training resulted in significantly lower mean resting pulse rate, diastolic blood pressure, depression, and body weight. There were no controls for comparison.

This section has reviewed the effectiveness of traditional broad-spectrum, controlled drinking, multiple risk factor reduction, self-control, relaxation, and exercise training treatments for alcoholic patients. Although some effectiveness has been found for each separate type of treatment, few have involved comprehensive assessment, especially involving personal, social, vocational, psychological, physical, and risk factor analyses. Because many of these techniques may have broad-ranging effects across categories, such assessment in controlled clinical trials would be helpful in treatment planning. In addition, more sophisticated studies of patient-treatment matches should lead to more effective treatment based on individual patient characteristics.

SUMMARY

The purpose of this chapter has been to demonstrate ways in which behavioral medicine approaches might be helpful in creating new means of assessment, prevention, and treatment of alcoholic and alcohol-related problems and behaviors. Because alcoholism is conceived as a multidetermined set of behaviors with complex etiology involving psychological, physiological, genetic, and interpersonal factors, comprehensive assessment of current problems of alcoholic patients should include evaluation of these spheres, as well as demographic, learning, and motivational factors. Similar broad-spectrum assessment should reveal a greater range of successful predictors or treatment outcome. Such developments should also produce more effective treatment plans for individual patients, depending on their assessed characteristics.

REFERENCES

Alberti, R. E., & Emmons, M. L. *Your perfect right*. San Luis Obispo, Calif.: Impact, 1974.
Baker, B. L., Cohen, D. C., & Saunders, J. T. Self-directed desensitization for acrophobia. *Behaviour Research and Therapy*, 1973, *11*, 79 – 82.
Blake, B. C. The application of behaviour therapy to the treatment of alcoholism. *Behaviour Research and Therapy*, 1965, *3*, 78 – 85.
Blake, B. C. A follow-up of alcoholics treated by behaviour therapy. *Behaviour Research and Therapy*, 1967, *5*, 89 – 94.
Blum, J., & Levine, J. Maturity, depression, and life events in middle-aged alcoholics. *Addictive Behavior*, 1975, *1*, 37 – 45.
Breslow, L. A quantitative approach to the World Health Organization definition of health: Physical, mental and social well-being. *International Journal of Epidemiology*, 1972, *1*, 4.
Brown, J. S., & Crowell, C. R. Alcohol and conflict resolution: A theoretical analysis. *Quarterly Journal of Studies on Alcohol*, 1974, *5*, 89 – 94.
Caddy, G. R., Addington, H. J., & Perkins, D. Individualized behavior therapy for alcoholics: A third year independent double-blind follow-up. *Behaviour Research and Therapy*, 1978, *16*, 345 – 362.
Cahalan, D. *Problem drinkers: A national survey*. San Francisco: Jossey – Bass, 1970.
Cahalan, D., & Cisin, I. H. American drinking practices: Summary of findings from a national probability sample. II. Measurement of massed versus spaced drinking. *Quarterly Journal of Studies on Alcohol*, 1968, *29*, 642 – 656.
Cahalan, D., & Cisin, I. H. Drinking behavior and drinking problems in the United States. In B. Kissin & H. Begleiter (Eds.), *The biology of alcoholism* Vol. 4: *Social aspects of alcoholism*. New York: Plenum, 1976.
Cahalan, D., Cisin, I. H., & Crossley, H. M. *American drinking practices: A national survey of behavior and attitudes*. New Brunswick, N.J.: Rutgers Center for Alcohol Studies, 1969.

Cameron, O. N., Campbell, A. R., & Cipywnyk, D. Alcoholism: A new approach to an old problem. *Canadian Journal of Public Health*, 1977, *68*, 483 – 485.

Cappell, H., & Herman, C. P. Alcohol and tension reduction — A review. *Quarterly Journal of Studies on Alcohol*, 1972, *33*, 33 – 64.

Cappiello, L. A. Prevention of alcoholism: A teaching strategy. *Journal of Drug Education*, 1977, *7*, 311 – 316.

Carnegie, D. *How to win friends and influence people*. New York: Simon and Schuster, 1936.

Chafetz, M. E. Alcoholism. *Psychiatric Annals*, 1976, *6*, 5 – 39.

Clark, F. Self-administered desensitization. *Behaviour Research and Therapy*, 1973, *11*, 335 – 338.

Clark, W. B., & Cahalan, D. Changes in problem drinking over a four-year span. *Addictive Behavior*, 1976, *1*, 251 – 259.

Conger, J. J. Alcoholism: Theory, problem and challenge. II. Reinforcement theory and the dynamics of alcoholism. *Quarterly Journal of Studies on Alcohol*, 1956, *17*, 291 – 324.

Davidson, R. S. Alcoholism: Experimental analyses of etiology and modification. In K. S. Calhoun, H. E. Adams, & K. M. Mitchell (Eds.), *Innovative treatment methods in psychopathology*. New York: Wiley, 1974.

Davidson, R. S. Experimental analysis and modification of pathological behavior. In R. S. Davidson (Ed.), *Modification of pathological behavior: Experimental analyses of etiology and behavior therapy*. New York: Gardner Press, 1979.

Davidson, R. S. *Discriminant validity of the AlcEval*. Unpublished manuscript, 1980.

Davidson, R. S. Behavioral medicine: Treatment of addictive behaviors. In D. M. Doleys, R. L. Meredith, & A. R. Ciminero (Eds.), *Behavioral psychology in medicine: Assessment and treatment strategies*. New York: Plenum, 1981.

Davidson, R. S., & Bremser, R. F. Controlled alcoholic drinking: Differential reinforcement of low rates of drinking. *Behavior Modification*, 1977, *1*, 221 – 234.

Docter, R., & Perkins, R. B. The effects of ethyl alcohol on autonomic and muscular responses in humans. I. Dosage of 0.5 milliliter per kilogram. *Quarterly Journal of Studies on Alcohol*, 1971, *22*, 374 – 387.

Doleys, D. M., Groves, J. A., & Davidson, R. S. Behavioral approaches to the assessment and modification of alcoholic behavior. In R. S. Davidson (Ed.), *Modification of pathological behavior: Experimental analyses of etiology and behavior therapy*. New York: Gardner Press, 1979.

Drew, L. R. H. Alcohol as a self-limiting disease. *Quarterly Journal of Studies on Alcohol*, 1968, *29*, 956 – 967.

Ellis, F. W., & Pick, J. R. Experimentally induced ethanol dependence in rhesus monkeys. *The Journal of Pharmacology and Experimental Therapeutics*, 1970, *175*, 88 – 93.

Emrick, C. D. A review of psychologically oriented treatment of alcoholism. I. The use and interrelationships of outcome criteria and drinking behavior following treatment. *Quarterly Journal of Studies on Alcohol*, 1974, 523 – 549.

Emrick, C. D. A review of psychologically oriented treatment of alcoholism. II. The relative effectiveness of different treatment approaches and the effectiveness of treatment versus no-treatment. *Journal of Studies on Alcohol*, 1975, *36*, 88 – 108.

Ewing, J. A., & Rouse, B. A. Outpatient group treatment to inculcate controlled drinking behavior in alcoholics. *Alcoholism*, 1973, *9*, 64 – 75.

Fensterheim, H., & Baer, J. *Don't say yes when you want to say no*. New York: McKay, 1975.

Fillmore, K. M. Drinking and problem drinking in early adulthood and middle age: An exploratory 20-year follow-up study. *Quarterly Journal of Studies on Alcohol*, 1974, *35*, 819 – 840.

Fox, R. A multidisciplinary approach to the treatment of alcoholism. *American Journal of Psychiatry*, 1967, *123*, 769 – 778.

Foy, D. W., Miller, P. M., Eisler, R. M., & O'Toole, P. H. Social skills training to teach alcoholics to refuse drinks effectively. *Journal of Studies on Alcohol*, 1976, *37*, 1340 – 1345.

Frank, C. W., Weinblatt, E., Shapiro, S., & Sager, R. V. Physical inactivity as a lethal factor in myocardial infarction among men. *Circulation*, 1966, *34*, 1022 – 1033.

Frankel, A., & Murphy, J. Physical fitness and personality in alcoholism: Canonical analysis of measures before and after treatment. *Quarterly Journal of Studies on Alcohol*, 1974, *35*, 1272 – 1278.

Franks, C. M. Alcohol, alcoholism and conditioning: A review of the literature and some theoretical considerations. *Journal of Mental Science*, 1958, *104*, 14 – 33.

Franks, C. M. Alcoholism. In C. G. Costello (Ed.), *Symptoms of psychopathology*. New York: Wiley, 1970.

French, S. W., & Morris, J. R. Ethanol dependence in the rat induced by non-intoxicating levels of ethanol. *Research Communications in Chemistry, Pathology, and Pharmacology*, 1972, *4*, 221 – 233.

Freund, G. Alcohol withdrawal syndrome in mice. *Archives of Neurology*, 1969, *21*, 315 – 320.

Gaitz, C. M., & Baer, P. E. Characteristics of elderly patients with alcoholism. *Archives of General Psychiatry*, 1971, *24*, 372 – 378.

Gary, V., & Guthrie, D. The effect of jogging on physical fitness and self-concept in hospitalized alcoholics. *Quarterly Journal of Studies on Alcohol*, 1972, *33*, 1073 – 1078.

Goodwin, D. W. Is alcoholism hereditary? A review and critique. *Archives of General Psychiatry*, 1971, *25*, 545 – 549.

Goodwin, D. W. *Is alcoholism hereditary?* New York: Oxford University Press, 1976.

Goodwin, D. W., David, D. H., & Robins, L. N. Drinking and abundant illicit drugs: The Vietnam case. *Archives of General Psychiatry*, 1975, *32*, 230 – 233.

Grant, M., & Gwinner, P. (Eds.). *Alcoholism in perspective*. Baltimore, Md.: University Park Press, 1979.

Hill, M. J., & Blane, H. T. Evaluation of psychotherapy with alcoholics. *Quarterly Journal of Studies on Alcohol*, 1967, *28*, 76 – 104.

Horn, J. L., Wanberg, K. W., Adams, G., Wright, S., & Foster, F. M. *The Alcohol Use Questionnaire*. Denver, Colo.: Fort Logan Mental Health Center, 1973.

Huber, H., Karlin, R., & Nathan, P. E. Blood alcohol discrimination by nonalcoholics. *Quarterly Journal of Studies on Alcohol*, 1976, *37*, 27 – 39.

Jellinek, E. M. Phases of alcohol addiction. *Quarterly Journal of Studies on Alcohol*, 1952, *13*, 673 – 684.

Jellinek, E. M. *The disease concept of alcoholism*. New Brunswick, N.J.: Hillhouse Press, 1960.

Kaij, L. *Alcoholism in twins*. Stockholm: Almquist & Wiksell, 1960.

Kendell, R. E., & Staton, M. C. The fate of untreated alcoholics. *Quarterly Journal of Studies on Alcohol*, 1965, *27*, 30 – 41.

Kissin, B., Platz, A., & Su, W. H. Selective factors in treatment choice and outcome in alcoholics. In N. K. Mello & J. K. Mendelson (Eds.), *Recent advances in studies of alcoholism: An interdisciplinary symposium*. Washington, D.C.: US Government Printing Office, National Institute of Alcohol Abuse and Alcoholism, 1971.

Lanyon, R. I., Primo, R. V., Terrell, F., & Wener, A. An aversion–desensitization treatment for alcoholism. *Journal of Consulting and Clinical Psychology*, 1972, *38*, 394 – 398.

Lazarus, A. A. Towards the understanding and effective treatment of alcoholism. *South African Medical Journal*, 1965, *39*, 736 – 741.

Lemere, F. What happens to alcoholics? *American Journal of Psychiatry*, 1953, *109*, 674 – 676.

Lloyd, R. W., & Salzberg, S. C. Controlled social drinking: An alternative to abstinence as a treatment goal for some alcohol abusers. *Psychological Bulletin*, 1975, *82*, 815 – 842.

Lovibond, S. H., & Caddy, G. R. Discriminated aversive control in the moderation of alcoholics' drinking behavior. *Behavior Therapy*, 1970, *1*, 437 – 444.

Ludwig, A. M., Bendfeldt, F., Wikler, A., & Cain, R. B. Deficits in the regulation of ethanol intake by alcoholics. *Diseases of the Nervous System*, 1977, *38*, 405 – 408.

Ludwig, A. M., & Wikler, A. Craving and relapse to drink. *Quarterly Journal of Studies on Alcohol*, 1974, *35*, 108 – 130.

Mahoney, M. J., & Thoresen, C. E. *Self-control: Power to the person*. Monterey, Calif.: Brooks/Cole, 1974.

Manson, M. P. *The Manson evaluation.* Beverly Hills, Calif.: Western Psychological Service, 1948.

Manson, M. P. *The Alcadd test.* Beverly Hills, Calif.: Western Psychological Service, 1949.

Marlatt, G. A. The drinking profile: A questionnaire for the behavioral assessment of alcoholism. In E. J. Mash & L. G. Terdal (Eds.), *Behavior therapy assessment: Diagnosis and evaluation.* New York: Springer, 1975.

Mash, E. J., & Terdal, L. G. (Eds.). *Behavior therapy assessment: Diagnosis and evaluation.* New York: Springer, 1976.

Masserman, J. H., & Yum, K. S. An analysis of the influence of alcohol on experimental neuroses in cats. *Psychosomatic Medicine,* 1946, *8*, 36 – 52.

McGuire, M. T., Stein, S., & Mendelson, J. H. Comparative psychosocial studies of alcoholic and nonalcoholic subjects undergoing experimentally induced ethanol intoxication. *Psychosomatic Medicine,* 1966, *28*, 13 – 26.

McNamee, M. B., Mello, N. K., & Mendelson, J. H. Experimental analysis of drinking patterns of alcoholics: Concurrent psychiatric observations. *American Journal of Psychiatry,* 1968, *124*, 81 – 87.

Mello, N. K. Animal models of alcoholism: Progress and prospects. In R. S. Davidson (Ed.), *Modification of pathological behavior: Experimental analyses of etiology and behavior therapy.* New York: Gardner Press, 1979.

Mendelson, J. H., LaDou, J., & Solomon, P. Experimentally induced chronic intoxication and withdrawal in alcoholics. Part 3. Psychiatric findings. *Quarterly Journal of Studies on Alcohol* (Suppl No. 2), 1964, 40 – 52.

Mendelson, J. H., & Mello, N. K. Natural history of alcohol dependence. In C. F. Gastineau, W. J. Darby, & T. B. Turner (Eds.), *Fermented food beverages in nutrition.* New York: Academic Press, 1979.

Mertens, G. C., & Fuller, G. B. *The manual for the alcoholic.* Willmar, Minn.: Willmar State Hospital, 1963.

Mertens, G. C., & Fuller, G. B. *The therapist's manual: A manual for assisting an alcoholic in his development of self-control.* Willmar, Minn.: Willmar State Hospital, 1964.

Miller, P. M., & Eisler, R. M. Alcohol and drug abuse. In W. E. Craighead, A. E. Kazdin, & M. J. Mahoney (Eds.), *Behavior modification principles, issues, and applications.* Boston: Houghton Mifflin, 1976.

Miller, W. R. Alcoholism scales and objective assessment methods: A review. *Psychological Bulletin,* 1976, *83*, 649 – 674.

Miller, W. R., & Munoz, R. F. *How to control your drinking.* Englewood Cliffs, N.J.: Prentice – Hall, 1976.

Millon, T. *Millon multiaxial clinical inventory manual.* Minneapolis, Minn.: National Computer Systems, Inc., 1977.

Mills, K. C., Sobell, M. B., & Schaefer, H. H. Training social drinking as an alternative to abstinence for alcoholics. *Behavior Therapy,* 1971, *2*, 18 – 27.

Morris, J. N., Heady, J. A., Raffle, P. A. B., Roberts, C. B., & Parks, J. W. Coronary heart disease and physical activity of work. *Lancet,* 1953, *2*, 105 – 111.

Morris, L. W., & Thomas, C. R. Treatment of phobias by a self-administered desensitization technique. *Journal of Behavior Therapy and Experimental Psychiatry,* 1973, *4*, 397 – 399.

Nathan, P. E., & O'Brien, J. S. An experimental analysis of the behavior of alcoholic and nonalcoholics during prolonged experimental drinking. *Behavior Therapy,* 1971, *2*, 455 – 476.

National Council on Alcoholism. Criteria for the diagnosis of alcoholism. *American Journal of Psychiatry,* 1972, *129*, 41 – 49.

National Institute on Alcohol Abuse and Alcoholism. *Facts about alcohol and alcoholism (DHEW Pub. No. ADM, 75 – 31).* Washington, D.C.: US Government Printing Office, 1974.

Neuringer, C., & Clopton, J. R. The use of psychological tests for the study of the identification, prediction and treatment of alcoholism. In G. Goldstein & C. Neuringer (Eds.), *Empirical studies of alcoholism.* Cambridge, Mass.: Ballinger, 1976.

Orford, J. A. Notes on ordering of onset of symptoms in alcohol dependence. *Psychological Medicine*, 1974, *4*, 281 – 288.

Paffenbarger, R. S., & Hale, W. E. Work activity and coronary heart mortality. *The New England Journal of Medicine*, 1975, *292*, 545 – 550.

Park, P. Developmental ordering of experiences in alcoholics. *Quarterly Journal of Studies on Alcohol*, 1973, *34*, 473 – 488.

Partanen, J., Bruun, K., & Markkanen, T. *Inheritance of drinking behavior.* New Brunswick, N.J.: Rutgers University Center of Alcohol Studies, 1966.

Phillips, R. E., Johnson, G. D., & Geyer, A. Self-administered systematic desensitization. *Behavior Research and Therapy*, 1972, *10*, 93 – 96.

Pomerleau, O. F., Pertschuk, M., Adkins, D., & Brady, J. P. A comparison of behavior and traditional treatment for middle income problem drinkers. *Behavior Therapy*, 1980.

Rosen, G. M. *The relaxation book: An illustrated self-help program.* Englewood Cliffs, N.J.: Prentice-Hall, 1976.

Ruggels, W. L., Armor, D. J., Polich, J. M., Mothershead, A., & Stephen, M. A. *A follow-up study of clients at selected alcoholism treatment centers funded by NIAAA. Final Report.* Menlo Park, Calif.: Stanford Research Institute, 1975.

Saward, E., & Sorensen, A. The current emphasis on preventive medicine. *Science*, 1978, *200*, 889 – 894.

Schaefer, H. H., Sobell, M. B., & Mills, K. C. Baseline drinking behavior in alcoholics and social drinkers: Kinds of drinks and sip magnitude. *Behaviour Research and Therapy*, 1971, *9*, 23 – 27.

Schuckit, M. A. Geriatric alcoholism and drug abuse. *Gerontologist*, 1977, *17*, 168 – 174.

Schuckit, M. A., Goodwin, D. W., & Winokur, G. A half-sibling study of alcoholism. *American Journal of Psychiatry*, 1972, *128*, 1132 – 1136.

Selzer, M. L. The Michigan Alcoholism Screening Test: The quest for a new diagnostic instrument. *American Journal of Psychiatry*, 1971, *128*, 89 – 94.

Shelton, J., Hollister, L. E., & Gocka, E. F. The drinking behavior interview: An attempt to quantify alcoholic impairment. *Diseases of the Nervous System*, 1969, *30*, 464 – 467.

Smart, R. G. Do some alcoholics do better in some types of treatment than others? *Drug and Alcohol Dependence*, 1978, *3*, 65 – 75.

Sobell, M. B., & Sobell, L. C. Individualized behavior therapy for alcoholics. *Behavior Therapy*, 1973, *4*, 49 – 72.

Sobell, M. B., & Sobell, L. C. Alternatives to abstinence: Time to acknowledge reality. *Addictions*, 1974, *21*, 2 – 29.

Sobell, L. C., Sobell, M. B., & Ward, E. (Eds.). *Evaluating alcohol and drug abuse treatment effectiveness: Recent advances.* New York: Pergamon Press, 1979.

Steffen, J. J. Electromyographically induced relaxation in the treatment of chronic alcohol abuse. *Journal of Consulting and Clinical Psychology*, 1975, *43*, 275.

Steffen, J. J., Nathan, P. E., & Taylor, H. A. Tension-reducing effects of alcohol: Further evidence and some methodological considerations. *Journal of Abnormal Psychology*, 1974, *83*, 542 – 547.

Strickler, D., Bigelow, G., Wells, D., & Liebson, I. Effects of relaxation instructions on the electromyographic responses of abstinent alcoholics to drinking-related stimuli. *Behaviour Research and Therapy*, 1977, *15*, 500 – 502.

Tamerin, J. S., & Mendelson, J. H. The psychodynamics of chronic inebriation: Observations of alcoholics during the process of drinking in an experimental group setting. *American Journal of Psychiatry*, 1969, *125*, 886 – 899.

Tamerin, J. S., Weiner, S., & Mendelson, J. H. Alcoholics' expectations and recall of experiences during intoxication. *American Journal of Psychiatry*, 1970, *126*, 1697 – 1704.

Trice, H. M., & Wahl, J. R. A rank order analysis of the symptoms of alcoholism. *Quarterly Journal of Studies on Alcohol*, 1958, *19*, 636 – 648.

Veterans Administration, evaluation of VA alcohol dependence treatment programs at 16 selected VA medical centers. Washington, D.C.: VA Pub. IL 11 – 79 – 10, 1979.

Voegtlin, W. L., & Broz, W. R. The conditioned reflex treatment of chronic alcoholism. X: An analysis of 3,125 admissions over a period of ten and one-half years. *Annals of Internal Medicine,* 1949, *30,* 580 – 597.

Vogler, R. E., Compton, J. V., & Weissbach, T. A. Integrated behavior change techniques for alcoholics. *Journal of Consulting and Clinical Psychology,* 1975, *43,* 233 – 2453.

Wallerstein, R. S. *Hospital treatment of alcoholism: A comparative experimental study.* New York: Basic Books, 1957.

Wallgren, H., & Barry, H. *Actions of alcohol,* Vol. 1. *Biochemical and physiological aspects.* Amsterdam: Elsevier Publishing Co., 1970.

Wikler, A., & Pescor, F. T. Classical conditioning of a morphine abstinence phenomenon, reinforcement of opioid-drinking behavior and "relapse" in morphine-addicted rats. *Psychopharmacologia (Berl.),* 1961, *10,* 255 – 284.

Wilkinson, R. *The prevention of drinking problems: Alcohol control and cultural influence.* New York: Oxford University Press, 1970.

Wilson, G. T., Leaf, R., & Nathan, P. E. The aversive control of excessive drinking by chronic alcoholics in the laboratory setting. *Journal of Applied Behavior Analysis,* 1975, *8,* 13 – 26.

World Health Organization. *Expert committee on mental health: Alcoholism subcommittee: Second report.* Geneva: World Health Organization, 1952.

15 Sexuality

C. Sue Carter
University of Illinois, Champaign-Urbana

INTRODUCTION

Direct experimentation on human sexuality is rare. Most of our information is derived from correlations among developmental, clinical, or pathological conditions and subsequent behavioral changes. Animal models also are valuable sources of experimental data. For both animal and human studies the generality of theories derived from existing data remains open to controversy. For example, male – male mounting behavior in rats and male human homosexuality may be viewed as analogous behavioral phenomena (Beach, 1979). However, before animal behavioral patterns can be accepted as valid models for human behavior it is necessary to discover whether parallels exist in the underlying causes and functions served by these behaviors.

It is obvious that a multitude of social and psychological factors influence human sexuality. In addition, individual differences are the rule, not the exception. Although discussion of these is generally beyond the scope of this chapter, they cannot be ignored. Successful attempts to understand biological processes such as sexuality within a psychosocial perspective (and vice versa) are rare. In addition, some avenues of research on sexuality remain relatively closed because they may be perceived as invasions of privacy or areas too sensitive for objective study. Although public attitudes toward sexual behavior have become somewhat more liberal, private and emotional responses around the issue of sexuality are available and continue to generate controversy. Against this background, this chapter will review some of the major concepts and issues in sexuality as an area of study within behavioral medicine.

BASIC CONCEPTS IN REPRODUCTIVE PHYSIOLOGY

The physiological regulation of the reproductive system depends on the action of *hormones*. Hormones are classically defined as chemical agents, produced by specialized tissues (endocrine organs) and released into the blood-stream, thus reaching target organs in other areas of the body. Hormones may be classified biochemically as either steroids or amino acid derivatives. Steroid hormones act on tissues by entering the target cells, where cellular *receptors* transport the hormones into the cell nucleus. The primary effects of steroids are believed to be due to their capacity to alter nuclear functions and thus influence protein synthesis. In general steroid hormones act slowly and have broad-ranging effects throughout the body. Hormones that are synthesized from amino acids (and therefore, considered amino acid derivatives) act by affecting cell surface receptors and do not enter the cell. In general the latter group of hormones produces relatively rapid effects and can have somewhat more localized actions than steroids.

Hormone production is regulated by endocrine organ secretion rates. In addition, a given hormone may be produced by the conversion of a precursor into a hormone at a site other than the endocrine organ. (For example, adipose tissue, the liver, etc., can provide sites for such conversions.) Circulating hormone levels are also controlled by the metabolic clearance rate of organs such as the liver and kidney. The proportion of free hormones versus those that are bound to protein carrier molecules is also of functional significance.

Reproductive Hormones

For the reproductive system several hormone-producing organs (Table 15.1) are involved including the gonads and adrenal cortices (capable of steroid hormone production), the pituitary gland (producing gonadotropins), and the preoptic — hypothalamic regions of the central nervous system (involved in the regulation of pituitary hormone synthesis and release). Reproductive hormones produced in both pituitary and neural tissues are amino acid derivatives.

In mammals, and presumably most other animals, males and females are capable of synthesizing identical hormones. However, distinct sex differences do occur in the concentrations of hormones available during the life cycle.

Other Biochemical Factors

Most of the behavioral effects of hormones are assumed to be due to biochemical changes within the nervous system. New compounds with potential behavioral effects are constantly being discovered. At present our knowledge of the interaction among hormones and other neural elements is largely restricted to the better known neurotransmitters, including the *catecholamines* (*dopamine* and *norepinephrine*), *serotonin*, and *acetylcholine*. There is also growing interest in the

TABLE 15.1
Sex Differences in Anatomy, Physiology, and Behavior

	Male	*Female*
Chromosomes	XY	XX
Gonads	Testes	Ovaries
Gametes	Sperm	Eggs
Hormones	*Androgens*	*Estrogens*
	Testosterone	Estradiol
	Dihydrotestosterone	Estrone
	Androstenedione	Estriol
		Progestins
		Progesterone
External genitalia	Phallus (penis)	Clitoris
	Scrotum	Labia
		Vagina
Accessory sex organs and secondary sexual characteristics	Epididymis (sperm storage)	Uterus or womb
		Cervix
	Vas Deferens (sperm duct)	Mammary glands (breasts)
	Seminal vesicles (sperm production)	
Reproductive pattern	Tonic sperm and hormone production	Cyclic or periodic egg production (Menstrual or estrous cycle)
Behavioral pattern	Mounting	Receptive posture
	Intromission	(Lordosis)
	Ejaculation	

behavioral effects of the endogenous opiates (including the endorphins and enkephalins). Each of these agents may have the potential to directly influence behavior and/or indirectly regulate behavioral processes through effects on the neuroendocrine system (as discussed in Chapters 4 and 5).

FEMALE REPRODUCTION

Sexual Physiology in the Female

A variety of stimuli can produce sexual arousal and may eventually lead to sexual intercourse. Initial activation can result from the visual, auditory, and chemical senses, and humans seem uniquely able to experience fantasy or emotionally induced arousal. Tactile stimulation of the genital area is typically necessary to initiate the events leading to the neuromuscular response termed *orgasm*.

The characteristics of a sexual response cycle were described by Masters and Johnson (1966). Four phases have been identified: excitement, plateau, orgasmic, and resolution. Inter- and intraindividual variations in the patterns of sexual responses are common.

The genital components of the sexual response include vaginal lubrication and vasocongestion, caused by dilatation of the blood vessels that enter and constriction of the vessels that drain the area. The vaginal cavity increases in size and darkens in color. The cervix and uterus are elevated and the clitoris becomes tumescent. In the plateau phase external vaginal changes become more pronounced and the clitoris may withdraw. In the orgasmic phase, rhythmic contractions of the genital area and the uterus are typically accompanied by psychic experiences that presumably reflect intense neurophysiological events. In the resolution phase the aforementioned changes revert to the resting condition. Many women are capable of multiple orgasms before experiencing the resolution phase.

The Menstrual Cycle and Steroid Hormones

The female primate reproductive cycle is defined by menstrual bleeding, due to the periodic shedding of the inner uterine wall. Ovulation occurs approximately 14 days prior to menstruation (Fig. 15.1). The preovulation portion of the menstrual cycle is called the *follicular* phase and the postovulatory period, prior to menstrual bleeding, is called the *luteal* phase. Individual variations in the length of the menstrual cycle are due mainly to differences in the follicular phase.

In adult female humans an egg (ovum) is expelled at roughly 28 – 29-day intervals. In addition, the ovarian *follicle* secretes *estrogens*. Following ovulation this follicle is transformed into the *corpus luteum*, an important source of *progestins*.

Estrogens and progestins (Table 15.1) are often described as "female reproductive hormones" because of their vital roles in all aspects of the female reproductive cycle. The most potent *estrogenic* hormone, produced primarily by the ovary, is *estradiol* (E2). This hormone increases in reproductively mature cycling females during the follicular phase of the menstrual cycle and shows a second peak following ovulation. A second estrogenic steroid, *estrone* (E1), is produced by either the ovary or as a result of extraovarian, peripheral conversion of other steroids (androstenedione, testosterone, or estradiol). Both estradiol and estrone levels are low during the menstrual period.

The ovary is also a primary source of *progestins*, of which *progesterone* and *17–OH progesterone* are the best known examples. Progestin levels are highest in the luteal phase of the menstrual cycle and decrease rapidly in the premenstrual period.

Appreciable concentrations of *androgenic* hormones, including *androstenedione* and *testosterone*, are also measured in women and show cyclic variations in levels. Approximately 40% of this testosterone is produced by the ovaries and adrenals, with the remainder contributed by peripheral conversion (Utian, 1980).

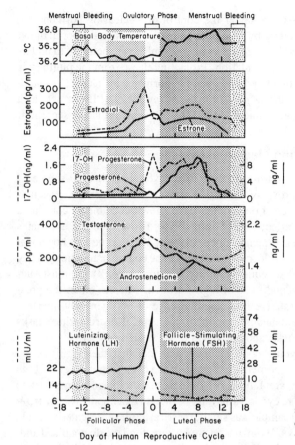

FIG. 15.1. Patterns of hormone secretion in a single menstrual cycle. Modified from Yen (1980) with permission.

Pituitary Hormones

The anterior lobe of the pituitary gland produces at least three hormones involved in reproductive function; *prolactin, luteinizing hormone* (LH), and *follicle stimulating hormone* (FSH). LH and FSH are known as *gonadotropins* and the collective effects of the pituitary hormones regulate cyclic steroid production and time ovulation. Excessive levels of prolactin (hyperprolactinemia) may prevent ovulation and interfere with menstrual cyclicity.

Hypothalamic Releasing Hormones

Pituitary function can be influenced by the central nervous system, providing a potential link between endocrine activities and external environmental cues such as photoperiod, stress, etc. Current animal research suggests that the pituitary gonadotropins, LH and FSH, are under the control of a releasing hormone (or hormones) carried to the pituitary by a vascular pathway known as the portal blood vessels. Pulses in *gonadotropin releasing hormone* (GnRH) are believed to underlie the surge of LH that preceeds ovulation. Prolactin release from the pituitary is under the inhibitory control of a hypothalamic hormone or factor. Research suggests that dopamine is either a *prolactin inhibiting factor* (PIF) or acts as a critical component of the biochemical system that prevents prolactin secretion.

Behavioral Changes in the Menstrual Cycle

Possible behavioral changes during the menstrual cycle have been a source of research (and political) controversy. Objective measures of performance (such as reaction times, test scores, etc.) only rarely have shown decrements correlated with the menstrual cycle (Parlee, 1973; Smith, 1975). Broverman and associates (Broverman, Vogel, Klaiber, Majcher, Shea, & Paul, 1981) argue that hormonal fluctuations in the menstrual cycle may in fact influence cognitive functions. They suggest that simple tasks that require rapidity ("automization") are most successfully performed under conditions of high estrogen, whereas either the presence of progesterone or a relative functional absence of estrogen may interfere with such abilities and simultaneously facilitate "perceptual-restructuring" tasks (such as embedded figures tests and the WAIS block design subtest).

Women often report cyclic mood changes and feel that their abilities are impaired in the premenstrual or menstrual phase of the cycle, when levels of both estrogen and progesterone are falling or low. Hysterectomized women (with ovaries intact) did not report cyclic variations in mood (Beaumont, Richards, & Gelder, 1975). Although the sample was small, these results if representative could be interpreted in several ways. Women who are hysterectomized do not bleed and, therefore, may not be able to identify or label cyclic phenomena. The findings may suggest that menstrual symptoms primarily reflect this labeling process. Possibly the dysmenorrhea (pain) associated with cyclic changes in the uterus is a primary source of the discomforts of the menstrual period and indirectly influences mood at this time. The surgical removal of the uterus also could have reduced ovarian function and therefore the physiological impact of ovarian hormone cycles.

It is possible that some of the negative behavioral phenomena associated with the premenstrual period result from sociocultural expectations. Support for this explanation of women's responses to the premenstruum is found in the experimental study of Ruble (1977). Women who were in fact premenstrual were told that the experimenter could accurately predict their next menstrual period. Those led to believe that they were in the intermenstrual period (7 to 10 days prior to menstruation) reported more positive feelings than those women who were told that they would begin to menstruate within a day or so, although all women were at approximately 6 to 7 days before the onset of menstrual bleeding. Paige (1973) also found support for cultural conditioning of responses to the menstrual cycle. Menstrual complaints were more pronounced in women from traditional religious and cultural backgrounds. In addition, several investigators have reported that both males and females have relatively clear ideas regarding emotional changes that can be expected in the premenstrual period. In fact men may view menstrual symptoms as more severe than do women (Parlee, 1974). Women who expect "debilitating" symptoms during the menstrual period are more likely to report retrospectively higher levels of personal distress during the menstrual cycle (Ruble, 1977).

Hormones and Behavior in the Menstrual Cycle

In spite of problems associated with documenting behavioral changes during the premenstrual and menstrual periods, it seems that at least some women experience marked cyclic behavioral changes including symptoms that are severe enough to require treatment. Medical theories and efforts to deal with these cyclic phenomena have focused recently on hormone-related processes. It has been proposed that deficiencies in estrogens and/or progesterone or withdrawal from these hormones may precipitate behavioral "irritability" or depression (Dalton, 1977; Smith, 1975; Steiner & Carroll, 1977). Dalton (1977) in particular has promoted the use of progesterone injections for the alleviation of menstrually related psychological disorders or dysphoria. However, Smith (1975) was unable to obtain improvements in premenstrual depression using progesterone injections.

A related group of theories regarding the origins of cyclic behavioral changes have involved cyclic hormonal effects on sodium and water retention. According to one version of these theories effects of estrogens and progestins on water balance are regulated through a complex of physiological events involving the kidney and adrenal systems. Behavioral changes can involve any of the aspects of physiology affected by this system, including renin and angiotensin (involved in kidney function), or aldosterone (an adrenal cortex hormone regulating electrolyte balance), or the edema resulting from fluid retention. Clinical attempts to prevent premenstrual symptoms through diuretic-induced water loss have not been generally successful and recent reviews of these theories (Smith, 1975; Steiner & Carroll, 1977) present contradictory evidence regarding the possible involvement of the renin-aldosterone system in premenstrual or menstrual discomfort.

Perhaps the most recent candidates for "causes" for premenstrual symptoms (including edema and mood changes) are the pituitary hormone, prolactin, and/or the dopaminergic system believed responsible for regulating prolactin release (Carroll & Steiner, 1978). Drugs that stimulate dopamine receptors inhibit prolactin release and may also reduce a variety of premenstrual symptoms (Benedek-Jaszmann & Hearn-Sturtevant, 1976). High levels of prolactin tend to be associated with irregular cycles and with at least one form of infertility. Drugs, such as bromocriptine used in the aforementioned study, may restore regular cycles and fertility. However, it is not possible at present to clearly identify whether such drugs may function behaviorally through prolactin inhibition, dopaminergic stimulation, or some alternative pathway.

Hormones and Female Sexual Behavior

The role of ovarian hormones in female sexual behavior has been difficult to demonstrate. There are indications that some women show cyclic variations in sexual activity with midcycle and/or pre- and postmenstrual increases in intercourse or autoerotic behaviors and luteal phase decreases in sexual activity (Adams, Gold, & Burt, 1978; Udry & Morris, 1968). However, because removal of the ovary does not eliminate female sexual behavior and some women report increases in sexual desire following ovariectomy, the role of ovarian hormones in the activation of female sexual behavior is not obligatory.

It was suggested some years ago that androgens (probably of adrenal origin) may play an important role in the activation of female sexual responses (Greenblatt, Mortara, & Torpin, 1942; Waxenberg, Drellich, & Sutherland, 1959). However, this continues to be an issue of controversy (Bancroft, 1978, 1980). Because of the anticipated virilizing effects of exogenous androgens, and perhaps also because of other nonmedical factors such as discomfort with the notion of giving women so-called "male" hormones, or issues regarding the desirability of intervening to enhance female sex drive, research on the clinical use of androgen treatments in women has been rare. We have collected recent pilot data on the physiological responses of two women who had elected to receive large amounts of exogenous androgen in preparation for female-to-male sex-change surgery. The vaginal blood flow responses of these women were exceptionally large (Morrell, Dixen, Davidson, & Carter, unpublished observation). These data may offer support for the hypothesis that androgens play an important role in female sexual behavior. An additional study of normal, cycling women has reported a correlation between female vaginal responses and endogenous testosterone levels (Schreiner-Engel et al., 1981).

Oral Contraceptives

There has been no general medical hesitance to treat women with exogenous steroids and in particular with hormones intended to prevent ovulation (i.e., oral contraceptives or the "pill"). Studies of the effects of oral contraceptives on sexual behavior have not produced unitary findings, probably due to the fact that sexual activity may be generally less inhibited in confident contraceptive users. However, several studies have suggested reductions in sexual interest in at least a portion of the population of women receiving oral contraceptives. In one carefully controlled study (Cullberg, 1972) in which all subjects maintained another form of contraception, the use of progestin–estrogen combination pills was associated with declines in both sexual interest and general feelings of well-being in some women. Cullberg concluded that the sexual effects in that study were secondary to mood changes.

Progestins are a component of most oral contraceptives and progesterone levels are high during the luteal phase of the menstrual cycle and during pregnancy (when sexual behavior may be depressed). In addition, progestins may have anti-androgenic and antiestrogenic effects. There are indications in both humans and animals that long-term exposures to progestins may inhibit sexual activity (Bancroft, 1978). Whether these effects of progestins are direct reflections of actions on systems regulating sexual behavior and/or indirect results of other actions of these hormones is not clear at present. However, the potential sexual side effects of progestin treatments cannot be ignored.

Some women receiving oral contraceptives may experience improvements in menstrual cycle-related symptoms; menstrual bleeding and accompanying pain are typically reduced. However, as mentioned there is also evidence of a form of psychological depression that may be related to the use of oral contraceptives in some women. Based on the latter findings, several other possible behavioral effects of sex steroids have been proposed (Parry & Rush, 1979). Current theories of depression (Maas, 1975) often focus on deficiencies in neurotransmitter systems that rely on either serotonin or norepinephrine. Steroid hormones may influence metabolic pathways responsible for both serotonin and norepinephrine synthesis. Deficiencies in the B vitamin complex (and in particular B6, B12, and folate acid) may result from oral contraceptive hormone treatments. There is clinical evidence supporting the value of B vitamin replacement therapy for the amelioration of hormone-related psychological disorders and it has been suggested that this mode of treatment acts indirectly by altering serotonin and/or norepinephrine production (Parry & Rush, 1979).

Puberty

Readily observable changes in anatomy, physiology, and behavior accompany adolescence. In fact the very existence of puberty constitutes evidence for a role for biological factors in the expression of sexuality.

In the United States, female puberty begins between the ages of 9 and 12, with menarche (first menstrual bleeding) occurring between the ages of 11 and 14. For the young female the first indications of puberty are increases in breast tissue. A general increase in height may anticipate breast development and the female growth surge takes about 2 − 2.5 years (Benson & Migeon, 1975). Pubic hair growth begins about 6 months after the onset of breast enlargement and axillary hair appears within about one year. Hormonal support for these early pubertal changes may come from the adrenal glands. Menarche typically occurs about 2 years after breast enlargement begins and by this time increases in skeletal growth are declining. Estrogens eventually act to terminate long-bone growth and further increases in height in girls are rare after about age 17.

Environmental factors are presumably important in the onset of puberty, as in industrial countries there appears to have been a decline in age of menarche over the last century (Frisch, 1972). It is proposed that the onset of the menstrual cycle is triggered either when the female achieves a critical body weight (about 46-47 kg) or when a critical ratio of fat to lean tissue is reached. A variety of evidence indicates that the pulsatile release of GnRH from the pituitary may be part of the mechanism for the onset of puberty. Ovulation and other events related to reproductive maturity can be elicited by pulsed injections of GnRH.

The Climacteric and Menopause

At approximately 50 years of age, with a range of between 35 and 55, many women experience the symptoms of the *menopause* or *climacteric*. The climacteric is a period of life characterized by the transition between reproductive and non-reproductive functions. The term menopause is medically defined as the last menstrual period during the climacteric (Utian, 1980). However, for epidemiological purposes menopause is often used to indicate a period of one year or longer following the last menstrual period and the term *perimenopause* can be used to refer to the several years just before and after the menopause.

The first symptoms of the climacteric often include a shortening of the follicular (preovulatory) phase of the menstrual cycle. In subsequent cycles abnormalities of the luteal phase may lead to a lengthening of the cycle and an eventual complete cessation of menstrual periods (Jones, 1980). Alternatively, some women experience an abrupt end to menstrual cycles. The hormonal consequences of this period are eventual declines in both progesterone and estrogen levels and elevations in gonadotropin concentrations (Utian 1980; Yen, 1980).

The most frequently reported symptom of the menopause is the "hot flash or flush" (Neugarten & Kraines, 1965). This symptom is described as a sensation of heat, typically accompanied by an increase in surface blood flow (vasodilatation). Perspiration and cold sweating may follow the "flush." It has recently been shown (Casper, Yen, & Wilkes, 1979) that hot flushes are correlated with surges in the pituitary release of LH. However, hot flushes occur in women even following surgical removal of the pituitary and elimination of the source of LH. Thus, it is likely that the cause of hot flushes is at a higher level of control, presumably located in the central nervous system. GnRH injections into the preoptic – hypothalamic area are capable of inducing rapid, temporary increases in body temperature in rats (Carter, unpublished observations) and it is possible that this temperature response to GnRH might be part of the basis for the physiological origins of the hot flush. In human females estrogen treatments provide relief from hot flushes.

A second "true" menopausal symptom is vaginal atrophy. After estrogen withdrawal, the walls of the vagina tend to become thin, causing painful intercourse in some women. Systemic or local estrogen treatments also prevent this problem.

Other tissues (Rakoff & Nowroogi, 1978), including the uterus and cervix, tend to decrease in size. Breasts may become flaccid. The urinary bladder, urinary tract, and epidermis of the skin become thinner in the absence of estrogen. One of the most detrimental symptoms of aging is the loss of calcium in bone tissue resulting in osteoporosis. As the bones soften they may become susceptible to injury, allowing spinal deformities (including the so-called "dowager's hump"), painful compression of the spinal cord, and an increased ease of fracture. The role of hormones in the prevention of these symptoms is not completely understood, but steroid hormones and/or dietary calcium and exercise may have therapeutic effects in the prevention and treatment of osteoporosis.

Medical treatments for climacteric symptoms most typically involve steroid hormone replacement therapies (Utian, 1980). Hormones may be given orally or by injection or subcutaneous pellet. Table 15.2 lists examples of estrogens, progestins, and androgens that are used alone or in combinations for the treatment of menopausally related symptoms. It has been estimated that about 80% of women taking estrogens for menopausal symptoms receive estrone sulfate ("Premarin", Marx, 1976). Diethyl stilbestrol (DES) is a nonsteroid synthetic estrogen that was widely used in the past for menopausal symptoms. (DES may also be given as a "morning-after" abortive, contraceptive treatment, or as a food supplement to fatten domestic animals.) In general DES is considered the least preferred source of estrogen, because it has been implicated in the ontogeny of vaginal cancer, in women exposed before birth.

Estrogen replacement therapy may be given either continuously or for a period of 3 weeks, followed by approximately a week of nontreatment. To reduce the possibility that estrogen therapy may promote uterine hypertrophy or cancer, it is also desirable to give a progestin during the last week or so of estrogen treatment (Gambrell, 1978; Greenblatt, Nezhat, & Karpas, 1980). When both the estrogen and progestin are stopped, withdrawal bleeding occurs. This menstrual like bleeding prevents the estrogen-dependent buildup of uterine tissue, believed to be a potential site for cancerous growths in postmenopausal women. The widespread

TABLE 15.2
Hormonal Preparations Available as Medical Treatments

Hormonal Classification	Examples
Estrogens	
Conjugated estrogens	Estrone sulfate ("Premarin")
	Estradiol valerate
Nonconjugated estrogens	Ethinyl estradiol
Synthetic nonsteroid estrogens	Diethyl stilbestrol (DES)
Progestins (progestagens)	Progesterone
	Medroxyprogesterone ("Provera")
	Norethindrone
Androgens	Testosterone
	Methyltestosterone

use of progestin treatments is relatively recent, primarily because their protective value was not widely recognized and also because many medical professionals believed that postmenopausal women would be intolerant of the resumption of menstrual like symptoms.

Hormonal Effects on Behavior During the Climacteric

A variety of behavioral symptoms and psychological disorders have been associated with the climacteric. For example, Neugarten and Kraines (1965) found that headaches, irritability, nervousness, and depression were more commonly described in menopausal than in nonmenopausal women. Jaszmann (1976) found similar results in perimenopausal women. A separate study of a sample of women between 40 and 50 years of age showed a higher than expected incidence of hypochondria, depression, and hysteria as measured by the Minnesota Multiphasic Personality Inventory (Kruskemper, 1975). However, other studies have failed to find any association between the menopause and psychological symptoms associated with depression or related disorders (Thompson, Hart, & Durno, 1973).

In general, controversy exists regarding the possibility that depression may accompany the climacteric, or in fact may actually be caused by hormonal changes experienced during that phase of the life cycle. In one survey of this literature (Christie Brown & Christie Brown, 1976) it was concluded that depression during the climacteric generally reflects a reaction to external life events and does not differ in form from depression experienced at other ages. A number of studies have examined the possible psychological benefits of estrogen replacement therapies and somewhat irrespective of the results of this research, it appears that many practicing physicians have confidence in the behavioral effectiveness of estrogen therapy (Rust, Langley, Hill, & Lamb, 1977).

Perhaps the most compelling evidence for behavioral effects of estrogens comes from the observation that estrogen therapies provide relief from hot flushes within a few days, whereas improvements in psychological symptomology have been reported 1 to 3 months or more following the onset of estrogen treatments (Durst & Maoz, 1979; Lauritzen & Van Keep, 1978). However, it is not uncommon for placebo-treated women to report improvements also in their psychological well-being (Campbell, 1976; Coope, 1976).

In an attempt to explain these somewhat contradictory findings, Klaiber and his associates (Klaiber, Broverman, Vogel, & Kobayashi, 1976) have proposed that severely depressed women are particularly resistant to the behavioral effects of estrogen. Thus, they suggest that the doses of estrogen used in routine treatment programs may be insufficient to influence serious behavioral disorders. Klaiber et al. recommend the use of high doses and prolonged treatment regimens for the alleviation of psychological problems that may be hormone related.

Hormone replacement therapies often involve both estrogens and progestins. Based on her own clinical experience, Dalton (1977) has advocated the psychological benefits of progesterone therapy (distinguishing in this case the natural form of progesterone, from synthetic progestins). However, because progesterone must be injected or implanted as a subcutaneous pellet, most clinicians have favored synthetic (and orally administerable) progestins in the treatment of menopausal symptoms. Thus, little is known regarding the behavioral effects of progesterone. One recent study of medroxyprogesterone ("Provera") indicated a transient dysphoric effect of this treatment (Bullock, Massey, & Gambrell, 1975). There are also indications that progestin treatments may ameliorate hot flushes (Dennerstein, Burrows, Hyman, & Wood, 1978). However, in general the behavioral effects of either natural or synthetic estrogens and progestins in humans remain open to investigation. It is particularly important that studies of the behavioral effects of progestins be conducted because of the growing tendency to prescribe progesterone to postmenopausal women.

Androgens are secreted endogenously (Utian, 1980) and may also be administered to postmenopausal women. However, androgens can have virilizing effects on hair growth or voice pitch and may stimulate libido (Waxenberg et al., 1959). Any or all of the changes may be viewed as undesirable in some women. Androgen therapy may be recommended for some postmenopausal women (Greenblatt et al., 1980), but the possible behavioral effects of these steroids have not been adequately explored. Probably because they are viewed as "male" sex hormones, androgens are not commonly given to women.

MALE REPRODUCTION

Sexual Physiology in the Male

The phases of the sexual response cycle in the male are similar to those described for the female. In the excitement phase erection results from vasocongestion of the penile vessels. The testes are elevated and increase in size. These changes progress in the plateau phase and a drop or more of a clear liquid from the Cowper's gland may pass through the penis. In the orgasmic phase rhythmic contractions expel the ejaculate (known as seminal fluid or semen). As in the female intense emotional changes are perceived. The resolution phase results in a loss of the erection and a return to the preexcitement phase. Most males must enter the resolution phase and experience a refractory period before they can again reach orgasm, although exceptions exist (Robbins & Jensen, 1977).

Neural Influences on Male Sexual Behavior

Peripheral Nervous System. The mechanisms of male sexual responses depend on neural input from the autonomic nervous system and are integrated and perceived through the spinal cord and central nervous system (Bancroft, 1980;

Hart, 1978; Tarabulcy, 1972). Specifically, the parasympathetic system, along with spinal (somatic) nerves, is necessary for ejaculation.

Animal studies have implicated the preoptic area (located near the base of the brain) in male sexual behavior. Damage to this region reduced or eliminated heterosexual responses in male rhesus monkeys but it was also noted that these animals continued to masturbate to ejaculation (Slimp, Hart, & Goy, 1978). In contrast, removal or damage to another brain region, the amygdala, may disinhibit or increase sexual responses in monkeys and other species. The effects in animals may partially reflect a loss of the ability to discriminate an appropriate sexual partner. However, there is some evidence that human sexual responses are also disinhibited following temporal lobe damage (Blumer, 1970). Electrical stimulation of related regions of the brain (known collectively as the limbic system) produces, in monkeys, peripheral indications of sexual arousal, such as erection (MacLean, 1975). In general, animal research tends to support the hypothesis that hypothalamic–limbic system regions are involved in the arousal and performance of male sexual behavior.

Drugs and Male Sexual Behavior

Drugs can influence sexual behavior through effects on: (1) sexual desire or subjective responses; (2) potency (as reflected by erections); (3) the ability to ejaculate, with or without changes in subjective pleasure; or (4) reproductive functions including hormone and gamete production (reviewed in Carter & Davis, 1976; Kaplan, 1974). Aphrodisiac properties have been attributed to various foods and other "love potions." Many of these agents probably have no advantages beyond their nutritional values and may gain their reputations primarily from their physical resemblance to parts of the reproductive anatomy. Among the more modern agents that have gained popularity as sexual stimulants are the drugs listed in Table 15.3. In general, these chemicals probably act either to alter sensory awareness and/or to reduce sexual inhibitions.

Marijuana or hashish (forms of cannabis) have popular reputations as aphrodisiacs. This class of drugs may in fact serve to reduce general social and sexual inhibitions. However, true aphrodisiac or sexual stimulant effects of these drugs have not been demonstrated, and there is evidence that long-term or chronic cannabis users may experience reductions in gonadal hormone levels, impotence, or infertility (Kolodny, Masters, Kolodner, & Toro, 1974). Other hallucinogen drugs such as LSD have had reputations as aphrodisiacs. However, again, sexual effects of these drugs may be transient and related to the sensory alterations induced by the drug.

There is some indication that central nervous system stimulants may facilitate either central or peripheral nervous system components of male sexual behavior. For example, intravenous injections of amphetamines or cocaine reportedly elicit spontaneous erections and orgasmic responses (Gay & Sheppard, 1972). In gen-

TABLE 15.3
Drugs with Reported Ability to Increase or Facilitate
Some Aspect of Sexual Activity

Drug	Reported Behavioral Effects
Alcohol	Reduced sexual inhibitions, vasodilation
Marijuana or hashish	Reduced sexual inhibitions, altered sensory awareness
LSD	Reduced sexual inhibitions, altered sensory awareness
MDA	Reduced sexual inhibitions, altered sensory awareness
Amylnitrite (poppers)	Altered sensory awareness, especially in genital area
Amphetamines	Altered sensory awareness, CNS stimulation, slight increase in potency
Yohimbine	Altered sensory awareness, CNS stimulation, slight increase in potency
Strychine (nux-vomica)	Altered sensory awareness, CNS stimulation, slight increase in potency
Cocaine	Altered sensory awareness, CNS stimulation
L-dopa	CNS stimulation, slight increase in potency, general improvement in health

eral, chemicals that promote erections also have been commonly viewed as aphrodisiacs. For example, urogenital irritants (such as "Spanish Fly," tincture of cantharides) or high doses of strychnine may cause priapism (sustained erections). Strychnine and yohimbine (a parasympathomimetic and vasodilator) have also been used as ingredients in contemporary medical preparations, prescribed for impotence (with names such as "afrodex" or "potensa-forte"). However, in general, these drug treatments do not provide effective relief from sexual disorders and they may have serious negative side effects.

Among the drugs that have become popular for the enhancement of sexual pleasure is amylnitrite. Originally available as an inhalant for relief from angina, this drug provides rapid vasodilation and smooth muscle relaxation. It has been suggested that amylnitrite may intensify the experience of orgasm and/or delay ejaculation (Hollister, 1975). Among the possible side effects of the drug are headaches and more rarely serious cardiovascular effects.

More easily documented are inhibitory drug effects (Table 15.4). Depressants, or sedatives including barbituates and large amounts of alcohol, may produce impotence. For alcohol, at least, this effect can be manifest as an inability to reach orgasm due to an inhibition of spinal reflexes. Alcohol-induced impotence may precipitate psychological problems and is a common trigger for the onset of male erectile disorders that can continue to appear even after the alcohol is discontinued.

Opiate users frequently report a loss of sexual interest and potency. Methadone treatment may have similar, although less pervasive and/or less severe effects on sexual behavior. These effects may reflect direct actions on the nervous system or may be due to a gradual decline in reproductive hormone production. (Chronic heroin use probably reduces both male and female fertility.)

TABLE 15.4
Drugs with Reported Ability to Decrease or Inhibit
Some Aspect of Sexual Activity

Drug	Reported Behavioral Effects
Heroin, morphine, or opium	Decreased libido and potency
Methadone	Temporary decrease in libido and potency
Barbiturates	Decreased libido and potency
Alcohol	Decreased potency after high doses
Phenothiazines (esp. Mellaril)	Decreased libido and potency, aspermia
Guanethidine	Aspermia
Pargyline	Aspermia
Phenoxybenzamine	Aspermia

Major tranquilizers, such as the phenothiazines (chlorpromazine, mellaril, etc.) can interfere with reproductive functions and fertility. In addition, in some cases these drugs inhibit the spinal reflexes responsible for preventing the flow of ejaculate into the urinary bladder, producing a condition termed "aspermia" (Shader, 1972). Phenothiazine users can experience dry ejaculations and concurrently note "white" urine, resulting from semen in the urine. Breast development (gynecomastia) and breast secretion (galactorrhea) may occur in males during phenothiazine treatment.

Male Reproductive Hormones

The male gonads or *testes* serve two major functions: sperm production and steroid hormone secretion. The predominant male sex steroids are the *androgens*, of which *testosterone* is the most abundant and best known example. Testosterone is secreted by the Leydig cells of the testes and acts within the testes itself to influence sperm production. In addition, testosterone enters the circulation and is carried throughout the body to target organs including the brain, spinal cord, pituitary, genitalia, and other tissues. It is believed that some of testosterone's actions may occur after that hormone has been converted to either *dihydrotestosterone* (another androgen with effects on genital anatomy) or *estradiol*. Animal research indicates that testosterone can be converted to estradiol in the nervous system and for some species (such as the rat) it is possible that the behavioral effects of androgens primarily occur after this conversion to an estrogenic hormone. It has been suggested that testosterone acts as a "prohormone" and provides a readily available substrate chemical that can be used by target organs. (These target organs may contain appropriate metabolic enzymes to break down the prohormone into active hormones.) In the case of testosterone the biologically active agent may be dihydrotestosterone or estradiol. Whether testosterone itself has direct behavioral effects is at present a point of theoretical controversy.

Pituitary Hormones

As in the female, LH and FSH are secreted by the anterior pituitary and act to regulate gonadal steroid and gamete production. LH in particular plays an essential role in the control of androgen synthesis by the Leydig (interstitial) cells. When it was originally discovered in males, LH was given the name interstitial cell-stimulating hormone (ICSH), reflecting this function. Prolactin is also produced in males and is under the inhibitory control of dopamine. Hyper- or hypoprolactinemia may interfere with male reproductive activities. (Phenothiazines, which block dopamine receptors, may produce hyperprolactinemia.)

Hypothalamic Releasing Hormones

GnRH (gonadotropin releasing hormone) also regulates the pituitary secretion of LH and FSH in males. GnRH actions in the male, as in the female, depend on the pulsatile release of this hormone, which in turn triggers episodic fluctuations in pituitary and gonadal hormone release. The functional importance of these surges is a matter of current investigation. For example, the female nervous system may be uniquely able to evoke or permit surges in GnRH and thus in LH, which in turn are apparently responsible for the cyclic events leading to ovulation. In contrast, in males, a more tonic or continuous pattern of hormone secretion sustains sperm production and other male reproductive activities.

Puberty

In males the first sign of sexual development is growth in the size of the testes, apparent at around 11 years of age with a range of 9–15 years considered as normal (Benson & Migeon, 1975). Within the next 2 years pubic hair develops and genital size increases. An increase in skeletal size, taking several years for completion, frequently follows the onset of pubic hair growth. Axillary and facial hair appear later, and complete body hair development may require several years. Seminal fluid production begins at approximately 13–14 years of age although sperm may not be present initially. Nocturnal emissions or "wet dreams" may begin at this age.

Hormones and Male Sexual Behavior

It is generally accepted that testicular hormones play a critical role in the activation and maintenance of male sexual arousal and behavior (Bancroft, 1978, 1980). Testicular activity at puberty is usually accompanied by increases in sexual interest and eventually by actual increases in sexual intercourse. If human males are castrated (i.e., testes removed) for medical, legal, or other reasons, declines in libido and potency are typical. Rare individuals may exhibit postcastrational sexual activity for years (in one case over 20 years), but most men experience declines in sexual behavior within a few months after castration (Bancroft, 1978; Bancroft & Skakkeback, 1979; Kinsey, Pomeroy, & Martin, 1948). Other hypogonadal conditions caused, for example, by testicular failure, are also usually accompanied by reduced levels of sexual activity. Hormone replacement therapies are often successful in instances in which testicular hormone levels are reduced.

In the male there typically is no discrete event (i.e., menopause equivalent) marking the end of the reproductive period. In fact, viable sperm may be produced throughout the entire life-span. However, gradual declines in sperm production and androgen secretion do occur and it appears that in some men declines in androgen levels may be rapid enough to create symptoms like the hot flushes experienced by women in the climacteric.

Attempts to control male sexual behavior have focused on individuals convicted of sexual offenses, including particularly rape or child molesting. Sex criminals have been treated with castration and more recently, particularly in Europe, have been offered chemical therapies, usually an antiandrogen. The most common of these antiandrogens, cyproterone acetate, is actually a progestin like compound. Reports support the conclusion that sexual thoughts and actions tend to decline during treatment, although the magnitude of this effect may not be very great (Bancroft, 1978).

In spite of the relatively consistent finding that lowering the availability of testicular hormones in adulthood is followed by declines in sexual arousal or activity, many questions regarding the role of hormones in male sexual behavior remain unresolved. For example, why do postcastrational changes not appear immediately? Why are individual variations in both behavior and hormone levels so great? Why are some individuals with apparently normal levels of hormones impotent? And more generally, what are the mechanisms through which testicular (or other) hormones activate and maintain male sexual function?

Suggestions regarding the answers to such questions involve various regulatory levels in the male reproductive system. Inter- and intraindividual variations in hormone secretion can be enormous. Sex hormone binding proteins may influence the relative availability of free versus bound hormones. The neural and other tissues that must respond to these hormones have wide individual, perhaps in part genetic, variations in sensitivity. Even following castration, steroid hormones may continue to be produced by the adrenals. The importance of adrenal hormones in the maintenance of male sexual function is not known. Finally, it is not clear which reproductive hormones mediate the role of the testicular secretions in male sexual behavior. Animal studies indicating that testosterone may be converted into other steroids (estradiol and dihydrotestosterone) have raised the question of which hormones are in fact biologically active. In addition, there has been support for a possible stimulatory role for the hypothalamic hormone, GnRH. There are recent reports that impotence may improve after GnRH treatment (Bancroft, 1978). It is not known at present whether GnRH is acting directly on behavior or through indirect effects on other aspects of the endocrine system.

SEXUAL DIFFERENTIATION

Genetic sex is established at the time of fertilization (Table 15.1). In mammals an XX sex chromosome pattern will typically result in female development; whereas an XY chromosome configuration (in which the father contributes the Y chromosome) leads to masculine development. In normal development, presumably through a series of biochemical events (Gordon & Ruddle, 1981; Haseltine & Ohno, 1981; Jost, 1979), the sex chromosomes instruct the body of the developing fetus to maintain genetically appropriate *gonadal* tissue. Undifferentiated gonadal tissue may give rise to either testicular or ovarian tissue, and tissue typical of the opposite sex regresses. (If one individual develops both ovarian and testicular tissue that individual may be considered a "true hermaphrodite.")

In the presence of androgenic hormones, tissues may develop that are responsible for physical characteristics that we identify as *masculine* (Wilson, George, & Griffin, 1981). For example, for normal male phallic and scrotal development genital tissue must be exposed to androgenic hormones. (These hormones are produced in the human male fetus as early as the second month of gestation.) If concentrations of these hormones are low or absent, presumably the case in the female, then a feminine pattern of genital anatomy results.

In a rare endocrine abnormality, known as *testicular feminization* or the *androgen insensitivity* syndrome, genetic males may fail to produce androgen receptors. These individuals have XY chromosome patterns and testes, capable of secreting androgens, but they lack the receptors necessary to respond to these hormones. The external genital anatomy and behavioral patterns of individuals with androgen insensitivity typically appear feminine (Money & Ehrhardt, 1972), suggesting a functional role for androgens in the development of the latter characteristics. An additional clinical syndrome suggesting the importance of androgens in masculine development appears in individuals with an XO chromosome pattern; no Y chromosome is present. This condition, called *Turner's syndrome*, is characterized by a feminine (although immature) anatomy, which results because the gonads in Turner's syndrome sufferers do not secrete either male or female hormones.

Further evidence for the importance of early androgens in masculine development comes from cases in which genetic females are prenatally exposed to abnormally high levels of androgens. These androgens can enter the system as a consequence of maternal hormone treatment or exposure. For example, hormones with androgenic properties have been used medically in an attempt to reduce spontaneous abortions. Alternatively, endogenously produced hormones can become elevated, as sometimes happens in a clinical condition known as the *adrenogenital syndrome*. Prenatal exposure to either exogenous or endogenous hormones may (depending on the time and length of exposure and potency of the available hormones) produce anatomical masculinization. Typically the exposure of a female fetus to excess androgenic hormones causes varying degrees of clitoral enlargement, scrotal development, and abnormalities of vaginal structure. The resultant ambiguities in genital anatomy, sometimes termed *pseudohermaphrodism*, (Money & Ehrhardt, 1972), are usually surgically corrected to appear feminine.

There is also experimental evidence from animal studies supporting a critical role for early androgens in masculine anatomical development (Jost, 1979; Wilson et al., 1981). In cases in which androgens are absent the pattern of development is typically feminine. Thus it is assumed that androgens facilitate or induce cellular changes leading to male anatomy. The *absence of androgens*, with or without accompanying female gonadal activity, may result in feminine anatomical features.

Considerably more controversial is the possible developmental role of androgens in the direction or "organization" (Phoenix, Goy, Gerall, & Young, 1959) of patterns of sexual behavior. Many laboratory studies of rodents suggest parallels between anatomical and behavioral development; that is, early androgen exposure promotes masculine sexual behavior and tends to inhibit feminine sexual behavior, when the animal is tested as an adult (MacLusky & Naftolin, 1981). However, in humans and other primates, the behavioral and neural effects of early androgens are less clear (Baum, 1979).

In animal studies, sexual behavior is routinely assessed by direct observations of sexual *performance*. In humans, more complex features of sexuality are usually studied. In addition to actual behavioral patterns (which are rarely observed), researchers have sought to understand the development of *gender*. The concept of gender may include the sex role an individual chooses publicly. In some cases sex roles may diverge from sexual or *gender identity*. The term gender identity is used to define the "private experience of gender role" (Money & Ehrhardt, 1972).

Based primarily on studies of various clinical cases or syndromes, including those already discussed, Money and Ehrhardt (1972; Ehrhardt & Meyer-Bahlburg, 1979) have concluded that early gender assignment plays a primary role in determining human gender identity and subsequent sexual orientation. Their findings suggest that gender identity is formed during the first 2–3 years of life and that later gender identity is primarily due to social factors experienced as a result of sex assignment during that period. Money and Ehrhardt have added the reservation that gender identity may be less firmly established or more labile to later change in cases in which confusion exists, particularly on the part of parents, regarding the sex of the child. Support for lability in gender identity also comes from the study of a remarkable genetic defect first observed in the Dominican Republic (Imperato-McGinley, Peterson, Gautier, & Sturla, 1979). A unique population of individuals was discovered in which prenatal masculinization of the external genitalia was incomplete, apparently due to a deficiency in an enzyme necessary for the production of the virilizing androgen, dihydrotestosterone. In the absence of dihydrotestosterone a relatively female anatomical pattern developed and, as children, these people were usually reared as girls. However, at puberty large amounts of androgens were presumably secreted by the testes and sufficient masculinization of the anatomy resulted to cause most of these "females" to change to male gender roles. These results suggest that gender roles may be changed well beyond the presumed sensitive period for gender identity formation. Imperato-McGinley et al. (1979) hypothesize: "that the extent of androgen (i.e., testosterone) exposure of the brain in utero, during the early postnatal period and at puberty has more effect in determining male-gender identity than does sex of rearing."

Information regarding the sexual behavior and orientation of individuals who have been exposed to discordant (with genetic sex) or abnormal levels of steroid hormones during development is also of theoretical interest. In the androgen-insensitivity syndrome, sexual identity and preferences are reportedly feminine and there are no indications that these individuals are as adults more likely than normal women to exhibit homosexuality or bisexuality (Lewis, 1977; Money & Ehrhardt, 1972). In addition, women who have experienced unusually high levels of prenatal androgen, due to excessive adrenal production (adrenogenital syndrome), have shown indications of difficulties in establishing sexual relationships with men (Schwartz, 1977). In both situations social or cultural learning explanations for these observations cannot be discounted. However, these results are also compatible with the hypothesis that prenatal hormones influence adult sexual orientations.

One of the most vocal advocates of a possible role for prenatal hormones in the development of adult sexual preferences, and specifically in the development of homosexuality, is the German physician Dörner (1979). Arguing from animal and human experiments Dörner has reported that predominantly homosexual male humans and neonatally castrated male rats have marked female like patterns of pituitary hormone (luteinizing hormone, LH) release in response to estrogen injections. Normal male and female rats that are exposed to early androgen show less distinct LH release patterns.

Sex differences in testosterone concentrations have been measured in human amniotic fluids. Dörner (1979) has postulated that differential levels of fetal androgens may contribute to male–female differences in sexual physiology and preference and also may explain, at least in part, the origins of homosexuality.

Homosexuality

Homosexuality can be defined in several ways, including: "a lasting sexual orientation towards the same sex, expressed in attraction, erotic imagery, and sociosocial experience [Meyer-Bahlburg, 1977]." Homosexual behavior may be viewed as a normal variation in behavioral preference or as deviance or perversity. Explanations for homosexuality range from total biological determination to the view that environmental or experimental factors are primarily responsible for sexual orientations. Most contemporary researchers maintain positions that blend these views. The present discussion highlights research describing biological or physiological factors that have been implicated in homosexuality, with the understanding that such factors probably offer at best only partial explanations for the countless diversities reflected in human sexual preferences.

Approaches to the biology of homosexuality have emphasized hormonal factors either acting during development (for example, prenatally) or in adulthood. Most homosexual men have normal levels of testosterone in adulthood (Meyer-Bahlburg, 1977). However, there is evidence that some "effeminized" predominantly homosexual men may have slightly lower levels of *free* testosterone. *Total* testosterone did not vary from levels measured in heterosexual or homosexual, but "noneffeminized," males. Dörner (1979) has observed that at least some effeminized homosexual males had relatively high levels of FSH and in a few cases LH levels were elevated beyond the range of heterosexual males in both effeminized and noneffeminized homosexuals. Dörner also has reported that homosexual males showed more pronounced LH responses (positive feedback) to estrogen injections than did bisexual or heterosexual males. There are also indications that some (perhaps one-third of those sampled) female homosexuals may have elevated testosterone levels (Meyer-Bahlburg, 1978) and that this effect is most likely to appear in physically virilized females (Dörner, 1979).

For all these endocrine parameters in both sexes it should be noted that there are wide individual variations, and many homosexuals show hormone levels that do *not* differ from those measured in heterosexuals. A further caution in interpreting these results, comes from the knowledge that hormone production may be influenced by external factors such as behavioral experiences, drug use, etc. Thus, even in cases in which there are apparently reliable correlations between endocrine factors and behavior, it is not possible to prove directional causation.

The potential effects of prenatal hormones on adult reproductive functions, including both behavioral and endocrine factors, have been discussed previously. Although it has been tempting to researchers to assume that developmental or genetic "abnormalities" may account for adult homosexuality (Dörner, 1979), current evidence supporting this view remains circumstantial (Bancroft, 1980). An alternative strategy is to accept considerable sexual variation as within the biological norms permitted by both male and female physiologies. Experiential and social factors (including those dictated by the evolutionary constraints of reproduction, life-styles, child-rearing practices, etc.) would function against this biological background, permitting the observed differences in sexual preferences and activities.

SEXUAL DYSFUNCTIONS

Behavioral and physiological interactions contribute to sexual dysfunctions or disorders in both sexes (Bancroft, 1980; Geer, O'Donohue, & Schorman, in press). It is possible to classify levels at which sexual problems exist, but it is rare that any individual will experience a difficulty that involves only one aspect of sexual functioning. In addition, because sexual interactions rely on and reflect social relationships, sexual dysfunction has proliferated over the last decade. Stimulated in particular by the work of Masters and Johnson (1970), journals and books largely devoted to this topic are available (*Journal of Sex and Marital Therapy*; Kaplan, 1974; LoPiccolo & LoPiccolo, 1978; Meyer, 1976). Most of this work focuses on the treatment of perceived sexual inadequacy. Hypersexual behavior may be viewed as desirable, although in those cases in which the behavior is seen as extreme or antisocial, legal and/or medical treatments may be applied.

Low levels of sexual activity can originate from physiological and psychogenic causes and may be manifest as: (1) sexual aversions; (2) declines in sexual interest or arousability; or (3) difficulties in sexual performance. It is accepted *in theory* that physical disorders should be excluded before a given problem is attributed to a psychological or psychogenic cause. However, in practice our understanding of the physiology of human sexuality is too incomplete and the interactions among physical and behavioral systems are too complex to assure that this approach will be successful.

Clinicians working with patients with reported or suspected sexual dysfunction can obtain suggestions for obtaining sexual histories in Masters and Johnson (1966, 1970), Hartman and Fithian (1972), or Green (1975). Physical examinations may of course prove useful in evaluating the sources of sexual dysfunction. Questionnaires intended for patient assessment and/or research have been prepared by (to list a few): Locke and Wallace (1959), Thorne (1965), Bentler (1968a, 1968b), Lief and Reed (1971), and Zuckerman (1973).

Common Sexual Complaints

For men *impotence* appears to be perceived as the most serious, although not necessarily the most common sexual disorder. Primary impotence has been described as erectile failure (the inability to achieve and/or maintain an erection) that occurs on the first and all subsequent attempts at sexual intercourse (Masters & Johnson, 1970). Secondary impotence is erectile failure after a prior history of successful vaginal penetrations. *Premature* or *retarded ejaculation* may also be considered as sexual dysfunction.

For women the most common disorders include *vaginismus* (involuntary contraction of the muscles surrounding the vaginal opening), *dyspareunia* (vaginal or pelvic pain during intercourse), and *anorgasmia* (inability to reach orgasm). These complaints may be primary (always present) or situational.

Causes and Treatments for Sexual Dysfunctions

In both sexes gonadal or reproductive tract malfunction due to congenital or anatomical abnormalities or disease or infection are relatively easily diagnosed. Infertility and/or more subtle behavioral difficulties may also arise due to neurological disorders including those associated with hypothalamic-pituitary dysfunction (such as hyperprolactinemia, hypothalamic or pituitary tumors, etc.), temporal lobe damage including epilepsy, spinal cord injuries, multiple sclerosis, or diabetes (Lundberg, 1977). In all these cases interventions are based on prevalent medical practice and rely on behavioral, pharmacological, and/or surgical treatments. The success of such treatment in restoring fertility or sexual performance varies widely depending on the origins and severity of the problem (Mooney, Cole, & Chilgren, 1975; Tarbulcy, 1972). Urological or gynecological abnormalities obviously should be corrected whenever possible.

One of the most common causes of sexual dysfunction is diabetes. There are indications that as many as 50% of male diabetics are impotent or have other sexual difficulties (Karacan, Salis, Ware, Dervent, Williams, Scott, Attia, & Beutler, 1978). In fact, impotence is considered an early symptom of diabetes. Diabetic patients may have hormonal abnormalities, but it is believed that the most important factor producing impotence is a progressive neuropathy of the autonomic nerves responsible for erection. Diabetic men also show reductions in the incidence of episodes of nocturnal (spontaneous) penile tumescence and it has been proposed that recordings of nocturnal erections can be used to differentiate physiologically based impotence (Karacan et al., 1978). However, at present because expensive and portable instrumentation is usually used to record nocturnal changes in penile circumference, this technique is not widely applied in clinical practice. Little has been reported regarding the sexual behavior of diabetic women.

Prostatectomy, colostomy, or surgeries of the genital area can also interfere with the erectile mechanism and may lead to impotence. In general, treatments to reverse erectile disorders due to diabetes or other chronic failures of peripheral neurovascular mechanisms are not very successful.

Prosthetic devices are sometimes used to simulate erections. These may involve either a synthetic penis or the surgical implantation of a baculum (usually silicone or metallic tubes) used to mechanically stiffen the penis. These devices are also used in congenital abnormalities, mechanical or disease-induced damage to the penis, and for the construction of phallic organs in female-to-male transsexuals (Noe, Laub, & Schulz, 1976).

In some cases medical treatments, and in particular tranquilizers and drugs used to control hypertension, may inhibit sexual behavior (see Table 15.4 and previous section on drugs and sexual behavior). Failure on the part of the clinician or patient to be aware of these sexual side effects can result in unnecessary anxiety and inappropriate treatments.

Behavioral Approaches to Sexual Dysfunctions

The primary treatments for most psychosexual problems depend on: (1) education; (2) attitudinal changes; and (3) methods of reducing performance anxiety. Most libraries and bookstores carry an assortment of "sex education" books, marriage manuals, etc. For example, the works of Comfort (1972, 1974), McCary (1973), Katchadourian and Lunde (1979), and many others contain useful basic information on human sexuality. Films, videotapes, or slide presentations can also provide valuable educational opportunities. Among the companies that supply films or slides dealing with human sexuality are Williams and Wilkins (Baltimore, Md.), Wiley and Sons (New York), McGraw-Hill (New York), EDCOA Productions (Englewood, N.J.), Behavioral and Educational Consulting Corporation (New Haven, Conn.), Audio-Digest Foundation (Glendale, Calif.), and Research Press (Champaign, Il.). These publishers tend to orient their products to sex education or marriage counseling audiences. A selection of highly sexually explicit audiovisual materials is also available from the Multi-Media Resource Center (San Francisco, Calif.).

Materials such as those listed may be useful in therapist training or in the treatment of sexual dysfunction. Group discussions following the reading or viewing of such materials seem to be particularly useful to encourage the restructuring of attitudes and the eventual reduction of sex-related anxieties.

Therapists tend to agree that facilitating openness between sexual partners is a valuable aid in dealing with sexual dysfunction. Therapist-led or group discussions seem to promote better communication. In general, the contemporary trend in sexual therapies has been to develop ways to encourage sexual intimacy. For example, compare Barbach's 1975 "For Yourself" to her 1982 "For Each Other" to see this movement away from "me"-oriented to "we"-oriented treatments of sexuality.

Behavioral therapies have been especially successful in the treatment of female sexual disorders including vaginismus, dyspareunia, and anorgasmia. For women for whom organic problems have been excluded as causes of sexual dysfunction (see Masters & Johnson, 1970) desensitization therapies have often proven effective. These therapies tend to focus on presenting symptoms, such as painful intercourse or orgasmic failure, and often are based on behavioral modification or relaxation procedures.

Muscle spasms in the pelvic floor may cause vaginismus and dyspareunia. One treatment for this problem is the use of successively larger vaginal dilators or manual stretching of the vagina (Masters & Johnson, 1970). Although this is a physical procedure it incorporates in many cases desensitization and increased relaxation in the presence of genital sensation.

Several therapists have recommended masturbatory training for women with difficulty experiencing orgasm (Barbach, 1975; LoPiccolo & LoPiccolo, 1978). Films are available from a number of the publishers listed previously that offer guided instruction in methods to increase genital awareness through self-stimulation.

Exercises of the muscles around the vagina have been suggested to improve muscle tone and increase genital feedback (Kegel, 1952). Kegel recommended the use of a mechanical pressure gauge for monitoring the effectiveness of these exercises. Alternatively, women may practice the use of muscles of the pelvic floor while urinating. Successfully being able to regulate the onset or offset of urination is an index of the use of these (pubococcygeus) muscles and can be used initially as a method for training this procedure. Subsequent exercise simply involves contracting and relaxing the pelvic floor muscles. Women are encouraged to practice the "Kegel" exercise on a daily basis throughout life.

A variety of other procedures have been proposed for the treatment of female sexual dysfunction. Among these are the use of vibrators and/or guided fantasy (Asirdas & Beech, 1975). Hypnosis has also been employed with success in some women. For example, under hypnosis women may be able to recall their own early sexual and nonsexual experiences and then can be encouraged to remember these experiences with fewer feelings of guilt (Cheek, 1976). Psychoanalysis and psychotherapy have also been used in the treatment of sexual disorders. In general, an important unifying principle for all these therapeutic methods is the reduction of sex-related guilt or anxiety.

For the male, many behavioral approaches to sexual dysfunction also focus on attitudinal changes and education. Premature ejaculation in the male is one disorder that is amenable to behavioral therapy. The most effective treatment for premature ejaculation is known as "squeeze technique" (Masters & Johnson, 1970). Males who wish to delay ejaculation can apply pressure to, or have their partner apply pressure to, the area just below the head of the penis (after erection, but prior to ejaculation).

Failure to ejaculate (in the apparent absence of physical dysfunction) is a more difficult problem to treat. Although guilt reduction or reeducation may be helpful in some cases, behavioral therapies for this condition have not been very successful. This may be because many apparently psychologically based cases of sexual dysfunction do in fact reflect some degree of physiological impairment that remains undiagnosed (Kaplan, 1974).

Many forms of sexual dysfunction seem to respond well to treatments that are centered around the relationship between sexual partners. The best known partner-based sexual therapies employ the Masters and Johnson method (1970) or are modifications of the procedures originally described by Masters and Johnson. As originally proposed, this therapy involved both partners and a male and female therapist team. A 2- to 3-week continuous behavioral treatment schedule is oriented to the sexual problems of the couple. Couples are encouraged to be alone together, when not with the therapists. They are trained to become more aware of and involved in learning to satisfy their own sexual needs and the sexual desires of their partner. Masters and Johnson reported that about 70–80% of the patients treated with this method showed a favorable response. Modifications of the Masters and Johnson method have also been reported to be successful (Schumacher, 1977). In general these modifications alter the timing of the therapy (using spaced therapy sessions), or expand the treatment program to encompass other problems or additional techniques, or alter the composition of the therapy group (using, for example, only one therapist). Strategies of behavioral intervention are discussed in Chapter 9 by Tapp.

Among these various behavioral approaches to sexual problems, success rates tend to range from about 50 to 85% (O'Connor, 1976; Schumacher, 1977). The patients in such samples may be preselected to eliminate obvious physiological abnormalities, but in the case of failures, undetected physical problems may not be excluded. In general, the success of a given therapeutic method depends heavily on the physical and mental health of the patient and some patients (and/or relationships) are not helped by any of the existing procedures.

CONCLUSION

Human sexual functions and dysfunctions are interactive. Even autoerotic stimulation is usually performed within a cognitive context that includes other individuals. The choice of a sexual partner or partners, the setting for sexual activity, the impact of sexual behavior on other aspects of life, and so forth are pivotal to our understanding of sexuality.

In *The Pleasure Bond, A New Look at Sexuality and Commitment* (1975) Masters and Johnson interviewed individuals from a variety of life situations, in an attempt to capture the essence of the psychosocial context that accompanies sexual activity in modern Western society. Unlike their earlier contributions to our knowledge of sexual physiology (1966) and sexual inadequacy (1970), *The Pleasure Bond* does not really shed new light on the problems of sexuality. However, it does serve to remind us that human sexual behavior manifests itself within personal and cultural constraints. The individuals interviewed by Masters and Johnson described their sexual activities and histories against a background of emotional needs and life stresses. It became clear that sexual interactions reflect these needs.

One of the major nonreproductive functions of sexual behavior is to develop or reinforce emotional bonds. It is not uncommon for individuals to engage in, either sequentially or simultaneously, sexual relationships with more than one partner. Such multiple interactions sometimes may be seen as positive. However, sexual activity in the absence of emotional involvement is typically perceived as unsatisfying and may lead to (and/or reflect) disorganization in many aspects of the individual's life.

Like many modern sources, Masters and Johnson (1975) conclude that the successful expression of sexuality requires the ability to assume responsibility for one's own behavior and the capacity to develop intimacy and emotional commitment. In the absence of commitment sexuality becomes a biological process with limited value and it is not uncommon for sexual dysfunction to eventually follow.

REFERENCES

Adams, D. B., Gold, A. R., & Burt, A. D. *New England Journal of Medicine*, 1978, *299*, 1145–1148.

Asirdas, S., & Beech, H. R. The behavioral treatment of sexual inadequacy. *Journal of Psychosomatic Research*, 1975, *19*, 345–353.

Bancroft, J. The relationship between hormones and sexual behavior in humans. In J. B. Hutchison (Ed.), *Biological determinants of sexual behaviour*. Chichester: J. Wiley & Sons, 1978.

Bancroft, J. Psychophysiology of sexual dysfunction. In H. M. van Praag (Ed.), *Handbook of biological psychiatry. Part II. Brain mechanisms and abnormal behavior*. New York: Marcel Dekker, 1980.

Bancroft, J., & Skakkeback, N. E. Androgens and human sexual behaviour. In Ciba Foundation Symposium 62, *Sex, hormones and behaviour*. Excerpta Medica: Amsterdam, 1979.

Barbach, L. G. *For yourself: The fulfillment of female sexuality*. New York: Doubleday, 1975.

Barbach, L. G. *For each other: Sharing sexual intimacy*. New York: Doubleday, 1982.

Baum, M. J. Differentiation of coital behavior in mammals: A comparative analysis. *Neuroscience and Biobehavioral Reviews*, 1979, *3*, 284.

Beach, F. A. Animal models for human sexuality. In Ciba Foundation Symposium 62, *Sex, hormones and behaviour*. Excerpta Medica: Amsterdam, 1979.

Beaumont, P. J. V., Richards, D. H., & Gelder, M. G. Study of minor psychiatric and physical symptoms during the menstrual cycle. *British Journal of Psychiatry*, 1975, *126*, 431–434.

Benedek-Jaszmann, L. G., & Hearn-Sturtevant, M. D. Premenstrual tension and functional infertility. *Lancet I*, 1976, 1095–1098.

Benson, R. M., & Migeon, C. J. Physiological and pathological puberty, and human behavior. In B. E. Eleftheriou & R. L. Sprott (Eds.), *Hormonal correlates of behavior*. New York: Plenum Press, 1975.

Bentler, P. M. Heterosexual behavior assessment—I: Males. *Behavior Research and Therapy*, 1968, *6*, 21–25. (a)

Bentler, P. M. Heterosexual behavior assessment—II: Females. *Behavior Research and Therapy*, 1968, *6*, 27–30. (b)

Blumer, D. Hypersexual episodes in temporal lobe epilepsy. *American Journal of Psychiatry*, 1970, *126*, 1099–1106.

Broverman, D. M., Vogel, W., Klaiber, E. L., Majcher, D., Shea, D., and Paul, V. Changes in cognitive task performance across the menstrual cycle. *Journal of Comparative and Physiological Psychology*, 1981, *95*, 646–654.

Bullock, J. L., Massey, F. M., & Gambrell, R. D. Use of medroxyprogesterone acetate to prevent menopausal symptoms. *Obstetrics and Gynecology*, 1975, *46*, 165–168.

Campbell, S. Double-blind psychometric studies on the effects of natural estrogens on post-menopausal women. In S. Campbell (Ed.), *The management of the menopause and post-menopausal years*. Baltimore: University Park Press, 1976.

Carroll, B. J., & Steiner, M. The psychobiology of premenstrual dysphoria: The role of prolactin. *Psychoneuroendocrinology*, 1978, *3*, 171–180.

Carter, C. S., & Davis, J. M. Effects of drugs on sexual arousal and performance. In J. K. Meyer (Ed.), *Clinical management of sexual disorders*. Baltimore: Williams & Wilkins, 1976.

Casper, R. F., Yen, S. S. C., & Wilkes, M. M. Menopausal flushes: A neuroendocrine link with pulsatile luteinizing hormone secretion. *Science*, 1979, *205*, 823–825.

Cheek, D. B. Short-term hypnotherapy for frigidity using exploration of early life attitudes. *American Journal of Clinical Hypnosis*, 1976, *19*, 20–27.

Christie Brown, J. R. W., & Christie Brown, M. E. Psychiatric disorders associated with menopause. In R. J. Beard (Ed.), *The menopause*. Baltimore: University Park Press, 1976.

Comfort, A. *The joy of sex*. New York: Crown Publishers, 1972.

Comfort, A. *More joy*. New York: Crown Publishers, 1974.

Coope, J. Double-blind cross-over study of estrogen replacement therapy. In S. Campbell (Ed.), *The management of the menopause and the post-menopausal years.* Baltimore: University Park Press, 1976.

Cullberg, J. Mood changes and menstrual symptoms with different gestagen/estrogen combinations. *Acta Psychiatrica Scandinavica Supplementum,* 1972, *236,* 1–86.

Dalton, K. *The premenstrual syndrome and progesterone therapy.* Chicago: Year Book Medical Publications, 1977.

Dennerstein, L., Burrows, G. D., Hyman, G., & Wood, C. Menopausal hot flushes: A double blind comparison of placebo, ethinyl oestradiol and norgestrel. *British Journal of Obstetrics and Gynaecology,* 1978, 852–856.

Dörner, G. Hormones and sexual differentiation of the brain. In Ciba Foundation Symposium 62, *Sex, hormones and behaviour.* Excerpta Medica: Amsterdam, 1979, 81–101.

Durst, N., & Maoz, B. Changes in psychological well-being during postmenopause as a result of estrogen therapy. *Maturitas,* 1979, *1,* 301–315.

Ehrhardt, A. A., & Meyer-Bahlburg, H. F. L. Psychosexual development: An examination of the role of prenatal hormones. In Ciba Foundation Symposium 62, *Sex, hormones and behaviour.* Excerpta Medica: Amsterdam, 1979, 41–50.

Frisch, R. E. Weight at menarche: Similarity for well-nourished and under-nourished girls at differing ages and evidence for historical constancy. *Pediatrics,* 1972, *50,* 445–450.

Gambrell, R. D. The prevention of endometrial cancer in postmenopausal women with progestogens. *Maturitas,* 1978, *1,* 107–112.

Gay, G. R., & Sheppard, C. W. Sex in the "drug culture." *Medical Aspects of Human Sexuality,* 1972, *6,* 28.

Geer, J. H., O'Donohue, W. T., & Schorman, R. H. T. Sexuality. In M. G. H. Coles, E. Donchin, & S. W. Porges (Eds.), *Psychophysiology: Systems, processes and applications — A handbook.* New York: Guilford Press, in press.

Gordon, J. W., & Ruddle, F. H. Mammalian gonadal determination and gametogenesis. *Science,* 1981, *211,* 1265–1271.

Green, R. (Ed.). *Human sexuality: A health practitioner's text.* Baltimore: Williams & Wilkins, 1975.

Greenblatt, R. B., Mortara, F., & Torpin, R. Sexual libido in the female. *American Journal of Obstetrics and Gynecology,* 1942, *44,* 658–663.

Greenblatt, R. B., Nezhat, C., & Karpas, A. The menopausal syndrome hormone replacement therapy. In B. A. Eskin (Ed.), *The menopause.* New York: Masson, 1980.

Hart, B. L. Hormones, spinal reflexes and sexual behaviour. In J. B. Hutchison (Ed.), *Biological determinants of sexual behaviour.* Chichester: J. Wiley & Sons, 1978.

Hartman, W. E., & Fithian, M. A. *Treatment of sexual dysfunction: A biopsychosocial approach.* Long Beach, Calif.: Center for Marital and Sexual Studies, 1972.

Haseltine, F. P., & Ohno, S. Mechanisms of gonadal differentiation. *Science,* 1981, *211,* 1272–1278.

Hollister, L. E. The mystique of social drugs and sex. In M. Sandler & G. L. Gessa (Eds.), *Sexual behavior: Pharmacology and biochemistry.* New York: Raven Press, 1975.

Imperato-McGinley, J., Peterson, R. E., Gautier, T., & Sturla, E. Androgens and the evolution of male-gender identity among male pseudohermaphrodites with 5-reductase deficiency. *New England Journal of Medicine,* 1979, *300,* 1233–1237.

Jaszmann, L. B. Epidemiology of the climacteric syndrome. In S. Campbell (Ed.), *The management of the menopause and post-menopausal years.* Baltimore: University Park Press, 1976.

Jones, G. S. Hormonal changes in perimenopause. In B. A. Eskin (Ed.), *The menopause.* New York: Masson, 1980.

Jost, A. Basic sexual trends in the development of vertebrates. In Ciba Foundation Symposium 62, *Sex, hormones and behavior.* Excerpta Medica: Amsterdam, 1979, 5–13.

Kaplan, H. S. *The new sex therapy.* New York: Brunner/Mazel, 1974.

Karacan, I., Salis, P. J., Ware, J. C., Dervent, B., Williams, R. L., Scott, F. B., Attia, S. L., & Beutler, L. E. Nocturnal penile tumescence and diagnosis in diabetic impotence. *American Journal of Psychiatry*, 1978, *135*, 191–196.

Katchadourian, A., & Lunde, D. *Human sexuality*. New York: Holt, Rinehart & Winston, 1979.

Kegel, A. Sexual functions of the pubococcygeus muscle. *Journal of Obstetrics and Gynecology*, 1952, *60*, 521–524.

Kinsey, A. C., Pomeroy, W. B., & Martin, C. E. *Sexual behavior in the human male*. Philadelphia: Saunders, 1948.

Klaiber, E. L., Broverman, M., Vogel, W., & Kobayashi, Y. The use of steroid hormones in depression. In T. M. Itil, G. Laudahn, & W. Herrmann (Eds.), *Psychotropic actions of hormones*. New York: Spectrum, 1976.

Kolodny, R. C., Masters, W. H., Kolodner, R. M., & Toro, G. Depression of plasma testosterone level after chronic intensive marihuana use. *New England Journal of Medicine*, 1974, *290*, 872–874.

Krouse, T. B. Menopausal pathology. In B. A. Eskin (Ed.), *The menopause*. New York: Mason, 1980.

Kruskemper, G. Results of psychological testing (MMPI) in climacteric women. *Frontiers in Hormone Research*, 1975, *3*, 105–115.

Lauritzen, C., & Van Keep, P. A. Proven beneficial effects of estrogen substitution in the post-menopause — A review. *Frontiers in Hormone Research*, 1978, *5*, 1–25.

Lewis, V. G. Androgen insensitivity syndrome: Erotic component of gender identity in nine women. In R. Gemme & C. C. Wheeler (Eds.), *Progress in sexology*. New York: Plenum Press, 1977.

Lief, H. I., & Reed, D. M. *Sex knowledge and attitude test*. Philadelphia: Center for the Study of Sex Education in Medicine, 1971.

Locke, H. J., & Wallace, K. M. Short marital adjustment and prediction tests: Their reliability and validity. *Marriage and Family Living*, 1959, *21*, 251–255.

LoPiccolo, J., & LoPiccolo, L. (Eds.). *Handbook of sex therapy*. New York: Plenum Press, 1978.

Lundberg, P. O. In R. Gemme & C. C. Wheeler (Eds.), *Progress in sexology*. New York: Plenum Press, 1977.

Maas, J. M. Biogenic amines and depression: Biochemical and pharmacological separation of two types of depression. *Archives of General Psychiatry*, 1975, *32*, 1357–1361.

MacLean, P. D. Brain mechanisms of primal sexual functions and related behavior. In M. Sandler & G. L. Gessa (Eds.), *Sexual behavior: Pharmacology and biochemistry*. New York: Raven Press, 1975.

MacLusky, N. J., & Naftolin, F. Sexual differentiation of the central nervous system. *Science*, 1981, *211*, 1294–1303.

Marx, J. L. Estrogen drugs: Do they increase the risk of cancer? *Science*, 1976, *191*, 838–882.

Masters, W. H., & Johnson, V. E. *Human sexual response*. Boston: Little, Brown, 1966.

Masters, W. H., & Johnson, V. E. *Human sexual inadequacy*. Boston: Little, Brown, 1970.

Masters, W. H., & Johnson, V. E. *The pleasure bond: A new look at sexuality and commitment*. Boston: Little, Brown & Company, 1975.

McCary, J. L. *Human sexuality*. New York: Van Nostrand, 1973.

Meyer, J. K. (Ed.). *Clinical assessment of sexual disorders*. Baltimore: Williams & Wilkins, 1976.

Meyer-Bahlburg, H. F. L. Sex hormones and male homosexuality in comparative perspective. *Archives of Sexual Behavior*, 1977, *6*, 297–325.

Meyer-Bahlburg, H. F. L. Sex hormones and female homosexuality: A documentation. *Archives of Sexual Behavior*, 1978.

Money, J., & Ehrhardt, A. A. *Man and woman, boy and girl*. Baltimore: Johns Hopkins University Press, 1972.

Mooney, T. Q., Cole, T. M., & Chilgren, B. A. *Sexual options for paraplegics and quadriplegics*. Boston: Little, Brown, 1975.

Neugarten, B. L., & Kraines, R. J. Menopausal symptoms in women of various ages. *Psychosomatic Medicine*, 1965, *27*, 266–273.

Noe, J. M., Laub, D. R., & Schulz, W. The external male genitalia: The interplay of surgery and mechanical prostheses. In J. K. Meyer (Ed.), *Clinical management of sexual disorders*. Baltimore: Williams & Wilkins, 1976.

O'Connor, J. F. Sexual problems, therapy and prognostic factors. In J. K. Meyer (Ed.), *Clinical management of sexual disorders*. Baltimore: Williams & Wilkins, 1976.

Paige, K. E. Women learn to sing the menstrual blues. *Psychology Today*, 1973, *7*, 4–46.

Parlee, M. B. The premenstrual syndrome. *Psychological Bulletin*, 1973, *80*, 454–465.

Parlee, M. B. Stereotypic beliefs about menstruation: A methodological note on the Moos menstrual distress questionnaire and some new data. *Psychosomatic Medicine*, 1974, *36*, 229–240.

Parry, B. L., & Rush, A. J. Oral contraceptives and depressive symptomatology: Biologic mechanisms. *Comprehensive Psychiatry*, 1979, *20*, 347–358.

Phoenix, C. H., Goy, R. W., Gerall, A. A., & Young, W. C. Organizing action of prenatally administered testosterone propionate on the tissues mediating mating behavior in the female guinea pig. *Endocrinology*, 1959, *65*, 369–382.

Rakoff, A. E., & Nowroogi, K. The female climacteric. In R. B. Greenblatt (Ed.), *Geriatric endocrinology*. New York: Raven Press, 1978.

Robbins, M. B., & Jensen, G. D. Multiple orgasm in males. In R. Gemme & C. C. Wheeler (Eds.), *Progress in sexology*. New York: Plenum Press, 1977.

Ruble, D. Premenstrual symptoms: A reinterpretation. *Science*, 1977, *197*, 291–292.

Rust, J. A., Langley, I. I., Hill, E. C., & Lamb, E. J. Estrogens: Do the risks outweigh the benefits? *American Journal of Obstetrics and Gynecology*, 1977, *128*, 431–439.

Schreiner-Engel, P., Schiavi, R. C., Smith, H., & White, D. Sexual arousability and the menstrual cycle. *Psychosomatic Medicine*, 1981, *43*, 199–214.

Schumacher, S. Effectiveness of sex therapy. In R. Gemme & C. C. Wheeler (Eds.), *Progress in sexology*. New York: Plenum Press, 1977.

Schwartz, M. F. Pair-bonding experience of 26 early treated adrenogenital females aged 17–27. In R. Gemme & C. C. Wheeler (Eds.), *Progress in sexology*. New York: Plenum Press, 1977.

Shader, R. L. *Psychiatric complications of medical drugs*. New York: Raven Press, 1972.

Slimp, J. C., Hart, B. L., & Goy, R. W. Heterosexual, autosexual and social behavior of adult male rhesus monkeys with medial preoptic-anterior hypothalamic lesions. *Brain Research*, 1978, *142*, 105–122.

Smith, S. L. Mood and the menstrual cycle. In E. J. Sachar (Ed.), *Topics in psychoendocrinology*. New York: Grune & Stratton, 1975.

Steiner, M., & Carroll, B. J. The psychobiology of premenstrual dysphoria: Review of theories and treatments. *Psychoneuroendocrinology*, 1977, *2*, 321–335.

Tarabulcy, E. Sexual function in the normal and paraplegia. *Paraplegia*, 1972, *10*, 202–208.

Thompson, B., Hart, S. A., & Durno, D. Menopausal age and symptomatology in a general practice. *Journal of Biosocial Science*, 1973, *5*, 71–75.

Thorne, F. C. *The sex inventory*. Brandon, Vt.: Clinical Psychology Publishing, 1965.

Udry, J. R., & Morris, N. M. Distribution of coitus in the menstrual cycle. *Nature*, 1968, *220*, 593–596.

Utian, W. H. *Menopause in modern perspective*. New York: Appleton–Century–Crofts, 1980.

Waxenburg, S. E., Drellich, M. G., & Sutherland, A. M. The role of hormones in human behavior. I. Changes in female sexuality after adrenalectomy. *Journal of Clinical Endocrinology and Metabolism*, 1959, *19*, 193–202.

Wilson, J. D., George, F. W., & Griffin, J. E. The hormonal control of sexual development. *Science*, 1981, *211*, 1278–1284.

Yen, S. S. C. Neuroendocrine regulation of the menstrual cycle. In D. T. Kreiger & J. C. Hughes (Eds.), *Neuroendocrinology*. Sunderland, Mass.: Sinauer Associates, 1980.

Zuckerman, M. Scales for sex experience for males and females. *Journal of Consulting and Clinical Psychology*, 1973, *41*, 27–29.

16 Coronary Prone Behavior

Charles S. Carver
University of Miami

Eric L. Diamond
University of Florida Health Science Center

Charlene Humphries
University of Miami

INTRODUCTION

Coronary heart disease (CHD) is a frequent cause of death in this country. Despite the fact that epidemiological research (Brand, Rosenman, Scholtz, & Friedman, 1976; Dawber & Kannel, 1961) has identified a number of risk factors for CHD, the importance of some of these factors is still a matter of considerable controversy (Friedman, 1969), and even the best combination of these factors fails to identify most new cases before they occur (Jenkins, 1971). This difficulty in predicting CHD has led to a broadening of the search for potential risk factors. One variable that has received a good deal of attention in recent years is a *psychological* variable: a behavioral style that has come to be known as the Type A coronary-prone behavior pattern.

TYPE A BEHAVIOR PATTERN

The Type A behavior pattern has been described as an "action-emotion complex" comprised of a competitive achievement orientation, time urgency, and hostility (Rosenman, 1974, p. 67; see also Friedman, 1969). Both retrospective and prospective research have identified this pattern as a risk factor for CHD (Blumenthal, Williams, Kong, Schlanberg, & Thompson, 1978; Haynes, Levine, Scotch, Feinleib, & Kannel, 1978; Jenkins, Rosenman, & Zyzanski, 1974; Rosenman, Brand, Jenkins, Friedman, Straus, & Wurm, 1975; Rosenman, Friedman, Straus, Wurm, Jenkins, & Messinger, 1966). One prospective study (Rosenman et al., 1975) found that Type A men had more than twice the incidence of heart disease

437

(over an 8 1/2-year follow-up period) as did Type B men (defined by the relative absence of A-type characteristics). This was true even when statistical adjustments were incorporated for traditional risk factors such as smoking and serum cholesterol.

These findings suggest that Pattern A exerts an influence on CHD that is independent of other risk factors. This is important because of the fact that Type A also has an association with certain traditional risk factors. Fully developed Type A's have been found to have higher levels of cholesterol and related substances in their blood than Type B's (Friedman & Rosenman, 1959; Rosenman & Friedman, 1974), even among subjects as young as 19 years of age (Glass, 1977). Type A's also show more lability in their blood pressure than do Type B's (Dembroski, Mac-Dougall, Shields, Petitto, & Lushene, 1978; Manuck, Craft, & Gold, 1978), although there apparently is no relationship between Pattern A and chronic hypertension (Shekelle, Schoenberger, & Stamler, 1976).

Coronary-Prone Behavior: A Pattern, or Components?

More recently, questions have been raised as to whether all aspects of Type A behavior contribute to the relationship between the pattern and heart disease. Is the total Type A action – emotion complex a risk factor? Or is perhaps a single facet of that complex uniquely predictive of CHD? Preliminary evidence on this questions suggests two answers. First, in a reanalysis of data from an extensive longitudinal study (Matthews, Glass, Rosenman, & Bortner, 1977) only seven of the more than 40 Type A attributes on which information was available discriminated (prospectively) between CHD cases and matched controls. Four items related to hostility, anger, and irritation; two concerned vigorousness of vocal stylistics. This suggests the possibility that hostility and aggressiveness represent the facet of Pattern A that is critical to the development of CHD.

In the Matthews et al. study, subjects were not separated according to their clinical manifestations of CHD. There are, in fact, several such manifestations: angina pectoris (constricting chest pains), acute myocardial infarction or MI (heart attack), and "silent" MI (heart attacks that are clinically unrecognized). A subsequent study (Jenkins, Zyzanski, & Rosenman, 1978) separated subjects into those three categories, based on each subject's initial manifestation of disease. An effort then was made to ascertain what psychological characteristics (measured years earlier) were associated with each syndrome. This study found considerable differences among the groups, particularly between angina subjects and MI subjects. Angina cases were the only group in this study who gave strong evidence of hostility. By contrast, the cases of acute MI were characterized by a strong sense of job involvement. Jenkins et al. concluded that there are at least two distinct behavioral patterns associated with the emergence of distinctly different clinical manifestations of CHD.

One result of studies such as these is a growing awareness that the two constructs from which this area of investigation has grown both require differentiation. That is, it is increasingly recognized that CHD comprises a cluster of disorders that may not occur together, and that Pattern A comprises a cluster of behaviors that may not occur together. In studying the Pattern A–CHD relationship, greater emphasis thus is being placed on the importance of investigating the relationships among the *components* of each construct. Though this theme recurs throughout the chapter, component analysis is relatively rare in the existing literature.[1] Most of the studies discussed in the following section have treated Pattern A as a global construct.

ASSESSMENT OF BEHAVIOR PATTERNS

The method first developed for classifying persons as Type A or Type B is a structured, stress-inducing interview (Friedman, 1969; Jenkins, Rosenman, & Friedman, 1968). The interviewee is asked questions about situations that would be expected to elicit competitiveness, time urgency, and hostile feelings. The content of the person's answers is one determinant of A–B classification, but the manner and tone of the answers are weighted somewhat more heavily. For example, Type A's use explosive vocal intonations more than do Type B's, and Type A's become impatient when the pace of the interview slows. Indeed, one recent study (Schucker & Jacobs, 1977) has shown that an index of voice volume and speed of speech yields much the same classifications as does the more standard scoring technique. Classification based on this structured interview (SI) typically makes use of four categories: A1 or fully developed Type A; A2 or incompletely developed Type A; X or indeterminate pattern; and Type B. Presumably, however, Type A characteristics are normally distributed in a given population. Thus most researchers do not regard the A − B division as really representing a typology.

Though the basic SI scoring yields only a global A − B classification, several factor analyses of interview data have been conducted (Matthews et al., 1977; Matthews, Krantz, Dembroski, & MacDougall, 1982). The first of these (Matthews et al., 1977) yielded factors of competitive drive, past achievement, non-job achievement, impatience, and speed. These factors appear to relate well to the initial conceptualization of the Type A style, except that hostility did not form a separate factor. Instead, data reflective of hostility loaded primarily on impatience or competitive drive. Subsequent analyses (Matthews et al., 1982) yielded a somewhat different pattern, at least in part because the SI has been altered over the years by the omission of several of its items. The factors of these more recent analyses have been labeled pressured drive, clinical ratings, anger, and competitiveness.

A second mechanism for classification is a self-report questionnaire called the JAS, or the Jenkins Activity Survey for Health Prediction (Jenkins, Rosenman, & Zyzanski, 1972). It consists of a series of items (derived from SI questions) such as

---

[1] Research published since the writing of this chapter has focused to a far greater extent on component analysis of Pattern A.

the following: (1) "How would your wife (or closest friend) rate you?" where "Definitely hard-driving and competitive" is an extreme Pattern A response and "Definitely relaxed and easy-going" is a Pattern B response. The JAS provides a continuous distribution of A−B scores, though research subjects are usually dichotomized by division at the median or selection of top and bottom segments of the distribution. The JAS has also been modified for use with college students (Krantz, Glass, & Snyder, 1974; see Glass, 1977, for greater detail). As is true of the SI, the adult version of the JAS has been validated as a predictor of CHD. Although it is somewhat less sensitive than the SI in prospectively identifying CHD cases (Brand, Rosenman, Jenkins, Sholtz, & Zyzanski, in press), its predictive validity is statistically reliable (Jenkins et al., 1974).

The JAS was designed to mimic aspects of the SI, and the weighting of its scoring was developed by reference to the SI. The JAS has also been subjected to several factor analyses in its various forms (see Glass, 1977, Appendix A; Zyzanski & Jenkins, 1970). These analyses typically yield separate factors characterized as "hard-driving and competitiveness" and "speed and impatience," which are similar to two of the defining attributes of Pattern A. The third attribute—hostility—regularly fails to emerge as a separate component in factor analyses of the JAS, as was true of the factor analysis of SI data using the original SI format (Matthews et al., 1977).

Several other self-report measures have also been used to assess Pattern A, including the Gough Adjective Checklist, the Thurstone Temperament Schedule (Chesney, Black, Feuerstein, Rosenman, Calligan, & Chadwick, 1978; Mac-Dougall, Dembroski, & Musante, 1979; Rosenman, Rahe, Borhani, & Feinleib, 1974), and the Framingham Type A schedule (Haynes et al., 1978). There is evidence that certain of these measures may show greater agreement than the JAS with diagnosis from the structured interview (cf. MacDougall et al., 1979). And one of them—the Framingham—has been validated as a predictor of CHD (Haynes et al., 1978). But very little behavioral validation research has been conducted using these alternative measures. Most such research has employed the JAS.

Indeed, there is a broader issue here that should receive our attention. Several researchers have raised serious questions as to whether or not the various methods of assessing Pattern A are actually measuring the same thing. Scores on the JAS and the SI are not always highly associated (Jenkins, 1971; Matthews et al., 1982). And the heavy reliance on response stylistics in scoring the SI obviously cannot be easily duplicated in any self-report measure. Matthews (1982; Matthews et al., 1982) has cautioned against treating the JAS and the SI as interchangeable. On the other hand, it should be noted that the literature of the field is anything but homogeneous in terms of use of various measures. The vast majority of the evidence of behavioral construct validity comes from studies using the JAS. The majority of studies examining cardiovascular reactivity have used the SI. Unless one assumes that the various measures tap some common central characteristic, one rapidly encounters a difficult dilemma in attempting to evaluate the literature.

VALIDITY OF BEHAVIORAL COMPONENTS OF PATTERN A

The assessment of Pattern A characteristics relies on subjects' statements about themselves, and—when the SI is used—on an interviewer's clinical judgment. Although the evidence is strong that these assessment techniques can predict increased risk of CHD, until the mid 1970s there was little systematic objective evidence of the existence of the behavioral characteristics believed to comprise the Type A behavior. Do Type A's actually behave in ways that reflect a competitive achievement orientation? Do they have a sense of time urgency? Are they easily incited to aggression? In recent years these questions have all received considerable research attention (see Matthews, 1982, for a more complete review).

Hostility and Aggression

The potential for hostility—not always apparent, but never too far beneath the surface—was an integral part of the Pattern A conceptualization from its inception. An early study provided suggestive evidence that Type A's become irritable when frustrated or impeded in their task attempts (Glass, Snyder, & Hollis, 1974, Experiment 3). In a systematic test of the hypothesis (Carver & Glass, 1978), subjects were induced to teach an ostensible cosubject (actually an accomplice of the experimenter) in a concept-formation task. As part of this procedure, subjects administered shocks to the accomplice as punishment for incorrect responses. Unbeknownst to the subject, the accomplice never actually received the shocks, but by a hidden device was able to monitor the shock intensity that the subject chose on any given trial. The mean shock intensity over a series of trials was the measure of aggression.

Before the presumed learning session, some participants were subjected to a procedure in which the accomplice denigrated their attempts to perform a difficult task. Others did not receive this provocation. The provocation increased aggression significantly among Type A's, but not among Type B's (Experiment 1). Subsequent research determined that the full instigation was not necessary to elicit aggression from Type A's. A simple task frustration (failure at the same task, but with no verbal harassment) actually yielded nearly as great an increase in aggression among A's as did the full provocation (Experiment 2). Among B's, however, the effect of frustration per se was negligible. Conceptually similar findings have been reported by others (Chesney, Black, Chadwick, & Rosenman, 1981; Dimsdale, Hackett, Hutter, Block, Catanzano, & White, 1978).

It is worth noting that in neither of the Carver and Glass (1978) studies did the aggression of the Type A's and Type B's diverge from each other in a control condition in which task mastery was not threatened. Type A's apparently are not *chronically* aggressive. Their hostility is a *potential*, which must be elicited by situational events. This general point—that Pattern A characteristics are elicited when the susceptible individual confronts suitably threatening circumstances— recurs numerous times in the literature discussed in the following sections.

Time Urgency

The second component of Pattern A as originally conceptualized is a sense of time urgency. Type A's prefer a fast pace and quickly become impatient with delay. Indeed, even their sense of the passage of time may differ from that of Type B's. In one study, for example, A's estimated that a time interval of 1 minute had elapsed reliably sooner than did B's (Burnam, Pennebaker, & Glass, 1975; see also Bortner & Rosenman, 1967). A more recent study (Gastorf, 1980) found that Type A's arrived earlier for scheduled appointments than did Type B's.

This sense of time urgency and impatience has other behavioral consequences. For example, it handicaps Type A's on tasks that require delayed responses. On such a task, the subject must wait for a fixed time interval before responding; a premature response resets a timer and the subject is not rewarded. This task is difficult and is mastered only with considerable patience. Glass et al. (1974) found that Type A's did significantly worse on such a task than did Type B's, because they were unable to wait long enough after receiving reinforcement before responding again. Observation also confirmed that A's openly displayed impatience with delayed responding. Nearly half the A's, but only 12% of the B's, were judged as having displayed tense and hyperactive movements during their sessions.

Competitive Achievement Striving

The third major component of the Type A behavior pattern is an exaggerated competitive achievement orientation. Indeed, in many ways this achievement orientation seems to be implicit in other facets of the pattern. The sense of time urgency, for example, probably arises as part of an attempt to do more and more within a shorter and shorter time span (cf. Matthews & Siegel, 1982). The hostility and aggressiveness are elicited by impediments in the Type A's activities, which presumably are often aimed at achieving instrumental goals.

Evidence that Type A's maintain a competitive achievement orientation comes from a number of sources (though the relationship between Pattern A and tradi-tional measures of achievement motivation is more complex—see, e.g., Glass, 1977; Matthews & Saal, 1978). In one laboratory study, for example, college students were given a series of arithmetic problems under moderately challenging instructions, which either did or did not indicate the presence of a time deadline

(Burnam et al., 1975). Type A's attempted more problems than did B's when a deadline had not been established. This difference disappeared, however, when the deadline was explicit, largely as a function of increased efforts among Type B's. Type A's, in contrast, did not require this salient deadline to engage their maximum efforts.

Other research investigated college students' reports of their academic achievements and future plans (Glass, 1977). Type A's reported having earned more honors than Type B's, and more A's than B's intended to go to graduate or professional school (see also Waldron, Hickey, McPherson, Butensky, Gruss, Overall, Schmader, & Wohlmuth, 1980, for more recent findings of this type). These relationships are consistent with other evidence: e.g., a small but reliable relationship between Pattern A and educational, occupational, and socioeconomic status (Mettlin, 1976; Shekelle et al., 1976; Stokols, Navaco, Stokols, & Campbell, 1978; Waldron, 1978; Waldron, Zyzanski, Shekelle, Jenkins, & Tannenbaum, 1977), and the recent finding that Type A social psychologists are cited more frequently in professional publications than are their Type B counterparts (Matthews, Helmreich, Beane, & Lucker, 1980).

Thus far, this description of Type A achievement behavior portrays achievement, but with no specific emphasis on competition with others. The competitive edge of this achievement orientation is revealed most plainly in a study by Van Egeren (1979) who paired subjects in a mixed-motive zero-sum game. Type A pairs emitted reliably more competitive responses in this situation than did Type B pairs. Moreover, when communications were permitted between partners, Type A pairs sent fewer cooperative or conciliatory messages, and more competitive and antisocial messages, than did either Type B pairs or mixed-Type pairs.

This competitive achievement orientation among Type A's has led to several additional hypotheses, extending this reasoning to new aspects of behavior. This research, in turn, has led to the discovery of what might be regarded as a wholly new reflection of Pattern A.

Symptom Suppression and Attentional Style

The picture of the Type A as a person who believes that with sufficient effort he can overcome any obstacle (Friedman & Rosenman, 1974) suggests the following question: Might Type A's, in an effort to achieve task mastery, attempt to suppress or ignore subjective states that threaten their best efforts? An example of such a potentially debilitating state is fatigue. The possibility that Type A's would suppress fatigue in order to persist at a tiring but challenging task was investigated using a paradigm designed to produce veridical fatigue (Carver, Coleman, & Glass, 1976). College-student subjects were required to walk continuously on a motorized treadmill at increasingly sharp angles of incline (cf. Balke, 1954; Balke, Grillo, Konecci, & Luft, 1954). While doing this, they rated their fatigue at 2-minute intervals, according to a labeled 11-point scale. Type A's were found to force themselves closer to the limits of their personal capabilities (as assessed by a measure of oxygen uptake) than did Type B's. Even while doing so, A's expressed less fatigue than did B's. These results have since been replicated with middle-aged adults (Graham, Ho, Thoresen, Levenkron, Vodak, Blair, Gelston, Terry, Moran, Haskell, & Wood, 1981).

The finding of fatigue suppression has subsequently been extended in several different ways. In one project (Carver, DeGregorio, & Gillis, 1981), college football coaches reported that injured Type A's exerted themselves closer to their limits than did injured Type B's, presumably reflecting efforts to ignore their injuries. Another project (Weidner & Matthews, 1978) examined a different sort of subjective experience. Subjects were presented with a series of noise bursts as they attempted a task. After a period of this, they rated the physical symptoms that they were experiencing in response to the noise. Type A's reported fewer symptoms than did Type B's, but only when they believed that a portion of the task remained to be attempted. This is consistent with the notion that symptoms are suppressed in order to focus on the task. Once a task is finished, there is no need to continue ignoring the symptoms (see also Stokols et al., 1978). The finding of symptom suppression has also recently been conceptually replicated in a study of perceived severity of menstrual symptoms (Matthews & Carra, 1982).

Matthews and Brunson (1979) pursued this phenomenon further, extending the research in a new and important way. Using paradigms from cognitive psychology, they provided a variety of evidence supportive of the notion that Type A's actively *suppress* their attention to intrusive, potentially disruptive, task-irrelevant stimuli. Type A's thus do not simply deny their fatigue for purposes of public display. Rather, when they are engaged in a focalized task, Type A's apparently are less *aware* of their fatigue than are Type B's.

The Matthews and Brunson findings suggest the following picture of the Type A: When confronting a task that has been defined as centrally important, Type A's enhance their degree of focus upon that central task and correspondingly diminish their focus on peripheral stimuli or events. These peripheral stimuli include internal sensations such as fatigue. They also include external stimuli associated with tasks that have been defined as being of secondary importance.

If correct, this reasoning also has implications for more *internal* cognitive events, such as category formation and use. An attentional difference of the form described previously should lead Type A's to form relatively restrictive mental representations of categories; said differently, they should form relatively "black and white" pictures of the way the world is organized. Support for this reasoning has been obtained in a study using yet a different cognitive paradigm (Humphries, Carver, & Neumann, 1983). This finding appears to lend important converging support to the Matthews and Brunson position. Once again, as in so many other cases, the Humphries et al. finding was dependent on elicitation by situational challenge.

PATTERN A AND CONTROL

The results of several studies conducted in the mid 1970s led Glass (1977) to characterize Pattern A as a response style aimed at gaining and maintaining control over significant aspects of the environment (see Matthews, 1982, for discussion of alternative formulations). In this view, Type A's wish to exercise personal control over their outcomes (cf. Dembroski & MacDougall, 1978); when elements of a situation appear to threaten that control, Pattern A behavior emerges. This conceptualization, taken together with another theoretical statement, has suggested additional behavioral predictions. Tests of these predictions, in turn, have often supported Glass' position.

The other theoretical statement relevant here is an attempt by Wortman and Brehm (1975) to account for the fact that exposure to uncontrollable outcomes sometimes leads to renewed efforts, and sometimes to giving up. In essence, Wortman and Brehm's argument was as follows. A *threat* to control—provided it does not entirely remove the perception of control—leads to reactance (Brehm, 1966; Wicklund, 1974) and an attempt to reassert control, reflected by such indices as increased efforts. If exposure to uncontrollable events is long enough or thorough enough to cause the perception that control has been *lost*, the result is giving up or helplessness (Seligman, 1975), reflected by such indices as decreased efforts or poorer performance. Glass (1977; see also Glass & Carver, 1980) has contended that these processes may be particularly pronounced among Type A's, given their need to maintain control. The results of several studies appear to support this contention.

Enhanced Responding After Threat to Control

Much of the research reviewed earlier in the chapter seems to reflect a kind of hyperresponsiveness among Type A's, appearing more concretely as intense competitiveness, time urgency, and aggressiveness. Two further studies have tested a more specific question about hyperresponsiveness: When exposed to a limited amount of an uncontrollable stressor, will Type A's reassert control by increasing their efforts at a subsequent task?

In one experiment (Krantz & Glass, reported in Glass, 1977), subjects were pretreated with noise bursts that were either escapable or inescapable. Immediately afterward, subjects were given a reaction time task with long intervals between trials. Type A's normally do more poorly than do Type B's at such a task, because having to wait causes restlessness among A's. Indeed, this was the outcome after exposure to escapable noise. But moderate exposure to *un*controllable noise apparently motivated A's to reassert control, which resulted in better reaction times.

Krantz and Glass (see Glass, 1977) conceptually replicated this finding, varying perceptions of control by providing either veridical or random feedback (i.e., "correct" or "incorrect") for attempts to solve two cognitive problems (taken from Hiroto & Seligman, 1975). Exposure to uncontrollable feedback enhanced the performance of Type A's (and had the opposite effect among Type B's) on a task requiring patience and low rates of responding. Presumably this reflected an increased motivation to reassert control among the Type A's, consistent with the Glass hypothesis.

Recall that Wortman and Brehm (1975) viewed response to threat to control as reflecting a state of reactance. If the hyperresponsiveness that Type A's display when their control is threatened is a reactance phenomenon, then one might also expect Type A's to be more sensitive than Type B's to more traditional manipulations of reactance. Indeed, recent studies of responses to coercive communications (Carver, 1980; Snyder & Frankel, 1980) and the elimination of choice alternatives (Rhodewalt & Comer, 1982) have verified this sensitivity.

Giving Up After Loss of Control

Enhanced efforts to reassert control are not always effective. If the person is confronting a stressor that is truly uncontrollable, at some point the perception will develop that control has been lost. This perception leads to a reduction in behavioral efforts: giving up, or helplessness. Though the data are mixed, there is at least some evidence that Type A's are more susceptible than Type B's to this sort of effect.

The pretreatment in one such study (Krantz et al., 1974) was an extensive series of noise bursts. Thus it did not merely *threaten* the subject's control, it should have induced the perception of complete *absence* of control. When the noise was both intense and inescapable, Type A's (but not B's) subsequently displayed a helplessness effect. When the noise was less intense, however, an opposite pattern emerged (see Krantz et al., 1974, or Glass & Carver, 1980, for more detail).

Similar results were obtained in a second experiment conducted by Hollis and Glass (reported in Glass, 1977). Subjects in this study were pretreated with either veridical feedback or random feedback (failure) on four cognitive problems. Type A's (but not Type B's) reacted to failures that were made highly salient by displaying helplessness.

Though findings of this sort have not always been obtained (Lovallo & Pishkin, 1980, found no evidence of greater helplessness among A's than among B's), at least one additional study yielded data that are very consistent with the Glass position. Subjects in this study (Brunson & Matthews, 1981) were presented with the same sort of cognitive problems as had been used by Hollis and Glass and were instructed to verbalize their thoughts while attempting the problems. When a consistent failure was made highly salient, the sophistication of the strategies used by Type A's deteriorated substantially (relative to those used by Type B's), and their verbalizations were characterized by self-blame and pessimism. These findings are consistent with the notion that a very salient loss of control hampers the Type A more than the Type B.

PATTERN A AND PHYSIOLOGICAL RESPONSES TO STRESS

The research outlined thus far focused on the *psychological* nature of Pattern A. It verifies the overt display of A-type characteristics and has indicated some of the conditions that elicit those behaviors. But overt action and cognition are not the only manifestations of Pattern A. When people confront stresses, they also experience *physiological* changes. Given that Type A's are behaviorally more responsive to stressful stimuli than are Type B's, the question arises as to whether they may also be more responsive physiologically. Recent research suggests that this is indeed the case. These studies have focused primarily on cardiovascular reactivity among A's and B's in laboratory situations designed to elicit A-type behavioral characteristics. In one of the first such studies (Dembroski, Mac-Dougall, & Shields, 1977) heart rate (HR), blood pressure (BP), and galvanic skin potential of interview-defined A and B college students were monitored during a choice reaction time task. The task instructions emphasized speed and accuracy of performance. Changes of both HR and BP from baseline to task period were markedly greater for A's than for B's.

Other researchers reported findings that were generally similar to these, but with some variations. For example, Manuck et al. (1978) found that Type A males (but not females) responded to a difficult cognitive task with greater elevations of systolic BP than did Type B's. Another study (Manuck & Garland, 1979) replicated this finding, although yielding no A – B difference in diastolic BP or HR changes.

Additional studies by Dembroski and his colleagues provide more evidence of A – B differences in cardiovascular responsivity. For example, Dembroski et al. (1978) asked subjects to respond rapidly and accurately on three tasks involving perceptual-motor and cognitive skills. Interview-defined fully developed A's showed the largest magnitude of systolic BP and HR changes, incomplete A's the next largest, and B's the least (averaged across tasks). Dividing subjects at the median JAS score yielded a significant A – B difference for diastolic BP, as well.

Dembroski, MacDougall, and Lushene (1979) extended this research to coronary patients. They monitored BP and HR among these and control patients, while administering both the structured interview and a challenging American history quiz. Type A coronary cases and Type A controls responded with greater elevations in systolic BP during both interview and quiz, compared to their Type B counterparts. Diastolic blood pressure differed between A's and B's only for the latter portion of the interview. No significant heart rate differences appeared in these data. But intercorrelations between physiological response measures showed a high correlation of HR and systolic (though not diastolic) BP among the Type A's, a pattern suggestive of general sympathetic arousal.

Role of Challenge

The tasks used in these studies were chosen implicitly on the basis of their likelihood of eliciting A-type psychological responses from susceptible individuals. Presumably it is the engagement of this psychological response that results in exaggerated cardiovascular responses. Additional research has explicitly tested the assumption that the Type A's physiological reactivity is a product of situational challenge.

Dembroski, MacDougall, Herd, and Shields (1979) investigated the effect of challenge by varying experimental instructions to male college students for cold pressor and reaction time tasks. Some were told that the tasks were commonly used procedures that would be accomplished with little difficulty. Others were told that the tasks were quite difficult and required considerable "will power" (for the cold pressor) and rapid, accurate performance (for the reaction time task). Across both tasks, Type A's had greater HR and systolic BP changes than did Type B's. The differences were largest under high challenge conditions, but the interaction between Type and condition was not statistically significant. In addition to these effects, there was evidence that A's who were particularly high in hostility differed from B's and other A's under conditions of low challenge. With this exception, A − B differences in the low challenge condition were minimal.

This study investigated degree of challenge with task held constant. Another study (Goldband, 1980) investigated the notion that some stressors elicit Pattern A whereas others do not. Goldband reasoned that Type A's should be hyperresponsive not to *all* stressors, but rather selectively to stressors that represent potentially manageable threats to control. To test this hypothesis, he presented JAS-classified male undergraduates with a reaction time task, under varying instructional sets, one of which emphasized speed, competitiveness, and time pressure. Additional subjects were exposed to a stressor that did not represent a challenge to their task mastery (blowing up balloons until they popped). All subjects were monitored for HR and pulse transit time (an analogue of blood pressure, considered an indicator of sympathetic activation). Excessive physiological responsivity emerged among Type A's only when they attempted the reaction time task under a challenging instructional set. No A − B difference emerged with this task in nonchallenging conditions, or in response to the mastery-irrelevant stressor.

A study conducted by Holmes, Solomon, and Spreier (1979) makes a related point. Subjects in this study completed two tasks: a challenging IQ test, and a rigidly paced exercise task. Type A males (but not females) experienced a heart rate acceleration while undertaking the IQ test. During the exercise period, however, no A − B difference emerged. The authors concluded that the exaggerated reactivity of the Type A does not reflect a physical makeup that overreacts to whatever demands are placed on it. Rather, it represents a psychologically mediated reaction to situational challenges.

Yet another project (Glass, Krakoff, Contrada, Hilton, Kehoe, Mannucci, Collins, Snow, & Elting, 1980) examined physiological responses of Type A and Type B adults who competed against a confederate in a video game. Half the subjects completed this procedure while being harassed and insulted by the confederate; for the remaining subjects there was no harassment. Dependent measures included HR, BP, and plasma catecholamine levels. The competitive challenge—even in the absence of harassment—produced marked increases in HR and systolic BP among both A's and B's, but no A − B difference. In the harassment condition, however, Type A's—but not Type B's—exhibited even more pronounced changes, including a marked elevation in plasma epinephrine. Similar findings for cardiovascular changes have been obtained by Diamond, Schneiderman, Schwartz, Smith, Vorp, and Pasin (1982).

There is one finding that cuts against the grain of this reasoning, however. Type A's have been found to exceed Type B's in systolic BP response while anesthetized in preparation for coronary bypass surgery (Kahn, Kornfeld, Frank, Heller, & Hoar, 1980), a result that has since been replicated (Krantz, Arabian, Davia, & Parker, 1982). This suggests the possibility of a more fundamental underlying autonomic hyperreactivity.

Component Analyses

Some of the research already discussed (Dembroski et al., 1979; Dembroski, MacDougall, & Lushene, 1979; Dembroski, MacDougall, Herd, & Shields, 1979) also examined the possibility that different aspects of Pattern A would vary in their relationship to cardiovascular reactivity. Dembroski et al. (1978) found that (interviewer-rated) potential for hostility had the strongest predictive relationship to physiological change. Within their Type A samples alone, there was a reliable correlation between this index and magnitude of systolic BP change under stress. Similar results were found in the study in which subjects' responses were monitored while completing the structured interview and the history quiz (Dembroski, MacDougall, & Lushene, 1979). Indeed, there is even some evidence that A's with a high potential for hostility experience cardiovascular hyperreactivity in stressful situations in which challenge is minimal (Dembroski, MacDougall, Herd, & Shields, 1979). This hostility-reactivity relationship has also been found recently among women (MacDougall, Dembroski, & Krantz, 1981), though it appears to be specific to *interpersonally* challenging situations.

These findings seem particularly intriguing in light of the suggestive evidence discussed earlier in the chapter that potential for hostility may be the best predictor of CHD of all the elements of Pattern A (Matthews et al., 1977). Taking these two sets of data together suggests the possibility of a link between Pattern A and CHD via hostility, which in turn induces exaggerated physiological responsiveness. Consistent with this possibility is the finding that hostility (assessed by an MMPI-derived scale) is independently a better predictor of atherosclerosis than Type A (Williams, Haney, Gentry, & Kong, 1978).

At least one other study is suggestive of the possibility that A − B differences in cardiovascular reactivity are based on a component rather than the totality of Pattern A. This study (Scherwitz, Berton, & Leventhal, 1978) found no overall A − B difference during a series of tasks including cold pressor, mental arithmetic, and generation of emotions. However, subdividing the sample of Type A's according to "self-involvement" (operationalized as the number of first-person pronouns uttered during the interview and generation of emotion) revealed marked differences between A's who were high and low in self-involvement. The highly self-involved A's exhibited reliable BP increases (compared to the less self-involved A's), which (paradoxically) were associated with HR decreases.

As this group of studies suggests, one goal of future research must be to specify what aspect or aspects of Pattern A are associated with cardiovascular lability in response to challenge. Not all A's are hyperreactive in the laboratory setting; and some B's are hyperreactive. Indeed, an even more pointed question in this context is whether hyperreactivity per se is what is important, as opposed to the presence of A-type psychological and behavioral characteristics.

Another goal will be to determine more specifically what environmental factors elicit inappropriately large physiological changes among susceptible individuals. It appears that harassment elevates responses among Type A's when presented in the context of competition (Glass et al., 1980; Diamond et al., 1982). But is harassment alone responsible for the effect, or is it the combination of harassment and competition?

Yet another goal will be to determine more precisely the nature of the physiological responses under investigation. That is, with few exceptions (e.g., Glass et al., 1980), research to this point has focused largely on HR and BP data. Among the questions arising now are to what degree peripheral resistance and cardiac output contribute separately to BP increases, and to what degree other factors covary with the responses that have been observed thus far. In the broader view, it remains to be determined whether such changes reflect the tendency to generate nonspecific sympathetic arousal; or a more general tendency to exaggerate a wide variety of physiological response patterns (cf. Williams, 1978); or perhaps even a more specific tendency to react to control-threatening stressors with a specific emotion (cf. Diamond, 1982).

At this point we should make explicit the rationale that underlies the effort to demonstrate differences in physiological responsiveness between A's and B's. The rationale is this: By demonstrating that A's and B's have different patterns of physical responses, we may thereby be one step closer to obtaining evidence of a physiological mechanism by which Pattern A is associated with heart disease. We turn now to a consideration of possible mechanisms of association.

MECHANISMS MEDIATING ASSOCIATION BETWEEN TYPE A AND CHD

It is often argued that repeated episodes of sympathetically mediated hyperarousal constitute the primary mechanism by which Pattern A is associated with CHD. A number of theorists (Charvat, Dell, & Folkow, 1964; Eliot, 1974; Herd, 1978; Obrist, 1976) have argued, in essence, that repeated arousal of the "defense reaction"—an integrated pattern of physiological changes involved in mobilization of the organism for action—has cardiovascular and biochemical consequences that are intrinsically damaging to the heart and blood vessels.

This argument is generally consistent with animal models of cardiovascular disease. Data from this area indicate that chronic "active coping"—which occurs when an animal is exposed to stressors in the presence of an available coping response—can lead to tachycardia, atherosclerosis, and myocardial damage (see Schneiderman, 1978). Such a model also seems to fit well with the characterization of the coronary-prone Type A as an active coper, aggressive and mastery-oriented. There are several ways in which chronic reactivity could lead to both atherosclerosis and acute clinical events. The following paragraphs describe some of these possible pathways, along with evidence implicating A-type behavior in their occurrence.

Atherosclerosis

An important consequence of the chronic activation of the mobilization response is atherosclerosis: the depositing of lipids in the lining of the coronary arteries that supply blood to the heart muscle, eventually resulting in arterial damage and occlusion. It is a long-term process. Current theory of atherogenesis (Friedman, 1969; Ross & Glomset, 1976) suggests a 4-stage process involving: (1) injury to the lining (endothelium) of the coronary arteries; (2) response to injury in the form of smooth muscle cell proliferation and aggregation of blood platelets; (3) accumulation of lipids leading to the formation of plaques; (4) eventual breakdown of tissue and occlusion of the artery, and also the release of thrombi composed of plaque material.

Consider the influence of stress on this process. Increased catecholamine output is a component of the stress response, being released both centrally from nerve terminals and from the adrenal medulla (cf. Schneiderman, 1982). Circulating catecholamines can alter cellular structure of endothelial cells, causing easier entry of lipids through the arterial wall (Shinamoto, 1974; Shinamoto, Kobayashi,

& Numano, 1975). Catecholamines can also cause focal necrosis of heart tissue (Eliot, Todd, Pieper, & Clayton, 1979) and accelerate the rate of arterial damage (Raab, Chaplin, & Bajusz, 1964; Raab, Stark, MacMillan, & Gigee, 1961). In addition, excitement of the heart through sympathetic nervous system input (mediated by catecholamines) may increase the speed, force, and turbulence of blood flow, thereby contributing further to the initial possibility of damage (Williams, 1978). Finally, there is evidence that catecholamines can induce arrhythmias (Schneiderman, 1982), which may lead to clinical complications and even sudden death (Sigler, 1967).

Evidence has accumulated that Type A's respond to stressors with excessive sympathetic responses, implying catecholamine secretion. A's have been shown to have higher serum levels of norepinephrine in response to competitive challenge (Friedman, Byers, Diamant, & Rosenman, 1975). More recently, the study by Glass et al. (1980) discussed above found marked epinephrine release among Type A's who were harassed during a competitive task. These findings fit the pattern of cardiovascular reactivity found in other studies. That is, a pattern of increases in both systolic BP and HR (Dembroski et al., 1978) suggests that the sympathetic arousal is mediated primarily by the action of epinephrine on the heart. The fact that this Type A response is selective to mastery-threatening situations also fits with the notion that the arousal represents an organismic mobilization or preparation for action (i.e., active coping).

Consider more closely now the process of plaque formation. Lipids form the plaques that bulge into the coronary artery, blocking the flow of oxygenated blood to the heart. There is evidence that catecholamines can break down fats, leading to elevated levels of circulating triglycerides and cholesterol (Carlson, Levi, & Oro, 1968), and this process increases as a function of increased stress (Wolf, McCabe, Yamamoto, Adsett, & Schottstaedt, 1961). In turn, high levels of circulating cholesterol have been implicated as a cause of endothelial damage (Ross & Harker, 1976).

And what of Pattern A? There is evidence that Type A's exceed B's in levels of both lipoproteins (carriers of lipids) and cholesterol (Friedman & Rosenman, 1959). Friedman, Rosenman, and Byers (1964) found elevated triglyceride levels among A's both before and after ingestion of a meal. Friedman (1977) reviews a series of studies of well-developed A's yielding evidence of abnormality in cholesterol metabolism. A – B differences in serum cholesterol have even been found among college students (Glass, 1977; Lovallo, 1978).

Blood-clotting mechanisms may also play an important role in the process of response to injury in the arterial lining and may be associated with the atherosclerosis and the formation of thrombi (Ardlie, Glew, & Schwartz, 1966). The platelet aggregation process is likely to be enhanced by the catecholamine norepinephrine (Davies & Reinert, 1965; Davis, 1974). It is suggestive in this regard that A's show less decrease in platelet aggregation after stressful treadmill exercise than B's (Simpson, Olewine, Jenkins, Ramsey, Zyzanski, Thomas, & Hames,

1974) and show more rapid blood clotting under stress (Rosenman & Friedman, 1974).

Pattern A and Atherosclerosis

Recent epidemiological research has confirmed a statistical relationship between Pattern A and the major endpoint of the events discussed in the preceding section: i.e., coronary atherosclerosis. Autopsy data from one longitudinal study revealed that Type A's had significantly greater degrees of atherosclerosis than did B's, regardless of actual cause of death (Friedman, Rosenman, & Straus, 1968).

Several investigators have subsequently examined the relationship between Type A and severity of atherosclerosis among persons undergoing coronary angiography. The results of these studies have been somewhat mixed, but generally consistent with the picture of a connection between Pattern A and the atherosclerotic process. For example, Blumenthal et al. (1978) found greater proportions of interview-defined A's among subjects with moderate to severe occlusion than among those with only mild occlusion. Subjects' JAS scores did not predict this relationship, however. Frank, Heller, Kornfeld, Sporn, and Weiss (1978) reported similar results for interview-defined A's and B's, Type A's again having greater proportions of heavily occluded arteries. At least one study (Dimsdale, Hackett, Catanzano, & White, 1979), on the other hand, has failed to replicate this relationship. One additional study has found a relationship between JAS scores and severity of atherosclerosis (Zyzanski, Jenkins, Ryan, Flessas, & Everist, 1976) and another has failed to find such a relationship (Dimsdale, Hackett, Hutter, Block, Catanzano, & White, 1978). Finally, at least one study has failed to find a relationship between severity of atherosclerosis and magnitude of cardiovascular response to situational challenge (Krantz, Schaeffer, Davia, Dembroski, MacDougall, & Shaffer, 1980).

One recent study has gone an important step further, by examining the *progression* of atherosclerosis (Krantz, Sanmarco, Selvester, & Matthews, 1979). In this research, male outpatients underwent repeated angiography over an average period of 17 months. When subjects were divided into thirds according to their JAS scores, Type A's were more likely than Type B's to show progression of the disease over the course of the study. Interview classifications (which were not available for all subjects) failed to predict progression in this study, however.

This study (along with the data discussed earlier) suggests that the depositing of arterial plaques may be an important mechanism linking Pattern A to recurrence of myocardial infarction (cf. Jenkins, Zyzanski, & Rosenman, 1976). However, Krantz et al. (1979) cautioned that their sample—patients with already diagnosed disease—may be biased by such factors as volunteering for inclusion in the study, survival of the testing interval without recommendation for surgery, and influence of medication on vocal stylistics. Despite these caveats, and the previously noted failures to replicate certain of the findings in this area, the evidence for a statistical association between Pattern A and atherosclerosis seems substantial.

Possible Behavioral Mechanisms

Besides its role in atherogenesis, there are other ways in which Type A can contribute to acute clinical events. Two possibilities are suggested by findings discussed earlier indicating that Type A's tend to actively suppress their awareness of physical symptoms (Carver et al., 1976; Matthews & Brunson, 1979; Weidner & Matthews, 1978). First, suppression of one's awareness of fatigue raises the possibility of continually driving oneself past normal points of exhaustion. Fatigue is, after all, an informative message telling one to slow down. The message must be noticed before it is heeded, however. Continued efforts once exhaustion has set in may seriously deplete one's resources.

A second possible link is suggested by the fact that fatigue is the most common symptom of a developing heart attack (Greene, Moss, & Goldstein, 1974). If Type A's suppress their attention to that symptom and persist in their activities despite it (cf. Matthews, Siegel, Kuller, Thompson, & Varat, 1983), they may thereby increase the chances of aggravating their condition, resulting in a heart attack of greater severity than would otherwise be the case.

A very different possibility is suggested by the findings that Pattern A is associated with a pronounced giving-up response when confronted by a very salient loss of control (Glass, 1977). A number of writers have suggested that the sense of helplessness and uncontrollability that is induced by certain types of negative life events may facilitate the onset of a variety of types of diseases (Engel, 1968; Paykel, 1974; Schmale, 1972). And it has been reported that sudden death is abnormally frequent among men who had had an immediately preceding period of depression (Greene, Goldstein, & Moss, 1972). Indeed, in one retrospective study (Glass, 1977), coronary patients reported an unusually high incidence of uncontrollable events during the year prior to their hospitalization (compared to controls). These data, of course, are far from being conclusive. But they suggest interesting possibilities for future study.

BEHAVIORAL INTERVENTION IN PATTERN A

With the role of Type A behavior as a risk factor for CHD firmly established (though mechanisms by which it exerts its influence being somewhat more speculative) researchers have begun to explore the possible utility of modifying Type A behavior, thus reducing associated CHD risk (Rosenman & Friedman, 1977; Roskies, Spevack, Surkis, Cohen, & Gilman, 1978; Suinn & Bloom, 1978). These approaches have been based for the most part on the notion that Type A's respond to environmental stressors with heightened physiological arousal, and the further assumption that heightened arousal eventually is pathogenic. Intervention strategies based on this reasoning attempt through a variety of methods to reduce the Type A's tendency toward heightened arousal. This may be accomplished either by changing subjects' perceptions of stressors, or by reducing physiological reactions to them (Roskies, 1980).

The relatively few studies conducted in this area to date seem to fall into two general groups. These are: (1) limited attempts at specific interventions; and (2) what may be termed "shotgun" studies, in which subjects are exposed to various combinations of therapy in an attempt to influence one or more elements of the Type A pattern.

In one study of the first type, Roskies et al. (1978) compared the effects on Pattern A (among men 39 − 57 years old) of psychoanalytic and behavioral therapy techniques, respectively. The rationale behind the psychoanalytic group was that the need of Type A's to master and control the environment results from unresolved childhood conflicts. Exposing those conflicts and working through them would reduce the needs, thus reducing Type A behaviors. The behavioral therapy had the more restricted goal of modifying Type As' reactions to challenging or stressful situations. Subjects learned progressive muscle relaxation and deep-breathing exercises, and how to use them to avoid physiological arousal during especially stressful periods. A third group was included in this study, consisting of men who had been unaware until the initial screening for the study that they had symptoms of CHD. This group, which received behavioral therapy, was included to examine whether learning that one has heart disease may influence motivation for treatment, hence treatment outcome. After 14 weeks of training, all groups showed pre to posttreatment reductions in mean systolic BP, serum cholesterol, self-reported time pressures, and number of self-reported psychological symptoms. Though no control group was included in the study, the researchers inferred that Type A behavior and resulting CHD risk may be amenable to change.

In a similar study, Suinn and Bloom (1978) taught Type A's deep muscle relaxation and had them engage in stressful imagery and pinpoint the physical symptoms of accompanying arousal. Subjects were encouraged to become proficient in identifying the physiological cues of arousal and to relax in response to them. After the 6-session 3-week training period, Type A's exhibited reduced scores on the hard-driving and the speed–impatience subscales of the JAS, compared to controls. The treatment group also reported lowered trait and state anxiety. However, significant reductions in lipid levels and BP—which were expected on the basis of prior studies using a similar treatment (Suinn, 1975a, 1975b)—did not occur.

Other projects have taken more eclectic approaches to intervention. Rosenman and Friedman (1977) suggested that acquisition and maintenance of Pattern A characteristics stem from the belief that such behaviors are essential for socioeconomic success. They further suggested that intervention incorporate an attempt to reorient subjects away from this belief, and also from the belief in the paramount importance of career success. In addition, they encouraged patients to engage in behavioral "drills" and environmental management strategies, to rid themselves of A-type habits. This approach was subsequently elaborated to include training in recognition of one's own Type A actions; practice in deceleration of motor activities; training in progressive muscle relaxation; development of skills to cope with challenging situations; and encouragement to minimize the presence of situational stimuli that would unnecessarily elicit A-type behavior.

Roskies has also expanded her behavioral treatment (Roskies & Avard, 1982) to include techniques for altering both the perception of stress and the Type A reactions to stressful stimuli. Specifically chosen were modification techniques that could fit easily into people's daily routines. Four separate types of therapy were offered to the participants in the study (Roskies & Avard, 1982). These included progressive muscle relaxation, rational–emotive therapy to increase awareness of feelings, training in problem-solving skills, and stress inoculation to deal with perceptions of and cognitive responses to stress. Subjects in this research reported feelings of enhanced well-being, success in controlling emotional outbursts, and so on, as a result of the training.

Criticisms of Intervention Studies

Intervention research has not been without its critics. Indeed, some of these projects represent "research" only in an exploratory or pilot sense, in that they comprise very small samples, have confounded several treatment procedures with each other, and have lacked necessary control groups. Even the more systematic projects confront difficulties, however.

Perhaps the most basic problem is defining and measuring "improvement" in an acceptable fashion. The ultimate criterion in this case is a reduction in risk for CHD. But evaluation with respect to this criterion is quite difficult, requiring long-term follow-up of many subjects. Thus, most researchers have settled instead for alternative criteria: changes in subjects' JAS or SI responses, or changes in physiological indices believed to be relevant to pathogenesis of CHD. Each of these alternatives has its own drawbacks.

Use of the SI or JAS to measure change in A-type characteristics has been criticized on the grounds that these instruments were designed as initial assessment techniques, and not as criteria for intervention. The JAS contains items that pertain to the person's past history and that therefore cannot change with intervention (Chesney, 1978). On the other hand, although the SI is effective in initial identification of Type A's and Type B's, it is somewhat insensitive to variation within those categories and may not detect changes less than a full-scale conversion from Type A to Type B (Roskies, 1980). Use of either of these measures may therefore mask real change.

Physiological measures are also occasionally used as criteria for assessing interventions. Sometimes these measures show changes (Suinn, 1975a, 1975b; Roskies, 1980); sometimes they do not (Suinn & Bloom, 1978). This form of examining Type A improvement confronts the fact that accurate physiological measures are difficult and expensive to carry out on a large scale (Roskies, 1980). Another problem with such measures is that Type A carries CHD risk independent of many physiological factors. Thus it may very well be possible to demonstrate physiological changes without eliminating Type A-related risk (Chesney, 1978).

A second major problem in intervention research stems from an issue that has reemerged several times in the chapter. That is, it is not at all clear whether the statistical relationship between Pattern A and CHD is based on the *entire* behavior pattern, or whether a single *component* of that pattern uniquely increases risk. Most attempts to alter Type A behavior have been broad-based interventions in virtually all aspects of the pattern. But much of that effort may be focused on changing aspects of the Type A style that are unrelated to pathogenesis of heart disease. Furthermore, there are potential costs to the subjects of grand-scale intervention efforts. Reengineering Type As' life-style may negatively influence their productivity, career advancement, and views of themselves. Workers in this area thus are beginning to question the wisdom of massive intervention, until it is clearer where the intervention should be focused (Chesney, 1978; Gentry & Suinn, 1978; Roskies, 1980).

Even if it were clear exactly what constitutes coronary-prone behavior, it is far from certain that individual or group therapy represents a cost-effective approach to the problem. That is, despite a statistically reliable association between A-type characteristics and eventual CHD, most Type A's never have any clinical manifestations of CHD (Scherwitz, Cleary, Leventhal, & Laman, 1978). Is it worth conducting behavioral interventions on large numbers of people who would not have had heart disease, in order to modify the behavior of the individual who would have developed heart disease? Indeed some Type *B's* have heart attacks. Should intervention, then, be aimed at an even broader set of people? These questions have not been answered. Perhaps screening techniques can ultimately pick out individuals whose behaviors can be modified successfully in a way that is not too disruptive to their lives. But the cost of doing so remains an important issue.

There are issues other than cost-effectiveness to consider in deciding upon a target population. For example, should one focus on persons at risk but without clinical symptoms, or on victims of heart attack? It would seem desirable in principle to *prevent* disease rather than simply reacting *to* disease. But success in an intervention program can be strongly influenced by motivational characteristics. And it may well be that persons with no clinical manifestations of CHD are less interested in altering their behavior patterns than are post-MI patients. The danger of heart disease probably seems much less real to the former than to the latter. The result may be differences in compliance and differences in long-term maintenance of the desired changes. This again raises the issue of cost-effectiveness.

It also brings to hand another problem. Attempts to influence voluntary behaviors such as diet and smoking are often unsuccessful over long time periods (Bernstein & McAllister, 1976; Kirschenbaum & Tomarken, 1982; Stunkard,

1977). Given that intervention in Pattern A typically bears on the person's total life-style, might it not be reasonable to expect a high degree of recidivism? Though this is a potentially serious problem, it is encouraging that Pattern A has been found in at least one study to be amenable to relatively long-term influences from intervention (Roskies, Kearney, Spevack, Surkis, Cohen, & Gilman, 1979). Possible ways to facilitate this long-term influence include having participants keep detailed records of their progress, report back for periodic "booster" sessions (Chesney, 1978; Roskies, 1980), and practice confronting the possibility of relapse, so that temptations of actual incidents of relapse could be dealt with constructively (Marlatt & Gordon, 1980; Roskies, 1980).

As suggested in the foregoing, research on alteration of Pattern A behavior faces serious difficulties. Some of these problems are shared by all evaluation research. And some of them are dictated by the fact that coronary-prone behaviors exert their pathogenic influence slowly, over long periods of time. Yet it seems likely that intervention research will continue to be planned and conducted. Indeed, if done properly, such studies are the only way to answer the questions just outlined.

CORONARY PRONE BEHAVIOR AND BEHAVIORAL MEDICINE

We conclude our discussion of the Type A behavior pattern by briefly addressing the relationship between this research area and the broader field of behavioral medicine. The study of coronary-prone behavior exemplifies at least two characteristics of the burgeoning field. First, research on Pattern A represents a fine example of the interweaving of psychological and medical research techniques. The procedures by which coronary-prone behavior has been studied have ranged broadly from the procedures of epidemiology, coronary angiography, and rheology to those of psychophysiology, and social and cognitive psychology. All these approaches have proven useful in gaining important insights into the nature and consequences of Pattern A behavior. The result is a truly interdisciplinary understanding of the phenomenon that is virtually unmatched by any other research area.

The second general theme illustrated by this research area is the delicate interplay between psychosocial variables and biomedical variables in the disease process itself. Ultimately coronary heart disease is a physiological phenomenon. Yet it seems clear that the developmental sequence of this phenomenon can be influenced by behavioral and cognitive events, both in terms of cardiovascular deterioration and in terms of precipitating incidents. This blend of biomedical and psychosocial variables involved in heart disease highlights what may be more general involvement of factors at many different levels of analysis on physical disorders.

REFERENCES

Ardlie, N. G., Glew, G., & Schwartz, C. J. Influence of catecholamines on nucleotide-induced platelet aggregation. *Nature*, 1966, *212*, 415 – 417.

Balke, B. Optimale koerperliche leistunsfaehigkeisihre messung und veraenderung infrolage arbeitsermuedung. *Arbeitsphysiologie*, 1954, *15*, 311 – 323.

Balke, B., Grillo, G. P., Konecci, E. B., & Luft, U. C. Work capacity after blood donation. *Journal of Applied Physiology*, 1954, *7*, 231 – 238.

Bernstein, D. A., & McAllister, A. L. The modification of smoking behavior: Progress, and problems. *Addictive Behavior*, 1976, *1*, 89 – 102.

Blumenthal, J. A., Williams, R. B., Kong, Y., Schlanberg, S. M., & Thompson, L. W. Type A behavior pattern and coronary atherosclerosis. *Circulation*, 1978, *58*, 634 – 639.

Bortner, R. W., & Rosenman, R. H. The measurement of Pattern A behavior. *Journal of Chronic Diseases*, 1967, *20*, 525 – 533.

Brand, R. J., Rosenman, R. H., Jenkins, C. D., Sholtz, R. I., & Zyzanski, S. J. Comparison of coronary heart disease prediction in the Western Collaborative Group Study using the Structured Interview and the Jenkins Activity Survey assessments of the coronary-prone Type A behavior pattern. *Journal of Chronic Diseases*, in press.

Brand, R. J., Rosenman, R. H., Sholtz, R. I., & Friedman, M. Multivariate prediction of coronary heart disease in the Western Collaborative Group Study compared to the findings of the Framingham Study. *Circulation*, 1976, *53*, 348 – 355.

Brehm, J. W. *A theory of psychological reactance*. New York: Academic Press, 1966.

Brunson, B., & Matthews, K. A. The Type A coronary-prone behavior pattern and reactions to uncontrollable stress: An analysis of learned helplessness. *Journal of Personality and Social Psychology*, 1981, *40*, 906 – 918.

Burnam, M. A., Pennebaker, J. W., & Glass, D. C. Time consciousness, achievement striving, and the Type A coronary-prone behavior pattern. *Journal of Abnormal Psychology*, 1975, *84*, 76 – 79.

Carlson, L. A., Levi, L., & Oro, L. Plasma liplids and urinary excretion of catecholamines in man during experimentally induced emotional stress, and their modification of nicotinic acid. *Journal of Clinical Investigation*, 1968, *47*, 1795 – 1805.

Carver, C. S. Perceived coercion, resistance to persuasion, and the Type A behavior pattern. *Journal of Research in Personality*, 1980, *19*, 467 – 481.

Carver, C. S., Coleman, A. E., & Glass, D. C. The coronary-prone behavior pattern and the suppression of fatigue on a treadmill test. *Journal of Personality and Social Psychology*, 1976, *33*, 460 – 466.

Carver, C. S., DeGregorio, E., & Gillis, R. Challenge and Type A behavior among intercollegiate football players. *Journal of Sport Psychology*, 1981, *3*, 140 – 148.

Carver, C. S., & Glass, D. C. Coronary-prone behavior pattern and interpersonal aggression. *Journal of Personality and Social Psychology*, 1978, *36*, 361 – 366.

Charvat, J., Dell, P., & Folkow, B. Mental factors and cardiovascular diseases. *Cardiologia*, 1964, *44*, 124 – 141.

Chesney, M. *Coronary-prone behavior and heart disease: Intervention strategies*. Paper presented at the annual meeting of the American Psychological Association, Toronto, Canada, 1978.

Chesney, M. A., Black, G. W., Chadwick, J. H., & Rosenman, R. H. Psychological correlates of the coronary-prone behavior pattern. *Journal of Behavioral Medicine*, 1981, *4*, 217 – 229.

Chesney, M. A., Black, G. W., Feuerstein, M., Rosenman, R. H., Calligan, M. D., & Chadwick, J. H. *Coronary-prone behavior: Characteristics and therapeutic implications*. Paper presented at the annual meeting of the American Psychological Association, Toronto, Canada, August 1978.

Davies, R. F., & Reinert, H. Arteriosclerosis in the young dog. *Journal of Atherosclerosis Research*, 1965, *5*, 181 – 188.

Davis, R. Stress and hemostatic mechanisms. In R. S. Eliot (Ed.), *Stress and the heart*. Mt. Kisco, N. Y.: Futura, 1974.

Dawber, T. R., & Kannel, W. B. Susceptibility to coronary heart disease. *Modern Concepts in Cardiovascular Disease*, 1961, *30*, 671 – 676.

Dembroski, T., & MacDougall, J. M. Stress effects on affiliation preferences among subjects possessing the Type A coronary-prone behavior pattern. *Journal of Personality and Social Psychology*, 1978, *36*, 23 – 33.

Dembroski, T., MacDougall, J. M., Herd, J. A., & Shields, J. L. Effects of level of challenge on pressor and heart responses in Type A and B subjects. *Journal of Applied Social Psychology*, 1979, *9*, 209 – 228.

Dembroski, T. M., MacDougall, J. M., & Lushene, R. Interpersonal interaction and cardiovascular response in Type A subjects and coronary patients. *Journal of Human Stress*, 1979, *5*, 28 – 36.

Dembroski, T. M., MacDougall, J. M., & Shields, J. L. Physiologic reactions to social challenge in persons evidencing the Type A coronary-prone behavior pattern. *Journal of Human Stress*, 1977, *3*, 2 – 10.

Dembroski, T. M., MacDougall, J. M., Shields, J. L., Petitto, R., & Lushene, R. Components of the Type A coronary-prone behavior pattern and cardiovascular responses to psychomotor performance challenge. *Journal of Behavioral Medicine*, 1978, *1*, 159 – 176.

Diamond, E. The role of anger and hostility in essential hypertension and coronary heart disease. *Psychological Bulletin*, 1982, *92*, 410–433.

Diamond, E., Schneiderman, N., Schwartz, D., Smith, J.C., Vorp, R., & Pasin, R.D. *Harassment, hostility, and Type A as determinants of cardiovascular reactivity during competition*. Unpublished manuscript, University of Miami, 1982.

Dimsdale, J. E., Hackett, T. P., Catanzano, D. M., & White, P. J. The relationship between diverse measures for Type A personality and coronary angiographic findings. *Journal of Psychomatic Research*, 1979, *23*, 289 – 293.

Dimsdale, J. E., Hackett, T. P., Hutter, A. M., Block, P., Catanzano, D., & White, P. Type A personality and extent of coronary atherosclerosis. *American Journal of Cardiology*, 1978, *42*, 583 – 586.

Eliot, R. S. (Ed.). *Stress and the heart*. Mt. Kisco, New York: Futura, 1974.

Eliot, R. S., Todd, G. L., Pieper, G. M., & Clayton, F. C. Pathophysiology of catecholamine-mediated myocardial damage. *Journal of the South Carolina Medical Association*, 1979, *75*, 513 – 518.

Engel, G. L. A life setting conducive to illness: The giving-up complex. *Annals of Internal Medicine*, 1968, *69*, 293 – 300.

Frank, K. A., Heller, S. S., Kornfeld, D. S., Sporn, A., & Weiss, M. Type A behavior and coronary angiographic findings. *Journal of the American Medical Association*, 1978, *240*, 761 – 763.

Friedman, M. *Pathogenesis of coronary artery disease*. New York: McGraw-Hill, 1969.

Friedman, M. Type A behavior pattern: Some of its pathophysiological components. *Bulletin of the New York Academy of Medicine*, 1977, *58*, 593 – 604.

Friedman, M., Byers, S. O., Diamant, J., & Rosenman, R. H. Plasma catecholamine response of coronary-prone subjects (Type A) to a specific challenge. *Metabolism*, 1975, *4*, 205 – 210.

Friedman, M., & Rosenman, R. H. Association of a specific overt behavior pattern with increases in blood cholesterol, blood clotting time, incidence of arcus senilis and clinical coronary artery disease. *Journal of the American Medical Association*, 1959, *169*, 1286 – 1296.

Friedman, M., & Rosenman, R. H. *Type A behavior and your heart*. Greenwich, CT: Fawcett, 1974.

Friedman, M., Rosenman, R., & Byers, S.O. Serum lipids and conjunctival circulation after fat ingestion in men exhibiting Type A behavior pattern. *Circulation*, 1964, *29*, 874 – 886.

Friedman, M., Rosenman, R., Straus, R., et al. The relationship of behavior pattern A to the state of the coronary vasculature: A study of 51 autopsied subjects. *American Journal of Medicine*, 1968, *44*, 525 – 537.

Gastorf, J. W. Time urgency of the Type A behavior pattern. *Journal of Consulting and Clinical Psychology*, 1980, *48*, 299.

Gentry, W. D., & Suinn, R. M. Section summary: Behavioral intervention. In T. M. Dembroski, S. M. Weiss, J. L. Shields, S. G. Haynes, & M. Feinleib (Eds.), *Coronary-prone behavior.* New York: Springer – Verlag, 1978.

Glass, D. C. *Behavior patterns, stress, and coronary disease.* Hillsdale, N. J.: Lawrence Erlbaum Associates, 1977.

Glass, D. C., & Carver, C. S. Helplessness and the coronary-prone personality. In J. Garber & M. E. P. Seligman (Eds.), *Human helplessness: Theory and application.* New York: Academic Press, 1980.

Glass, D. C., Krakoff, L. R., Contrada, R., Hilton, W. F., Kehoe, K., Mannucci, E. G., Collins, C., Snow, B., & Elting, E. Effects of harassment and competition upon cardiovascular and plasma catecholamines responses in Type A and Type B individuals. *Psychophysiology,* 1980, *17,* 453 – 463.

Glass, D. C., Snyder, M. L., & Hollis, J. F. Time urgency and the Type A coronary-prone behavior pattern. *Journal of Applied Social Psychology,* 1974, *4,* 125 – 140.

Goldband, S. Stimulus specificity of physiological response to stress and the Type A coronary-prone behavior pattern. *Journal of Personality and Social Psychology,* 1980, *39,* 670 – 679.

Graham, L. E., Ho, P., Thoresen, C. E., Levenkron, J. C., Vodak, P., Blair, S. N., Gelston, M., Terry, R. B., Moran, J. A., Haskell, W. L., & Wood, P. D. *Predicting treadmill fatigue suppression with various measures of Type A behavior.* Annual meeting of the American Psychological Association, Los Angeles, August 1981.

Greene, W. A., Goldstein, S., & Moss, A. J. Psychosocial aspects of sudden death: A preliminary report. *Archives of Internal Medicine,* 1972, *129,* 725 – 731.

Greene, W. A., Moss, A. J., & Goldstein, S. Delay, denial, and death in coronary heart disease. In R. S. Eliot (Ed.), *Stress and the heart.* Mt. Kisco, N. Y.: Futura, 1974.

Haynes, S. G., Levine, S., Scotch, N., Feinleib, M., & Kannel, W. B. The relationship of psychosocial factors to coronary heart disease in the Framingham study: I. Methods and risk factors. *American Journal of Epidemiology,* 1978, *107,* 362 – 383.

Herd, J. A. Physiological correlates of coronary-prone behavior. In T. M. Dembroski, S. M. Weiss, J. L. Shields, S. G. Haynes, & M. Feinleib (Eds.), *Coronary-prone behavior.* New York: Springer– Verlag, 1978.

Hiroto, D. S., & Seligman, M. E. P. Generality of learned helplessness in man. *Journal of Personality and Social Psychology,* 1975, *31,* 311 – 327.

Holmes, D. S., Solomon, S., & Spreier, B. J. *Cardiac and subjective response to cognitive challenge and to controlled physical exercise by male and female coronary-prone (Type A) and non-coronary-prone persons.* Unpublished manuscript, 1979.

Humphries, C., Carver, C. S., & Neumann, P. G. Cognitive characteristics of the coronary-prone behavior pattern. *Journal of Personality and Social Psychology,* 1983, *44,* 177 – 178.

Jenkins, C. D. Psychologic and social precursors of coronary disease. *New England Journal of Medicine,* 1971, *284,* 244 – 255.

Jenkins, C. D., Rosenman, R. H., & Friedman, M. Replicability of rating the coronary-prone behavior pattern. *British Journal of Preventive and Social Medicine,* 1968, *22,* 16 – 22.

Jenkins, C. D., Rosenman, R. H., & Zyzanski, S. J. *The Jenkins Activity Survey for Health Prediction.* Boston: Published by the Authors, 1972.

Jenkins, C. D., Rosenman, R. H., & Zyzanski, S. J. Prediction of clinical heart disease by a test for the coronary-prone behavior pattern. *New England Journal of Medicine,* 1974, *23,* 1271 – 1275.

Jenkins, C. D., Zyzanski, S. I., & Rosenman, R. H. Risk of new myocardial infarction in middle-aged men with manifest coronary heart disease. *Circulation,* 1976, *53,* 342 – 347.

Jenkins, C. D., Zyzanski, S. J., & Rosenman, R. H. Coronary-prone behavior: One pattern or several? *Psychosomatic Medicine,* 1978, *40,* 25 – 43.

Kahn, J. P., Kornfeld, D. S., Frank, K. A., Heller, S. S., & Hoar, P. F. Type A behavior and blood pressure during coronary artery by-pass surgery. *Psychosomatic Medicine,* 1980, *42,* 407 – 414.

Kirschenbaum, D. S., & Tomarken, A. J. On facing the generalization problem: The study of self-regulatory failure. In D. C. Kendall (Ed.), *Advances in cognitive – behavioral research and therapy* (Vol. 1). New York: Academic Press, 1982.

Krantz, D. S., Arabian, J. M., Davia, J. E., & Parker, J. S. Type A behavior and coronary artery bypass surgery: Intraoperative blood pressure and perioperative complications. *Psychosomatic Medicine*, 1982, *44*, 273–284.

Krantz, D. S., Glass, D. C., & Snyder, M. L. Helplessness, stress level and the coronary-prone behavior pattern. *Journal of Experimental Social Psychology*, 1974, *10*, 284–300.

Krantz, D. S., Sanmarco, M. E., Selvester, R. H., & Matthews, K. A. Psychological correlates of progression of atherosclerosis in men: A preliminary report. *Psychosomatic Medicine*, 1979, *41*, 467–475.

Krantz, D. S., Schaeffer, M. A., Davia, J. E., Dembroski, T. M., MacDougall, J.M., & Shaffer, R.T. *Investigation of the extent of coronary atherosclerosis, Type A behavior, and cardiovascular response to social interaction.* Paper presented at the meeting of the Society for Psychophysiological Research, Vancouver, B. C., October 1980.

Lovallo, W. R. The role of stress in the development of heart disease: Theory and research. *Biological Psychology Bulletin*, 1978, *5*, 70–95.

Lovallo, W. R., & Pishkin, V. Performance of Type A (coronary-prone) men during and after exposure to uncontrollable noise and task failure. *Journal of Personality and Social Psychology*, 1980, *38*, 963–971.

MacDougall, J. M., Dembroski, T. M., & Krantz, D. S. Effects of types of challenge on pressor and heart rate responses in Type A and B women. *Psychophysiology*, 1981, *18*, 1–9.

MacDougall, J. M., Dembroski, T. M., & Musante, L. The structured interview and questionnaire methods of assessing coronary-prone behavior in male and female college students. *Journal of Behavioral Medicine*, 1979, *2*, 71–83.

Manuck, S. B., Craft, S. A., & Gold, K. J. Coronary-prone behavior pattern and cardiovascular response. *Psychophysiology*, 1978, *15*, 403–411.

Manuck, S. B., & Garland, F. N. Coronary-prone behavior pattern, task incentive and cardiovascular response. *Psychophysiology*, 1979, *16*, 136–147.

Marlatt, G., & Gordon, J. Determinants of relapse: Implications for the maintenance of behavior change. In P. O. Davidson & S. M. Davidson (Eds.), *Behavioral medicine: Changing health lifestyles*. New York: Brunner/Mazel, 1980.

Matthews, K. A. Psychological perspectives on the Type A behavior pattern. *Psychological Bulletin*, 1982, 91, *2*, 293–323.

Matthews, K. A., & Brunson, B. I. The attentional style of Type A coronary-prone individuals: Implications for symptom reporting. *Journal of Personality and Social Psychology*, 1979, *37*, 2081–2090.

Matthews, K. A., & Carra, J. Suppression of menstrual distress symptoms: A study of Type A behavior. *Personality and Social Psychology Bulletin*, 1982, *8*, 146–151.

Matthews, K. A., Glass, D. C., Rosenman, R. H., & Bortner, R. W. Competitive drive, Pattern A, and coronary heart disease: A further analysis of some data from the Western Collaborative Group Study. *Journal of Chronic Diseases*, 1977, *30*, 489–498.

Matthews, K. A., Helmreich, R. L., Beane, W. E., & Lucker, G. W. Pattern A, achievement-striving, and scientific excellence: Does Pattern A help or hinder? *Journal of Personality and Social Psychology*, 1980, *39*, 962–967.

Matthews, K. A., Krantz, D. S., Dembroski, T. M., & MacDougall, J. M. The unique and common variance in the Structured Interview and the Jenkins Activity Survey measures of the Type A behavior pattern. *Journal of Personality and Social Psychology*, 1982, *42*, 303–313.

Matthews, K. A., & Saal, F. E. The relationship of the Type A coronary-prone behavior pattern to achievement, power, and affiliation motives. *Psychosomatic Medicine*, 1978, *40*, 631–636.

Matthews, K. A., & Siegel, J. M. The Type A behavior pattern in children and adolescents: Assessment, development, and associated coronary-risk. In A. Baum & J. E. Singer (Eds.), *Handbook of psychology and health* (Vol. 2). Hillsdale, N. J.: Lawrence Erlbaum Associates, 1982.

Matthews, K. A., Siegel, J. M., Kuller, L. H., Thompson, M., & Varat, M. Determinants of decisions to seek medical treatment by patients with acute myocardial infarction symptoms. *Journal of Personality and Social Psychology*, 1983, *44*, 1144–1156.

Mettlin, C. Occupational careers and the prevention of coronary-prone behavior. *Social Science and Medicine*, 1976, *10*, 367–372.

Obrist, P. A. The cardiovascular—behavioral interaction—as it appears today. *Psychophysiology*, 1976, *13*, 95–107.

Paykel, E. S. Life stress and psychiatric disorder: Applications of the clinical approach. In B. S. Dohrenwend & B. P. Dohrenwend (Eds.), *Stressful life events: Their nature and effects*. New York: Wiley, 1974.

Raab, W., Chaplin, J. P., & Bajusz, E. Myocardial necroses produced in domesticated rats and in wild rats by sensory and emotional stresses. *Proceedings of the Society of Experimental Biology and Medicine*, 1964, *116*, 665–669.

Raab, W., Stark, E., MacMillan, W. H., & Gigee, W. R. Sympathetic origin and antidrenergic prevention of stress-induced myocardial lesions. *American Journal of Cardiology*, 1961, *8*, 203–211.

Rhodewalt, F., & Comer, R. Coronary-prone behavior and reactance: The attractiveness of an eliminated choice. *Personality and Social Psychology Bulletin*, 1982, *8*, 152–158.

Rosenman, R. H. The role of behavior patterns and neurogenic factors in the pathogenesis of coronary heart disease. In R. S. Eliot (Ed.), *Stress and the heart*. Mt. Kisco, N.Y.: Futura, 1974.

Rosenman, R. H., Brand, R. J., Jenkins, C. D., Friedman, M., Straus, R., & Wurm, M. Coronary heart disease in the Western Collaborative Group Study: Final follow-up experience of 8 1/2 years. *Journal of the American Medical Association*, 1975, *233*, 872–877.

Rosenman, R. H., & Friedman, M. Neurogenic factors in pathogenesis of coronary heart disease. *Medical Clinics of North America*, 1974, *58*, 269–279.

Rosenman, R. H., & Friedman, M. Modifying Type A behavior pattern. *Journal of Psychosomatic Research*, 1977, *21*, 323–333.

Rosenman, R. H., Friedman, M., Straus, R., Wurm, M., Jenkins, C. D., & Messinger, H. B. Coronary heart disease in the Western Collaborative Group Study: A follow-up experience of 2 years. *Journal of the American Medical Association*, 1966, *195*, 130–136.

Rosenman, R. H., Rahe, R. N., Borhani, N. O., & Feinleib, M. Heritability of personality and behavior pattern. *Proceedings of the First International Congress on Twins*, Rome, Italy, November 1974.

Roskies, E. Considerations in developing a treatment program for the coronary-prone (Type A) behavior pattern. In P. O. Davidson & S. M. Davidson (Eds.), *Behavioral medicine: Changing health life-styles*. New York: Brunner/Mazel, 1980.

Roskies, E., & Avard, J. Teaching healthy managers to control their coronary-prone (Type A) behavior. In K. Blankstein & J. Polivy (Eds.), *Self-control and self-modification of emotional behaviors*. New York: Plenum, 1982.

Roskies, E., Kearney, H., Spevack, M., Surkis, A., Cohen, C., & Gilman, S. Generalizability and durability of treatment effects in an intervention program for coronary-prone (Type A) managers. *Journal of Behavioral Medicine*, 1979, *2*, 195–207.

Roskies, E., Spevack, M., Surkis, A., Cohen, C., & Gilman, S. Changing the coronary-prone (Type A) behavior pattern in a non-clinical population. *Journal of Behavioral Medicine*, 1978, *1*, 201–217.

Ross, R., & Glomset, J. A. The pathogenesis of atherosclerosis: Part I. *New England Journal of Medicine*, 1976, *295*, 369–377.

Ross, R., & Harker, L. Hyperlipidemia and atherosclerosis. *Science*, 1976, *193*, 1094–1100.

Schmale, A. H. Giving up as a final common pathway to changes in health. *Advances in Psychosomatic Medicine*, 1972, *8*, 18–38.

Scherwitz, L., Berton, K., & Leventhal, H. Type A behavior, self-involvement and cardiovascular response. *Psychosomatic Medicine*, 1978, *40*, 593–609.

Scherwitz, L., Cleary, P., Leventhal, H., & Laman, C. Type A behavior: Consideration for risk modification. *Health values: Achieving high level wellness*, 1978, *2*, 291–296.

Schneiderman, N. Animal models relating behavioral stress and cardiovascular pathology. In T. M. Dembroski, S. M. Weiss, J. L. Shields, S. G. Haynes, & M. Feinleib (Eds.), *Coronary-prone behavior*. New York: Springer–Verlag, 1978.

Schneiderman, N. Behavior, autonomic function and animal models of cardiovascular pathology. In T. Dembroski & T. Schmidt (Eds.), *Biological basis of coronary-prone behavior.* New York: Harper, 1982.

Schucker, B., & Jacobs, D. R., Jr. Assessment of behavioral risk for coronary disease by voice characteristics. *Psychosomatic Medicine,* 1977, *39,* 219 – 228.

Seligman, M. E. P. *Helplessness: On depression, development, and death.* San Francisco, CA.: W. H. Freeman, 1975.

Shekelle, R. B., Schoenberger, J. A., & Stamler, J. Correlates of the JAS Type A behavior pattern score. *Journal of Chronic Diseases,* 1976, *29,* 381 – 394.

Sigler, L. H. Emotion and arteriosclerotic heart disease. I. Electrocardiographic changes observed on the recall of past emotional disturbances. *British Journal of Medical Psychology,* 1967, *30,* 55 – 64.

Shinamoto, T. Injury and repair in arterial tissue. *Angiology,* 1974, *25,* 682 – 699.

Shinamoto, T., Kobayashi, M., & Numano, F. Immunoflorescent demonstration of plasma protein entry into arterial wall by cholesterol, epinephrine, norepinephrine, and angiotension II. *Acta Pathologica Japonica,* 1975, *25,* 51 – 67.

Simpson, M. T., Olewine, D. A., Jenkins, C. D., Ramsey, F. H., Zyzanski, S. J., Thomas, G., & Hames, C. G. Exercise-induced catecholamines and platelet aggregation in the coronary-prone behavior pattern. *Psychosomatic Medicine,* 1974, *36,* 476 – 487.

Snyder, M. L., & Frankel, A. *Reactance and the Type A.* Unpublished manuscript, 1980.

Stokols, D., Novaco, R. W., Stokols, J., & Campbell, J. Traffic congestion, Type A behavior, and stress. *Journal of Applied Psychology,* 1978, *63,* 467 – 480.

Stunkard, A. Behavioral treatment of obesity: Failure to maintain weight loss. In R. B. Stuart (Ed.), *Behavioral self-management: Strategies, techniques and outcome.* New York: Brunner/Mazel, 1977.

Suinn, R. Anxiety management training for general anxiety. In R. Suinn & R. Weigel (Eds.), *The innovative psychological therapies: Critical and creative contributions.* New York: Harper, 1975. (a)

Suinn, R. The cardiac stress management program for Type A patients. *Cardiac Rehabilitation,* 1975, *5,* 13 – 15. (b)

Suinn, R., & Bloom, L. Anxiety management training for Pattern A behavior. *Journal of Behavioral Medicine,* 1978, *1,* 25 – 35.

Van Egeren, L. F. Cardiovascular changes during social competition in mixed motive game. *Journal of Personality and Social Psychology,* 1979, *37,* 858 – 864.

Waldron, I. Sex differences in the coronary-prone behavior pattern. In T. M. Dembroski, S. M. Weiss, J. L. Shields, S. G. Haynes, & M. Feinlieb (Eds.), *Coronary-prone behavior.* New York: Springer– Verlag, 1978.

Waldron, I., Hickey, A., McPherson, C., Butensky, A., Gruss, L., Overall, K., Schmader, A., & Wohlmuth, D. Type A behavior pattern: Relationship to variation in blood pressure, parental characteristics, and academic and social activities of students. *Journal of Human Stress,* 1980, *6,* 16 – 27.

Waldron, I., Zyzanski, S. J., Shekelle, R. B., Jenkins, C. D., & Tannenbaum, S. The coronary-prone behavior pattern in employed men and women. *Journal of Human Stress,* 1977, *3,* 2 – 19.

Weidner, G., & Matthews, K. A. Reported physical symptoms elicited by unpredictable events and the Type A coronary-prone behavior pattern. *Journal of Personality and Social Psychology,* 1978, *36,* 213 – 220.

Wicklund, R. A. *Freedom and reactance.* Potomac, MD.: Lawerence Erlbaum Associates, 1974.

Williams, R. B. Psychophysiological processes, the coronary-prone behavior pattern, and coronary heart disease. In T. M. Dembroski, S. M. Weiss, J. L. Shields, S. G. Haynes, & M. Feinlieb (Eds.), *Coronary-prone behavior.* New York: Springer – Verlag, 1978.

Williams, R. B., Haney, T., Gentry, W. D., & Kong, Y. Relation between hostility and arteriographically documented coronary atherosclerosis. *Psychosomatic Medicine,* 1978, *40,* 88.

Wolf, S., McCabe, W. R., Yamamoto, J., Adsett, C. A., & Schottstaedt, W. W. Changes in serum lipids in relation to emotional stress during rigid controls of diet and excerise. *Transactions of the American Clinical and Climatological Association*, 1961, *73*, 162 – 175.

Wortman, C. B., & Brehm, J. W. Responses to uncontrollable outcomes: An integration of reactance theory and the learned helplessness model. In L. Berkowitz (Ed.), *Advances in experimental social psychology*. New York: Academic Press, 1975.

Zyzanski, S. J., & Jenkins, C. D. Basic dimensions within the coronary-prone behavior pattern. *Journal of Chronic Diseases,* 1970, *22,*781 – 795.

Zyzanski, S. J., Jenkins, C. D., Ryan, T. J., Flessas, A., & Everist, M. Psychological correlates of angiographic findings. *Archives of Internal Medicine*, 1976, *136*, 1234 – 1237.

V BEHAVIORAL ASPECTS OF HEALTH DISORDERS

17 Behavioral Medicine Approaches to Cardiovascular Disorders

Neil Schneiderman

David Hammer
University of Miami

INTRODUCTION

Cardiovascular diseases pose the most serious health problem to developed nations in terms of mortality and morbidity. Approximately half of all deaths in the United States are attributable to these disorders; *ischemic* or *coronary heart disease* (CHD) alone accounts for about 38% and strokes for nearly 10% (National Center for Health Statistics, 1979). More than half of the 4 million Americans with chronic illness due to CHD are under age 65. And of the nearly 1 million people in the United States partially or completely disabled by *cerebrovascular disease* nearly a quarter of a million persons per year under the age of 65 are afflicted by strokes.

Epidemiological research has established cigarette smoking, elevated levels of low-density lipoproteins in the blood, hypertension, advancing age, the presence of diabetes mellitus, and a family history of heart disease as risk factors for CHD (Brand, Rosenman, Sholtz, & Friedman, 1976; Kannel, McGee, & Gordon, 1976). Knowledge about these risk factors, alone or in combination, however, does not predict most new cases of CHD (Jenkins, 1976). This has led to a search for other, nontraditional risk factors. One of these, the Type A coronary-prone behavior pattern (see Carver, Diamond, & Humphries, Chapter 16), was identified in the Western Collaborative Group Study as an independent risk factor for CHD (Brand et al., 1976; Rosenman, Brand, Jenkins, Friedman, Strauss, & Wurm, 1975). In addition, evidence has accumulated that chronic stressors such as job dissatisfaction and burdensome responsibilities (Haynes, Feinleib, & Kannel, 1980; Jenkins, 1976) are associated with an increased risk of CHD, as are stressful life events such as the death of a spouse (Dohrenwend & Dohrenwend, 1974;

Engel, 1971), or a major change in occupation (Shekelle, Ostfield, & Paul, 1969) or place of residence (Syme, Borhani, & Buechley, 1965).

It would thus appear that a number of psychosocial and behavioral factors may contribute to the development of CHD. These include life-style variables such as cigarette smoking and diet, stressful environmental variables such as the loss of a job or spouse, and personality variables such as those evinced in the Type A coronary-prone behavior pattern. Presumably, by eliminating or minimizing those psychosocial and behavioral factors that convey risk, it should be possible to impede the development of CHD and its manifestations. The major problem, here, is that the causal mechanisms relating any risk factor (e.g., cigarette smoking, diet, coronary-prone behavior) to CHD are not yet adequately understood. Therefore, for most risk factors having a behavioral component, it is not apparent exactly what needs to be modified.

The exact nature of the relationship between diet and serum cholesterol, for example, is still not entirely clear. In the case of smoking, it has not yet been determined whether it is nicotine, tar, or carbon monoxide that conveys coronary risk. Certainly, with regard to the Type A coronary-prone behavior pattern, which is said to involve competitiveness, achievement striving, time urgency, and hostility, it is not evident which behavioral component(s) increase risk. In spite of these formidable obstacles, however, knowledge has been accumulating that suggests that behavioral approaches to prevention and treatment may prove useful in reducing morbidity and mortality from cardiovascular diseases. With these considerations in mind, the present chapter examines the biobehavioral and psychosocial aspects of cardiovascular disease in terms of pathogenesis, treatment, prevention, and rehabilitation. (i.e., secondary prevention).

HYPERTENSION

Hypertension is a major risk factor for CHD and for cerebrovascular disease (Kannel, 1975; Paul, 1971). This is because high levels of blood pressure maintained over many years are associated with increased risk of target-organ damage and life-threatening disorders of the heart, kidneys, and blood vessels (Kannel, Gordon, & Schwartz, 1971). The risk conveyed by hypertension in these disorders appears to be directly proportional to mean arterial pressure and the length of time blood pressure has been elevated.

Although the exact mechanisms underlying hypertension are presently unknown, there are several important reasons for believing that the study of hypertension is directly relevant to behavioral medicine. First, sodium intake and obesity appear to be significant behavioral factors in the pathogenesis of hypertension. Second, behavioral stress appears to be capable of interacting with other variables to produce or exacerbate chronic hypertension. Third, a major problem in achieving hypertension control has been the behavioral problem of maintaining *ad-*

herence to antihypertensive medications. Fourth, there is some evidence that behavioral treatments may have some therapeutic effects in dealing with hypertension. Let us consider some of the issues involved in relationships between hypertension and behavior.

Etiology and Pathogenesis

Hypertension reflects a disruption of regulatory physiologic mechanisms that normally operate to keep blood pressure at healthy levels. Although some cases of hypertension are secondary to known kidney, endocrine, or other specific physical disorders, approximately 85% of cases are classified as *primary* or *essential hypertension,* in which the exact regulatory disruption leading to the elevated pressure can not be specified (Julius, 1977). According to Page's (1949, 1977) mosaic theory, the origins and development of hypertension in most instances are multifactorily determined. Heredity, environmental, and psychological factors have all been implicated. Before examining behavior as an interactive variable in the genesis of hypertension, however, let us briefly consider it as a putative main effect.

Noncontingent Stimulation.   At present there is scant evidence to suggest that behavioral factors alone can produce chronic hypertension. Reports emerging from World War II indicate that battlefield or siege conditions can lead to increased blood pressure levels, but that the effects are relatively transient (Graham, 1945). Blast victims of the Texas City disaster in the United States also showed transient but pronounced elevations in blood pressure, when an explosion aboard a ship triggered major explosions in nearby Monsanto chemical plants (Ruskin, Beard, & Schaffer, 1948).

Experiments using noncontingent auditory (Farris, Yeakel, & Medoff, 1945; Rothlin, Cerletti, & Emmenegger, 1956) and multimodal sensory stimuli (e.g., Buckley & Smookler, 1970; Perhach, Ferguson, & McKinney, 1976) in animals have provided evidence of increased blood pressure changes that persisted past the time of direct stimulation, but relatively little evidence that the elevated pressures might have some permanence. For a more complete discussion of this issue see Schneiderman (1983b).

Contingent Stimulation.   Animal behavior experiments examining the effects of operant (contingent) conditioning upon the development of hypertension have been of two kinds. In one, changes in pressure have been observed as concomitants of the performance of an instrumental response such as lever pressing to avoid shock (Forsyth, 1969; Herd, Morse, Kelleher, & Jones, 1969). In the second kind of experiment, rewards and/or punishments have been made contingent upon prespecified increases in blood pressure (Benson, Herd, Morse, & Kelleher, 1969; Harris, Gilliam, Findley, & Brady, 1973). Although both procedures have evoked large increases in blood pressure during the course of many months of training, the evidence is convincing that these procedures alone do not lead to sustained hypertension.

Psychosocial Stimulation. Studies in which occupational stress (e.g., Cobb & Rose, 1973) or living in a stressful residential neighborhood (Harburg, Erfurt, Hauenstein, Chape, Schull, & Schork, 1973) have been related to hypertension suggest that psychological variables may contribute to the development of hypertension. In the Harburg et al. study, blacks living in high stress (high crime rates, high population density, low socioeconomic status) neighborhoods of Detroit had higher blood pressure levels than blacks living in low stress areas. Furthermore, the blood pressure of blacks living in low stress neighborhoods is comparable to that of nonblacks also living in low stress areas. Although studies such as this suggest that the cultural environment can play a role in the etiology of hypertension, other cross-cultural research has not uniformly demonstrated clear relationships between environmental stress and hypertension. Differences in dietary salt intake, genetic background, and access to medical care have confounded much of the research.

The animal behavior experiments conducted by Henry and his collaborators upon colonies of Agouti CBA (brown) mice appear to provide the most convincing evidence that psychosocial variables can lead to sustained hypertension (Henry, Ely, & Stephens, 1972; Henry, Ely, Stephens, Ratcliffe, Santisteban, & Shapiro, 1971; Henry, Stephens, & Santisteban, 1975). In these experiments experimental animals were isolated shortly after birth and then introduced into a complex population environment several months later. The complex environment, which was designed to maximize confrontation, consisted of boxes joined by narrow interconnecting tubes to a single feeding and watering place. In contrast to control animals raised in social groups and not subjected to the complex environments, the experimental animals experienced repeated confrontations leading to vigorous fighting that produced epilation and scarring.

After several months in the complex environment the experimental mice developed evidence of sustained hypertension, whereas the control animals remained normotensive. Hypertension in the experimental animals was accompanied by interstitial nephritis, increased heart weight, myocardial fibrosis, and arteriosclerosis of the intramural coronary vessels and aorta (Henry et al., 1971, 1972, 1975). The sustained hypertension and degenerative effects observed as a function of psychosocial stress appear to have been at least in part related to increased sympathetic nervous system (SNS) activation and to the release of catecholamines into the circulation. Increases were seen, for example, in the adrenal medullary enzymes, tyrosine hydroxylase and phenylethanolamine N-methyltransferase (Henry, Stephens, Axelrod, & Mueller, 1971) and in plasma renin activity (Vander, Henry, Stephens, Kay, & Mouw, 1978).

Although the experiments conducted by Henry and his collaborators strongly suggest that emotional behavior can contribute to the development of hypertension, the role of genetic susceptibility in these experiments also needs to be considered. Agouti CBA mice, for instance, are known to be more agressive and active than many other mouse strains. When Alexander (1974) performed experiments on rats, which were similar to those conducted on mice by Henry and his coworkers, only a third of the rats showed elevated blood pressures, and the elevations were relatively small. Because the disparities between the Henry and Alexander experiments include a species difference, it would be useful to determine whether psychosocial stress can produce sustained hypertension in mouse strains other than the CBA.

Genetic-Behavioral Interactions. The mosaic theory proposed by Page (1949, 1977) implies that the hereditary factors underlying hypertension consist of a spectrum of variants more or less haphazardly mixed in the genetic coding of human reproduction. Development of selectively bred strains of rats has provided a useful tool for isolating putative genetic variants that might contribute to human hypertension. It has also provided a valuable tool for examining the extent to which genetic variants are influenced by environmental factors.

The *spontaneously hypertensive rat* (SHR) developed by Okamoto and Aoki (1963) is the most extensively used experimental model. Hypertension in the SHR appears to be due to a relatively few genetic components acting in concert (Hansen, 1972). Pronounced increases in tonic blood pressure begin shortly after birth and develop rapidly during the next several months. During the early accelerating phase of the hypertension, young SHRs, like relatively young borderline or early stage hypertensive humans, display a "hyperkinetic" circulation with increased cardiac output related to enhanced sympathetic discharge. This pattern of responses is reminiscent of the defense reaction (Folkow & Hallback, 1977; Julius & Esler, 1975). In contrast, more mature SHRs, like relatively older, chronic hypertensive humans, have a normal or subnormal cardiac output, but a high peripheral resistance. At this stage, sympathetic tone seems to be reduced, but secondary structural changes such as arteriosclerosis are apparent.

A very large number of experiments have demonstrated that young SHRs show greater increases in SNS and cardiovascular reactivity than normotensive control rats when subjected to environmental stimulation (Yamori, Matsumoto, Yamabe, & Okamoto, 1969; see Schneiderman, 1983b, for additional references and discussion). In general, the experimental findings indicate that exposure to aversive stimulation facilitates the development of hypertension in SHRs; whereas, reduced environmental stimulation impedes its development. The neural and cardiovascular hyperreactivity to environmental stimulation in SHRs seems to be central in origin, and it appears likely that the hyperreactivity plays an important role in the development of hypertension.

A limitation of the SHR as an experimental model is that, unlike the human, the SHR will invariably develop severe hypertension unless it is socially isolated. In order to minimize this problem, Lawler, Barker, Hubbard, and Allen (1980) mated SHRs with normotensive rats and studied the offspring. These latter animals developed more moderate levels of hypertension (borderline hypertension), unless subjected to environmental stimulation. The borderline hypertensive rat is therefore a potentially interesting experimental model. This is especially true in light of human research indicating that persons having at least one hypertensive parent show greater heart rate and blood pressure reactivity on experimental tasks involving mental arithmetic or shock avoidance than do the offspring of normotensive parents (Falkner, Onesti, Angelakos, Fernandes, & Langman, 1979; Manuck, Giordani, McQuaid, & Garrity, 1981; Obrist, 1981).

Another valuable genetic model for hypertensive research was developed by Dahl and his colleagues (Dahl, Heine, & Tassinari, 1962, 1963, 1965). This model consists of two lines of rats having opposite, genetically determined predispositions toward hypertension. One line, the *Dahl hypertension-sensitive (S) strain*, shows increasing levels of hypertension as a function of an increasing amount of sodium chloride in the diet. The second line, or *Dahl hypertension-resistant (R) strain*, is relatively insensitive to sodium chloride intake in terms of blood pressure. Both strains remain normotensive at relatively low dietary sodium levels. Although the difference between the R and S strains in terms of hypertension is most pronounced with regard to salt load, the S strain is also more prone to become hypertensive in response to deoxycorticosterone-sodium chloride, cortisone, renal artery clamping, or aversive stimulation (Dahl et al., 1963, 1965; Friedman & Dahl, 1975; Friedman & Iwai, 1976, 1977). These experiments suggest that genetic predisposition, diet, and emotional behavior can interact systematically to produce sustained increases in blood pressure. Furthermore, genetic predispositions may not manifest themselves unless environmental factors challenge the organism.

Salt-Stress Interaction.   A possible synergism between sodium ingestion and behavioral stress in the development of hypertension has begun to receive attention. In one study, Anderson, Kearns, and Better (1983) infused isotonic saline into an arterial catheter in dogs while subjecting the animals to multiple daily sessions of unsignaled avoidance training. Within 2 weeks of exposure to this dual challenge the dogs became hypertensive between as well as during the avoidance session. In contrast, control animals exposed either to saline infusion alone or to avoidance conditioning alone revealed negligible changes in blood pressure. In another study, Anderson, Kearns, and Worden (1983) found that avoidance-saline hypertension in their dogs was attenuated by increasing the intake of potassium. This suggests that it is the ratio of sodium to potassium, rather than simply level of sodium intake, that may be important in blood pressure regulation. It also suggests that further research is needed to examine the synergism between behavioral stress and diet because of its implications for treatment as well as pathogenesis.

Comment. The experimental data do not convincingly support the hypotheses that emotional behavior alone can produce sustained hypertension. These data do indicate, however, that behaviors associated with pronounced increases in SNS activity (i.e., emotional behaviors) can interact with diet (e.g., sodium), renal infection (Lipman & Shapiro, 1967) or genetic predisposition (Dahl et al., 1962, 1963, 1965; Friedman & Iwai, 1976, 1977; Okamoto & Aoki, 1963; Yamori et al., 1969) to produce hypertension. It therefore would be reasonable for future behavioral research into the causes of hypertension to examine interactions between behavior on the one hand and atherogenic or high sodium diets or genetic predispositions on the other.

Treatment

Hypertension, for the most part, is a disorder with very few signs or symptoms. Furthermore, treatment can be costly, inconvenient and disruptive in terms of unpleasant and/or debilitating side effects. Consequently, adherence to treatment regimes can be a problem. Nevertheless, there is reason to believe that even moderate levels of hypertension deserve treatment. The Framingham study, for example, clearly showed that a casual systolic blood pressure above 160 mmHg or a diastolic blood pressure above 100 mmHg are significantly related to increased morbidity and mortality (Kannel, 1974). More recently, the report of the Hypertension Detection and Follow-up Program Cooperative Group (1979a, 1979b) contended that aggressive treatment of systolic blood pressure above 140 mmHg or a diastolic blood pressure above 90 mmHg (140/90 mmHg) can significantly reduce morbidity and mortality.

Current pharmacologic treatment of hypertension is based on the "stepped-care" approach used in the Hypertension Detection and Follow-up Program. Briefly, when blood pressure remains consistently above 140/90 mmHg over the course of several weeks, the patient is placed on a thiazide diuretic. The lowering of blood pressure by the diuretic is achieved by decreasing blood volume largely through increased sodium excretion. If the diuretic does not reduce blood pressure below 140/90 mmHg, the patient is stepped to a sympathetic blocking agent (e.g., propranolol, methyldopa) either alone or in conjunction with a diuretic. If the second step does not normalize the blood pressure, a third step is taken in which a vasodilator, which works directly upon vascular smooth muscle, is added to the diuretic and sympathetic blocking agents. With these combinations of drugs, almost all cases of hypertension can be controlled.

Although drug therapy is highly effective in the control of hypertension, it is conceivable that behavioral approaches (e.g., diet, exercise, relaxation) may be useful as an initial step in minimally hypertensive patients. Because the casual blood pressure of millions of American adults is in the vicinity of 140/90 mmHg, drugs may produce unpleasant or as yet unknown side effects, and the taking of antihypertensive drugs usually requires a lifetime commitment, research into behavioral alternatives to drug treatment for these people appears reasonable.

Similarly, because antihypertensive medications can produce side effects, behavioral approaches may have use as adjuncts to standard pharmacologic therapy. This might result in either lowering drug dosages required to control the hypertension or in increasing drug options. Before turning to these behavioral treatment approaches, let us briefly consider some of the basic behavioral issues in the adherence of patients to antihypertensive medication.

Adherence.   A major problem in achieving control over hypertension is lack of patient adherence to antihypertensive medications. It has been estimated that, in clinical practice, only about half of all hypertensive patients take as much as 80% of their prescribed medication (Sackett, Gibson, Taylor, Haynes, Hackett, Roberts, & Johnson, 1975).

Blackwell (1979) reviewed the literature that has addressed patient compliance with prescribed medical regimens and concluded that several factors may be the source of poor adherence. Factors such as the complexity of the regimen, amount of behavior change required, and the amount of painful side effects of the therapy were inversely related to adherence. Factors such as viewing the disease as serious, family stability, close supervision, and compliance with other aspects of treatment were noted to be associated with better compliance. Overall, there appear to be several things that the physician, the patient, and others may do to improve compliance.

Physicians who work to reduce client waiting room time, schedule individual rather than block appointment times, and take care to check patient expectations and satisfaction, while providing close personal supervision of treatment, are likely to observe greater compliance in their patients (Blackwell, 1976; Dunbar & Stunkard, 1979). Although elaborate education programs regarding the nature of hypertension, its risks, and the efficacy of medical treatment have proven relatively unsuccessful (Caplan, Robinson, French, Caldwell, & Shinn, 1976; Sackett et al., 1975), simple procedures such as combining medications in a single tablet (Clark & Troop, 1972; David, Welborn, & Pierce, 1975), utilizing pill dispenser packets (Eshelman & Fitzloff, 1976), associating medication taking with daily activities (Haynes et al., 1976), and prescribing less potent medications when possible (Haynes, Gibson, Taylor, Bernholz, & Sackett, 1982) have been useful in increasing adherence rates. More demanding practices such as patient self-monitoring, reviews by nonprofessional counselors, plus praise and monetary incentives have also been shown to improve adherence (Haynes et al., 1976). In addition, there are data to indicate that programs designed to engender social support and reinforcement for regimen compliance both in the home (Becker & Green, 1975) and in the work setting (Alderman & Schoenbaum, 1975) may have beneficial effects. Counseling new patients about the detection and management of possible side effects in their medication also seems to be useful. Thus, McKeeney, Slining, Henderson, Devins, and Beer (1973) found a 78% adherence rate in counseled hypertensive patients as opposed to a 16% rate in patients not receiving early counseling.

Diet and Exercise. There has been some support for the contention that life style changes such as restriction of salt intake, weight loss in obese individuals, and regular aerobic exercise can reduce existing hypertension. As yet, however, this contention is unsupported by controlled clinical trials.

The evidence that a decrease in sodium intake in the diet will lower blood pressure in humans is derived mostly from the proven effectiveness of diuretic drugs and from studies in which hypertensive patients were placed on relatively low sodium diets. In one study, reduction in sodium intake to 75 − 100 milli-equivalents (mequiv)/day led to decreases of 5 mmHg systolic and 10 mm Hg diastolic pressure (Parijs, Joossens, Van der Linden, Verstreken, & Amer, 1973). Another study showed that reducing sodium intake, as reflected in a urinary sodium decrease from 190 mequiv to 157 mequiv/day, led to a decrease in diastolic pressure of 7 mmHg (Morgan, Gillies, Morgan, Adam, Wilson, & Carney, 1978). The decrease in sodium intake and the concomitant reduction in blood pressure were maintained throughout the 2-year study period.

The decreases in sodium intake achieved in the Parijs et al. (1973) and Morgan et al. (1978) studies were accomplished by not adding salt to food at the table or during cooking, and by not eating foods that are high in sodium. Refraining from eating foods that are unusually high in sodium, however, requires some patient education, as many foods that do not taste obviously salty (e.g., chocolate pudding; cottage cheese) are quite high in sodium.

Another form of diet restriction that appears to have an impact on hypertension is that of limiting caloric intake to reduce excess body weight. Based on an association between blood pressure and weight among hypertensive patients, a number of studies have attempted to evaluate the effects of weight loss without sodium restriction upon blood pressure level (Ramsay, Ramsay, Hettiarachi, Davies, & Winchester, 1978; Reisin, Abel, Modan, Silverberg, Eliahow, & Modan, 1978). These studies have demonstrated that weight loss in hypertensive patients can produce a moderate but significant reduction in blood pressure.

Another life style change that has been recommended for hypertensive patients is that of routine physical exercise. Several studies have supported the ability of regular 30 − 40 minute exercise sessions to produce a moderate reduction in blood pressure levels over a period of several months (Boyer & Kasch, 1970; Choquette & Ferguson, 1973). These effects were noted only for subjects exhibiting elevated blood pressures. Normotensive subjects showed no such decline in blood pressure throughout the exercise sessions. The typical exercise activities employed in the studies were of an aerobic nature including jogging or riding a bicycle ergometer.

In addition to its direct effects upon blood pressure, a regular program of aerobic exercise appears to have a synergistic effect in terms of weight control. Weight loss is more likely to occur (Epstein & Wing, 1980) and is reportedly maintained better when diet modification is combined with increased exercise than when changes occur only in diet (Dahlkoetter, Callahan, & Linton, 1979). Although the reasons for this are not entirely clear, exercise appears to influence weight loss not only by burning up calories, but also by suppressing appetite

(Mayer, Roy, & Mitra, 1956) and by offsetting decreases in metabolic rate associated with caloric restriction (Wooley, Wooley, & Dyrenforth, 1979).

Blood Pressure Biofeedback and Relaxation-Based Treatments. Several studies have trained hypertensive patients to reduce blood pressure by providing the patient with feedback about their blood pressure levels (Benson, Shapiro, Tursky, & Schwartz, 1971; Elder & Eustis, 1975; Kristt & Engel, 1975). In general, it could be concluded from these studies that: (1) decreases of about 10–15 mmHg can be obtained in some patients; (2) results are transferable to the home setting; (3) the decreases in pressure can be obtained in patients already taking hypertensive medication; and (4) the results can be sustained if the patients continue to practice.

Because behavioral stress has been linked to the pathogenesis of hypertension, several studies have examined the effects of behavioral treatments aimed at a reduction in behavioral arousal and/or SNS activity. These studies have used a variety of procedures including progressive relaxation (Jacobson, 1939), autogenic training (Schultz & Luthe, 1969), biofeedback-assisted relaxation (Patel, 1973), meditation (Benson, 1975), and hypnosis (Friedman & Taub, 1977, 1978). Procedures such as meditation and progressive relaxation training have demonstrated clinically significant success in controlled studies (Patel & North, 1975; Stone & DeLeo, 1976; Taylor, Farquhar, Nelson, & Agras, 1977) and have been shown to generalize to settings outside the laboratory (Graham, Beiman, & Ciminero, 1977).

Direct comparisons between *blood pressure biofeedback* and the various *relaxation* procedures indicate comparable reductions in blood pressure (Blanchard, Miller, Able, Haynes, & Wicker, 1979; Surwit, Shapiro, & Good, 1978). Several of the relaxation-based studies also reported reductions of blood pressure in patients who had already received their maximal pressure decreases on medication (Benson, Rosner, Marzetta, & Klemchuk, 1974; Patel, 1973; Patel, Marmot, & Terry, 1981; Southam, Agras, Taylor, & Kraemer, in press). For some patients this allowed a lowering of medication dosage while the newly acquired lower blood pressure was maintained for at least 8 months after treatment (Patel et al., 1981).

In general, the behavioral treatment of hypertension seems to be promising for select (i.e., highly motivated) patients, at least as an adjunct to pharmacologic treatment. It should be pointed out, however, that most of the behavioral studies have used small numbers of patients who were studied for relatively short periods of time. Large-scale controlled trials are needed in which comparisons are made with known effective pharmacologic treatments. Cost – benefit analyses are also in order.

At least one clinical expert in the area of hypertension has also raised the issue of whether prescribing behavioral interventions such as dietary restriction, exercise, biofeedback, or relaxation training may adversely affect adherence to pharmacotherapy (Solomon, 1982). The logic of this argument is that: (1) stepped-care pharmacologic treatment can effectively control hypertension; and (2) the physician can therefore make the simplest of behavioral contracts with the patient. The contract is that: (1) if the patient takes a couple of pills a day, the physician will control the hypertension; and (2) if the patient reports adverse side effects, the physician will remedy the situation immediately. According to Solomon, anything that places an added burden on the patient (e.g., dietary sodium restriction) or can lead to a patient's perception of failure (e.g., not losing weight; discontinuation of exercise or meditation) is likely to affect adherence adversely and decrease the likelihood of the patient returning to the physician's office to be monitored.

Comment. There can be no doubt that a stepped-care program of drug treatment can reduce morbidity and mortality in patients with *severe* hypertension. For such patients, Solomon's (1982) caution deserves consideration. To the extent that behavioral treatments can lower drug dosages and reduce disturbing side effects, however, further investigation of behavioral treatment with such patients is warranted. Although drug treatment is necessary in cases of servere hypertension, a good case can be made that in the range of diastolic blood pressures between 90 and 99 mmHg, behavioral treatments including dietary restriction, relaxation training, etc., may actually be preferable.

Of the 60 million people in the United States with hypertension, approximately 40 million have diastolic pressures of 90 − 99 mmHg (United States Department of Health and Human Services, 1981). Problems of drug toxicity, unpleasant or incapacitating side effects, and the enormous expense of exposing such a large proportion of the population to drugs for years at a time, suggest that caution is in order, given our current state of information.

First, there are many individuals with mild hypertension whose blood pressure declines over time. In the Australian Hypertension Trial (Management Committee of the Australian Hypertension Trial, 1979), for example, 48% of the patients in the placebo control group with diastolic pressures initially in the range of 95 to 109 mmHg revealed diastolic pressures below 95 mmHg after 3 years. In contrast, 32% stayed in the initial range, and only 12% of untreated individuals progressed to a more severe stage.

A second reason for suggesting caution in recommending drug treatment for patients with uncomplicated, mild hypertension, is that the data suggesting the benefits of treatment are at best inconclusive. The Oslo study, for instance, which was a 5-year controlled drug trial, found no evidences that reducing blood pressure of mildly hypertensive individuals reduced morbidity or mortality (Helgelland, 1980). Moreover, the Hypertension Detection and Follow-up (1979a, 1979b) study, which is the only trial to have reported a significant reduction of total CHD with the treatment of mild hypertensives, was flawed in design. In this study the experimental group received complete, intensive, free medical care in special University Medical Center clinics. The control group received whatever medical care they could find or afford in the community. Availability, cost, and quality of medical care were therefore quite different in the two groups. Although cardiovascular-related mortality was 26% lower in the experimental group relative to the control group, noncardiovascular mortality was also 14% lower in the experimental group. It is therefore not possible to determine from this study whether improved mortality from CHD was due to the antihypertensive stepped-care drug treatment per se or to better general medical care.

Based on current evidence, Freis (1982) has suggested that stepped-care drug treatment for patients with diastolic pressures in the 90 to 99 mmHg range should only be considered if multiple risk factors are present. However, if we consider that a person who smokes heavily and has mild hypertension can reduce risk of CHD as well by quitting smoking as by spending a life-time on medication, behavioral approaches to reducing risk may actually be preferable. For those with uncomplicated mild hypertension, monitoring, dietary restriction, and in some cases exercise and/or relaxation training, may be the preferred couse.

It would therefore appear that behavioral interventions may be useful in the treatment of hypertension, although large-scale controlled clinical trials are needed to test the hypothesis rigorously. Such trials could determine: (1) efficacy of alternate procedures; (2) which patients are likely to benefit from specific interventions; (3) adherence rates with different treatments; and (4) the likely cost of time and effort for specific interventions.

CORONARY HEART DISEASE

The term CHD refers to cardiac disorders that result from inadequate delivery of blood to the heart muscle (myocardium). In the vast majority of cases CHD is associated with severe damage (i.e., *atherosclerosis*) of the coronary arteries. The resultant limitation of blood flow to the heart muscle restricts its supply of oxygen and nutrients and interferes with the heart's ability to remove the waste products of metabolism.

The major clinical manifestations of CHD are myocardial infarction, angina pectoris, and sudden cardiac death. Congestive heart failure can also result from myocardial ischemia, but is not uniquely a complication of coronary atherosclerosis. Briefly, *acute myocardial infarction (MI)* refers to the death of heart muscle. Usually, an MI is due to the abrupt occlusion of one or more coronary arteries. Frequently, the occlusion is attributable to a *thrombus* (blood clot) forming on an atherosclerotic plaque. *Angina pectoris* is a syndrome of periodic chest pain resulting from inadequate coronary blood flow, and consequently an insufficient oxygen supply to heart muscle. In most, but not all cases, angina attacks can be triggered by exertion. *Sudden cardiac death* often occurs in people who have no overt symptoms of CHD. Death follows from a fatal *arrhythmia*, which is thought in many cases to be due to a transient interruption of blood flow to muscle or to an imbalance between oxygen supply and demand. In most cases, autopsy reveals the presence of severe coronary atherosclerosis.

Congestive heart failure is generally a chronic condition. It occurs when the heart becomes unable to pump an adequate quantity of blood to meet the normal metabolic demands of the body. The result is the accumulation of excess fluid in body tissues including the lungs, abdomen, and limbs. A common cause of congestive heart failure is coronary atherosclerosis leading to MI. There are other causes of congestive heart failure, however, besides coronary atherosclerosis. These include infections of heart muscle, rheumatic valvular defects, or severe chronic hypertension. In this last instance, the continually elevated blood pressure places a severe burden on the pumping requirements of the heart muscle.

As previously indicated, increased risk of CHD has been associated with hypertension, high levels of serum cholesterol, cigarette smoking, advancing age, male sex, diabetes mellitus, a family history of CHD, and Type A coronary-prone behavior (Brand et al., 1976; Kannel et al., 1976). Stressful life events have also been implicated (e.g., Dohrenwend & Dohrenwend, 1974). Because risk factors are based on associations uncovered in epidemiologic studies, they may be causative agents, secondary manifestations of the disease process, early symptoms of the disease, or correlates of as yet unspecified variables. Therefore, direct experimentation, in conjunction with prospective studies, is necessary to establish risk factors as causative agents. In this section we look at the possible role played by behavioral factors in the development of atherosclerosis, CHD, and sudden death, and then look at the role of behavior in the prevention (including secondary prevention) and treatment of CHD.

Atherosclerosis and CHD

The term *arteriosclerosis* means hardening of the arteries and includes a variety of conditions that cause the artery wall to become thick and hard. Atherosclerosis is a specific type of arteriosclerosis in which the inner layer of the arterial wall becomes thick and irregular due to a lesion called an *atheromatous plaque*. This plaque usually has a lipid core of cholesterol covered by a cap of fibrous tissue. The mechanisms by which plaques grow and progressively narrow the arterial lumen are not fully known, but lipid and lipoprotein accumulation in the lesion, hemorrhage into the plaque, and fibrous organization of thrombi on the plaque wall have all been implicated. Once the lumen of a coronary artery is narrowed by at least 75%, regional blood flow to the heart may be compromised (Hollander, 1977).

The exact manner by which emotional stress promotes atherogenesis is not known, but the SNS is strongly implicated. Under conditions of emotional upheaval, for example, the resulting increase in blood pressure may produce damage to the thin inner (endothelial) lining of arterial vessels due to turbulence and shear stress. According to Ross and Glomset (1976), for example, the initiating event in the atherosclerotic process involves injury to the arterial endothelium. The catecholamines, norepinephrine (N) and epinephrine (E), released during prolonged stress reactions, might also insult the endothelium directly (Fuller & Langner, 1970; Raab, 1971; Schade & Eaton, 1977). For fuller discussions of the role of catecholamines and other agents (e.g., free fatty acids, cortisol) in the development of atherosclerosis, consult Schneiderman (1983a, 1983b).

Although the exact mechanisms by which emotional stresses induce arteriosclerosis and atherosclerosis remain speculative, there is evidence that such associations exist. Ratcliffe (1968) related an increase in the prevalence of arterial lesions among birds and mammals dying at the Philadelphia Zoo to intraspecies social pressures. Similar arterial lesions were experimentally induced in chickens (Ratcliffe & Snyder, 1967) and swine (Ratcliffe, Luginbuhl, Schnarr, & Chacko, 1969) by subjecting the animals to psychosocial stress. Henry et al. (1971) also found arteriosclerosis in the intramural coronary arteries and in the aorta of psychosocially stressed mice. In addition, rats (Uhley & Friedman, 1959) and squirrel monkeys (Lang, 1967) subjected to atherogenic diets and to psychological stress (e.g., escape-avoidance situations) have shown higher levels of serum cholesterol and more severe intramural coronary atherosclerosis than control animals.

There is some indication that cynomolgus monkeys, who are highly reactive to aversive behavioral challenges, may be more prone to atherosclerosis than monkeys who are less highly reactive. Manuck, Kaplan, and Clarkson (1983) examined heart rate reactivity in monkeys during a standard challenge involving threatened capture and handling of the animals. The monkeys had previously been fed a moderately atherogenic diet for 22 months. At necropsy high heart rate reactors were found to have more severe atherosclerosis of the coronary arteries and thoracic aorta than did low heart rate reactors. High heart rate reactors were also significantly more aggressive than low heart rate reactors in group situations.

The study by Manuck et al. (1983) is of interest with regard to atherosclerotic CHD in humans, because Type A relative to Type B individuals reveal: (1) greater heart rate reactivity in challenging behavioral situations (Dembroski, Mac-Dougall, Herd, & Shields, 1979; Glass, Krakoff, Contrada, Hilton, Kehoe, Mannucci, Collins, Snow, & Elting, 1980); (2) more severe coronary atherosclerosis when studied at autopsy (Friedman, Rosenman, Strauss, Wurm, & Kositchek, 1968); and (3) more pronounced atherosclerosis when studied by coronary angiography (Blumenthal, Williams, Kong, Schlanberg, & Thompson, 1978; Krantz, Sanmarco, Selvester, & Matthews, 1979).

The Manuck et al. (1983) study is of further interest with regard to atherosclerotic CHD in humans, because it linked aggression as well as heart rate reactivity to severity of atherosclerosis. Interestingly, Glass (1977) has reported that when frustrated, Type A's are more likely than Type B's to engage in aggressive behavior. Type A behavior pattern appears to involve a "high potential for hostility" (Friedman, 1969). When assessed as a component of the Type A pattern, "potential for hostility" was found to be predictive of CHD in the data of the Western Collaborative Group Study (Matthews, Glass, Rosenman, & Bortner, 1977). Persons scoring high on an MMPI-derived hostility scale have also been found to have more severe coronary occlusion than individuals scoring low on the scale, based on the results of coronary angiography (Williams, Haney, Lee, Kong, Blumenthal, & Whalen, 1980).

Still other findings have linked physiological reactivity to CHD. In a prospective study Keys, Taylor, Blackburn, Brozek, Anderson, and Simonson (1971) reported that magnitude of diastolic blood pressure response to a cold pressor test (i.e., the subject is asked to place a limb in ice water) was a significant predictor of CHD. In a case-control study Schiffer, Hartley, Schulman, and Abelman (1976) reported that patients with angina pectoris or hypertension had higher mean and maximal heart rate and systolic blood pressures than a healthy control group during a challenging history quiz. Subsequently, Sime, Buell, and Eliot (1980) found that postinfarct patients with clinical symptons (e.g., angina, electrocardiographic changes, hypertension) had higher elevations in diastolic pressure and, unexpectedly, lower heart rate changes during a challenging quiz compared to asymptomatic post infarct patients or healthy control subjects. Preliminary data indicate that those patients who tended to show the most cardiovascular reactivity were also the most likely to suffer reinfarction (Sime, Buell, & Eliot, 1979).

In general, then, the data suggest that aversive environmental stress and personality characteristics (e.g., Type A, potential for hostility, aggressiveness) may contribute to the development of atherosclerosis. The exact mechanisms are presently unknown, but SNS activity and the release of catecholamines and other chemicals into the circulation have been implicated. Physiological reactivity to behavioral challenges has also been linked to atherogenesis and various manifestations of CHD, but the mechanisms involved here are also obscure.

Aside from not distinguishing among the various manifestations of CHD, most of the studies linking physiological reactivity to atherosclerosis and CHD have not adequately taken hypertension into account. Elevated blood pressure is a major risk factor for CHD, and many borderline hypertensives (Julius & Esler, 1975) and their offspring (Falkner et al., 1979; Manuck et al., 1981; Obrist, 1981) are physiologically hyperreactive. Thus, the risk for CHD may be carried by the hypertension rather than by the reactivity per se, and the hyperreactivity may be genetic in origin. It would therefore appear that further research is needed to examine the exact roles of psychological, constitutional, and genetic factors relating physiological reactivity to the development of atherosclerosis and CHD.

Arrhythmias and Sudden Cardiac Death

Approximately 60% of fatalities attributable to CHD occur in ambulatory individuals within 24 hours after the onset of symptoms (American Heart Association, National Academy of Sciences, and National Research Council, 1974; Cobb, Werner, & Trobaugh, 1980; Lown & Graboys, 1977). Most of these deaths occur within the first 2 hours. In most instances the terminal event is ventricular fibrillation (Cobb, Baum, Alvarez, & Schaffer, 1975; Friedman, Manwaring, Rosenman, Donlon, Ortega, & Grube, 1973). Usually, but not inevitably, the victim can be shown to have had a background of CHD. Although myocardial ischemia associated with atherosclerotic CHD appears to create the biochemical and metabolic conditions that set the stage for ventricular fibrillation, most often acute changes in atherosclerotic lesions or obstructing thrombi are not evident (Titus, 1978). Furthermore, in a large number of cases, the heart disease is no worse than that found in comparable individuals dying of trauma, and in approximately 15% of sudden cardiac deaths, no underlying pathology is evident (Kuller & Lillenfield, 1966; Moritz & Zancheck, 1946; Schwartz & Gerrity, 1975). Undetectable sources of acute ischemia, however, have not been ruled out as precipitating causes (e.g., coronary spasm, platelet aggregation, metabolic overdrive of the myocardium).

Although myocardial ischemia appears to be an important predisposing factor for a fatal arrhythmia, it appears that other factors associated with autonomic functioning and the central nervous system (CNS) may be necessary to precipitate ventricular fibrillation by transiently destabilizing the heart. Total cardiac denervation, for example, can prevent the initiation of ventricular fibrillation following coronary artery occlusion (Ebert, Vanderveek, Allgood, & Sabiston, 1970) as can CNS lesions (Skinner & Reed, 1981) or habituation to psychological stress (Skinner, Lie, & Entman, 1975).

Animal studies have indicated that either exposure to behaviorally defined states of stress (Corley, Shiel, Mauck, & Greenhoot, 1973; Johansson, Jonsson, Lannek, Blomgren, Lindberg, & Poupa, 1974; Skinner et al., 1975) or electrical stimulation of the SNS (Corr & Gillis, 1978; Malliani, Schwartz, & Zanchetti, 1980) will enhance the susceptibility of the heart to ventricular fibrillation. The neural mechanisms that may link environmental stressors to deleterious autonomic outflows are also in reach of being understood. Electrical stimulation of neocortical, hypothalamic, and brainstem structures have been shown to produce, in the normal heart, both a variety of arrhythmias (Delgado, 1960; Hockman, Mauck, & Hoff, 1966; Manning & Cotten, 1962; Melville, Blum, Shister & Silver, 1963; Ulyaninsky, Stepanyan, & Krymsky, 1977) including ventricular fibrillation (Garvey & Melville, 1969) and diffuse myocardial injury (Hall, Livingston, & Bloor, 1977; Hall, Sybers, Greenhoot, & Bloor, 1974; Ulyaninsky et al., 1977). Similar patterns of lethal arrhythmias and diffuse myocardial injury have been produced by environmental and psychological stressors (Johansson et al., 1974; Corley et al., 1973, 1977).

The animal experiments just cited are consistent with a growing body of information showing that psychosocial emotional stressors are significant predictors of sudden cardiac death in human populations (Jenkins, 1976; Parkes, 1967; Rahe, Bennet, Romo, Seltanen, & Arthur, 1973; Rees & Lutkins, 1967; Reich, DeSilva, Lown, & Murawski, 1981; Rissanen, Romo, & Seltanen, 1978; Vikhert, Velisheva, & Matova, 1977; Wolf, 1969). Although retrospective in nature, these studies conducted upon humans suggest that acute emotional trauma may precipitate ventricular fibrillation in persons with atherosclerotic CHD, and may even be the causal event in those relatively few cases where underlying pathology is not evident.

Research Strategies.   The major objectives in studying cardiovascular pathology are to identify those persons at risk, and to identify the mechanisms leading to pathology so that interventions can be instituted to reduce morbidity and mortality. One important problem that has not been solved with regard to sudden cardiac death has been the identification of unequivocal prodromata or precipitating events for the letal ventricular fibrillation. A related problem involves the differential prediction of events leading to sudden cardiac death versus myocardial infarction; traditional risk factors such as hypertension, hypercholesterolemia, and cigarette smoking do not discriminate between the two. Still another problem that awaits solution is whether there are particular psychosocial and/or psychophysiological characteristics that make some individuals more susceptible than others to lethal arrhythmias. If, as previous research suggests, sudden cardiac death may be precipitated by behavioral factors leading to deleterious autonomic activity, then reasearch should address the issue of the potentially most efficacious treatments. These could be pharmacological interventions targeted at either the autonomic effectors or at various levels of the CNS. In some instances behavioral interventions such as relaxation training or biofeedback may be appropriate.

Pathogenesis.   Both retrospective clinical investigations (Myers & Dewar, 1975; Reich et al., 1981) and animal experimentation (Rosenfeld, Rosen, & Hoffman, 1978; Skinner et al., 1975) have implicated acute emotional traumas as precipitating events for life-threatening arrhythmias. Although these studies suggest that increases in SNS activity associated with emotional behavior may precipitate lethal arrhythmias in susceptible individuals, the relationship between increases in SNS activity and the elicitation of arrhythmias is not a simple one. Situations actually occur in which increases in heart rate and/or myocardial contractions are associated with reductions rather than increases in ventricular arrhythmias. Some patients with ventricular extrasystoles, for example, show a suppression of these arrhythmias during exercise (Lamb & Hiss, 1962; Pickering, Johnston, & Honour, 1978), and patients with premature ventricular contractions (PVCs) during rest can learn to suppress their arrhythmias by means of operantly conditioned (biofeedback training) increases in heart rate (Pickering & Miller, 1977). In an aversive Pavlovian conditioning experiment conducted upon rhesus monkeys, Randall and Hasson (1978) have shown that if coronary occlusion takes place after the monkeys have been thoroughly trained to make conditioned responses, the frequency of ventricular arrhythmias is sometimes reduced below basal levels on conditioning trials even though the conditioned responses include increases in cardiac contractility, heart rate, and systemic arterial pressure.

Animal experiments that have shown behavioral procedures to increase (Skinner et al., 1975) or decrease (Randall & Hasson, 1978) the frequency of ventricular arrhythmias have typically differed from one another in important respects. One difference has been in species; a second in the nature of the psychological stimulus; a third in the period of the experiment when the coronary artery was ligated. Although differences in species cannot be ruled out, the most important factors involved may have been in the stimulus situation and in the period during the experimental protocol when the coronary artery was ligated.

The pigs in the Skinner et al. (1975) experiment were subjected to the acute, severe, unexpected stress of being bound and transported to an unknown place, whereas the monkeys in the Randall and Hasson (1978) experiments were subjected to a predictable, Pavlovian conditioned stimulus in a situation with which the animal was already familiar. Previously, Mason, Mangan, Brady, Conrad, & Rioch (1961) found that during novel, unpredictable, threatening situations, pronounced increases in E as well as NE occur; whereas, during predictable situations such as in Pavlovian conditioning, increases occur in NE but not E. Interestingly, Lawler, Botticelli, and Lown (1976) found that the effective refractory period (i.e., time following a paced beat before stimulation elicits an extrasystole) is shortest at the outset of the first session of a signaled avoidance situation, when novelty, uncertainty, and perceived threat are likely to be greatest.

It is conceivable that the differences in the frequency of ventricular arrhythmias triggered during exercise versus emotional behavior as well as similar differences obtained in well-established Pavlovian conditioning versus novel, highly aversive situations may be related to the differential release of catecholamines. In Chapter 5 of this volume McCabe and Schneiderman review evidence suggesting that plasma NE is preferentially released during exercise or well-learned situations; whereas, plasma E is preferentially released during emotional stress. They also review evidence suggesting that the release of E is more likely than the release of NE to trigger ventricular arrhythmias.

These findings would appear to have important implications for the study of arrhythmias by stress testing. Although Kosowski, Lown, Whiting, and Guiney (1971), as well as other investigators, have found that treadmill exercise testing is more effective than the resting ECG in detecting ventricular arrhythmias, research would appear to be needed in which the effects of exercise are specifically compared with the effects of various standardized behavioral-emotional challenges in their ability to uncover potentially lethal ventricular arrhythmias. In this regard, it is important that such investigations be carried out upon appropriate clinical populations. Thus, for example, the clinical significance of PVCs is to a large extent determined by the type, extent, and severity of underlying cardiac disease. Whereas PVCs appear to have little if any pronostic meaning in overtly normal people, they appear to have considerable prognostic value for patients in whom ischemic, fibrotic, or infarctive processes complicate CHD (Moss, 1981). For patients having such complications, the results of ambulatory ECG (i.e., Holter) monitoring and behavioral stress ECG testing in conjunction with psychosocial examination (e.g., Type A structured interview; hostility measures) may improve upon predictions based primarily on exercise stress tests. Such comprehensive testing would also provide new information relating types and durations of arrhythmias elicited by behavioral challenges with increased risk.

CARDIOMYOPATHIES

Cardiomyopathy refers to heart disease in which there is a functional impairment of muscle that is not specifically related to damage of other cardiac structures. Coronary artery disease, for example, may occur in conjunction with cardiomyopathy, but is not a sign of the disorder. Similarly, diffuse myocardial damage related to emotional stress is not classified as cardiomyopathic disease, because it has not been associated with functional impairment. Most classifications of cardiomyopathy also exclude inflammatory heart disease (i.e., myocarditis) caused by viruses, bacteria, fungi, or protozoa (Brandenburg, Chazov, Cherian, Falasen, Grosgogeat, Kawai, Loogen, Judez, Orinius, Goodwin, Olsen, Oakley, & Pisa, 1981).

The three major subgroups of cardiomyopathy are dilated, hypertrophic, and restrictive (Brandenburg et al., 1981). In *dilated cardiomyopathy* the left ventricle, or occasionally the right or both ventricles, becomes dilated. The walls of the ventricle seem thin although because of the overall enlargement of the heart there may actually be an increase in muscle mass. The ventricle is hypocontractive so that the amount of blood ejected on each beat is reduced. Congestive heart failure can supervene. Risk factors for this disease include alcoholism, pregnancy, and hypertension.

Hypertrophic cardiomyopathy is characterized by a disproportionate enlargement of the muscle mass of the left ventricle, decreased cavity size, and an impaired volume of blood ejected on each heart beat. The major form of hypertrophic cardiomyopathy is called asymmetric septal hypertrophy because the septum between the ventricles is more affected than the free wall. This cardiomyopathy is usually related to the presence of an autosomal dominant gene. In other forms of hypertrophic cardiomyopathy the increase in muscle mass is concentric. This can occur from hypertension.

The last major subgroup of the cardiomyopathies is restrictive cardiomyopathy. In this subgroup, characterized by endomyocardial fibrosis, or amyloid or other deposits, the ability of the ventricles to contract is impaired so that a decreased stroke volume results. In contrast to hypertrophic cardiomyopathy, "athlete's" hypertrophy is characterized by an enlarged cavity, and an increase rather than a decrease in the volume of blood ejected on each beat.

Pathogenesis

There is relatively little evidence to link behavioral factors to most forms of cardiomyopathy. Life-style factors such as alcoholism, however, have been linked to dilated cardiomyopathy. Also, increased SNS activity and the excessive release of catecholamines has been linked to dilated cardiomyopathy and to concentric hypertrophic cardiomyopathy.

An important set of findings relating SNS hyperreactivity to hypertrophic cardiomyopathy has been found in SHRs (Sen, Tarazi, Khairallah, & Bumpus, 1974). These findings suggest that it is the release of catecholamines by the SNS rather than the hypertension per se that produces the hypertrophy. First, ventricular weight increases dramatically in the SHR before the development of significant hypertension. Second, administration of methyldopa, which acts upon the CNS to decrease the release of catecholamines by the SNS, can reduce ventricular weight in the SHR. Third, administration of vasodilators, which reduce blood pressure but increase SNS activity and heart work, produce augmented hypertrophy.

Evidence suggests that the excessive release of catecholamines in SNS hyperreactivity not only causes hypertrophic cardiomyopathy, but also a decrease in beta-adrenergic receptors at the heart (Watanabe, Jones, Manalin, & Besch, 1982). Such a decrease in receptors has been documented in the hypertrophic cardiomyopathy seen in the discarded hearts of transplant patients (Bristow, Ginsburg, Sagemen, Billingham, & Stinson, 1981). It is therefore conceivable that the diminished contractility associated with ventricular hypertrophy related to hypertension may in part be due to a decreased population of beta-adrenergic receptors. Interestingly, the mechanisms responsible for the increased pumping capacity of the "athlete's" heart at rest (e.g., Starling's "law of the heart") do not rely upon the release of large quantities of catecholamines into the circulation for prolonged periods, and hence should not lead to the down-regulation of receptors.

Arrhythmias in Patients with Cardiomyopathy

The occurrence of PVCs does not convey increased risk of sudden death unless other cardiac complications are present (Moss, 1981). However, PVCs and other ventricular arrhythmias are fairly common in patients with cardiomyopathy and are prognostic. Although dilated and restrictive cardiomyopathies arise from diverse etiologies, they tend to share in common a deteriorating clinical course, a high prevalence of ventricular arrhythmias, and an increased incidence of sudden death. Thus far, little research has been done relating specific ventricular arrhythmias to increased risk of sudden death in such patients, and no research has yet assessed the possible role that behavioral factors might play in precipitating potentially lethal arrhythmias. There is evidence, however, that the SNS is involved, as survival in dilated cardiomyopathy patients is prolonged by beta-receptor blockage (Swedberg, Hjalmarson, Waagstein, & Wallentin, 1979).

The occurrence of ventricular arrhythmias is also common in patients with hypertrophic cardiomyopathy. It is conceivable, but not yet shown definitively, that ventricular arrhythmias may play a causal role in the relatively high incidence of sudden cardiac death in such patients.

The high prevalence of potentially serious arrhythmias and the hemodynamic vulnerability of patients with hypertrophic cardiomyopathy suggest that emotional factors associated with SNS activation and the release of E from the adrenal medulla may precipitate potentially lethal arrhythmias (see McCabe & Schneiderman, this volume). In this regard it is interesting that ambulatory ECG (Holter) monitoring appears to be superior to exercise testing for exposing these arrhythmias (Savage, Seides, Maron, Myers, & Epstein, 1979).

Ambulatory ECG monitoring in conjunction with the supervised keeping of a behavioral diary; the use of behavioral challenge tests in conjunction with the monitoring of ECG, systemic blood pressure responses, and plasma catecholamines; and psychosocial assessment of Type A behavior pattern and various measures of anger-proneness might help in the identification of patients who are at high risk. Similarly, relaxation-based therapies may be useful in reducing the incidence of sudden cardiac death in such patients.

OTHER CIRCULATORY DISORDERS

A number of circulatory disorders have been related to SNS activity that, although not life-threatening, are severely discomforting. Among the most important of these are migraine headache and Raynaud's disease. Both of these disorders appear to be amenable to interventions directed at reducing general sympathetic tone.

Migraine

The class of headaches known to be associated with vascular dysfunction is commonly referred to as migraine. These headaches have been classified into various groupings based on variations in symptomology. However, the general course of the headache seems to be similar in most cases. Dalessio (1972) has listed a number of parameters common to the migraine headache. Typically, the headache is preceded by a period of intense constriction of the intra and extracranial arteries in the temporal region. Often this produces mild sensory hallucinations and photophobia in the patient. This phase is most notable in the classic migraine syndrome. Following the initial constriction phase there is a rebound dilation of the vasculature that is frequently unilateral. The patient usually reports an intense throbbing pain in the temporal region. The rebound dilation is followed by a sterile inflammation and edema of the arteries causing them to become rigid and thickened. At this point, a shift occurs from painful throb to constant pain.

Medication typically employed for treating migraine headaches consists of vasoconstrictors such as Sansert or Cafergot. However, these interventions are often only marginally successful in controlling the frequency and intensity of the headaches. This has prompted the investigation of nonpharmacological forms of intervention.

One of the first attempts at using biofeedback for migraines was conducted by Sargent, Green, and Walters (1973). They used feedback of finger skin temperature combined with an autogenic procedure requiring the patient to imagine warmth in the hands and fingers to produce a vasodilation in peripheral blood vessels. Basic research had suggested that dilation in the hands is associated with constriction of cranial arteries. Although the investigators reported considerable success, the outcome was based upon subjective clinical opinions rather than upon objective data.

A better controlled study examining the effects of finger temperature feedback for migraine patients was subsequently conducted by Turin and Johnson (1976). Separate groups of patients were trained either to increase or decrease finger temperature. The subjects taught to increase finger temperature via biofeedback reported fewer headaches, shorter durations of headache, and fewer pain pills taken. The patients taught to decrease finger temperature showed no such improvement in headaches until subsequently trained to increase finger temperature. An important aspect of this study was that the researchers instructed the patients to practice hand warming at home. Thus, they did not require the use of elaborate biofeedback instrumentation by the end of the study to produce a hand warming response.

Another form of biofeedback that has been used with migraine patients is direct feedback on the relative state of constriction of the temporal extracranial arteries. Friar and Beatty (1976) trained some patients to constrict their temporal artery, while other patients received training to constrict their finger vasculature. The outcome of the study showed a moderate improvement in those patients trained to constrict extracranial arteries. A subsequent study by Bild and Adams (1980) compared the effects of extracranial blood volume feedback or EMG frontalis feedback to a waiting-list control group. By the end of the 10 biofeedback sessions both experimental groups demonstrated that they had learned control over the targeted physiological responses. Following training, both EMG and vascular feedback groups reported decreases in headache activity relative to the waiting-list control group. However, the group receiving temporal artery feedback reported significantly greater improvement compared to the EMG feedback group. An 18-week follow-up session indicated that the difference between groups was no longer statistically significant, although the authors claimed that the vascular feedback group continued to report decreased use of sedatives and vasoconstrictive medications compared to the other groups.

Treatment of migraines with relaxation training to reduce general sympathetic tone was first reported to be successful by Hay and Madders (1971). Subsequently, Paulley and Haskel (1975) evaluated the efficacy of relaxation training with over 800 migraine patients. Their success rate, based on anecdotal information, was impressive. Three-quarters of their patients apparently claimed to have experienced long-term success using relaxation.

Mitchell and Mitchell (1971) reported that systematic desensitization appears to augment the effects of relaxation training in the control of migraine headaches. They reasoned that this approach allowed each individual patient to identify and reduce stress responses to particular environmental events unique to that individual's life situation. Thus, this provided a more direct means of controlling sympathetic activity compared to generalized relaxation training. A subsequent study by Mitchell and White (1977) showed that an intervention package utilizing cue-controlled progressive relaxation, mental and differential relaxation, and self-desensitization could produce a large reduction in the frequency of migraine headaches. These effects were reportedly maintained a year following treatment. The efficacy of relaxation and desensitization procedures relative to interventions such as medication and direct biofeedback has yet to be determined. More and better controlled studies will be necessary before a clearly superior intervention package can be recommended for migraine patients.

Raynaud's Disease

Severe forms of Raynaud's disease are relatively uncommon, but approximately 20% of young people experience it in some mild form. In general, it occurs five times more frequently in females than males and has its onset during the first or second decade of life (Lewis, 1949). The disorder is characterized by the following sequence of events: a sudden local blanching and numbness of fingers and/or toes; cyanosis causing the digit pallor to change to a bluish color associated with deoxygenation of the tissue; and a reactive hyperemia that produces the spread of red oxygenated blood throughout the surface layers of the epidermis, causing a reddish coloration. This final stage of the Raynaud's sequence is often accompanied by a burning or tingling sensation that lasts until the skin returns to normal color. In severe cases, gangrene or ulcerations can eventually appear at the ends of the digits. Although these symptoms are typically reported for the fingers and toes, they can also occur in facial regions. Any stimulus that normally produces peripheral vasoconstriction appears capable of producing such an episode in Raynaud patients. Thus, extreme cold or emotional stress are often reported to be a source of Raynaud attacks. Raynaud-type symptoms can be ideopathic in origin or can appear in conjunction with some identifiable pathological process such as Lupus or scleroderma. In the case of the latter, they are referred to as Raynaud phenomenon (Spittell, 1972).

The typical medical treatment of Raynaud's disease in the past has mostly been preventive. Patients are typically instructed to dress warmly, avoid excessive cold, and occasionally to move to a warmer climate (Pratt, 1949). Other medical interventions such as surgical procedures in the form of sympathectomy and administration of medications such as reserpine, guanethidine, and methyldopa, have been used with some success. Severe side effects are often experienced by the patients, however, as most of these medications have their effect by reducing alpha-adrenergic activity. This has motivated some researchers to investigate behavioral interventions aimed at decreasing sympathetic tone in Raynaud disease patients.

A number of early case studies have in fact suggested a positive therapeutic effect for procedures such as finger temperature biofeedback, autohypnosis, and assertiveness training for a number of Raynaud's patients (Jacobson, Hackett,

Surman, and Silverberg, 1973; Surwit, 1973). A subsequent study conducted by Blanchard and Haynes (1975) demonstrated that biofeedback of finger temperature can be a significant hand-warming intervention procedure. Although most of these studies have dealt with idiopathic Raynaud's disease, Freedman, Ianni, Hale, and Lynn (1979) demonstrated in two case studies of patients with scleroderma and associated Raynaud's phenomena that biofeedback training could be effective and generalize to outside the training setting. Telemetric recordings of hand temperature in various natural settings showed maintenance of temperature control for these patients, and they reported a decrease in the number of attacks following the biofeedback training.

Recognizing the validity problems that exist with patients' self-report data, a number of investigators have attempted to improve their assessment of treatment effects by incorporating cold stressor situations during and after the training sessions. Taub (1977), for instance, used a specially designed thermal suit worn by the patient through which cold water was flushed and the patient's ability to maintain digital temperature was recorded. Others have used the procedure of reducing ambient room temperature while monitoring hand temperature (Surwit, Pilon, & Fenton, 1978). Such assessment procedures should be helpful in assessing the course and outcome of treatment.

Other procedures aimed at reducing sympathetic activity also have been shown to be effective in treating Raynaud's disease. Autogenic and progressive muscle relaxation training procedures practiced at home have been shown to be equally efficacious when compared to hand temperature feedback practiced in the laboratory or at home. Each of the three techniques produced reductions in vasospastic attacks by approximately 40% (Keefe, Surwit, & Pilon, 1980; Surwit et al., 1978). Similar results have been demonstrated by Jacobson, Manschreck, and Silverberg (1979). In this latter study, 12 patients suffering from idiopathic Raynaud's disease received training in muscle relaxation. Half the subjects also received skin temperature feedback training sessons. Both groups demonstrated increases in skin temperature during the training session. Interestingly the larger increases were recorded for the group that did not receive the feedback. After one month of training, all subjects reported moderate or marked improvement in Raynaud symptoms. At 2-year follow-ups, seven of the twelve subjects continued to report maintained improvement.

The issue of maintenance of treatment effects has been addressed in several studies. The study by Keefe et al. (1980), which evaluated the ability of patients to maintain hand temperature increases in the presence of ambient room temperature decreases, is particularly notable. A 1-year reassessment was conducted with all patients who had demonstrated improved capabilities by the end of treatment and who reported a maintenance of improvement in Raynaud's symptoms after 1 year. Upon reassessment at 1-year follow-up, most subjects were unable to maintain hand temperature in the face of ambient room temperature decreases. Surwit, Williams, and Shapiro (1982) suggest that this is not necessarily a contradictory finding. They speculate that temperature control necessary to abort a typical Raynaud's episode may not be as great as that required to compete against this stringent form of assessment.

Comment. The overall outcome of the studies conducted with Raynaud's disease and migraine headaches appears to indicate that interventions based on relaxation, autogenic training, and biofeedback are all effective means of reducing patients' symptoms. The relatively cumbersome and costly procedures involved in temperature biofeedback seem to argue against it as a treatment of choice. Easily implemented procedures such as relaxation or autogenic training can be practiced at home or in the work setting. Thus, they may be the treatment of choice as nonpharmacological and nonsurgical intervention procedures. More work is necessary, however, to assess effective procedures for the maintenance and generalization of treatment effects to other settings in the patient's everyday life. As Mitchell and White (1977) have suggested, the more an intervention package can be tailored to the individual patient's life situation, the more benefits may be derived from the behavioral intervention approach.

PREVENTION OF ATHEROSCLEROTIC CHD

During the past decade, there have been several large-scale studies conducted in the United States and other countries to evaluate the impact of various intervention procedures to reduce cardiovascular risk factors in the general population. The end goal of these attempts has been to promote a significant decrease in atherosclerotic CHD and the morbidity and mortality rates associated with it. Most of the interventions involved public education concerning risk factors, personal or group counseling, and various behavior modification procedures for changing lifestyles.

The Stanford Heart Disease Prevention Program

An interdisciplinary team of researchers conducted a study involving three comparable communities near Stanford University (Farquhar, 1978; Farquhar, Maccoby, Wood, Brietrose, Haskell, Meyer, Maccoby, Alexander, Brown, McAlister, Nash, & Stern, 1977; Meyer, Nash, McAlister, Maccoby, & Farquhar, 1980). The basic intent of the study was to assess the effects of a media-based health education program designed specifically to target cardiovascular risk factors. One community received radio and television programs, newspaper columns, and direct mailings regarding risk factors and their reduction. Another community received the same media educational program plus a direct behavior modification intervention program that provided face-to-face counseling for risk factor reduction. The third community served as a no-treatment control group. Over 500 high risk subjects were sampled in each community to obtain base-line and annual follow-up data regarding individual risk factors and a multiple risk factor score was derived for each subject. Physiological data was also obtained during each assessment session.

After 3 years, the subjects receiving media education plus face-to-face behavioral counseling showed a 28% reduction in their multiple risk factor scores. The media education-only sample showed a 25% reduction after 2 years, which deteriorated to a 15 − 20% reduction level by the end of the third year. The control community fluctuated by plus or minus 5% of base-line levels during this time. The largest change noted was the reduction in smoking for the media plus counseling subjects. Both experimental groups showed significant reductions in intake of dietary saturated fat. Measures of blood pressure and physical activity levels showed no consistent results. This study has recently been updated to include five rather than three communities, morbidity and mortality data, and more reliance on community organizations for program development and implementation.

The North Karelia Project

Beginning in 1972, a community-based risk factor reduction program was established in North Karelia, Finland (McAlister, Puska, Salonen, Tuomilehto, & Koskela, 1982; Puska, Tuomilehto, Salonen, Neittaanmaki, Maki, Virtamo, Nissinen, Kottke, & Tuomilehto, 1981; Salonen, Puska, & Mustaniemi, 1979). This project adopted a broader approach to providing social interventions than did the Stanford study, reasoning that life-style behavior changes might be effectively introduced by modifying social influences in many segments of the community. The intervention package used mass media and general health education, provision of practical services, installation of communication and information networks, training programs for local personnel, and a number of environmental changes. Subjects from the intervention community were contrasted with matched subjects who had not experienced such a change in social context. More than 10,000 subjects were initially assessed and followed up after 5 years. Measures were taken on smoking habits, cholesterol levels, and blood pressure, and a multiple risk factor score was computed for each subject.

After 5 years, the results showed significant reductions of the combined multiple risk factor scores by 17.4% for men and 11.5% for women compared to the matched control sample. As in the Stanford study, the largest change was noted in smoking behavior. Morbidity and mortality were also significantly reduced in the intervention community as reflected in a myocardial infarction decrease of 16.7% in men and 10.2% in women. Cerebrovascular accidents (i.e., strokes) also decreased by 12.7% in men and 35.5% in women.

The results of the North Karelia project would seem to indicate that social networks can effectively disseminate information and induce and maintain behavior changes in a community-based intervention program. Additionally such a program appears to have a significant effect on cardiovascular mortality and morbidity. This may in fact be due to the largely positive reception the project received from both the community and government officials, which no doubt aided in implementing the intervention procedures and in obtaining the cooperation of the target population.

The Oslo Study

A large-scale project to assess the effects of direct individual counseling and group instruction to stop smoking and change eating habits was conducted in Oslo (Hjermann, 1980; Hjermann, Velve-Byre, Home, & Leren, 1981). This randomized, controlled clinical trial included over 12,000 high risk, middle-age males studied over a 5-year period. High risk was determined on the basis of serum cholesterol levels and smoking habits. Counseling procedures produced a 13% reduction in cholesterol, a 20% reduction in triglycerides, and 45% reduction in tobacco use in the intervention group compared to the control group. Furthermore, the rate of myocardial infarction and sudden death was 47% lower in the intervention group. These data were most highly correlated with cholesterol levels and to a lesser degree with smoking habits among the subjects in this group. Thus, the Oslo study seems to indicate that reductions in the risk factors of elevated cholesterol and smoking can have a significant preventive effect for cardiovascular mortality and morbidity.

MRFIT

The Multiple Risk Factor Intervention Trial (MRFIT) was initiated in 1972 by the National Heart and Lung Institute to determine the benefits of a risk factor reduction program in preventing cardiovascular-related morbidity and mortality in middle-age American males (The Multiple Risk Factor Intervention Trial, 1982). Over 366,000 men were initially screened for the study in 20 centers across the United States. Nearly 13,000 men were selected for the study based upon: (1) a multiple risk factor score in the upper 15% mortality risk category; (2) absence of significant, related diseases; and (3) subject agreement to participate in the program. Selected individuals were randomly assigned to one of two groups. One group, labeled the Usual Care Group, received encouragement to seek assistance from a private physician for treatment of their risk factors, and underwent annual physical examinations at the local MRFIT center. The Special Intervention Group also underwent annual physical examination and received a systematically administered risk factor reduction program at the MRFIT center. All subjects were followed for 6 years after beginning the program.

The general treatment package used in the Special Intervention Group included treatment of hypertension (e.g., stepped-care medication, salt restriction, and weight reduction) and counseling for life-style changes to reduce serum cholesterol and to help individuals to stop smoking. Counseling began with 10 weeks of intensified training sessions, which included the subjects's wives. Subsequently, subjects were closely followed by case managers and specialists to maintain progress or modify programs for subjects who were falling short of their treatment goals.

A number of ancillary intervention procedures were systemically incorporated into this project. These included motivational techniques aimed at improving compliance, assertiveness training, role-playing, and rehearsal techniques.

Although the Special Intervention and the Uusal Care groups were originally nearly identical in terms of risk with regard to blood pressure, serum cholesterol, and smoking behavior, significant differences were found between groups for each of these risk factors during the six annual follow-up visits. Based upon calculated risk factor estimates determined from the Framingham study (Kannel, 1975; Kannel et al., 1971), the reduction in risk factors for the combined groups resulted in a decrease from otherwise expected mortality of about 20%. Unfortunately, the differences in mortality from CHD (i.e., 7.1%) and from cardiovascular disease in general (4.7%) between the Special Intervention and Usual Care groups were not significant.

The MRFIT (1982) investigators have suggested that the failure to achieve significant differences was in large part due to greater than expected risk factor reduction in the Usual Care group. They suggest that contributing factors may have included: (1) the psychological impact on the Usual Care group of being enrolled in a trial limited to persons at high risk; (2) the likelihood that individuals volunteering for a 6-year clinical trial are unusually health conscious and motivated; (3) sensitization of the Usual Care group to their risk factor status due to the annual visits; and (4) the general effects of health education in the United States that have been aimed at modifying risk.

Comment. In general the large-scale studies that have been conducted in several different countries since 1970 have unequivocally shown that behavioral interventions can reduce cardiovascular risk factors in the general population. The results of the North Karelia and Oslo studies indicate that such interventions can also reduce morbidity and mortality. The outcome of the MRFIT study highlights the difficulties that can be encountered in directly linking risk factor reduction to decreased mortality. These include both: (1) ethical considerations that rule out the use of "no-treatment" control groups; and (2) dealing with decreased mortality that may be due to improved medical care and improved health education that have characterized the past two decades.

CORONARY REHABILITATION

Approximately 1.25 millon people in the United States have MI's each year (Seventh report of the director of the National Heart, Lung, and Blood Institute, 1979). About half of these individuals survive through the course of recovery. Of those who do not survive, approximately half die within an hour or so of symptom onset. For those who survive the acute phase of MI, posthospital mortality is about 10% the first year and 3 to 5% thereafter (Moss, 1980). Survivorship rates are best for patients under age 60, especially for those experiencing their first MI.

Prehospital Behavior

The average time period between symptom onset of MI (e.g., chest pains, shortness of breath, fatigue) and admission to a medical facility is about 3 hours and may extend up to several days (Gentry & Haney, 1975; Moss & Goldstein, 1970). Delay in seeking help is greatest when symptoms are denied or attributed to other than heart problems. Hackett and Cassem (1969), for example, found that patients who used denial minimally, more often attributed their symptoms to the heart and sought help themselves than did "major deniers." The major deniers most frequently listed indigestion as the cause of their chest pain and shortness of breath. They also required persistent urging from those about them before they would seek medical advice. In this regard, the social context in which symptoms occur influences the temporal delay before help is sought. Symptoms of acute MI at work, during a weekday, in the presence of others is more likely to generate prompt action than symptoms occurring at other times when fewer people are about.

The life-saving effectiveness of rapidly responsive mobile units in helping to save cardiac patients is well documented (Moss, 1980). Cardiopulmonary resuscitation by bystanders has also been shown to reduce mortality (Cobb, Hallstrom, Thompson, Mandel, & Copas, 1980).

Acute Care Phase

Care for the MI patient traditionally involved extended bed rest with strict curtailment of ambulation in the hospital and severe restriction of activities requiring exertion after hospital release. Recent trends have been toward early ambulation and discharge, with relatively early resumption of moderate activity after hospital release. In one study, patients with uncomplicated MI's, who were released from the coronary care unit (CCU) after 4 days and from the hospital after 7 days showed no difference in morbidity or mortality when compared with similar control patients discharged after 11 days (McNeer, Wagner, Ginsburg, Wallace, McCants, Conley, & Rosati, 1978).

Most emotional problems seen during the early acute stage of hospitalization appear to be short-lived and center around the fear of death (Hackett, Cassem, & Wishnie, 1968, 1969). After the first day or so in the CCU this anxiety becomes less evident, either because of denial (Hackett et al., 1968, 1969) or because the patient, with the reassurance of hospital staff, has been able to work through his or her concerns (Surwit, Williams et al., 1982). During a second phase of the CCU experience, anxiety often gives way to depression (Cassem & Hackett, 1971). This depression characteristically increases when the patient is transferred to a less intensive hospital ward (Klein, Kliner, Zipes, Troyer, & Wallace, 1968).

There is some indication of an association between affective states in MI patients and the physical complications of recovery, but the conclusion is based on a limited number of studies. In the study by Klein et al. (1968) an increased release in catecholamines was detected in patients facing the stress of transfer from the CCU into the general hospital population. The increased release of catecholamines was associated with ventricular arrhythmias, reinfarction, and even death. Other studies have also linked extreme emotional upset to an increased incidence of arrhythmias (Gruen, 1975; Leigh, Hofen, Cooper, & Reiser, 1972). Garrity and Klein (1975) have further observed that patients who remain upset throughout the CCU experience reveal increased mortality during the 6 months after MI relative to patients who show a pattern of low or diminishing upset in the CCU. These results were reported to be independent of MI severity or history of coronary events.

Counseling of patients in the CCU has been reported to have beneficial effects. Gruen (1975) randomized 70 MI patients into brief-psychotherapy and no-psychotherapy groups. The therapy consisted of daily half-hour sessions aimed at facilitating coping and identifying areas of psychological strength. Gruen found that treated patients had fewer days in the CCU, fewer supraventricular arrhythmias, and less emotional upset.

Posthospital Phase

More than 80% of first MI patients under 65 years of age have been reported to survive for more than 4 years after their attack (Mulcahey, Hickey, Graham, & McKenzie, 1975; Zukel, Cohen, Mattingly, & Hrubec, 1969). Although little is known about the exact role of psychological factors in influencing reinfarction and mortality, preliminary results from a 5 year (1978 – 1983) prospective study at Mt. Zion hospital in San Francisco suggest that behavior modification of Type A behaviors may reduce rates of reinfarction and death (Friedman, Thoresen, Gill, Ulmer, Thompson, Powell, Price, Elek, Rabin, Breall, Piaget, Dixon, Bourg, Levy, & Tasto, 1982).

In the Mt. Zion study 1035 consecutive postinfarction patients were studied. About 300 patients were enrolled in small groups and received cardiologic counseling on the usually accepted coronary risk factors. Approximately 600 patients received cardiologic counseling, and also advice and instructions specifically designed to reduce Type A behaviors. This involved procedures such as cognitive behavior modification aimed at altering perceptions of the interpersonal environment and reducing confrontational attitudes. It also taught relaxation procedures and self-reinforcement for such Type B behaviors as taking walks. The remaining patients served as controls, as did those who dropped out of the counseling groups. The controls received no counseling but were examined and interviewed annually.

Preliminary data obtained after 1 year indicated that rates of infarction and cardiovascular mortality were significantly lower among patients who received both behavior modification and cardiologic counseling than among control subjects. The rate of nonfatal infarction was also significantly lower among those who received behavior modification than among those who received only cardiologic counseling or those who dropped out of either group.

To the extent that the Type A behavior pattern consists of several diverse behaviors, it seems reasonable to question just which behaviors should be modified during coronary rehabilitation. The outcome of several studies conducted upon postinfarction patients has shown improved survival when beta-adrenergic blocking agents are given for the first 2 years after MI (Ahlmark, Saetre, & Korsgren, 1974; Beta-blocker Heart Attack Trial Research Group, 1982; Multicenter International Study, 1975; Wilhelmsson, Vedin, Wilhelmsson, Tiblin, & Werko, 1974). This link between post-MI mortality and SNS activity suggests that behaviors leading to the excessive release of catecholamines into the circulation (e.g., angry confrontation) would be the most in need of modification. Because type A individuals show an excessive release of plasma catecholamines when excessively challenged (Glass et al., 1980), it would seem that psychological treatments aimed at reducing the high incidences of perceived threat, confrontational behavior, and concomitant SNS activation might play a useful role, especially among Type A individuals, in decreasing reinfarction and mortality after a first MI.

Although there have been relatively few studies relating psychological factors to reinfarction and mortality, there have been numerous studies describing the impact of psychological factors upon the course of rehabilitation (Doehrman, 1977; Garrity, 1981; Gulledge, 1975). In general, the literature suggests that with a few conspicuous exceptions (e.g., effects of depression on sexual behavior), psychological factors are fairly minimally involved in determining to what extent patients resume a healthy and productive life. More important factors appear to be severity of the MI, number of previous MIs, physical complications, and age.

Following MI, approximately 50% of patients are back at work at the end of 3 months, 75% by 6 months, and 90% at the end of 1 year. Although there is little evidence that psychological interventions or exercise reconditioning has much impact on the percentage of MI patients who ultimately return to work, there is some indication that such interventions can increase the rapidity of return to the work force (Throckloth, Ho, Wright, & Seldon, 1973).

Return of sexual activity, as well as return to work, is generally high after an initial uncomplicated MI in patients who were sexually active in the period just prior to the attack. Hellerstein and Friedman (1970), for instance, have reported that level of sexual activity returns to about 80% of what it was before illness within 1 year after MI. In another study, approximately 70% of MI patients returned to normal sexual activity during the first year after infarction (Stern, Pascale, & McLoone, 1976). However, only 58% of depressed patients resumed some level of sexual intercourse, whereas 93% of nondepressed patients resumed sexual activity. It would thus appear that treatment interventions, including exercise reconditioning, that help to counteract depression (Kellerman, 1975) may play a useful role in coronary rehabilitation.

CONCLUSIONS

Reasonable evidence now exists relating psychosocial and biobehavioral factors to the pathogenesis of CHD. Adequate biobehavioral models are now at hand to invite the study of specific mechanisms by which behavior contributes to pathogenesis. It would also seem that behavioral and psychological assessment techniques are now appropriate for helping to identify prognostically homogeneous subgroups in the areas of hypertension and CHD. Enough is also known now about dietary behavior, smoking, adherence to medical regimes, Type A behavior pattern and other psychological factors in the development of CHD to warrant the incorporation of behavioral interventions into large-scale intervention studies aimed at eliminating hypertension, preventing CHD, and providing coronary rehabilitation to MI patients. To a limited extent, behavioral interventions also seem justifiable in the clinical treatment of cardiovascular disorders, if applied cautiously with an appropriate understanding of the underlying pathophysiology. It would thus appear that the biopsychosocial approach to behavioral medicine has much to commend it and has a bright future in the study and treatment of some major cardiovascular disorders.

REFERENCES

Ahlmark, G., Saetre, H., & Korsgren, M. Reduction of sudden deaths after myocardial infarction. *Lancet,* 1974, *2,* 1563.

Alderman, M., & Schoenbaum, E. Detection and treatment of hypertension at the work site. *New England Journal of Medicine,* 1975, *293,*65 – 68.

Alexander, N. Psychosocial hypertension in members of a Wistar rat colony. *Proceedings of the Society of Experimental Biology and Medicine,* 1974, *146,* 163–169.

American Heart Association, National Academy of Sciences, and National Research Council. Standards for cardiopulmonary resuscitation (CPR) and emergency cardiac care (ECC). *Journal of the American Medical Association,* 1974, *227,* 833 – 868.

Anderson, D. E., Kearns, W. D., & Better, W. E. Progressive hypertension in dogs by avoidance conditioning and saline infusion. *Hypertension,* 1983, *5,* 286–291.

Anderson, D. E., Kearns, W. D., & Worden, T. J. Potassium infusion attenuates avoidance-saline hypertension in the dog. *Hypertension,* 1983, *5,* 415–421.

Becker, M. H., & Green, L. W. A family approach to compliance with medical treatment: A selective review of the literature. *International Journal of Health Education,* 1975, *18,* 2 – 11.

Benson, H. *The relaxation response.* New York: William Morrow, 1975.

Benson, H., Rosner, B. A., Marzetta, B. R., & Klemchuk, H. M. Decreased blood pressure in pharmacologically treated hypertensive patients who regularly elicited the relaxation response. *Lancet,* 1974, 289 – 291.

Benson, H., Shapiro, H., Tursky, B., & Schwartz, G. E. Decreased systolic blood pressure through operant conditioning techniques in patients with essential hypertension. *Science*, 1971, *173*, 740 – 742.

Benson, H., Herd, J., Morse, W., & Kelleher, R. The behavioral induction of arterial hypertension and its reversal. *American Journal of Physiology*, 1969, *217*, 30 – 34.

Beta-blocker Heart Attack Trial Research Group. A randomized trial of propranolol in patients with acute myocardial infarction. I. Mortality results. *Journal of the American Medical Association*, 1982, *247*, 1707 – 1714.

Bild, R., & Adams, H. E. Modification of migraine headache by cephalic blood volume pulse and EMG biofeedback. *Journal of Consulting and Clinical Psychology*, 1980, *48*, 51 – 57.

Blackwell, B. Treatment adherence in hypertension. *American Journal of Pharmacology*, 1976, *148*, 75 – 85.

Blackwell, B. The drug regimen and treatment compliance. In R. B. Haynes, D. W. Taylor, & D. L. Sackett (Eds.), *Compliance in health care*. Baltimore: John Hopkins Press, 1979.

Blanchard, E. B., & Haynes, M. R. Biofeedback treatment of a case of Raynaud's Disease. *Journal of Behavior Therapy and Experimental Psychiatry*, 1975, *6*, 230 – 234.

Blanchard, E. B., Miller, S. T., Able, G. G., Haynes, M. R., & Wicker, R. Evaluation of biofeedback in the treatment of borderline essential hypertension. *Journal of Applied Behavioral Analysis*, 1979, *12*, 99 – 109.

Blumenthal, J. A., Williams, R. B., Jr., Kong, Y., Schlanberg, S. M., & Thompson, L. W. Type A behavior pattern and coronary atherosclerosis. *Circulation*, 1978, *58*, 634–639.

Boyer, J. L., & Kasch, F. W. Exercise therapy in hypertensive men. *Journal of the American Medical Association*, 1970, *211*, 1668 – 1671.

Brand, R. J., Rosenman, R. H., Sholtz, R. I., & Friedman, M. Multivariate prediction of coronary heart disease in the Western Collaborative Group Study compared to the findings of the Framingham Study. *Circulation*, 1976, *53*, 348 – 355.

Brandenburg, R. O., Chazov, E., Cherian, G., Falasen, A. O., Grosgogeat, Y., Kawai, C., Loogen, F., Judez, V. M., Orinius, E., Goodwin, J. F., Olsen, E. G. J., Oakley, C. M., & Pisa, Z. Report of the WHO/ISFC Task Force on definition and classification of cardiomyopathies. *Circulation*, 1981, *64*, 437A – 438A.

Bristow, M. R., Ginsburg, R., Sageman, M., Billingham, E., & Stinson, E. B. Analysis of the beta-adrenergic receptor pathway in myocardial disease. *Circulation*, 1981, *64*, 1091.

Buckley, J. P., & Smookler, H. H. Cardiovascular and biochemical effects of chronic intermittent neurogenic stimulation. In H. Welch & W. Welch (Eds.), *Physiological effects of noise*. New York: Plenum, 1970.

Caplan, R. D., Robinson, E. A. R., French, J. R. P., Caldwell, J. R., & Shinn, M. *Adhering to medical regimens: Pilot experiments in patient education and social support*. Ann Arbor: University of Michigan, 1976.

Cassem, N. H., & Hackett, T. P. Psychiatric consultation in a coronary care unit. *Annals of Internal Medicine*, 1971, *75*, 9 – 39.

Choquette, C., & Ferguson, R. J. Blood pressure reduction in "borderline" hypertensives following physical training. *Canadian Medical Association Journal*, 1973, *108*, 699.

Clark, G. M., & Troop, R. One tablet combination drug therapy in the treatment of hypertension. *Journal of Chronic Disease*, 1972, *25*, 57 – 64.

Cobb, L. A., Baum, R. S., Alvarez, H., & Schaffer, W. A. Resuscitation from out-of-hospital ventricular fibrillation: 4 year follow up. *Circulation* (Suppl. 3), 1975, *52*, 223 – 235.

Cobb, L. A., Hallstrom, A. P., Thompson, R. C., Mandel, L. P., & Copas, M. K. Community cardiopulmonary resuscitation. *Annual Review of Medicine*, 1980, 453 – 462.

Cobb, L. A., Werner, J. A., & Trobaugh, G. B. Sudden cardiac death. I. A decade's experience with out-of-hospital resuscitation. *Modern Concepts of Cardiovascular Disease*, 1980, *49*, 31 – 36.

Cobb, S., & Rose, R. M. Hypertension, peptic ulcer and diabetes in air traffic controllers. *Journal of American Medical Association*, 1973, *224*, 489–492.

Corley, K. C., Shiel, F. O'M., Mauck, H. P., Clark, L. S., & Barker, J. V. Myocardial degeneration and cardiac arrest in squirrel monkeys: Physiological and psychological correlation. *Psychophysiology*, 1977, *14*, 322 – 328.

Corley, K. C., Shiel, F. O'M., Mauck, H. P., & Greenhoot, J. Electrocardiographic and cardiac morphological changes associated with environmental stress in squirrel monkeys. *Psychosomatic Medicine*, 1973, *35*, 361 – 364.

Corr, P. B., & Gillis, R. A. Autonomic neural influences on the dysrhythmias resulting from myocardial infarction. *Circulation Research*, 1978, *43*, 1–9.

Dahl, L. K., Heine, M., & Tassinari, L. J. Role of genetic factors in susceptibility to experimental hypertension due to chronic excess salt injection. *Nature* (London), 1962, *194*, 480–482.

Dahl, L. K., Heine, M., & Tassinari, L. J. Effects of chronic excess salt ingestion: Role of genetic factors in both Doca-salt and renal hypertension. *Journal of Experimental Medicine*, 1963, *118*, 605–617.

Dahl, L. K., Heine, M., & Tassinari, L. J. Effects of chronic salt ingestion. Further demonstration that genetic factors influence the development of hypertension: Evidence from experimental hypertension due to cortisone and to adrenal regeneration. *Journal of Experimental Medicine*, 1965, *122*, 533–545.

Dahlkoetter, J., Callahan, E. J., & Linton, J. Obesity and the unbalanced energy equation: Exercise versus eating habit change. *Journal of Consulting and Clinical Psychology*, 1979, *47*, 898–905.

Dalessio, D. *Wolff's headache and other head pain* (3rd ed.). New York: Oxford University Press, 1972.

David, N. A., Welborn, W. S., & Pierce, H. I. Comparison of multiple and combination tablet drug therapy in hypertension. *Current Therapeutic Research*, 1975, *18*, 741–754.

Delgado, J. M. R. Circulatory effects of cortical stimulation. *Physiological Review*, 1960, *40* (Suppl. 4), 146–171.

Dembroski, T. M., MacDougall, J. M., Herd, J. A., & Shields, J. L. Effect of level of challenge on pressor and heart rate responses in type A and type B subjects. *Journal of Applied Social Psychology*, 1979, *9*, 209–228.

Doehrman, S. R. Psycho-social aspects of recovery from coronary heart disease: A review. *Social Science and Medicine*, 1977, *11*, 199–218.

Dohrenwend, B. S., & Dohrenwend, B. P. *Stressful life events: Their nature and effects.* New York: Wiley (Interscience), 1974.

Dunbar, J. M., & Stunkard, A. J. Adherence to diet and drug regimens. In R. Levy, B. Rifkind, B. Dennis, & N. Ernst (Eds.), *Nutrition, lipids and coronary heart disease.* New York: Raven, 1979.

Ebert, P. A., Vandeerveek, R. B., Allgood, R. J., & Sabiston, D. C., Jr. Effect of chronic cardiac denervation of arrhythmias after coronary artery ligation. *Cardiovascular Regulation*, 1970, *4*, 141–147.

Elder, S. T., & Eustis, N. K. Instrumental blood pressure conditioning in outpatient hypertensives. *Behavior Research and Therapy*, 1975, *13*, 185–188.

Engel, G. Sudden and rapid death during psychological stress. *Annals of Internal Medicine*, 1971, *74*, 771–782.

Epstein, L. H., & Wing, R. R. Aerobic exercise and weight. *Addictive Behaviors*, 1980, *5*, 371–388.

Eshelman, F. N., & Fitzloff, J. Effect of packaging on patient compliance with an antihypertensive medication. *Current Therapeutic Research*, 1976, *20*, 215–219.

Falkner, B., Onesti, G., Angelakos, E. T., Fernandes, M., & Langman, C. Cardiovascular response to mental stress in normal adolescents with hypertensive parents. Hemodynamics and mental stress in adolescents. *Hypertension*, 1979, *1*, 23–30.

Farquhar, J. W. The community-based model of life-style intervention trials. *American Journal of Epidemiology*, 1978, *108*, 103–111.

Farquhar, J. W., Maccoby, N., Wood, P. D., Brietrose, H., Haskell, W. L., Meyer, A. J., Maccoby, N., Alexander, J. K., Brown, B. W., McAlister, A. L., Nash, J. D., & Stern, M. P. Community education for cardiovascular health. *Lancet*, 1977, 1192–1195.

Farris, E. J., Yeakel, E. H., & Medoff, H. Development of hypertension in emotional gray Norway rats after air blasting. *American Journal of Physiology*, 1945, *144*, 331–333.

Folkow, B., & Hallback, M. Physiopathology of spontaneous hypertension in rats. In J. Genest, E. Koiw, & O. Kuchel (Eds.), *Hypertension: Physiopathology and treatment.* New York: McGraw-Hill, 1977.

Forsyth, R. P. Blood pressure response to long-term avoidance schedules in the retrained rhesus monkey. *Psychosomatic Medicine*, 1969, *31*, 300–309.

Freedman, R., Ianni, P., Hale, P., & Lynn, S. Treatment of Raynaud's phenomenon with biofeedback and cold desensitization. *Psychophysiology*, 1979, *16*, 182. (Abstract)

Freis, E. D. Should mild hypertension be treated? *New England Journal of Medicine*, 1982, *307*, 306–309.

Friar, L. R., & Beatty, J. Migraine: Management by trained control of vasoconstriction. *Journal of Consulting and Clinical Psychology*, 1976, *44*, 46–53.

Friedman, H., & Taub, H. A. The use of hypnosis and biofeedback procedures for essential hypertension. *International Journal of Clinical and Experimental Hypnosis*, 1977, *25*, 335 − 347.

Friedman, H., & Taub, H. A. A six-month follow-up of the use of hypnosis and biofeedback procedures in essential hypertension. *American Journal of Clinical Hypnosis*, 1978, *20*, 184 − 188.

Friedman, M. *The pathogenesis of coronary artery disease*. New York: McGraw-Hill, 1969.

Friedman, M., Manwaring, J. H., Rosenman, R. H., Donlon, G., Ortega, P., & Grube, S. M. Instantaneous and sudden deaths. *Journal of the American Medical Association*, 1973, *225*, 1319 − 1328.

Friedman, M., Rosenman, R. H., Straus, R., Wurm, M., & Kositchek, R. The relationship of behavior pattern A to the state of the coronary vasculature: A study of 51 autopsied subjects. *American Journal of Medicine*, 1968, *44*, 525-537.

Friedman, M., Thoresen, C., Gill, J., Ulmer, D., Thompson, L., Powell, L., Price, V., Elek, S., Rabin, D., Breall, W., Piaget, G., Dixon, T., Bourg, E., Levy, R., & Tasto, D. Feasibility of altering type A behavior pattern after myocardial infarction. *Circulation*, 1982, *66*, 83 − 92.

Friedman, R., & Dahl, L. K. The effect of chronic conflict on the blood pressure of rats with genetic susceptibility to experimental hypertension. *Psychosomatic Medicine*, 1975, *37*, 402 − 416.

Friedman, R., & Iwai, J. Genetic predisposition and stress-induced hypertension. *Science*, 1976, *193*, 161 − 172.

Friedman, R., & Iwai, J. Dietary sodium, psychic stress, and genetic predisposition to experimental hypertension. *Proceedings of the Society of Experimental and Biological Medicine*, 1977, *155*, 449-452.

Fuller, G., & Langer, R. Elevation of aortic proline hydroxylase: A biochemical defect in experimental atherosclerosis. *Science*, 1970, *168*, 987-989.

Garrity, T. F. Behavioral adjustment after myocardial infarction: A selective review of recent descriptive, correlational, and intervention research. In S. M. Weiss, J. A. Herd, & B. H. Fox (Eds.), *Perspectives on behavioral medicine*. New York; Academic Press, Inc., 1981.

Garrity, T., & Klein, R. Emotional response and clinical severity as early determinants of six-month mortality after myocardial infarction. *Heart and Lung*, 1975, *4*, 730 − 737.

Garvey, J. L., & Melville, K. I. Cardiovascular effects of lateral hypothalamic stimulation in normal and coronary-ligated dogs. *Journal of Cardiovascular Surgery*, 1969, *10*, 377 − 385.

Gentry, W. D., & Haney, T. L. Emotional and behavioral reaction to acute myocardial infarction. *Heart and Lung*, 1975, *4*, 738 − 745.

Glass, D. C. *Behavioral patterns, stress, and coronary disease*. Hillsdale, N.J.: Lawrence Erlbaum Associates, 1977.

Glass, D. C., Krakoff, L. R., Contrada, R., Hilton, W. F., Kehoe, K., Mannucci, E. G., Collins, C., Snow, B., & Elting, E. Effect of harassment and competition upon cardiovascular and plasma catecholamine responses in Type A and Type B individuals. *Psychophysiology*, 1980, *17*, 453 − 463.

Graham, J. D. P. High blood pressure after battle. *Lancet*, 1945, *1*, 239 − 242.

Graham, L. E., Beiman, I., & Ciminero, A. R. The generality of the therapeutic effects of progressive relaxation training for essential hypertension. *Journal of Behavioral Therapy and Experimental Psychiatry*, 1977, *8*, 161 − 164.

Gruen, W. Effects of brief psychotherapy during the hospitalization period on the recovery period in heart attacks. *Journal of Consulting and Clinical Psychology*, 1975, *43*, 223.

Gulledge, A. D. The psychological aftermath of a myocardial infarction. In W. D. Gentry & R. B. Williams (Eds.), *Psychological aspects of myocardial infarction and coronary care*. St. Louis: Mosby, 1975.

Hackett, T. P., & Cassem, N. H. Factors contributing to delay in responding to the signs and symptoms of acute myocardial infarction. *American Journal of Cardiology*, 1969, *24*, 651 − 659.

Hackett, T. P., Cassem, N. H., & Wishnie, H. A. The coronary care unit. An appraisal of its psychologic hazards. *New England Journal of Medicine*, 1968, *279*, 1365 − 1369.

Hall, R. E., Livington, R. R., and Bloor, M. D. Orbital cortical influences on cardiovascular dynamics and myocardial structure in conscious monkeys. *Journal of Neurosurgery*, 1977, *46*, 638 − 647.

Hall, R. E., Sybers, H. D., Greenhoot, J. H., & Bloor, C. M. Myocardial alterations after hypothalamic stimulation in the intact conscious dog. *American Heart Journal*, 1974, *88*, 770 − 776.

Hanson, J. P., Larson, M. E., & Snowden, C. T. The effects of control over high intensity noise on plasma cortisol levels in rhesus monkeys. *Behavioral Biology*, 1976, *16*, 333-340.

Harburg, E., Erfurt, J. C., Havenstein, L. S., Chape, C., Schull, W. J., & Schork, M.A. Socio-ecological stress, suppressed hostility, skin odor, and black-white male blood pressure: Detroit. *Psychosomatic Medicine*, 1973, *35*, 276–296.

Harris, A. H., Gilliam, W. J., Findley, J. D., & Brady, J. V. Instrumental conditioning of large-magnitude, daily, 12-hour blood pressure elevations in the baboon. *Science*, 1973, *182*, 175–177.

Hay, K. M., & Madders, J. Migraine treated by relaxation therapy. *Journal of the Royal College of General Practitioners*, 1971, *21*, 664–669.

Haynes, R. B., Gibson, E. S., Taylor, D. W., Bernholz, C. D., & Sackett, D. L. Process versus outcome in hypertension: A positive result. *Circulation*, 1982, *65*, 28–33.

Haynes, R. B., Sackett, D. L., Gibson, E. S., Taylor, D. W., Hackett, B. C., Roberts, R. S., & Johnson, A. L. Improvement of medication compliance in uncontrolled hypertension. *Lancet*, 1976, *1*, 1265–1268.

Haynes, S. G., Feinleib, M., & Kannel, W. B. Psychosocial factors and CHD incidence in Framingham: Results from an 8-year follow-up study. *American Journal of Epidemiology*, 1980, *108*, 229.

Helgeland, A. Treatment of mild hypertension: A five-year controlled drug trial: The Oslo study. *American Journal of Medicine*, 1980, *69*, 725–732.

Hellerstein, H. K. & Friedman, E. H. Sexual activity and the postcoronary patient. *Archives of Internal Medicine*, 1970, *125*, 987.

Henry, J. P., Ely, D. L., & Stephens, P. M. Changes in catecholamine-controlling enzymes in response to psychosocial activation of the defense and alarm reactions. Physiology, emotion and psychosomatic illness. *Ciba Foundation Symposium*, 1972, *8*, 225–251.

Henry, J. P., Ely, D. L., Stephens, P. M., Ratcliffe, H. L., Santisteban, G. A., & Shapiro, A. P. The role of psychosocial factors in the development of arteriosclerosis in CBA mice. *Atherosclerosis*, 1971, *14*, 203–218.

Henry, J. P., Stephens, P. M., Axelrod, J., & Mueller, R. A. Effect of psychosocial stimulation on the enzymes involved in the biosynthesis and metabolism of noradrenaline and adrenaline. *Psychosomatic Medicine*, 1971, *33*, 227–237.

Henry, J. P., Stephens, P. M., & Santisteban, G. A. A model of psychosocial hypertension showing reversibility and progression of cardiovascular complications. *Circulation Response*, 1975, *36*, 156–164.

Herd, J., Morse, W., Kelleher, R., & Jones, L. Arterial hypertension in the squirrel monkey during behavior experiments. *American Journal of Physiology*, 1969, *217*, 24–29.

Hjermann, I. Smoking and diet intervention in healthy coronary high risk men. Methods and 5-year follow-up of risk factors in a randomized trial. The Oslo Study. *Journal of the Oslo City Hospital*, 1980, *30*, 3–17.

Hjermann, I., Velve-Byre, K., Home, I., & Leren, P. Effect of diet and smoking intervention on the incidence of coronary heart disease. Report from the Oslo Study Group of a randomized trial in healthy men. *Lancet*, 1981, 1303–1310.

Hockman, C. H., Mauck, H. P., & Hoff, E. C. ECG changes resulting from cerebral stimulation. II. A spectrum of ventricular arrhythmias of sympathetic origin. *American Heart Journal*, 1966, *71*, 695–701.

Hollander, W. Biochemical pathology of atherosclerosis and relationship to hypertension. In J. Genest, E. Koiw, & O. Kuchel (Eds.), *Hypertension: Physiopathology and treatment*. New York: McGraw-Hill, 1977.

Hypertension Detection and Follow-up Program Cooperative Group. Five-year findings of the hypertension detection and follow-up program. I. Reduction in mortality of persons with high blood pressure, including mild hypertension. *Journal of the American Medical Association*, 1979, *242*, 2562–2571. (a)

Hypertension Detection and Follow-up Program Cooperative Group. Five-year findings of the hypertension detection and follow-up program. II. Mortality by race, sex, and age. *Journal of the American Medical Association*, 1979, *242*, 2572–2577. (b)

Jacobson, A. M., Manschreck, T. C., & Silverberg, E. Behavioral treatment for Raynaud's disease: A comparative study with long-term follow-up. *Journal of American Psychiatry*, 1979, *136*, 844–846.

Jacobson, A. M., Hackett, T. P., Surman, O. S., & Silverberg, E. L. Raynaud's disease phenomenon: Treatment with hypnotic and operant technique. *Journal of the American Medical Association*, 1973, *225*, 739–740.

Jacobson, E. Variation of blood pressure with skeletal muscle tension and relaxation. *Annals of Internal Medicine*, 1939, *12*, 1194 – 1212.

Jenkins, C. D. Recent evidence supporting psychosocial risk factors for coronary disease. *New England Journal of Medicine*, 1976, *294*, 987 – 1033.

Johansson, G., Jonsson, L., Lannek, N., Blomgren, L., Lindberg, P., & Poupa, O. Severe stress – cardiopathy in pigs. *American Heart Journal*, 1974, *87*, 451 – 457.

Julius, S., & Esler, M. D. Autonomic nervous system regulation in borderline hypertension. *American Journal of Cardiology*, 1975, *36*, 685 – 696.

Julius, S. Classification of hypertension. In J. Genest, E. Koiw, & O. Kuchel (Eds.), *Hypertension: Physiopathology and treatment*. New York: McGraw – Hill, 1977.

Kannel, W. B. Role of blood pressure in cardiovascular morbidity and mortality. *Progress in Cardiovascular Disease*, 1974, *17*, 5.

Kannel, W. B. Role of blood pressure in cardiovascular disease: The Framingham study. *Angiology*, 1975, *26*, 1 – 14.

Kannel, W. B., Gordon, T., & Schwartz, M. J. Systolic versus diastolic blood pressure and risk of coronary heart disease. *American Journal of Cardiology*, 1971, *27*, 335 – 343.

Kannel, W. B., McGee, D., & Gordon, T. A general cardiovascular risk profile: The Framingham study. *American Journal of Cardiology*, 1976, *38*, 46 – 51.

Keefe, F. J., Surwit, R. S., & Pilon, R. N. Biofeedback, autogenic training and progressive relaxation in the treatment of Raynaud's disease. *Journal of Applied Behavior Analysis*, 1980, *13*, 3 – 11.

Kellerman, J. Rehabilitation of patients with coronary heart disease. *Progress in Cardiovascular Diseases*, 1975, *17*, 303 – 328.

Keys, A., Taylor, H. L., Blackburn, H., Brozek, J., Anderson, J. T., & Simonson, E. Mortality and coronary heart disease among men studied for 23 years. *Archives of Internal Medicine*, 1971, *128*, 201 – 214.

Klein, R. F., Kliner, V. A., Zipes, D. P., Troyer, W. G., Jr., & Wallace. A. G. Transfer from a coronary-care unit: Some adverse responses. *Archives of Internal Medicine*, 1968, *122*, 104 – 110.

Kosowski, B. O., Lown, B., Whiting, R., & Guiney, T. Occurrences of ventricular arrhythmias with exercise as compared to monitoring. *Circulation*, 1971, *44*, 826 – 832.

Krantz, D. S., Sanmarco, M. E., Selvester, R. H., & Matthews, K. A. Psychological correlates of progression of atherosclerosis in men. *Psychosomatic Medicine*, 1979, *41*, 467 – 475.

Kristt, D. A., & Engel, B. T. Learned control of blood pressure in patients with high blood pressure. *Circulation*, 1975, *51*, 370 – 378.

Kuller, L., & Lillenfield, A. Epidemiological study of sudden and unexpected death due to arteriosclerotic heart disease. *Circulation*, 1966, *34*, 1056.

Lamb, L. E., & Hiss, R. G. Influences of exercise on premature contractions. *American Journal of Cardiology*, 1962, *10*, 209 – 216.

Lang, C. M. Effects of psychic stress on atherosclerosis in the squirrel monkey. *Proceedings of the Society of Experimental Biological Medicine*, 1967, *126*, 30 – 34.

Lawler, J. E., Barker, G. F., Hubbard, J. W., & Allen, M. T. The effects of conflict on tonic levels of blood pressure in the genetically borderline hypertensive rat. *Psychophysiology*, 1980, *17*, 363 – 370.

Lawler, J. E., Botticelli, L. J., & Lown, B. Changes in cardiac refractory period during signalled avoidance in dogs. *Psychophysiology*, 1976, *13*, 373 – 377.

Leigh, H., Hofen, M. A., Cooper, J., & Reiser, M. F. A psychological comparison of patients in "open" and "closed" coronary care units. *Journal of Psychosomatic Research*, 1972, *16*, 449 – 456.

Lewis, T. *Vascular disorders of the limbs: Described for practitioners and students*. London: Macmillan, 1949.

Lipman, R. L., & Shapiro, A. Effects of a behavioral stimulus on the blood pressure of rats with experimental pyelonephritis. *Psychosomatic Medicine*, 1967, *29*, 612 – 618.

Lown, B., & Graboys, T. B. Sudden death: An ancient problem newly perceived. *Cardiovascular Medicine*, 1977, *2*, 219 – 233.

Malliani, A., Schwartz, P. J., & Zanchetti, A. Neural mechanisms in life-threatening arrhythmias. *American Heart Journal*, 1980, *100*, 705 – 715.

Management Committee of the Australian Hypertension Trial. The Australian therapeutic trial in hypertension. *Lancet*, 1979, *57* (Suppl. 5), 4498 – 4528.

Manning, J. W., & Cotten, M. de V. Mechanisms of cardiac arrhythmias induced by diencephalic stimulation. *American Journal of Physiology*, 1962, *203*, 1120 – 1124.

Manuck, S. B., Giordani, B., McQuaid, K., & Garrity, S. J. Behaviorally induced cardiovascular reactivity among sons of reported hypertensive and normotensive parents. *Journal of Psychosomatic Research*, 1981, *25*, 261 – 269.

Manuck, S. B., Kaplan, J. R., & Clarkson, T. B. Behaviorally induced heart rate reactivity and atherosclerosis in cynomolgus monkeys. *Psychosomatic Medicine*, 1983, *45*, 95–108.

Mason, J. W., Mangan, G. F., Brady, J. V., Conrad, D., & Rioch, D. M. Concurrent plasma epinephrine, norepinephrine, and 17-hydroxycorticosteroid levels during conditioned emotional disturbances in monkeys. *Psychosomatic Medicine*, 1961, *23*, 344 – 353.

Matthews, K. A., Glass, D. C., Rosenman, R. H., & Bortner, R. W. Competitive drive, pattern A, and coronary heart disease. A further analysis of some data from the Western Collaborative Group Study. *Journal of Chronic Disease*, 1977, *30*, 489 – 498.

Mayer, J., Roy, P., & Mitra, K. P. Relation between caloric intake, body weight, and physical work: Studies in industrial male population in West Bengal. *American Journal of Clinical Nutrition*, 1956, *4*, 169 – 175.

McAlister, A., Puska, P., Salonen, J., Tuomilehto, J., & Koskela, K. Theory and action for health promotion: Illustrations from the North Karelia Project. *American Journal of Public Health*, 1982, *72*, 43 – 50.

McKeeney, J. M., Slining, J. M., Henderson, H. R., Devins, D., & Beer, M. The effect of clinical pharmacy services on patients with essential hypertension. *Circulation*, 1973, *48*, 1104 – 1111.

McNeer, J., Wagner, G., Ginsburg, P., Wallace, A., McCants, C., Conley, M., & Rosati, R. Hospital discharge one week after acute myocardial infarction. *New England Journal of Medicine*, 1978, *298*, 229 – 232.

Melville, K. I., Blum, B., Shister, H. E., & Silver, M. D. Cardiac ischemic changes in arrhythmias induced by hypothalamic stimulation. *American Journal of Cardiology*, 1963, *12*, 781 – 791.

Meyer, A. J., Nash, J. D., McAlister, A. L., Maccoby, N., & Farquhar, J. W. Skills training in a cardiovascular health education campaign. *Journal of Consulting and Clinical Psychology*, 1980, *48*, 129 – 142.

Meyers, A., & Dewar, H. A. Circumstances attending 100 sudden deaths from coronary artery disease with coroner's necropsies. *British Heart Journal*, 1975, *37*, 1133 – 1143.

Mitchell, K. R., & Mitchell, D. M. Migraine: An exploratory treatment application of programmed therapy techniques. *Journal of Psychosomatic Research*, 1971, *15*, 137 – 157.

Mitchell, K. R., & White, R. G. Behavioral self-management: An application to the problem of migraine headaches. *Behavior Therapy*, 1977, *8*, 213 – 221.

Morgan, T., Gillies, A., Morgan, G., Adam, W., Wilson, M., & Carney, S. Hypertension treated by salt restriction. *The Lancet*, 1978, *1*, 227.

Moritz, A. R., & Zancheck, N. Sudden and unexpected death of young soldiers. *Archives of Pathology*, 1946, *42*, 459 – 494.

Moss, A. J. Clinical significance of ventricular arrhythmias in patients with and without coronary artery disease. In E. H. Sonnenblick & M. Lesch (Eds.), *Sudden cardiac death*. New York: Grune & Stratton, 1980.

Moss, A. J., & Goldstein, S. The pre-hospital phase of acute myocardial infarction. *Circulation*, 1970, *41*, 737.

Mulcahey, R., Hickey, N., Graham, I., & McKenzie, G. Factors influencing long-term prognosis in male patients surviving a first coronary attack. *British Heart Journal*, 1975, *37*, 158 – 165.

Multicenter International Study. Improvement in prognosis of myocardial infarction by long-term beta-adrenoreceptor blockade using practolol. *British Medical Journal*, 1975, *3*, 735 – 740.

Multiple Risk Factor. Intervention trial, risk factor changes and mortality results. Multiple Risk Factor Intervention Trial Research Group. *The Journal of the American Medical Association*, 1982, *248*, 1465 – 1477.

National Center for Health Statistics. *Chartbook for the conference on the decline in coronary heart disease mortality*. Department of Health, Education, and Welfare, 1979.

Obrist, P. A. *Cardiovascular psychophysiology*. New York: Plenum, 1981.

Okamoto, K., & Aoki, K. Development of a strain of spontaneously hypertensive rat. *Japanese Circulation Journal*, 1963, *27*, 282–293.

Page, I. H. Pathogenesis of arterial hypertension. *Journal of the American Medical Association*, 1949, *140*, 451–458.

Page, I. H. Some regulatory mechanisms of renovascular and essential hypertension. In J. Genest, E. Koiw, & O. Kuchel (Eds.), *Hypertension: Physiopathology and treatment*. New York: McGraw-Hill, 1977.

Parijs, J., Joossens, J. V., Van der Linden, L., Verstreken, G., & Amer, A. K. P. C. Moderate sodium restriction and diuretics in the treatment of hypertension. *American Heart Journal*, 1973, *85*, 22.

Parkes, C. M. Bereavement. *British Medical Journal*, 1967, *4*, 13.

Patel, C. H. Yoga and biofeedback in the management of hypertension. *Lancet*, 1973, *7837*, 1053 – 1055.

Patel, C., Marmot, M. G., & Terry, D. J. Controlled trial of biofeedback-aided behavioral methods in reducing mild hypertension. *British Medical Journal*, 1981, *282*, 2005 – 2008.

Patel, C. H., & North, W. R. S. Randomized controlled trial of yoga and biofeedback in management of hypertension. *Lancet*, 1975, *7925*, 93 – 95.

Paul, O. Risks of mild hypertension: A ten-year report. *British Heart Journal*, 1971, *33* (Suppl.), 116 – 121.

Paulley, J. W., & Haskel, D. A. L. The treatment of migraine without drugs. *Journal of Psychosomatic Research*, 1975, *19*, 367 – 374.

Perhach, J. L., Ferguson, H. C., & McKinney, G. R. Evaluation of antihypertensive agents in the stress-induced hypertensive rats. *Life Science*, 1976, *16*, 1731–1736.

Pickering, T. G., Johnston, J., & Honour, A. J. Suppression of ventricular extrasystoles during sleep and exercise, and effects of autonomic drugs. In P. J. Schwartz, A. M. Brown, A. Malliani, & A. Zanchetti (Eds.), *Neural mechanisms in cardiac arrhythmias*. New York: Raven, 1978.

Pickering, T. G., & Miller, N. E. Learned voluntary control of heart rate and rhythm in two subjects with premature ventricular contractions. *British Heart Journal*, 1977, *49*, 152 – 159.

Pratt, G. H. *Surgical management of vascular disease*. Philadelphia: Lea & Febiger, 1949.

Puska, P., Tuomilehto, J., Salonen, J., Neittaanmaki, L., Maki, J., Virtamo, J., Nissinen, A., Kottke, & Tuomilehto. *The North Karelia Project: Evaluation of a comprehensive community programme for control of cardiovascular diseases in 1972 – 77 in North Karelia, Finland*. Geneva: WHD Monograph Series, 1981.

Raab, W. Cardiotoxic biochemical effects of emotional-environmental stressors—fundamentals of psychocardiology. In L. Levi (Ed.), *Society stress and disease*. London: Oxford University Press, 1971.

Rahe, R. H., Bennett, L., Romo, M., Seltanen, P., & Arthur, R. S. Subject's recent life changes and coronary heart disease in Finland. *American Journal of Psychiatry*, 1973, *130*, 1222–1226.

Ramsay, L. E., Ramsay, M. H., Hettiarachi, J., Davies, D. L., & Winchester, J. Weight reduction in a blood pressure clinic. *British Medical Journal*, 1978, *2*, 224.

Randall, D. C., & Hasson, D. M. Incidence of cardiac arrhythmias in monkey during classic aversive and appetitive conditioning. In D. J. Schwartz, A. M. Brown, A. Malliani, & A. Banchetti (Eds.), *Neural mechanisms in cardiac arrhythmias*. New York: Raven, 1978.

Ratcliffe, H. L. Environment, behavior, and disease. In E. Stellar & J. Sprague (Eds.), *Physiological psychology*, Vol. 2. New York: Academic Press, 1968.

Ratcliffe, H. L., Luginbuhl, H., Schnarr, W. R., & Chacko, K. Coronary arteriosclerosis in swine. *Journal of Comparative and Physiological Psychology*, 1969, *68*, 385–392.

Ratcliffe, H. L., & Snyder, L. *Arteriosclerotic stenosis of the intramural coronary arteries of chickens: Further evidence of a relation of social factors*. Penrose Research Laboratory, Zoological Society of Philadelphia and the Department of Pathology, University of Pennsylvania, 1967, 357–365.

Rees, W. D., & Lutkins, S. G. Mortality of bereavement. *British Medical Journal*, 1967, *4*, 13.

Reich, P., DeSilva, R. A., Lown, B., & Murawski, J. Acute psychological disturbances preceding life-threatening ventricular arrhythmias. *Journal of the American Medical Association*, 1981, *246*, 233 – 235.

Reisin, E., Abel, R., Modan, M., Silverberg, D. S., Eliahow, H. E., & Modan, B. Effect of weight loss without salt restriction in the reduction of blood pressure. *New England Journal of Medicine*, 1978, *298*, 1.

Rissanen, V., Romo, M., & Seltanen, P. Premonitory symptoms and stress factor preceding sudden death from ischemic heart disease. *Acta Medica Scandinavica*, 1978, *204*, 389.

Rosenfeld, J., Rosen, M. R., & Hoffman, B. F. Pharmacologic and behavioral effects on arrhythmias that immediately follow abrupt coronary occlusion: A canine model of sudden coronary death. *American Journal of Cardiology*, 1978, *41*, 1075 – 1082.

Rosenman, R. H., Brand, R. J., Jenkins, C. D., Friedman, M., Strauss, R., & Wurm, M. Coronary heart disease in the Western Collaborative Group study: Final follow-up experience of 8 1/2 years. *Journal of the American Medical Association*, 1975, *233*, 872 – 877.

Ross, R., & Glomset, J. A. The pathogenesis of atherosclerosis. *New England Journal of Medicine*, 1976, *295*, 369–377.

Rothlin, E., Cerletti, A., & Emmenegger, H. Experimental psychoneurogenic hypertension and its treatment with hydrogenated ergot alkaloids (hydergine). *Acta Medica Scandinavia*, 1956, *312*, 27–35.

Ruskin, A., Beard, O. W., & Schaffer, R. L. Blast hypertension: Elevated blood pressures in the victims of the Texas City disaster. *American Journal of Medicine*, 1948, *4*, 228 – 230.

Sackett, D. L., Gibson, E. S., Taylor, D. W., Haynes, R. B., Hackett, B. C., Roberts, R. R., & Johnson, A. L. Randomized clinical trial of strategies for improving medication compliance in primary hypertension. *Lancet*, 1975, 1205 – 1207.

Salonen, J. T., Puska, P., & Mustaniemi, H. Changes in morbidity and mortality during comprehensive community programme to control cardiovascular diseases during 1972 – 77 in North Karelia. *British Medical Journal*, 1979, *2*, 1178 – 1183.

Sargent, J. D., Green, E. E., & Walters, E. D. Preliminary report on the use of autogenic feedback training in the treatment of migraine and tension headaches. *Psychosomatic Medicine*, 1973, *35*, 129 – 135.

Savage, D. D., Seides, S. F., Maron, B. J., Myers, R., & Epstein, S. E. Prevalence of arrhythmias during 24-hour electrocardiographic monitoring and exercise testing in patients with obstructive and nonobstructive hypertrophic cardiomyopathy. *Circulation*, 1979, *59*, 866 – 875.

Schade, D., & Eaton, R. The regulation of plasma ketone body concentration by counter regulatory hormones in man. I. Effect of norepinephrine in diabetic man. *Diabetes*, 1977, *26*, 989.

Schiffer, H., Hartley, L. H., Schulman, C. L., & Abelman, W. H. The quiz electrocardiogram: A new diagnostic and research technique for evaluating the relation between emotional stress and ischemic heart disease. *American Journal of Cardiology*, 1976, *37*, 41 – 47.

Schneiderman, N. Animal behavior models of coronary heart disease. In D. Krantz, A. Baum, & J. E. Singer (Eds.), *Handbook of psychology and health* (Vol. 3). Hillsdale, N.J.: Lawrence Erlbaum Associates, 1983. (a)

Schneiderman, N. Behavior, autonomic function and animal models of cardiovascular pathology. In T. Dembroski & T. Schmidt (Eds.), *Biologic basis of coronary-prone behavior: Behavioral approaches to a 20th century epidemic*. Basel: Karger, 1983. (b)

Schultz, J. H., & Luthe, W. *Autogenic therapy* (Vol. 1). New York: Grune & Stratton, 1969.

Schwartz, C. J., & Gerrity, R. G. Anatomical pathology of sudden unexpected cardiac death. *Circulation*, 1975, *52*, 18 – 26.

Sen, S., Tarazi, R. C., Khairallah, P. A., & Bumpus, F. M. Cardiac hypertrophy in spontaneously hypertensive rats. *Circulation Research*, 1974, *35*, 775 – 783.

Seventh report of the director of the National Heart, Lung and Blood Institute. U.S. Department of Health, Education, and Welfare, Public Health Service, National Institutes of Health (NIH Publication No. 80 – 1672), 1979.

Shekelle, R. B., Ostfield, A. M., & Paul, O. Social status and incidence of coronary heart disease. *Journal of Chronic Disease*, 1969, *22*, 281 – 294.

Sime, W. E., Buell, J. C., & Eliot, R. S. Psychophysiological (emotional) stress testing: A potential means of detecting the early reinfarction victim. *Circulation*, 1979, *59 and 60* (Suppl. 2), II – 56 (Abstract).

Sime, W. E., Buell, J. C., & Eliot, R. S. Cardiovascular responses to emotional stress (quiz interview) in postinfarct cardiac patients and matched control subjects. *Journal of Human Stress*, 1980, *6* (3), 39 – 46.

Skinner, J. E., Lie, J. T., & Entman, M. L. Modification of ventricular fibrillation latency following coronary artery occlusion in the conscious pig: The effects of psychological stress and beta-adrenergic blockade. *Circulation*, 1975, *51*, 656 – 667.

Skinner, J. E., & Reed, J. C. Blockade of a frontocortical-brainstem pathway prevents ventricular fibrillation of the ischemic heart in pigs. *American Journal of Physiology*, 1981, *240*, H156 – H163.

Solomon, H. *Paper presented at a plenary symposium on physiological bases of preventive medicine*. Presented at the annual meeting of the Academy of Behavioral Medicine Research, Bolton Valley, Vermont, 1982.

Southam, M. A., Agras, W. S., Taylor, C. B., & Kraemer, H. C. Relaxation training: Blood pressure lowering during the working day. *Archives of General Psychiatry*, in press.

Spittell, J. A., Jr. Raynaud's phenomenon and allied vasospastic conditions. In J. F. Fairbairn, J. C. Juergens, & J. A. Spittell (Eds.), *Allen – Banker – Hines peripheral vascular diseases* (4th ed.). Philadelphia: Saunders, 1972.

Stern, M., Pascale, L., & McLoone, J. Psychosocial adaptation following an acute myocardial infarction. *Journal of Chronic Disease*, 1976, *29*, 513 – 526.

Stone, R. A., & DeLeo, J. Psychotherapeutic control of hypertension. *New England Journal of Medicine*, 1976, *294*, 80 – 84.

Surwit, R. S. Biofeedback: A possible treatment for Raynaud's disease. *Seminars in Psychiatry*, 1973, *5*, 483 – 490.

Surwit, R. S., Pilon, R. N., & Fenton, C. H. Behavioral treatment of Raynaud's disease. *Journal of Behavioral Medicine*, 1978, *1*, 323 – 335.

Surwit, R. S., Shapiro, D., & Good, M. I. A comparison of cardiovascular biofeedback, neuromuscular biofeedback, and meditation in the treatment of borderline essential hypertension. *Journal of Consulting and Clinical Psychology*, 1978, *46*, 252 – 263.

Surwit, R. S., Williams, R. B., & Shapiro, D. *Behavioral approaches to cardiovascular disease*. New York: Academic Press, 1982.

Swedberg, K., Hjalmarson, A., Waagstein, F., & Wallentin, I. Prolongation of survival in congestive cardiomyopathy by beta-receptor blockade. Preliminary communication. *Lancet*, 1979, *1*, 1374 – 1376.

Syme, S. L., Borhani, N. O., & Buechley, R. W. Cultural mobility and coronary heart disease in an urban area. *American Journal of Epidemiology*, 1965, *82*, 334 – 346.

Taub, E. Self-regulation of human tissue temperature. In G. E. Schwartz & J. Beattay (Eds.), *Biofeedback: Theory and research*. New York: Academic Press, 1977.

Taylor, C. B., Farquhar, J. W., Nelson, E., & Agras, W. S. Relaxation therapy and high blood pressure. *Archives of General Psychiatry*, 1977, *34*, 339 – 342.

Throckloth, R., Ho., S., Wright, H., & Seldon, W. Is cardiac rehabilitation really necessary? *Medical Journal of Australia*, 1973, *2*, 669 – 674.

Titus, J. L. Pathology of sudden cardiac death. In *USA – USSR, first symposium on sudden death*. Yalta, USSR, 1978, 309 – 318.

Turin, A., & Johnson, W. G. Biofeedback therapy for migraine headache. *Archives of General Psychiatry*, 1976, *33*, 517 – 519.

Uhley, H. N., & Friedman, M. Blood lipids, clotting and coronary atherosclerosis in rats exposed to a particular form of stress. *American Journal of Physiology*, 1959, *197*, 396–398.

Ulyaninsky, L. S., Stepanyan, E. P., & Krymsky, I. P. Cardiac arrhythmias of hypothalamic origin in sudden death. In *Proceedings USA – USSR joint symposium on sudden death*. DHEW No. (NIH) 78 – 1472, US Government Printing Office. Washington, D.C.: 1977.

United States Department of Health and Human Services, Public Health Service. *Health United States 1980 with prevention profile*. Washington, D.C.: US Government Printing Office, 1981 (DHHS publication No. (PHS) 81 – 1232).

Vander, A., Henry, J., Stephens, P., Kay, L., & Mouw, D. Plasma renin activity in psychosocial hypertension of CBA mice. *Circulation Research*, 1978, *42*, 496 – 502.

Vikhert, A. M., Velisheva, L. A., & Matova, E. E. Geographic distribution and pathology of sudden death in the Soviet Union. In *USA – USSR first symposium on sudden death*. DHEW No. (NIH) 78 – 1470, US Government Printing Office. Washington, D.C.: 1977, 19 – 40.

Watanabe, A. M., Jones, L. R., Manalin, A. S., & Besch, H. R. Cardiac autonomic receptors: Recent concepts from radio-labeled ligand-binding studies. *Circulation Research*, 1982, *50*, 161 – 174.

Wilhelmsson, C., Vedin, J. A., Wilhelmsson, L., Tiblin, G., & Werko, L. Reduction of sudden deaths after myocardial infarction by treatment with alpreholol. *Lancet*, 1974, *2*, 1157 – 1164.

Williams, R. B., Haney, T. L., Lee, K. L., Kong, Y., Blumenthal, J. A., & Whalen, R. E. Type A behavior, hostility, and coronary atherosclerosis. *Psychosomatic Medicine*, 1980, *42*, 539 – 550.

Wolf, S. Psychosocial forces in myocardial infarction and sudden death. *Circulation*, 1969, *40* (Suppl. 4), 74 – 83.

Wooley, S. C., Wooley, O. W., & Dyrenforth, S. R. Theoretical, practical, and social issues in behavioral treatments of obesity. *Journal of Applied Behavioral Analysis*, 1979, *12*, 3 – 25.

Yamori, Y., Matsumoto, M., Yamabe, H., & Okamoto, K. Augmentation of spontaneous hypertension by chronic stress in rats. *Japanese Circulation Journal*, 1969, *33*, 399–409.

Zukel, W., Cohen, B., Mattingly, T., & Hrubec, Z. Survival following first diagnosis of coronary heart disease. *American Heart Journal*, 1969, *78*, 159 – 170.

18

Behavioral Medicine Approaches to Diabetes Mellitus

Susan S. Hendrick
University of Miami

INTRODUCTION

History

General descriptions of diabetes mellitus were recorded by the Egyptians as long ago as 1550 B.C., while Chinese of the same period described "polyuria," a condition where the urine was abundant and where its sweet taste attracted animals. As early as 400 B.C., Charak and Susrut in India noted a sweetness in the urine as well as a correlation between such sweetness and obesity. They pointed out the tendency of the disease to be passed from generation to generation and were the first to describe two types of the disease, one with symptoms of emaciation and dehydration and the other manifesting obesity and drowsiness. It remained for Aretaeus (A.D. 70) to give the disease its name, diabetes mellitus, or a "running-through of sugar." The extravagant life-style of 16th and 17th century England added to accumulated knowledge. Although Paracelsus boiled patients' urine and thought the residue was salt, Dobson proved it to be sugar. Morton (1686) noted the hereditary nature of the disease, and Claude Bernard (1859) delineated hyperglycemia as a primary manifestation of the disorder.

About that time, a chain of discoveries began that has resulted in much of our present knowledge about diabetes. First, Paul Langerhans, a German physician and anatomist, in 1868 described the islet cell formation in the pancreas, thereafter referred to as the "islets of Langerhans." Diabetes was finally recognized as a disease associated with the pancreas as a result of the 1889 experiments of Minkowski and von Mering in Strassbourg, who induced diabetes in dogs by pancreatectomy. In 1902, Opie and Sobolew related diabetes directly to the islets of Langerhans and established that the beta cells within the islets functioned abnormally, precipitating diabetes. Nearly two decades passed, however, before Frederick Banting and Charles Best, two Canadians, discovered the antidiabetic hormone, insulin, in 1921. This discovery more than any other initiated modern medical treatment of diabetes. In 1939, Hagedorn developed the first long-acting insulin, and in 1955, Franke and Fuchs in Germany produced the first of the oral hypoglycemic drugs that are widely used today. Although insulin and oral hypoglycemics have revolutionized the treatment for diabetics, the number of diabetics is steadily increasing, and medicine's intervention with the disease is presently through diagnosis and treatment rather than through prevention or cure.

Epidemiological Data

Prevalence in the Population.   There are an estimated 10 million diabetics in the United States, and the number grows as 600,000 new cases of diabetes are diagnosed annually. There are several reasons for the increasing number of diabetics. The first is sheer population growth. People in general live longer, so the natural tendency of the disease to appear with age is thereby accelerated. Diagnosed diabetics are living longer and having more children, so the hereditary factors relating to the disease are more widespread. In addition, obesity, a predisposing factor to diabetes, is rapidly increasing in the United States.

Who Gets Diabetes?   No simple answers to this question now exist, as the disease can develop in anyone, anywhere, at any time. Some predisposing factors have been isolated, however, and these include obesity, being of middle age or older, or having a family history of diabetes. Although diabetes was traditionally thought to be inherited from a single recessive gene, multifactorial inheritance of the disease has more recently been acknowledged. Scientists believe that diabetes develops from a complex interaction between genetic predisposition and environmental factors (Notkins, 1979; Steinke & Soeldner, 1977). The possible combinations of viral agents (e.g., the Coxackie virus) affecting the pancreas, various gene pairs predisposing to diabetes, and assorted nongenetic factors, as well as the often considerable time lag between the genetic predisposition to diabetes (genotype) and the clinical manifestation and diagnosis of the disease (phenotype), make prediction of the disease's occurrence virtually impossible. Heredity appears to be a more important factor for insulin-dependent than noninsulin-dependent diabetes.

Classification of Diabetes

Diabetes has recently been reclassified by both national and international groups of diabetologists into the following types: insulin-dependent diabetes mellitus; non-insulin-dependent diabetes mellitus (nonobese and obese); impaired glucose tolerance; gestational diabetes; previous abnormality of glucose tolerance; potential abnormality of glucose tolerance; and diabetes mellitus associated with other conditions or syndromes. A detailed description of the new names, the old names, and the clinical manifestations is given in Table 18.1.

TABLE 18.1
Classification of Diabetes and Glucose Intolerance
(Adapted from Hamburg, Lipsett, Inoff, & Drash, 1979, pp. 372-373)

New Classification	Old Classification	Clinical Symptoms
Type I: Insulin-Dependent Diabetes Mellitus (IDDM)	Juvenile Diabetes Ketosis-prone Diabetes Brittle Diabetes	No endogenous insulin. Younger patients. Multiple causes.
Type II: Non-Insulin Dependent Diabetes Mellitus (NIDDM) a. nonobese b. obese	Adult-onset Diabetes Ketosis-resistant Diabetes Stable Diabetes	Some endogenous insulin. Usually over 40. Obese
Impaired Glucose Tolerance (IGT) a. nonobese b. obese	Asymptomatic Diabetes Chemical Diabetes Borderline Diabetes Latent Diabetes	Glucose levels between normal and diabetic. Tendency to atherosclerosis.
Gestational Diabetes (GDM)	Gestational Diabetes	Diabetes begins in pregnancy. May reoccur.
Previous Abnormality of Glucose Tolerance (PrevAGT)	Latent Diabetes Prediabetes	History of hyperglycemia but presently normal.
Potential Abnormality of Glucose Tolerance (PotAGT)	Potential Diabetes Prediabetes	No glucose intolerance but predisposition to diabetes, e.g., relatives with diabetes, islet cell antibodies, obesity.
Diabetes Mellitus Associated with other Conditions or Syndromes	Secondary Diabetes	Other conditions cause diabetes, e.g., pancreatic or hormonal disease, drug toxicity, certain genetic syndromes.

Diagnosis

An emphasis on early detection of diabetes has resulted in recent decades in an increase in diabetes screening and detection drives, usually sponsored by local branches of the American Diabetes Association. Although such drives can and do uncover previously undiagnosed diabetics, wide criteria for positive diagnosis will necessarily result in some false positives, whereas rigid criteria will mean that some true diabetics will go unrecognized. Although some physicians do not believe early diagnosis and treatment will positively affect the course of the disease, most physicians nevertheless support such screening. Checking for sugar in the urine is a first step in diagnosis, but a more specific technique is the glucose tolerance test, which documents the individual's fasting blood sugar and then proceeds to document the blood sugar at various intervals after the ingestion of 75 or 100 grams of glucose. Although blood sugar varies, levels of 200 mg/dl after a meal or of 140 mg/dl on a fasting blood glucose test would probably indicate diabetes. Though age and physical factors such as infection, liver disease, and myocardial infarction can cause elevated blood sugar levels that are not indications of true diabetes, the glucose tolerance test is a fairly good diagnostic instrument, overall.

Pathophysiology of Diabetes

General Structure.   Diabetes is a metabolic disorder. We can briefly define metabolism as the process by which an organism secures the fuel it needs to expend energy and replenish the cell systems. Diabetes occurs when there is a metabolic imbalance between the body's requirements for insulin during either the fed or fasting state and the beta cells' production and release of insulin from the islets of Langerhans in the pancreas.

In the nondiabetic, insulin is produced in conjunction with rising blood glucose levels, allowing sugar to enter muscle and fat cells to meet energy needs, and also stimulating the liver to make and store glycogen, an animal starch derived from sugar. These actions result in lowered blood sugar. In addition, insulin inhibits "glycogenolysis," the liver's reconversion of glycogen to sugar, as well as "gluconeogenesis," the liver's creation of new sugar. Thus insulin fosters certain processes that lower blood sugar and inhibits other processes that raise it.

In addition, insulin has a significant metabolic relationship to fat and protein tissues. It stimulates the incorporation of amino acids into muscle protein for tissue growth and allows sugar to enter the protein cell for energy purposes. It also stimulates lipogenesis (fat formation) and triglyceride synthesis in the adipose cells, the sites for long-term energy storage. Insulin's augmenting effects in fat and protein tissue are balanced by its inhibition of biochemical processes that would reverse this augmentation and release stored fats and amino acids back into the blood.

Another hormone in addition to insulin is vitally important to diabetes, and that is "glucagon," produced by the alpha cells in the islets of Langerhans. Although glucagon was discovered shortly after the advent of insulin, only recently has it been determined that it has the diabetogenic effect of raising blood sugar. The relative balance of insulin and glucagon in the blood determines whether glucose derivatives listed earlier are used for tissue building and storage (high insulin, anabolic activity) or whether they will circulate in the blood and possibly go unused (high glucagon, catabolic activity). It is not surprising that glucagon is a stimulator for insulin production, so that in the nondiabetic, the two hormones functionally balance to help maintain metabolic homeostasis.

So far, we have discussed the *physiology* of insulin production and concomitant processes rather than the *pathophysiology* occurring in diabetes. In the diabetic, there is not the delicate metabolic balance previously described. Rather, as glucose is ingested, little or no insulin is available for anabolic cell activity, so the blood sugar rises, glucose spills over into the urine, and both glycogenolysis and gluconeogenesis take place, raising the blood sugar levels even further. The next step in this process of glucose increase in the absence of insulin depends on the severity of an individual's diabetes.

Noninsulin-Dependent Diabetes.   This type of diabetes can be diagnosed at any age but is usually discovered in an individual after age 40. Although it may have some of the typical diabetic symptoms such as polyuria (increased urine output), polydipsia (increased thirst), and polyphagia (increased appetite), it has some unique properties. In the normal-weight diabetic of this type, insulin production may be reduced but does exist to some degree. In the overweight maturity-onset diabetic, insulin may be produced in normal or even supranormal quantities, but because the fat cells of the obese person are enlarged and are resistant to insulin's actions, the quantities of insulin do not have the stabilizing effect they would have in the normal person. When the obese maturity diabetic is tested for circulating insulin levels in the blood, these levels are found to be normal or above normal, though insulin's *effects* are below normal. There occurs then hepatic overproduction of glucose products as well as release of fatty acids and amino acids from adipose and muscle tissue. However, there is enough insulin available to prevent major catabolism of fatty tissues and the production of ketones.

Insulin-Dependent Diabetes.   This type of diabetes is typically diagnosed in childhood or adolescence and describes a situation in which the beta cells are virtually inactive, and endogenous insulin is simply not produced. Although there may be occasional temporary remission of the disease after diagnosis, the remission is usually short, and the individual quickly becomes fully dependent on exogenous insulin. If insulin needs are not met, ketoacidosis will occur. In the process of overproduction and underutilization of sugar, in addition to impaired triglyceride synthesis, fatty acids are released into the blood from fatty tissue, and part of these acids is metabolized in the liver into ketone bodies. Although the ketones can be used by muscle tissues, an overabundance of ketones will cause them to spill over into the urine. As the kidney prepares to excrete these strong acids it must suspend them in a fixed base, which then means substantial sodium, potassium, and water loss to the body. Because the kidney is already excreting massive amounts of water to rid the body of the excess sugar accumulating in the blood and spilling over into the urine, dehydration is a major accompaniment of the process. Eventually, urine output drops, wastes formerly secreted now pile up in the body, and nausea, vomiting, abdominal pain, and hunger for air, also called Kussmauls' breathing, can precede coma and death. Total lack of beta cell function, represented by the ability of the disease to proceed to ketoacidosis, is the prime differentiating factor for insulin-dependent as opposed to noninsulin-dependent diabetes (Brothers, 1976).

The general pathophysiology of diabetes mellitus has been documented for a number of years, and much has been written about the disastrous effects of *hyper*glycemia (overabundance of sugar) and insufficient insulin in the body. But what of the opposite situation, the *over*production of insulin and the accompaniment of too little sugar, called *hypo*glycemia?

Hypoglycemia.   Hypoglycemia has become a popular target for blame in the past decade, largely because it can produce a wide variety of symptoms such as faintness, weakness, trembling, heart palpitations, profuse sweating, and nervousness. More severe symptoms can include headache, visual impairment, staggering or even paralysis, confusion, and sometimes personality changes (Boylan & Weller, 1976). Hypoglycemia is a condition opposite that of diabetes and is characterized by high insulin levels and lower than desirable glucose levels. Inadequate amounts of blood sugar result in glucose shortages, particularly in the brain, and the nervous system disruption resulting from the brain's inadequate energy supply brings on the various symptoms already described. Functional hypoglycemia results most often from inadequate diet, excess exercise, lack of sleep, or from physical or psychological stress; and it tends to develop from an underavailability of glucose. Ford, Bray, and Swerdloff (1976) believe that preexisting psychological problems (not precipitated by the functional hypoglycemia) may be falsely attributed to the medical condition and may thus not receive the psychological treatment warranted.

Organic hypoglycemia, on the other hand, is caused by an overabundance of insulin in the bloodstream, usually resulting from a physical disorder of one of the endocrine glands, the abdomen, or the brain. An overdose of injected insulin can also put a diabetic into a hypoglycemic state. The typical etiology of and treatment for a diabetic's hypoglycemic reaction will be discussed later in the chapter. In addition to its short-term metabolic effects, diabetes can have significant long-term effects on both the vascular system and on several major body organs.

Macroangiopathy

Diabetes manifests itself in the large blood vessels (primarily arteries) by accelerating the occurrence of atherosclerosis, a narrowing of the arteries due to fatty deposits called atheroma, which thicken the arteries' inner walls and inhibit blood flow. When atherosclerosis occurs in the coronary arteries, the result can be an insufficient supply of blood to the heart (angina pectoris), which causes cardiac pain, or an actual blockage of blood to the heart (coronary occlusion), which results in a myocardial infarction or heart attack.

In diabetics, variability in insulin levels will affect lipase in its ability to metabolize fats, so various authors have proposed a direct link between atherosclerosis and diabetes (Brothers, 1976). However, high lipid levels and progressive atherosclerosis are common to much of the nondiabetic population, so there is some tendency to minimize diabetes' role in macroangiopathic complications.

Microangiopathy

Diabetic Nephropathy.   Microangiopathy is a disease of the small blood vessels, and one of the most serious types of diabetic microangiopathy occurs in the kidneys and is called "nephropathy." As in the coronary complications discussed earlier, there is a thickening of tissue, this time the basement membrane of the capillaries of the glomerulus, the major functional unit of the kidneys. In addition, nodules may form on the glomerulus. Because a primary task of the glomerular capillaries is to selectively filter wastes and water out of the blood and into the urine while retaining substances needed for proper body function, thickening of capillary walls results in loss of permeability and resultant loss of needed materials, most notably protein, from the kidney into the urine. Symptoms of diabetic nephropathy include heavy proteinuria, albumin loss, edema, hypertension, and low creatinine clearance (Steinke & Thorn, 1970). Tendency toward urinary infections increases with nephropathy and must be carefully monitored.

Diabetic Neuropathy.   Diabetic neuropathy usually involves the peripheral nervous system and/or the autonomic nervous system. It is again a case of membrane thickening (Schwann cell basement membrane) and segmental demyelinization of the nerves (Cahill, 1975). After demyelinization occurs, there is reduced ability of the nerve cell to conduct impulses. In the peripheral nervous system, there may be sensory loss in the extremities manifested by impaired deep tendon reflexes, loss of proprioception and pain, and some numbness in the extremities. There may also be neuromuscular weakness. Neuropathy involving the autonomic nervous system, on the other hand, manifests itself in hypotension, dysfunctional pupil constriction in the eye, gastrointestinal disorders, genitourinary disturbances, and certain skin disorders.

Peripheral vascular disease is a combined microangiopathic/macroangiopathic complication of diabetes and basically results in poor circulation to the extremities, particularly lower legs and feet. Foot ulcer and gangrene of the foot are serious neuropathic complications for diabetics.

Diabetic Retinopathy.   Diabetic retinopathy is the microangiopathic involvement of the tiny blood vessels in the retina of the eye. Diabetic retinopathy is the second leading cause of blindness among all adults in the United States and the leading cause for young adults. The exact cause of retinopathy is not known, but retinal hypoxia (caused by a variety of factors) and resulting endothelial and mural cell dysfunction has been posited as a probable cause (Blankenship & Skyler, 1978). The thickening of the capillary basement membrane is also part of the process. The pathophysiology of retinopathy is complex, and the extent of its progression determines whether a diabetic will have essentially normal vision, impaired vision, or even blindness. Nearly every diabetic has some degree of background retinopathy, which includes microaneurysms, small hemorrhages, and hard exudates on the back of the retina. There are also dilated capillary shunt vessels that develop to ensure perfusion of the retina when normal vessels are inoperative because of membrane thickening or other pathology. Background retinopathy will not diminish vision to any great extent unless there is involvement of the macula, an extremely sensitive portion of the retina responsible for central visual acuity, or unless the routine retinopathy increases.

Proliferative retinopathy is dangerous to sight and occurs when there is accelerated growth of many capillary shunts to form a network of blood vessels on the back of the eye, usually on the inner retinal surface or on the back of the formed vitreous. This network or neovascularization is dangerous because the vessels are thin-walled and delicate and are subject to rupture and hemorrhage inside the vitreous. Although hemorrhages usually do clear in time, excessive hemorrhage will cloud the vitreous, inhibiting light from passing through it, thereby greatly reducing visual acuity. In addition, the vessel network, often attached to both the vitreous and the retina, can be pulled by the vitreous into the vitreous cavity and can thereby elevate and detach sections of the retina. Again, vision is lost. Proliferation near the macula can impair central vision, whereas peripheral retinal involvement affects only peripheral vision. However, involvement of the optic disc usually signals inexorable progression to major visual impairment (Blankenship & Skyler, 1978). Although there is no known prevention of diabetic retinopathy, in recent years there have been several innovative treatments used (e.g., laser treatment) to restore some vision and retard further visual loss in many diabetics (Blankenship & Skyler, 1978).

Diabetes in Children—Physical Factors

Juvenile diabetes has customarily been described as insulin-dependent or ketoacidosis-prone diabetes that has its onset before full adulthood, usually by age 20. Although both adults and children who suffer from ketoacidosis-prone diabetes experience many of the same problems, in this section we discuss this type of diabetes as it is experienced by children and adolescents.

The peak year for onset of diabetes in children is age 11, and infection is a frequent precursor of the disease. The disease can begin much more dramatically in children than in adults, with acute thirst, urination, and weight loss occurring over a few days or weeks. In addition, children may exhibit fatigue and irritability. A diagnosis is usually made quite readily by blood and urine analyses, and although a period of remission may occur after the diagnosis is made, this remission is of short duration, and customarily the youngster becomes fully dependent on exogenous insulin. Thus most children are insulin-dependent.

Oral hypoglycemics are not used, as the child has no appreciable beta cell function, but diet, exercise, and insulin treatment have daily relevance to the youthful diabetic. The importance and the difficulties of dietary management are magnified for the youth with diabetes. Insistence on sugar-free diet is maintained by some diabetologists, though Schmitt (1975) speaks strongly for an unmeasured diet (with restrictions on types of food allowed), as he believes that the over-emphasis on diet may cause more problems of psychological stress, family disruption, and noncompliance than it is worth. Most authorities still take a more conservative approach, however, and urge diet limitations, while allowing enough flexibility and total calorie intake to account for the juvenile's activity pattern and growth rate.

Exercise is encouraged but also must be carefully managed, as hypoglycemic reactions may occur if unplanned or particularly strenuous exercise is not compensated for by decreased insulin or, preferably, increased calorie intake. Insulin must be carefully and constantly evaluated, as exogenous insulin requirements change with growth (Klam, Rohn, & Heald, 1975). Although need for exogenous insulin may drastically decrease during the remission phase described previously, most authorities continue administration of very small insulin doses during this period, believing that continuity of treatment is important and that a start – stop – start pattern can cause psychological stress.

STANDARD MEDICAL TREATMENTS

Diet

Although there are differing views regarding the specifics of diabetic diet, nearly all medical authorities view diet as extremely important in treating diabetes (Brothers, 1976; Steinke & Soeldner, 1977). Achievement of normal body weight is a high priority, as there is a growing number of overweight, obese diabetics. Obesity is often accompanied by ingestion of high amounts of glucose, clearly an unhealthy commodity, and also by enlarged fat cells that are resistant to insulin's actions. Diet for the obese diabetic must be two-pronged, aimed at both weight reduction and regularity and balance of food intake. A diabetic's reducing diet is similar to any other reducing diet and must be correlated carefully with insulin or oral hypoglycemic agents. When an acceptable weight is achieved, the diabetic can eat a more substantial but only slightly more varied diet. For many years, carbohydrates were considered anathema, but current medical regimes include carbohydrates as 40 – 60% of the diabetic's average daily caloric intake. Starches rather than purer sugars (cake, jelly, candy, etc.) are recommended because they are absorbed more slowly and do not cause the sharp peak in sugar levels brought on by pure glucose. In addition, reduction in dietary cholesterol is usually recommended. Diabetics are often encouraged to eat frequent, small meals in order to keep glucose at a constant level and avoid sharp peaks and dips, which can result in either sugar spillage or hypoglycemic reactions. In addition to careful selection of foods and timing of meals, diabetics must control their portions and keep accurate account of the calories they ingest.

In keeping with our modern society of fast living and fast foods, the American Diabetes Association has prepared exchange lists, which list the foods on a typical diabetic diet and their equivalent exchanges in popular or fast food. An example of an exchange list is shown in Fig. 18.1. Diet is a major concern in diabetic therapy because many diabetics can be maintained with careful diet alone and no oral hypoglycemics or insulin. In addition, good diet linked with good diabetic control is believed by many authorities to inhibit the development of secondary diabetic complications (Boylan & Weller, 1976; Steinke & Thorn, 1970).

Exercise

Most diabetic individuals can engage in exercise. Exercise complements diet, potentiating the weight loss of the reducing diet for the overweight diabetic and contributing to overall fitness and good health for the normal weight diabetic. Nearly all types of exercise and sports are appropriate for the otherwise healthy diabetic (excluding flying, skydiving, and other sports where a diabetic reaction of some kind could jeopardize safety). However, a diabetic must compensate for exercise by reduced insulin or by ingestion of some sugar before the activity, as accelerated physical activity reduces glucose levels and can result in hypoglycemic reactions.

Insulin Treatment

Exogenous insulin has been widely used since 1921 to supplement or replace endogenous insulin. The majority of insulin manufactured in the United States is bovine insulin, drawn from the pancreas of slaughtered cattle. Porcine insulin, a purer insulin drawn from pigs, is less available and more expensive. Most commercial insulin preparations are a combination of bovine and porcine insulin, though pure insulins can be obtained. In addition to different sources of insulin, there are also different types. These range from rapid-action (crystalline, regular) insulin to intermediate-action (globin, NPH, lente) to prolonged-action (ultralente, protamine zinc). Because the goal of diabetic control is to keep glucose and insulin levels in harmony, many experts now urge that a combination of rapid-acting and intermediate insulin be administered twice daily, before breakfast and before dinner. This allows the glucose-insulin balance to be better maintained around the clock.

A recent innovation in diabetic care is home monitoring of blood sugar levels. The patient is taught to obtain a blood sample and test it for glucose, either "reading" it on a monitor or visually. This can be done once or several times daily and allows the patient to titrate insulin dosages more exactly. Urine testing,

Exchange Values for Fast Foods

	The exchange system		
	Bread	(Med) Meat	Fat
ARTHUR TREACHER'S (fish, chips, coleslaw)			
3-piece dinner	6	4	9
2-piece dinner	3½	2½	8
BURGER CHEF			
Hamburger	1½	1	1½
Double Hamburger	2	2½	1
Super Chef	2½	3½	2
Big Chef	3	3	3
French Fries	2	—	2
BURGER KING			
Hamburger	1½	1½	½
Double Hamburger	2	3	—
Whopper	3	3	4
Whopper, Jr.	1½	2	1
French Fries	2	—	2½
KENTUCKY FRIED CHICKEN (Fried chicken, mashed potatoes, coleslaw, rolls)			
3-piece dinner—Original	4	6	2½
—Crispy	5	6	6½
2-piece dinner—Original	3½	2	1½
—Crispy	3	4½	3½
LONG JOHN SILVER'S (fish, chips, coleslaw)			
3-piece dinner	7	6	7
2-piece dinner	6	4	6
McDONALD'S			
Hamburger	1½	1	1½
Double Hamburger	2	2	1
Quarter Pounder	2½	3	1
Big Mac	3	2	4
French Fries	1½	—	2
PIZZA HUT (Cheese pizza)			
Individual—Thick crust	9½	7½	—
—Thin crust	8½	6	—
½ of 13-inch—Thick crust	7½	7	—
—Thin crust	7	5	—
½ of 15-inch—Thick crust	10	9	—
—Thin crust	9½	7	—

FIG. 18.1 Exchange list of regular and fast foods (Midgley, W., 1979).

frequently performed by diabetics on a daily basis, continues to be necessary to check for the presence of ketones in the urine.

The recently introduced Hemoglobin AlC test also makes monitoring of blood sugar more effective. This test is done in a physician's office and reflects the diabetic's sugar levels for the preceding 3 months. Thus the diabetic and the physician can monitor diabetic control on a continuing basis.

Adjusting an individual's insulin dosage to correlate well with body chemistry and life-style can be a difficult, time-consuming task. If there is too little insulin, there will be hyperglycemia. If there is too much insulin, a hypoglycemic reaction can occur.

A diabetic's hypoglycemic reaction is usually caused by excess insulin dosage, delayed food intake, or strenuous exercise. Reactions may vary, as typical reaction to crystalline insulin involves hunger, sweating, tremor, palpitation, tachycardia, weakness, irritability, and pallor, whereas a reaction to excessive lente insulin may manifest headache, blurred vision, tremor, sleepiness, hypothermia, and confusion (Steinke & Thorn, 1970). A beginning reaction can be halted by ingestion of pure sugar from cubes or packets (something the diabetic should carry at all times), whereas for a serious reaction involving an unconscious or nearly unconscious diabetic, a knowledgeable bystander can inject a glucagon mixture directly into the bloodstream to raise the glucose level quickly. Because hypoglycemic reactions can mimic drunken or other stuporous states, many diabetics carry identification cards so that a hypoglycemic reaction can be recognized and treated accurately.

Because hypoglycemic reactions resulting in coma can be confused with the very different state of ketoacidosis, we will briefly differentiate the two. In a hypoglycemic reaction, there is too much insulin for existing sugar levels, and the symptoms are some combination of those listed in the preceding paragraph. When ketoacidosis occurs, there is too little insulin available, and symptoms include nausea, vomiting, abdominal pain, dehydration, and Kussmaul breathing. The two reactions can be differentiated by symptoms and more definitely by blood analyses, with treatment for hypoglycemia consisting of glucose, and treatment for ketoacidosis consisting of insulin and i.v. solutions to replenish lost sodium and potassium (Steinke & Thorn, 1970).

An additional reaction frequent in older persons is hyperglycemic nonketonic coma, manifesting glucose elevation but no ketones. The treatment of choice is insulin and intravenous hypotonic saline solution (Steinke & Thorn, 1970).

Some possible complications of insulin treatment include localized allergic reactions at the injection site, insulin lipodystrophy of tissue at the injection site, or insulin resistance, all of which can usually be ameliorated. Even after type and quantity of insulin have been regulated and any adverse reactions overcome, the issue of administering the insulin remains.

Insulin is available in two strengths, U40 and U100, and is administered on a routine basis by injection. Although various injection techniques have been advocated, Brothers' (1976) suggestion of rapid penetration at right angles to the skin appears quite reasonable. Although some people consider injections to be aversive, insulin-dependent diabetics become adept at administering their own insulin and proceed to do it as simply as someone else might swallow a vitamin. Someone in the diabetic's family should also know how to administer an injection so that glucagon can be given if the diabetic has a severe hypoglycemic reaction.

Oral Hypoglycemics

The oral hypoglycemic agents are extremely useful with many maturity-onset diabetics who produce some quantity of insulin but cannot be controlled by diet therapy alone. The sulfonylureas (related to sulfa compounds) consist of tolbutamide (orinase), acetohexamide (dymelor), chlorpropamide (diabinase), and tolazamide (tolinase), which differ primarily in their length of action and in some potential side effects. The sulfonylureas, given in tablet form, appear to increase hepatic glucose output, but more importantly, they stimulate secretion of endogenous insulin by the beta cells. Thus they can be used only in patients who have some functional beta cells. The other type of oral hypoglycemic, the biguanides, has been taken off the market by the Food and Drug Administration because of its potentially serious gastrointestinal side effects.

There are some problems that must be noted with all the oral hypoglycemics. Perhaps the major problem is the tendency of some diabetics and their physicians to depend on the medications to replace adequate dietary control. In fact, medication is intended to supplement, not replace good diet. There are also risks of hypoglycemic reactions with these drugs, alcohol intolerance, possible kidney disturbance, and increased risk of heart disease. The last finding resulted from a well-known study by the University Group Diabetes Program (UGDP) (Steinke & Soeldner, 1977). Thus the oral hypoglycemic agents must be used with great caution.

Health Care Problems of the Diabetic

The diabetic patient really needs to be his or her own physician; no one else has as much control over total health care. The habits of good foot care such as daily washing, careful nail trimming, well-fitting shoes, etc., are potentially very important if a long-term diabetic wishes to prevent gangrene in lower extremities afflicted with vascular lesions or neuropathy. Infection or other systemic illness is particularly problematic, as metabolism may be thrown off, and typical eating schedules may change. In this situation, the diabetic is usually advised to take the customary medication, monitor himself or herself closely, and perhaps consult a physician. Although surgery was at one time rather risky for the diabetic, surgical risks for the diabetic and nondiabetic are now comparable. A diabetic may be admitted to the hospital earlier than normal, however, so that the diabetes can be carefully controlled throughout surgery and recovery.

Pregnancy, once considered difficult to achieve and risky to maintain for diabetic women, is now more common. Careful control of diabetes is viewed as the best way to insure good health for both mother and child, and this usually requires increased amounts of insulin during the third trimester. Most babies formerly were delivered by Caesarian section, though more normal deliveries are now done. Careful teamwork by the patient, the diabetologist, the obstetrician, and later the pediatrician, is required. (As pregnancy is a stress situation, note that some women develop "stress" diabetes during pregnancy but return to normoglycemia after the pregnancy is over.)

We have discussed diabetes mellitus as a disease entity and have reviewed its classification, diagnosis, treatment, and complications. In the remainder of the chapter, we address the psychological and social ramifications of the disease.

PSYCHOSOCIAL CONSIDERATIONS

Psychological Theories

Although researchers have attempted to identify emotional or stress factors that precipitate the occurrence of diabetes and have even tried to delineate a "diabetic personality," such research has not offered firm data, and the level of interest in this area has declined somewhat in recent years (Treuting, 1962). Mirsky surveyed emotional factors in diabetes many years ago (1948) and singled out chronic psychological tension that results in chronic physiological arousal as a logical precipitating factor in diabetes. He also pointed to eating disturbances in the diabetic's infancy as possibly related to the obesity that is a major precipitating factor in adult diabetes. A few years later, Hinkle and Wolf (1952) posited a relationship between life stress and diabetes, believing that loss of security or an intimate relationship caused a pathological physical reaction in predisposed or strongly conditioned adults. More recently, Grant, Kyle, Teichman, and Mendels (1974) have discussed the relationship between stressful life events and fluctuations in diabetes, finding at least a strongly "suggestive" relationship between negative life events and diabetic lability. On the other hand, Koh and Molnar (1974) found no uniform personality profile in unstable diabetes, no evidence of preexisting stress precipitating diabetic onset, and no change in blood glucose level for one patient monitored during an emotional stress period. There does not appear to be an unequivocal link between stress and either diabetes onset or lability.

Anxiety and depression have been found in many adult diabetics as well as in their families (Sanders, Mills, Martin, & Horne, 1975). Though there is often denial or disbelief after the initial diagnosis, this may give way to anger or to passive resignation. The patient may feel overwhelmed and anxious at assuming responsibility for his or her disease control, while depression may occur because of repressed anger about the disease, fear of long-term complications, or feelings of grief and loss that frequently accompany a physical disability.

Although all diabetologists have observed some diabetics who use their illness to display hysterical, dependent, or aggressive personality features, most diabetics are as emotionally healthy as nondiabetics. Most research studies on the psychological precursors as well as concomitants of diabetes are severely methodologically flawed, and much more precise research is needed.

Sexual Dysfunction and Marital Stress

Sexual dysfunction is a topic too often ignored. For men who have been diabetic over 6 years, 48% may have impotence problems (Renshaw, 1975). This figure is much higher than for a comparable group of nondiabetic males. Although there may indeed be reduced pituitary gonadotropin as well as sterility in diabetics, there are also likely to be various psychosocial problems that can be completely masked by a too hasty diagnosis of functional impotence. Renshaw notes the existence of possible neurological or vascular problems but is also careful to give considerable weight to the possible effects of depression, alcohol, anxiety, and anger on male (and female) sexual performance. Females may have functional problems because of decreased genital sensitivity, orgasmic capacity, and vaginal lubrication, but may also be affected by psychogenic factors. In a study of wives of diabetic men, Katz (1969) found that in this sample of couples with identified marriage problems, the wives complained bitterly about their husbands' sexual difficulties yet did little to ameliorate the problem. For these couples, the diabetes in part served as a "medium" for acting out longstanding marital conflicts. In looking at the impact of physical disability (including diabetes) on overall marital adjustment, Peterson (1979) found that there is indeed a relationship between marital stress and a spouse's physical handicap, but the actual extent of the stress is less related to the severity of the handicap than to the partners' role flexibility and realistic expectations of their own and each other's behavior. Thus the actual severity of diabetes, including possible sexual dysfunction, will impact a couple less if they have a realistic idea of what can be expected from the disorder and what control they can have over disease-related occurrences.

Employability and Economics

The employment pattern of diabetics is not given great attention in the literature, though career counseling is frequently part of the diabetic's rehabilitation.Most experts believe that diabetics can be employed in nearly all careers and professions. Well-controlled diabetics do not show a higher rate of absenteeism from work, and though they are often hard to insure, most diabetics will not develop the serious and costly medical complications outlined earlier in this chapter. Restrictions on employment do exist, however, as no diabetic can be a commercial airline pilot, and insulin-dependent diabetics are discouraged from operating dangerous heavy machinery or driving commercial vehicles. In most cases, diabetics perform comparably to nondiabetics.

Economically, diabetes is an expense to us all. Although estimates vary, Entmacher (1976) reports that the cost of diabetes in the United States in 1973 was four *billion* dollars. This figure is achieved by adding the direct costs due to the illness itself (i.e., prevention, physicians' care, medications, rehabilitation), indirect costs due to morbidity (lost earnings because of lowered productivity due to illness and disability), and indirect costs due to mortality (discounted present value of normal lifetime earnings of deceased diabetics) (p. 33). Although some would argue with this method of cost computation, if we assume that the costs of diabetes even approached four billion dollars in 1973, we must acknowledge that diabetes mellitus is a costly disease in terms of both human welfare and economics.

Counseling Approaches

The diabetic who receives counseling has traditionally been a patient with secondary complications who looks for aid within a rehabilitation counseling setting. In such a setting, the diabetic can receive acceptance and support, be presented with a "health-improvement" rather than a "sickness" approach to his or her disabilities, and, after testing and possible work evaluation, can look at both work and recreational possibilities. This type of counseling is typically available through a state's department of vocational rehabilitation, and special help targeted to the blind diabetic comes from the state's services for the visually handicapped.

More attention is gradually being paid to the psychosocial needs of the diabetic and his or her family. Rehabilitation is clearly still needed, but there is a commensurate need for early intervention. Supportive counseling, clear and repetitive education, and family communication training can be useful in teaching newly diagnosed diabetics and their families to be realistic and clear about their behavioral expectations of themselves and each other. Learning to handle diabetes in healthy ways may even influence the family's handling of problems unrelated to the disease. Virginia Satir says about families that when one family member hurts, all family members hurt (Satir, 1967), so the diagnosis of diabetes has implications for every family member. Family group therapy with diabetic families may thus be useful.

Diabetics can also profit from the newly developing area of sex therapy. First of all, just talking about the problem can be the first step in a couple's coping with sexual dysfunction. If functional impotence is the problem, sexually satisfactory alternatives to intercourse can be taught, or in some cases, a male may obtain an implant to achieve a partial, if permanent, erection. Comparable alternatives can be offered the sexually impaired female. And along with the tangible solutions go education and improved communication about sexuality in general. The best way to insure that the diabetic gets all the help he or she needs is to make diabetic education programs available to everyone.

Outpatient Educational Programs

Though some diabetologists favor an intensive inpatient diagnostic and educational experience for a newly diagnosed diabetic, the need for *continuing* education has been stressed and can best be implemented in an outpatient setting. Several investigators (Ludvigsson, 1977; Simon & Stewart, 1976) report that diabetics are poorly educated about their disorder and its control, and the authors stress the need for nonphysician medical personnel to assume a greater share in diabetic education. An innovative program at Detroit General Hospital (Power, Bakker, & Cooper, 1973) employs a nurse–clinician with special diabetic training who sees patients on a regular basis and uses the backup of a physician only when necessary. In addition, a health care team of nurses, dieticians, social workers, and various aides attempts to meet the continuous and total health care needs of the over 3000 patients who frequent the facility. Visual aids and written materials are used in most educational programs (Hassell & Medved, 1975), and group training plus audiovisual materials may be more effective than traditional one-to-one education with a dietician. The trend for diabetic education seems to be toward outpatient facilities, group instruction, and greater use of nonphysician health-care personnel, particularly the nurse–clinician. Because most education programs have only been evaluated from a patient-satisfaction basis, there is a great need for research on program effectiveness.

Compliance

Many professionals have found that merely making good health care available in no way assures that people will use it to their best advantage (Ryan & Dutton, 1977), so compliance is a major issue in behavioral medicine. Although various factors influence compliance, one study explored the phenomenon as a patient–doctor interaction rather than as only the patient's problem (Hulka, Cassel, Kupper, & Burdette, 1976). These researchers found that of the medication errors that occurred in their sample of over 350 diabetics, 19% of the errors were due to "omissions" (not taking medication), 19% to "commissions" (taking too much or the wrong medications), 17% to "misconceptions" (not knowing what medication to take), and only 3% to "scheduling noncompliance." In addition, the more medications an individual was taking and the more complex the administration schedule, the more errors occurred. Errors were reduced when the patient had a thorough knowledge of why he or she was taking the medications and what each medication was for. The medication errors in this study were not so much of "compliance" as of "communication" between doctor and patient and again demonstrate the need for thorough education.

One of the issues in compliance that has emerged recently is locus of control. Although certain studies have shown that subjects with an internal locus of control (self-responsibility) were more likely to engage in specific health behaviors than subjects with external locus of control (Straits & Sechrest, 1963), other studies have had different results (Best & Steffy, 1971). One step in improving compliance is to assess a patient's perceived locus of control in order to choose a therapeutic regime most appropriate for that patient. Wallston, Wallston, and DeVellis (1978) have had some success in developing a health-related locus of control scale that offers specificity of content not found in more general locus of control scales. Compliance is clearly a major issue for diabetics (Becker & Maiman, 1975; Simonds, 1979).

Diabetes in Children—Psychosocial Factors

Emotional Factors. Children who receive a diagnosis of diabetes may experience the same resistance or denial that is common to adults but, in addition, may construct explanations for the disease. They may see it as a punishment for negative behavior or a failure by their parents to adequately protect them from harm (Prazar & Felice, 1975). In order to avoid the development of mythology about diabetes, children must be given clear, accurate, and repetitive information about the etiology and the management of the disorder. Because of their ability to influence their own health (via diet, exercise, and insulin), children and adolescents must be involved in planning and care. Young diabetics are encouraged to exert control over what and when they eat and should be taught to administer their own insulin as soon as it is practical (usually by age 11 or 12). The assumption of responsibility for their own care may be an onerous task for some youth, though diabetic children demonstrate a normal ego structure (Fallstrom, 1975) and are likely to develop stronger inner controls for behavior than nondiabetic youth as long as they, not their parents, are primarily responsible for care. Academic and social skills are usually acquired fairly normally, though many diabetic youth feel the stigma of being different from their peers and may have an abnormal body image because of their handicap (Fallstrom, 1975).

Adolescence is a time of disruption for most youth, and diabetics are no exception. Anger and rebellion toward authority and particularly parents may cause the diabetic to eat forbidden foods or alter insulin dosage in order to test limits. The adolescent's need for peer acceptance and sexual identity may be exacerbated by the diabetes, though parental understanding and outside supportive counseling mitigate some of the adolescent's distress. Basically, teenage stresses are not so much altered as magnified for the youthful diabetic.

Family Aspects. The family is an important ingredient in treatment. If the diabetic's parents are educated about the disease, offer help and support, encourage independence, stress a "health-care" orientation to the disease (what is healthy) rather than a "sickness" orientation (what is unhealthy) (Cull & Hardy, 1974), and in general focus on the child rather than the disease, normal family development and interaction should ensue. However, this optimum level of behavior is extremely difficult to achieve. In fact, poor family coping with diabetes is fairly common. Obsessive concern with diabetic control by parents can result in either rebelliousness or in almost overcompliance by a child, neither extreme a healthy one. On the other hand, denial of or uninvolvement with the diabetes by parents can be disastrous. Delbridge (1975) examined juvenile diabetics with varying amounts of control and found that poor diabetic management was related to less understanding and less acceptance of the disorder by the family as well as lower overall family adjustment. If management is poor, there is greater incidence of ketoacidosis, more frequent hospitalizations, and then even greater family disruption. When parents, especially mothers (who are usually more involved with diabetes management) focus on the "burden" aspects of the child's disease, guilt and anger may be important factors for both child and parents. In addition, the diabetic's siblings may experience rejection and anger because of the energy focused by the parents on the ill child (Prazar & Felice, 1975).

Salvador Minuchin and his colleagues have done innovative work with extremely labile diabetic children and their families. Using family interviews, Minuchin has looked at interaction patterns, while also measuring free fatty acid levels in blood samples of subjects. He has found that free fatty acid levels of labile diabetics as compared to levels of controls rose dramatically when the child was placed in a conflictive family situation. Such conflict-prone families appeared to be poorly differentiated, with family members, especially the diabetic, overinvolved in other members' conflicts and communication. In a very real sense, the family displaced its conflicts onto the diabetic child and showed both rigidity and an inability to resolve difficult issues (Segal, 1977). The goals of family treatment with such a family include clarifying communication, bringing conflict into the open, and removing the diabetic child as the focus of family problems.

Bauer and Kenny (1975) believe that diabetes reflects physiologic vulnerability of the patient, a series of stressful events, and dysfunctional family interaction. They delineate various types of pathological family qualities such as enmeshment, overprotectiveness, lack of conflict resolution, rigidity, and involvement of the child in parental conflict. They describe a treatment model that employs ongoing individual therapy for the patient and family therapy for the total family group. Anderson and Auslander (1980) stress the need for a systems approach to family treatment that takes into account the family's personal and social supports as well as the medical setting in which the youth receives ongoing treatment.

Diabetic Camps.   There are approximately 50 summer camps that conduct programs for diabetic youth (White, 1974). Although some camps offer primarily a "safe" camp experience for the diabetic child, other camps offer educational experiences and specific interventions in diabetic treatment. There may be special lectures and instruction, and sometimes a child's therapeutic regimen may be changed. Although improved management and greater understanding of diabetes may result, the primary benefit from camps is the opportunity for juvenile diabetics to observe and share experiences with other young diabetics. Frequently the camps are staffed by diabetics who serve as effectively functioning role models for the youngsters. In addition, classic camping activities such as sports and overnight camp-outs offer excellent opportunities for diabetic children to try new things and feel both competent and "normal." A list of diabetic camps can be obtained from the American Diabetes Association.

We have paid more than cursory attention in this section to the psychosocial aspects of diabetes. Because medicine has yet found no cure for diabetes and because, in the meantime, diabetics and their families encounter psychosocial problems on a daily basis, professionals in the area are beginning to take a broader look at the disease and its ramifications.

The Future

Improved treatment and ultimate cure are contemporary goals in diabetic research. Although beta cell transplants and total pancreatic transplants have been performed, such operations show a low success rate because of rejection problems.

More promising developments are in the areas of insulin manufacture and delivery. Biosynthetic human insulin has been successfully manufactured and is chemically identical to pancreatic human insulin. It is being used in large clinical trials (Skyler, Pfeiffer, Raptis, & Viberti, 1981) and will hopefully be fully available in the near future. A newly developed insulin pump is now used by many diabetics. The pump is about the size of a hand calculator and is worn on a belt. Continuous base levels of regular insulin are released from the pump through a subcutaneous needle usually implanted in the individual's thigh. This is called an *open-loop* insulin feedback system because the insulin is dispensed at a consistent rate regardless of the body's fluctuating blood sugar levels. A *closed-loop* feedback system that monitors the individual's glucose level and releases insulin accordingly has been developed but is large and unwieldy, and is presently used only in medical centers. If this can be miniaturized and implanted, it would function as an artificial pancreas. The technology of diabetic treatment is progressing rapidly and offers great promise for the future.

Summary

We have seen that diabetes mellitus is a disease of ancient origin that is still prevalent and problematic today. The discovery of insulin in 1921 marked the beginning of modern medical treatment of diabetes. There are several million diagnosed diabetics in the United States, and there may be fully as many undiagnosed. Although increased age and obesity are predisposing factors in diabetes, the disease has a polygenetic heredity pattern and may even be precipitated by a virus. Diabetes can be classified into insulin-dependent, noninsulin-dependent, and several related categories. Diagnosis of diabetes mellitus can sometimes be made from physical symptoms alone or with a urine test, but most often it is made from a glucose tolerance test.

Diabetes results when an individual's beta cells do not produce enough insulin to metabolize all the glucose in the individual's system. Insulin is important also in metabolizing fats and protein, so an insulin deficiency thus causes many body processes to malfunction. Such malfunctioning results in symptoms of polydipsia, polyuria, and polyphagia. Diabetics who are totally or almost totally dependent on exogenous insulin are prone to ketoacidosis if the need for insulin is not met. This serious condition is characterized by nausea, dehydration, abdominal pain, increased acids in the urine, and labored or Kussmaul breathing, and is remedied by insulin and fluids. Hypoglycemia, a condition where there is too much insulin for existing glucose, is easily remedied on a short-term basis by the administration of sugar.

Long-term complications to diabetes can develop as vascular microangiopathy or macroangiopathy, or as diabetic retinopathy. We have discussed various types of complications within these categories, and their treatments. General treatment for diabetes consists of diet, exercise, insulin, and oral hypoglycemic agents. Though some physicians do not emphasize strict diabetic control, most diabetologists urge that the disease be as well controlled as possible.

We have surveyed the special problems of the youthful diabetic, noting the interaction of particular physical and emotional aspects of the disease with the child or adolescent's various developmental stages. A healthy and well-functioning family unit is of great importance to diabetic management. Diabetic summer camps are beneficial for juvenile diabetics.

Various stress factors have been identified in the course and possibly also in the onset of diabetes, and emotional health, marital satisfaction, and family stability all can affect diabetic control. Counseling of both patient and family can ameliorate some of the emotional concomitants of the disease. Compliance in treatment is poor, and great need exists for more comprehensive education programs for diabetics. Technological advances in diabetic treatment offer great promise for the future.

REFERENCES

Anderson, B. J., & Auslander, W. F. Research on diabetic management and the family: A critique. *Diabetes Care*, 1980, *3*, 696–702.

Bauer, R., & Kenny, T. J. Psychologic management of juvenile diabetes. *Pediatric Annal*, 1975, *4*(6), 72–78.

Becker, M. H., & Maiman, L. A. Sociobehavioral determinants of compliance with health and medical care recommendations. *Medical Care*, 1975, *13*, 10–24.

Best, J. A., & Steffy, R. A. Smoking modification tailored to subject characteristics. *Behavior Therapy*, 1971,*2*, 177–191.

Blankenship, G. W., & Skyler, J. S. Diabetic retinopathy: A general survey. *Diabetes Care*, 1978, *1*, 127–137.

Boylan, B., & Weller, C. *The new way to live with diabetes*. Garden City, N.Y.: Dolphin, 1976.

Brothers, M. *Diabetes: The new approach*. New York: Grosset & Dunlap, 1976.

Cahill, G. F. Diabetes mellitus. In P. B. Beeson & W. McDermott (Eds.), *Textbook of medicine* (14 ed.) Philadelphia: W.B. Saunders, 1975.

Cull, J. G., & Hardy, R. E. (Eds.). *Counseling and rehabilitating the diabetic*. Springfield, Ill.: Charles C. Thomas, 1974.

Delbridge, L. Educational and psychological factors in the management of diabetes in children. *Medical Journal of Australia*, 1975, *2*, 737–739.

Entmacher, P. S. Economic impact of diabetes. In S. S. Fajans (Ed.), *Diabetes mellitus* (DHEW Pub. No. NIH 76–854). Bethesda, Md.: Department of Health, Education, and Welfare, 1976.

Fallstrom, K. On the personality structure in diabetic school children aged 7–15 years. *Acta Paediatrica Scandinavica*, 1975, Supplement 251.

Ford, C. V., Bray, G. A., & Swerdloff, R. S. A psychiatric study of patients referred with a diagnosis of hypoglycemia. *American Journal of Psychiatry*, 1976, *133*, 290–294.

Grant, I., Kyle, G. C., Teichman, A., & Mendels, J. Recent life events and diabetes in adults. *Psychosomatic Medicine*, 1974, *36*, 121–128.

Hamburg, B. A., Lipsett, L. F., Inoff, G. E., & Drash, A. L. (Eds.). *Behavioral and psychosocial issues in diabetes: Proceedings of the national conference* (NIH No. 80–1993). Washington, D.C.: United States Department of Health and Human Services, 1979.

Hassell, J., & Medved, E. Group/audiovisual instruction for patients with diabetes. *Journal of the American Dietetic Association*, 1975, *66*, 465–470.

Hinkle, L. E., & Wolf, S. A summary of experimental evidence relating life stress to diabetes mellitus. *Journal of the Mount Sinai Hospital*, 1952, *19*, 537–570.

Hulka, B. S., Cassell, J. C., Kupper, L. L., & Burdette, J. A. Communication, compliance, and concordance between physicians and patients with prescribed medications. *American Journal of Public Health*, 1976, *66*, 847–853.

Katz, A. M. Wives of diabetic men. *Bulletin of the Menninger Clinic*, 1969, *3*, 279–294.

Klam, W. P., Rohn, R. D., & Heald, F. Care of the diabetic adolescent. *Pediatric Annal*, 1975, *4*(6), 38–47.

Koh, M. F., & Molnar, G. D. Psychiatric aspects of patients with unstable diabetes mellitus. *Psychosomatic Medicine*, 1974, *36*, 57–68.

Ludvigsson, J. Socio-psychological factors and metabolic control in juvenile diabetes. *Acta Paediatrica Scandinavica*, 1977, *66*, 431–437.

Midgley, W. On the fast food trail. *Diabetes Forecast*, 1979, *32*(4), 20–23.

Mirsky, I. A. Emotional factors in the patient with diabetes mellitus. *Bulletin of the Menninger Clinic*, 1948, *12*, 187–194.

Notkins, A. L. The causes of diabetes. *Scientific American*, 1979, *241*(5), 62–73.

Peterson, Y. The impact of physical disability on marital adjustment: A literature review. *Family Coordinator*, 1979, *28*, 47–51.

Power, L., Bakker, D. L., & Cooper, M. I. *Diabetes outpatient care through physicians' assistants*. Springfield, Ill.: Charles C. Thomas, 1973.

Prazar, G., & Felice, M. The psychologic and social effects of juvenile diabetes. *Pediatric Annal*, 1975, *4*(6), 59–70.

Renshaw, D. C. Impotence in diabetics. *Diseases of the Nervous System*, 1975, *36*, 369–371.

Ryan, L. K., & Dutton, C. B. Utilization of a nutrition service in a neighborhood health center. *American Journal of Public Health*, 1977, *67*, 565–567.

Sanders, K., Mills, J., Martin, F., & Horne, I. Emotional attitudes in adult insulin-dependent diabetics. *Journal of Psychosomatic Research*, 1975, *19*, 241–246.

Satir, V. *Conjoint family therapy.* Palo Alto, Calif.: Science and Behavior Books, 1967.

Schmitt, B. D. An argument for the unmeasured diet in juvenile diabetes mellitus. The physical and emotional risks of the measured diet. *Clinical Pediatrics,* 1975, *14,* 68–73.

Segal, J. *Psychosomatic diabetic children and their families* (DHEW Pub. No. ADM 74–477). Bethesda, Md.: Department of Health, Education, and Welfare, 1977.

Simon, J. W., & Stewart, M. M. Assessing patient knowledge about diabetes. *Mt. Sinai Journal of Medicine,* 1976, *43,* 189–202.

Simonds, J. F. Emotions and compliance in diabetic children. *Psychosomatics,* 1979, *20,* 544–551.

Skyler, J. S., Pfeiffer, E. F., Raptis, S., & Viberti, G. C. Biosynthetic human insulin: Progress and prospects. *Diabetes Care,* 1981, *4,* 140–143.

Steinke, J., & Soeldner, J. S. Diabetes mellitus. In G. W. Thorn, R. D. Adams, E. Braunwald, K. J. Isselbacher, & R. G. Petersdorf (Eds.), *Harrison's principles of internal medicine* (8th ed.). New York: McGraw–Hill, 1977.

Steinke, J., & Thorn, G. W. Diabetes mellitus. In M. M. Wintrobe, G. W. Thorn, R. D. Adams, I. L. Bennett, Jr., E. Braunwald, K. J. Isselbacher, & R. G. Petersdorf (Eds.), *Harrison's principles of internal medicine* (6th ed.). New York: McGraw–Hill, 1970.

Straits, B., & Sechrest, L. Further support of some findings about the characteristics of smokers and nonsmokers. *Journal of Consulting Psychology,* 1963, *27,* 282.

Treuting, T. F. The role of emotional factors in etiology and course of diabetes mellitus: A review of the recent literature. *American Journal of the Medical Sciences,* 1962, *244,* 93–109.

Wallston, K. A., Wallston, B. S., & De Vellis, R. Development of the multi-dimensional health locus of control (MHLC) scales. *Health Education Monographs,* 1978, *6,* 160–169.

White, P. Programs for the child with diabetes. In J. G. Cull & R. E. Hardy (Eds.), *Counseling and rehabilitating the diabetic.* Springfield, Ill.: Charles C. Thomas, 1974.

19 Psychological Considerations in Cancer

Paul H. Blaney
University of Miami

INTRODUCTION

Cancer is often viewed by laymen as a single disease. It is not. It is a class of conditions, generally classified by body site, though different disease processes may be found at any given site, and cancerous conditions at diverse sites may have strong commonalities.

All cancerous conditions reflect a proliferation of cells that do not contribute to the functioning of the organism as a whole and that displace cells that do. Ill health results from this displacement and from the attendant waste of nutritional resources on the noncontributing cellular life. The presence of such alien, probably mutant cells is apparently a common phenomenon, the effects of which are usually countered by the body's defenses (e.g., the immune system). Proliferating cancer suggests that bodily defenses have been unsuccessful, either because they are in a weakened state or because they have been outwitted or overwhelmed (cf. Fox, 1981; Keast, 1981). The diversity of oncological diseases presumably reflects the highly differentiated nature of the body's cells, the diversity of carcinogenic processes, and the multifaceted nature of the body's defenses.

The most common sites of appearance for cancers include the lungs, colon, stomach, bones, larynx, and, in women, breasts and cervix. A distinction can be drawn between the primary site—that body part whose cells are the first to become malignant—and the secondary site—any part to which the cancer has spread. The spread can be directly to adjacent tissue or by migration of malignant cells through the circulatory system to distant tissue (metastasis). Death is most likely when there is metastatic spread such that there is extensive tissue involvement and/or when one of the affected sites (primary or secondary) involves a vital organ.

The major topics covered in this chapter are psychosocial risk factors in the etiology of cancer, psychological reactions to having cancer, and related interventions. One's reaction to having cancer depends in part on the prognosis—likelihood of early death, pain, loss of function, disfigurement—associated with the particular site and extent of cancer, though simply knowing that one "has cancer" probably has a general emotional impact apart from prognostic specifics.

In considering psychosocial risk factors for cancer, there are compelling reasons *not* to assume that all cancers are as one. The known epidemiological risk factors for various cancers are divergent from one another, as are current biological explanations for the development of various cancers. In addition, some demonstrations of differences among cancer groups on psychosocial variables exist (Lehrer, 1980). Though it is possible that certain psychosocial variables pertain to risk for cancer-in-general, it is safer to assume that most or all do not. Unfortunately, the prevailing practice in the psychological literature has been to employ mixed-cancer samples, or to take findings on single-site samples as reflective of cancer-in-general. In the present chapter, when possible, findings are presented by site, and even when the original researcher presumed single-site findings to be generalizable to all cancer, the summary of these findings avoids this presumption.

PSYCHOLOGICAL RISK FACTORS

The two major classes of risk factors on which there has been research and speculation are: (1) enduring psychological characteristics such as personality and behavioral variables; and (2) stressful events. Strong conclusions can be drawn on questions of etiology only from prospective studies, in which subjects are first assessed before cancer is suspected. These are not common. Moreover, even prospective studies can give ambiguous results. When it is shown that persons assessed as showing a psychological characteristic at Time 1 show a high frequency of cancer at Time 2, this may mean; (1) that the characteristic predisposes individuals to cancer; (2) that the characteristic is an early symptom of cancer or of a precancerous biological state; or (3) that the characteristic and cancer are both predisposed by common genetic factors but are otherwise unrelated (cf. Eysenck, 1980; Fox, 1981).

The simplest alternative to prospective studies—cross-sectional comparison of already ill cancer patients with noncancer controls—is seriously limited, because the person's reaction to having cancer may influence the results. This distortion cannot be ruled out even when enduring personality traits are targeted or when reports of prior events are sought. Accordingly, most findings from such studies will be omitted from the selective review of research that follows.

However, a slight modification of this cross-sectional strategy enhances its usefulness: Obtaining data from persons who are being evaluated medically for cancer but who do not yet have the diagnostic verdict allows assignment to "cancer" and "control" groups subsequent to data collection. This provides a degree of control for whatever biasing effects are associated with the state of cancer dread.

Fortunately, a number of studies have used this design, and they deserve cautious attention. The need for caution arises from two considerations: (1) Differences between cancer subjects and controls cannot be presumed to have antedated cancer onset, as the presence of cancer, though undiagnosed, may have some subtle psychological effect, which may in turn be exaggerated by the stress of impending diagnosis; in fact, there is evidence that cancer patients may have different expectations regarding disease likelihood before being diagnosed than do such controls (Chesser & Anderson, 1975; Engelman, 1981). (2) In the case of several cancers, persons who emerge as "controls" (e.g., women with cervical dysplasia or benign breast masses) may be at high risk for cancer and may be viewed as having a precancerous condition; possible psychological risk factors would remain undetected if their role lay in instigating the precancerous state (as opposed to instigating movement from that state to true cancer).

The review that follows covers English-language reports of prospective studies and of cross-sectional studies that are judged to have employed control groups and assessment procedures having some merit. A number of widely-cited, "classic" studies were judged inadequate and are thus not mentioned. Prospective studies are so labelled; all others are cross-sectional. This is not a particularly critical review and most of these studies' numerous shortcomings are not mentioned. For a more selective, critical review of risk factor research, see Fox (1978).

Epidemiological Factors

It is beyond the scope of this chapter to review the large body of research on risk factors. Though risk factors are often labeled "epidemiological" rather than "psychological," many are behavioral. That is, a person's exposure to the risk factor is not something that happens to him or her, it results from something that he or she *does*.

Moreover, in a number of cases, the risk behavior is one that, in other contexts, some theorists have reckoned to be of special importance in understanding a person's psychological makeup, reflecting needs, salient traits, or conflicts. Two examples will suffice to make the point: the relation between smoking and lung cancer, and the relation between precocious, promiscuous sex and cervical cancer. Researchers tend to prefer nonpsychological explanations for these linkages, because sex and smoking do have direct effects on the body. But the fact that psychologically oriented explanations are logical alternatives should not be forgotten. For instance, it is possible that both cervical cancer and related sexual history arise in part from personality characteristics present at an early age.

Stress in Childhood

Recent reports by Thomas and associates (Duszynski, Shaffer, & Thomas, 1981; Thomas, Duszynski, & Shaffer, 1979) hold special interest, as subjects were queried about their childhoods while they were healthy medical students and then followed for cancer outcome for a period of 14 − 32 years. Duszynski et al. found no significant differences reflective of early trauma or aloneness between subjects who developed cancer and controls. However, Thomas et al. reported that subjects who developed major cancer had reported poorer family relationships during childhood, particularly between self and father. A similar but weaker pattern was evident for skin cancer and benign tumors. Both reports are limited by the heterogeneity of the major cancer category and by the absence of cervical and breast cancer in the sample.

There are data on early trauma and breast cancer. Reznikoff (1955) reported a relation between breast cancer: and (1) an elevated frequency of sibling death in infancy; and (2) being the nonfavored child, burdened with excessive household responsibilities. LeShan and Reznikoff (1960) reported data from two samples indicating that breast cancer patients show a family history of a shorter time lapse to the birth of the next younger child than controls, suggesting briefer time of being the primary focus of parental nurturance. Muslin, Gyarfas, and Pieper (1966), however, reported no difference between breast cancer patients and controls with respect to early loss or separation. Wheeler and Caldwell (1955) failed to find an elevated incidence of insufficient love and attention as a child among breast cancer subjects.

Wheeler and Caldwell (1955) reported a pattern of insufficient childhood nurturance among cervical cancer patients, a finding that may relate to the oft reported association between cervical cancer and early marriage (cf. Deeley, 1976); that is, subjects may have married young to escape home (Paloucek & Graham, 1960). In studies of lung cancer (Horne & Picard, 1979; Kissen, 1967), evidence has emerged of an elevated incidence of parental absence. In a study of children with various cancers, Jacobs and Charles (1980) found an elevated incidence of reports that the child had been the result of an unplanned pregnancy.

Personality Characteristics

Perhaps the most widely stated generalization in the area of personality-cancer relationships is drawn from the work of LeShan (e.g., 1969), who concluded that cancer develops against a backdrop of personal malaise and depression, often involving unresolved grief and emotional constriction. There are studies that bear on this claim, but they must be examined with an appreciation of the difficulty of assessing something like "undischarged grief resulting in an undercurrent of depression" in a reliable fashion. One could argue that an individual for whom this applied would be unlikely to appear depressed on a psychological test.

Work in the area of personality variables is extensive, and some discussion relating these variables to site is possible. There are also a number of studies that involve mixed cancer samples and that, in spite of this drawback, are important because of their prospective nature. They are discussed first.

Prospective Studies.   H. M. Voth (1976) alluded to an apparently unpublished study by A. C. Voth in which a large number of psychiatric patients who had been given a test of autokinesis (perceived movement of a point of light in a dark context) were followed up for cancer outcome. Those who later developed cancer showed less autokinesis than other psychiatric patients or normal controls. This result was interpreted as reflecting repression, vulnerability to feelings of despair, and unpsychological-mindedness among these persons. Another prospective study of psychiatric patients (Watson & Schuld, 1977) failed to obtain any premorbid differences on the Minnesota Multiphasic Personality Inventory (MMPI) between eventual cancer patients and matched controls. There are questions, of course, regarding whether such data on psychiatric samples can be generalized to non-psychiatric groups (cf. Kellerman, 1978; Watson & Schuld, 1978). Findings on the relation between psychiatric diagnosis and cancer risk are discussed in a subsequent section.

There are prospective findings from nonpsychiatric samples. Hagnell (1966) studied a diverse Swedish sample and found that women (but not men) who developed cancer had earlier tended to be described as "substable," a term implying sociability, industriousness, and naivete. Thomas and McCabe (1980) reported that several items on a checklist of signs of emotional tension yielded modest differences between a cancer-outcome group of medical students and a still healthy group (e.g., higher incidence of exhaustion and of the tendency to recheck one's work for accuracy). No differences were reported on variables particularly relevant to emotional distress (e.g., depression, anxiety), though an earlier report on a subgroup of these cancer subjects (Thomas, Ross, Brown, & Duszynski, 1973) indicated an elevated incidence of Rorschach responses involving disease or physical trauma. In a similar study in which persons assessed as undergraduates were followed up (Morrison, 1981), a composite group consisting of those who developed any kind of cancer did not differ from the source population.

Dattore, Shontz, and Coyne (1980), McCoy (1978), and Shekelle, Raynor, Ostfeld, Garron, Bieliauskas, Liu, Maliza, and Paul (1981) have all reported data on cancer patients and controls on whom premorbid MMPIs had been obtained. In the Dattore et al. study, the cancer-outcome group was reported to have greater repression and less depression. In the Shekelle et al. study *greater* depression was seen in the cancer-outcome group. In the McCoy study, the relevant finding was of greater introversion among cancer-outcome women (but not men).

Finally, Grossarth-Maticek (1980) has reported the results of a 10-year follow-up of a large number of persons, most of them elderly, and 15% of whom developed cancer. Subjects were initially assessed on a questionnaire formulated to tap stress responses characterized by blocked emotionality, hopelessness, rationality, and interpersonal harmony at the expense of self-negation. A scale based on these characteristics successfully predicted 78% of those who developed cancer and 96% of those who developed other diseases or remained healthy. Questionnaire items indicating rationality and antiemotionality stood out as contributing to the effectiveness of this discriminative success.

The lack of consistency of findings among these studies may derive from several sources, among them the divergent mixes of kinds of cancer among mixed-cancer groups, and the divergent nature of the control groups. Moreover, the differences reported were typically small in magnitude, and the variables on which they appeared comprised a small minority of those examined. Four of the nine studies reported in this section (Dattore et al., 1980; Shekelle et al., 1981; Thomas & McCabe, 1980; Watson and Schuld, 1977) employed only male subjects, so any factors associated with breast or cervical cancer would not have influenced their results. Fox (1982b) has noted that one anomalous finding—the relation between cancer and low depression in Dattore et al.—quite likely reflects the use of an inappropriate control group and is misleading if taken as revealing anything about cancer per se; indeed, his consideration of Dattore's findings has led Fox (1982a) to count them as indicating that depression *elevations* are predictive of cancer.

Grossarth-Maticek's (1980) results deserve special comment. Fox (in press) has described them as "hard to believe." Indeed they are, because they suggest an effect that is not only stronger than is suggested by other studies but stronger than even the most avid of proponents of psychosocial precursors would probably have anticipated. Moreover, it is not certain that the subjects were disease-free when initially assessed, nor is the procedure reported in the detail one would desire. It is possible, however, that the distinctive success of this study arises from the fact that it is the only prospective one in which subjects were assessed on an instrument formulated on the basis of the findings of earlier clinical and retrospective studies of cancer patients. That is, the weaker findings of other studies may reflect poorly tuned assessment procedures.

Breast Cancer.   Reznikoff (1955) reported that, in comparison with controls, breast cancer subjects tended to have a very household-oriented life, with few interests outside the home. They tended to harbor considerable ambivalence and resentment about the housewife/mother role but apparently lacked the assertiveness needed to act on this dissatisfaction and reject this role. Voth (1976) reported findings on a series of women who were at least 6 months postmastectomy on autokenesis and embedded figures tests. Results were viewed as suggesting emotional constrictedness and psychological undifferentiation. Coppen and Metcalfe (1963) presented data suggesting elevations on extroversion in breast cancer patients. However, Greer and Morris (1975) found that breast cancer subjects were not distinguishable from controls with respect to extraversion, or, for that matter, with regard to neuroticism or inward or outward hostility. The breast cancer group did show an elevated incidence of persons who rarely expressed strong feelings, particularly anger. Morris, Greer, Pettingale, and Watson (1981) replicated the Greer and Morris finding regarding anger expression but found cancer subjects to have especially *low* neuroticism scores. Somewhat similarly, Schonfield (1975) failed to find breast cancer/control differences with respect to depression, overt anxiety, or well-being, but there were suggestions in the data of denial of negative emotionality; in particular, among younger breast cancer subjects, a tendency to evidence more covert anxiety emerged. On the other hand, Jansen (1981) reported *elevated* scores on self-reported hostility in a sample of diagnosed breast cancer patients, though these patients did emerge as less assertive than controls.

Some of the inconsistency may be accounted for by a subsidiary finding reported by Greer and Morris (1975) and emphasized in Bagley's (1979) reanalyses of some of the same data. In addition to the high prevalence of emotional suppression, there was a less marked but significantly elevated incidence of persons given to frequent emotional outbursts among the breast cancer patients. That is, both extremes seemed more prominent among them, in comparison with nonmalignant breast patients, all assessed prior to medical diagnosis. Somewhat similarly, Wirsching, Stierlin, Hoffmann, Weber, and Wirsching (1982), in a comparison of breast cancer with benign lump patients all interviewed while awaiting biopsy, found the incidence both of extreme pessimism and of overoptimism to be elevated among the cancer group. This group also was distinguished by a higher percentage of women who: (1) showed initial denial of emotions followed by extreme expression of negative emotion; (2) were emotionally very distant during the interview; (3) tended to cope by means of being rational; (4) described themselves as having no fear regarding the biopsy; and (5) described themselves as especially self-sufficient and altruistic or self-sacrificing.

There have been preliminary but noteworthy attempts to specify the biological mediator between personality factors and breast cancer. On the basis of earlier findings suggesting a role of serum immunoglobulin A (IgA) in the development of breast cancer, Pettingale, Greer, and Tee (1977) studied the relationship between IgA and anger suppression in their (Greer & Morris, 1975) sample of benign and malignant breast mass subjects. A clear relation was obtained, lending credence to—though by no means demonstrating—that IgA may mark the path through which anger suppression is related to breast malignancy. Of probable indirect relevance are unpublished findings by Jemmott and coworkers (cf. Locke, 1982) indicating that salivary IgA is, in normal males, related to external stress and to the personality characteristics of inhibited power motivation. Note, however, that serum IgA did not distinguish benign from malignant breast patients in the Greer and Morris (1975) subjects (Pettingale, Merrett, & Tee, 1977), though there was some evidence of a relation between serum IgA elevation and metastatic spread.

Katz, Ackman, Rothwax, Sachar, Weiner, Hellman, and Gallagher (1970) employed a similar rationale to study the relation between the ratio of excreted corticosteroids-to-androgens and the adequacy of psychological defenses, measured as interview-based judgments of affective distress, disruption of function, and impairment of defensive reserve. Subjects, most of whom were eventually shown to have malignancies, were awaiting biopsy when assessed. Results suggested relations between hydrocortisone metabolite excretion and all aspects of defensive sufficiency, particularly affective sufficiency. The interest of this finding is limited by the absence of any demonstration that defensive adequacy is related to malignant status. Also, the relation between defensive adequacy (Katz et al., 1970) and anger suppression (Greer & Morris, 1975) is unclear. Ten-year follow-up assessment of a subsample of the Katz et al. sample (Gorzynski, Holland, Katz, Weiner, Zumoff, Fukushima, & Levin, 1980) has not added substantively to the original findings.

Finally, Nieburgs, Weiss, Navarrete, Strax, Teirstein, Grillione, and Siedlecki (1979) have reported findings regarding proportions of various kinds of lymphocytes in the blood. Though their report was rather unclear, it appears that, among noncancer women awaiting breast screening, those who indicated inhibition of negative emotions were more like women who emerged with a breast cancer diagnosis on the lymphocyte variables than like other noncancer women who did not show this emotional style.

In an earlier section of this chapter, the use of a design was advocated in which psychological evaluation of cancer patients is carried out before diagnosis is known, with those subjects who turn out not to have any malignancy then designated as controls. Given that several of the studies cited in this section used this design, it should be noted that women with benign breast masses may be especially prone to manifesting tension and depression, perhaps independent of knowledge of the breast mass (Kosch, 1981). Inasmuch as a history of such nonmalignancies constitutes a risk factor for cancer, this may suggest a role for emotional style very early in the cancer onset process. On the other hand, this also means that comparisons between malignant and nonmalignant breast patients may yield differences that, while appearing to reflect unemotionality among cancer patients, reflect excessive emotionality among those with the benign condition. Indeed, in a comparison among breast cancer, fibrocystic disease, and healthy control groups (Jansen, 1981), the fibrocystic disease subjects could be differentiated from both other groups on several variables (they appeared particularly restless, demanding, and competitive).

Finally, in her prospective study, Morrison (1981) found that neither persons who had died of, or who were alive with, breast cancer were distinguishable from controls. Although the fact that evaluations were completed well before disease onset may seem to render this finding especially deserving of attention, the actual assessment was minimal and, for instance, did not provide measures of emotional style variables that the foregoing literature suggests may be important.

Malignant Melanoma.   Rogentine, van Kammen, Fox, Docherty, Rosenblatt, Boyd, and Bunney (1979) have recently reported a prospective study on a group of persons all of whom, pursuant to a diagnosis of melanoma, had recently undergone surgery. Assuming that the surgery had achieved its purpose, they were thus disease-free when evaluated psychologically. Outcome was judged in terms of whether or not relapse occurred in the year following. Among a number of variables considered, one distinguished relapsers from nonrelapsers. In response to a query as to how much personal adjustment was needed to handle or cope with the recent illness, nonrelapsers gave substantially *higher* ratings. The predictive value of this variable was independent of any physical variable. The authors favor a view of the relapsers' unconcern as reflecting the use of denial and repression, though they note that this relative unconcern may be regarded less pathologically. It is noteworthy that the groups did not differ on measures of self-reported distress or depression (see also Fox, 1982a). Preliminary results of a study by Temoshok (1981) are generally supportive of Rogentine et al.'s findings. A tendency to view one's melanoma in an accepting fashion—one in which the self is viewed as capable of coping—was associated with medical indices of severity of melanoma in a cross-sectional study.

Abdominal Cancers. A study by Fras, Litin, and Pearson (1967) compared pancreas cancer patients with colon cancer patients and with a mixed disease group, on the basis of interview and MMPI. The pancreas group was most distinguished by a high incidence of reports of depression and related symptoms (particularly loss of ambition) in the months prior to physical disease symptoms, an "anger-in" personality style, and a mean elevation of the MMPI depression scale. Though some of these patients knew their diagnosis, degree of depression appeared not to be a function of this knowledge.

Given that the Fras et al. study is sometimes cited as suggesting that depression is commonly the first symptom of cancer of the pancreas, it should be noted that Jacobsson and Ottosson (1971), in a study of matched samples of 50 pancreas and stomach cancer patients, found that depression was the first symptom in only one case of each (according to information provided retrospectively by relatives). Indeed, in 68% of the pancreas cases, somatic symptoms (only) were first to appear, and the most prominent early emotional symptom was irritability. When depression does emerge prior to a diagnosis of pancreatic cancer, it may comprise the patient's response to the realization that his physician is not able to account for—or even willing to take seriously—his elusive physical complaints (cf. Salmon, 1967).

There are two longitudinal studies relating to abdominal cancers. In Morrison's (1981), men who later died of colorectal cancer had as youths described themselves as tense, anxious, self-conscious, and somatically reactive more often than did other youths. This finding did not emerge for men who were alive with colorectal cancer at follow-up or for men who had died of pancreatic cancer. These two groups were undistinguishable at initial evaluation from the population from which they were drawn. In Greenberg and Dattore's study (1981), men who eventually developed prostate cancer were not distinguishable on a number of MMPI-based indices of dependency from a variety of control groups.

Lung Cancer.   In the 1960s Kissen published a number of influential papers (e.g., 1967) in which he argued that lung cancer patients are characterized by restricted outlets for emotional discharge. Because much of Kissen's data (e.g., Maudsley neuroticism scale) involved self-report of past and current distress, Huggan (1968) has suggested that they are consistent with another explanation: that these patients are disinclined to admit to distress or weakness (see also Fox, 1978).

More recently, Grissom, Weiner, and Weiner (1975) have reported a comparison of lung cancer patients, many of whom knew their diagnosis, with controls. Self-report personality inventory data were generally supportive of Huggan's position: Cancer patients tended to report themselves as being psychologically healthier than controls, but their responses suggested relatively unintegrated and conflicted self-concepts. On the other hand, a report by Abse, Wilkins, van de Castle, Buxton, Demars, Brown, and Kirschner (1974) of a study of lung cancer patients and controls, assessed prediagnosis, yielded a finding more consistent with Kissen's presumption of defensive constriction: Cancer patients reported markedly less dream recall.

Gynecological Cancer.   An oft cited study by Schmale and Iker (1966a, 1966b, 1971) is the only one that addressed cervical cancer specifically. Though employing a design in which cancer and control (cervical dysplasia) subjects were evaluated prediagnosis, the study has a major weakness: Virtually all the "cancer" subjects merely had carcinoma in situ, a condition often classed as precancerous rather than cancerous. Conclusions regarding invasive cervical cancer, for instance, cannot be drawn from the study. In any case, these cancer patients, when evaluated by personality test and interview, appeared to be particularly perfectionistic, to show nonspecific indications of psychological distress, and to have an elevated incidence of psychological "giving-up" reaction (see also Spence, Scarborough, & Ginsberg, 1978).

Mastrovito, Deguire, Clarkin, Thaler, Lewis, and Cooper (1979) reported a study of hospitalized women admitted with a diagnosis of some kind of gynecological cancer. Subjects were given an adjective checklist personality evaluation before further medical assessment, and a minority were eventually found to have no malignancy. When these were compared with those whose cancer was confirmed, the latter were found to have given checklist reponses that portrayed them as significantly more controlled, deferent, and oriented to stability and conformity, and less emotionally labile, aggressive, or likely to view themselves as having emotional problems. Several qualifications must be noted. Groups were not necessarily alike with regard to perceived symptom severity or perceived prognosis when evaluated. Nor were the differences noted large in magnitude. Finally, the cancer group was regrettably diverse; the cervical subgroup was the largest, but it comprised just 39% of the sample and included in situ cases.

Psychiatric Disorder. If one assumes that personality functioning is of importance in the etiology of cancer, one would anticipate that the incidence of cancer in persons with psychiatric disorders might be different from that in the general population. These studies can be viewed as involving a specialized approach to the prospective study of the relation between personality variables and cancer.

The simplest summary of this literature is that markedly conflicting results are reported. For instance, although Rassidakis, Kelepouris, Goulis, and Karaiossefidis (1973) estimated that the incidence of death due to cancer was about half that to be expected from age-corrected population estimates among their hospitalized schizophrenics, a comparable study reported by Tsuang, Woolson, and Fleming (1980) reported a rate among schizophrenics almost identical to that based on population expectancy. (The percentage of deaths attributable to cancer was low, but that appeared merely to reflect the relatively high percentage of suicides and accidental deaths; percentage of deaths, employed in a number of such studies, is an inappropriate descriptive statistic.)

Turning to affective disorders, although there has been recent support for earlier findings suggestive that affective disorder incurs an increased likelihood of subsequent death by cancer (Whitlock & Siskind, 1979), a number of recent studies that have examined the issue have failed to find any relationship (Evans, Baldwin, Gath, 1974; Niemi & Jaaskelainen, 1978; Tsuang et al., 1980). Kerr, Schapira, and Roth (1969) reported such a relationship in males, but not in females. However, a particularly large-sample, long-term, well-controlled follow-up of males diagnosed as psychoneurotic (including depressed) yielded a rate of death by malignancy similar to that shown by controls (Keehn, Goldberg, & Beebe, 1974).

The conflicting results may be related to the use in some studies of sample sizes that are smaller than desirable for the purpose of establishing cancer rates. Moreover, even if results were more consistent than they are, such findings suffer the ambiguities of prospective studies noted earlier. For instance, if depressives show an elevated incidence of cancer, this may merely reflect a state of affairs in which depression is a very early symptom of some cancers (cf. Whitlock & Siskind, 1979). And any reduced cancer rate in schizophrenia might reflect something as irrelevant as the unavailability of cigarettes to psychiatric patients (cf. Fox & Howell, 1974).

A related issue is the possibility that certain classes of drugs given therapeutically to psychiatric patients may increase cancer risk. Specifically, the possibility that rauwolfia derivatives and antipsychotic agents may increase the risk of breast cancer has been raised, on the grounds that these drugs result in an increase of serum prolactin, which in turn may foster growth of these tumors. Studies addressing this possibility among psychiatric patients, though mixed, currently favor the conclusion that these drugs do not increase the cancer risk (Goode,

Corbett, Schey, Suh, Woodie, Morris & Morrisey, 1981; Schyve, Smithline, & Meltzer, 1978). Moreover, there is animal evidence suggesting that antipsychotic drugs may inhibit tumor growth (Sklar & Anisman, 1981b). Note that possible cancer – drug relationships and possible cancer – psychiatric disorder relationships are difficult to separate in human epidemiological studies, as the widespread use of neuroleptic drugs with psychiatric patients results in a confounding of variables.

Recent Stress

There has been a tendency to view findings of associations between personality factors suggestive of *dis*tress and cancer (cf. studies reviewed in prior sections) as relevant to a putative stress – cancer link (e.g., Bahnson, 1980, 1981). Because, however, personal distress may or may not be in response to a stressor, this practice invites conceptual confusion. Accordingly, the present section considers only research on recent stressful *events* (i.e., those occurring prior to cancer onset), during a time frame consistent with a possible role in cancer development. Only psychosocial stressors are considered, in constrast to physical stressors, some of which are presumably carcinogenic.

The research described here can be viewed in the context of a larger body of research on life stress and physical disease (Rabkin & Struening, 1976). That research, although generally suggesting a modest but reliable association between magnitude of stressors (usually number of events, weighted for seriousness) and subsequent illness, leaves open the possibility that specific illnesses may be very strongly linked, others not at all. The issue can be addressed only by studies of specific illnesses, such as those on cancer reviewed here.

Note that there is reason to believe that personality variables moderate the effects of life stress on illness—that some persons have coping resources that serve as buffers against the negative effects of stressors. Writers dealing with the role of personality and childhood stress variables in cancer (see earlier sections) have often proposed that these variables act not alone but in interaction with recent stress (Bahnson, 1980, 1981). However, although there is evidence for such an interaction where the outcome is ill health in general (Kobasa, Maddi, & Kahn, 1982), no study addresses this question satisfactorily with respect to cancer specifically. In the human research reviewed later, stress is always considered as an isolated variable.

Animal Studies.   For reviews of the considerable research on stress and cancer in animals, see Peters and Mason (1979), Riley (1981), or Sklar and Anisman (1981a, 1981b). Although the relevance of animal models to humans should always be questioned, and although in some studies the "stressors" were quite unlike those presumed to be important for humans, in other studies the stressors were of probable human relevance (e.g., removal from a social to an isolated environment). To summarize Sklar and Anisman's (1981b) observations, in animals exposed to a carcinogen or implanted with a tumor, stress induction sometimes increases malignant proliferation, sometimes inhibits it, and sometimes has no effect. Variables that influence which outcome will occur include: chronicity of the stress, maturity of the animal, timing of the stress vis-à-vis the cancer induction, opportunity for coping behaviors, and the nature of the stress itself. Parallels between the effects of stress on tumor growth and the effects of stress on hormonal, neurochemical, and immune system functioning render plausible any and all of these systems as links in the stress – cancer relationship.

Prospective Studies. Most studies of humans rely on retrospective reports from already ill persons versus controls, and most are specific as to site of cancer. The exceptions are quasi-prospective studies by McNeil (cited in Jacobs & Ostfeld, 1977), by Moss (1980), and by Parkes, Benjamin, & Fitzgerald (1969), which considered mortality rates among persons who had undergone a specific stress: recent death of spouse. In the Parkes et al. study, which considered only widowers, and in the Moss study, though subjects showed an increased risk of mortality following bereavement, little of the increase was attributable to death by cancer. However, in the McNeil study, malignant neoplasm was a source of increased rate of death among *widows*. Other data (Ernster, Sacks, Selvin, & Petrakis, 1979) confirm the relationship between widowed status and cancer incidence and suggest that site, gender, and race differences qualify this relationship; unfortunately, recency of spouse death was not considered in the Ernster et al. study, rendering it unclear if the findings reported can be viewed as related to recent stress. Moss (1980) did report prospective data showing that marital separation and recent divorce were associated with subsequent cancer development. For a more extensive discussion, see Joseph and Syme (1982).

Childhood Cancer. Jacobs and Charles (1980) studied a series of children with cancer, a majority of whom were leukemic. Parental reports indicated markedly elevated prior stress levels among the cancer patients, in comparison with levels obtained on a carefully matched group of children with other, less serious illnesses. Although the groups differed with respect to a number of events, the most striking was with respect to moves. In the year prior to symptom appearance, 60% of the cancer patients' families had moved, versus 12% of the controls'.

Breast Cancer. Four studies (Greer & Morris, 1975; Muslin et al., 1966; Schonfield, 1975; Snell & Graham, 1971) have sought a relation between recent stress and breast cancer, and none has found it. Given this consistency across diverse samples and research criteria, and given the fact that Schonfield actually found a reversal—breast cancer patients showed less stress than benign tumor controls—the conclusion that breast cancer is not precipitated by stress may appear secure. However, all these studies used control groups that, though ideal in some respects, may be contributing to a misportrayal: Snell and Graham used controls who had diseases (including cancer) of organs other than breast and genitalia. If there is an elevated stress level with many of these other diseases, an elevation in breast cancer would be obscured. The problem is similar with regard to the three remaining studies. All used as controls benign breast mass patients, a group that has recently been shown to have an elevated stress level (Kosch, 1981). It is thus possible that breast cancer patients would show higher stress levels than healthy controls. It is also possible that the role of stress in breast cancer is through stimulation of benign mass development, which in turn is a risk factor for cancer.

Perhaps consistent with this last speculation is a finding reported by Bagley (1979) based on analyses of the Greer and Morris subjects. Although cancerous and benign breast patients did not differ in stress during the prior 5 years, the cancer patients did have high levels of reports (unsolicited) of stress during the 10-year period previous to that. That is, there may be a role of life stress, and if so, it is probably quite early in the sequence of events culminating in clinical cancer.

Lung Cancer.   Findings on lung cancer are conflicting. Grissom et al. (1975) found no difference between lung cancer patients and controls with respect to recent life stress, whereas Horne and Picard (1979) presented data indicating a strong relation between significant loss in the prior 5 years and lung cancer. In the latter study, however, the possibility of an age confound was not ruled out. Kissen (1967, 1969) concluded that lung cancer patients showed an elevation in life stress, but his definition appears to have been rather broad, and not restricted to specific stressors.

Malignant Melanoma.   Temoshok (1981) has reported an association between recent stress and the severity of disease in a sample of malignant melanoma patients.

Abdominal Cancers.   Lehrer (1980) compared the life stress reports of colorectal cancer patients, gastric cancer patients, and healthy controls. The colorectal group did not differ from controls, but gastric cancer showed a significantly higher level than did the colorectal and the control groups. Fras et al. (1967) reported an elevated incidence of loss of a significant relationship during the years prior to disease identification in a group of patients with cancer of the pancreas, in comparison with colon cancer and mixed disease groups.

Cervical Cancer.   There are two major studies: Schmale and Iker's (1966a, 1966b, 1971) and Graham, Snell, Graham, and Ford's (1971). Their results differ, perhaps as a function of control group. Graham et al. found no elevation of prior stress in cervical cancer patients, but this was in comparison with ill controls, who may also have had an elevated stress level. Schmale and Iker's findings are widely cited as implicating a hopelessness reaction in cervical cancer (noted previously), but a careful examination of their 1966b paper (corrected version) reveals as strong a relationship between cancer and one specific stress—recent serious illness in a family member—as between cancer and the hopelessness reaction. In this case, controls were women with cervical dysplasia.

Stress and the Immune System

Finally, there has emerged in recent years research on the relation in humans between stress and certain immunological parameters of likely relevance to cancer (see Fox, 1981; Locke, 1982; and Rogers, Dubey, & Reich, 1979, for reviews). Briefly, there do appear to be such relationships, and, along with the parallel animal literature already mentioned, this research may point the way to a specification of paths through which any stress – cancer relationship may pass. A recent instance is that presented by Locke, Jemmott, Kraus, Hurst, Heisel, McClelland, and Williams (1981). They assessed, among other things, recent life stress, self-reported symptoms of distress, and natural killer cell activity in undergraduate volunteers. Interestingly, life stress was related to natural killer cell activity only in interaction with self-reported distress. Specifically, when the sample was grouped in terms of high versus low stress crossed with high versus low distress, the high stress – high distress group showed the lowest level of natural killer cell activity, the high stress – low distress group the highest, with both low stress groups showing intermediate levels. This result relates to two points raised in the opening paragraphs of this section: (1) the fact that stress sometimes enhances, sometimes inhibits tumor growth in animals; and (2) the lamentable fact that stress-cancer studies in humans have not been designed to consider the role of possible moderating variables. That is, Locke et al.'s findings are consistent with the widely held but unresearched tenet that stressors are important in the onset of cancer, but only in interaction with personal and situational variables that influence the stress response. Other aspects of the Locke et al. study point to stress having divergent effects upon various components of the immune system.

General comments regarding research on the psychological antecedents of cancer follow the next major sections, which deal with the consequences of having cancer and with interventions.

REACTIONS TO CANCER

Documentation of the high prevalence of emotional distress among cancer patients is ample (Craig & Abeloff, 1974). The knowledge that one has cancer can, in itself, rouse powerful, negative emotional states, regardless of the exact nature of the cancer. Beyond that are a number of more specific threats that many but not all cancer patients face, among them: (1) disfigurement (the importance of which is presumably linked to the personal meaning of whatever is disfigured; cf.

Meyerowitz, 1980); (2) impending death; (3) handicaps resulting directly from the disease or from surgery; (4) extreme physical discomfort either as a direct effect of disease or as a side effect of radiation or chemotherapy; (5) chronic hospitalization and invalid status; and (6) increased dependency upon and/or rejection by important others. Any cancer patient not confronting one of these threats may nonetheless be burdened by an awareness that it may lie ahead and, by the unpredictability of his or her fate with respect to any of them. Gordon, Freidenbergs, Diller, Hibbard, Wolf, Levine, Lipkins, Ezrachi, and Lucido (1980) and Ross, Stockdale, and Jacobs (1978) have described comprehensive assessment procedures tailored for cancer patients, to evaluate the extent to which these and related issues are of concern to a particular patient.

It is impossible to do justice to all these threats in this chapter, especially as in a number of cases there is a large, relevant literature not bounded by a focus on cancer. For instance, the extensive literature on terminal illness and death relies very heavily on cancer patients and obviously pertains to the experience of the terminal cancer patient, but no review of that literature is possible. The present section deals with an assortment of topics specific to cancer to which attention has been given in recent years. For reviews of some relevant literature not covered here, see Freidenbergs, Gordon, Hibbard, Levine, Wolf, and Diller (1982), Lloyd (1979), or Meyerowitz (1980).

Cancer in Children

Note that the threats commonly experienced by cancer patients are likely to be compounded in the case of children (Brunnquell & Hall, 1982). Primary dependency ties are likely to be disrupted by the prolonged separation that hospitalization often involves, by the intimate intrusions of numerous strangers (i.e., caregivers), and by the fact that the parents also are severely stressed. The boredom and restriction of activity that are part of some medical regimens may be especially difficult for children to tolerate. Children may be especially prone to unrealistic, morbid fantasies about the course of the disease and treatment and to notions that the disease represents punishment for past misdeeds. Being prevented from engaging in age-appropriate responsibilities and being sidetracked from the progress that peers are making are often hard on the child's self-image.

Predictors of Adjustment

There is a research literature on the psychological predictors of coping with cancer in adults. The import of these studies is unclear, as the typical results (Hinton, 1975; Sobel & Worden, 1979; Worden & Sobel, 1978) can be distilled to the following conclusion: Persons who are functioning relatively well at a given time on a given measure also function relatively well at a later time on another measure. Such studies may say little that pertains to cancer specifically; rather they comprise demonstrations of the cross-situational consistency of personality and interpersonal functioning. Accordingly, this literature is not reviewed further here.

Predictors of Medical Outcome

Personality variables have been assessed as predictors of response to treatment (e.g., survival), among cancer patients. It may or may not be that psychological factors in vulnerability to the onset of cancer are the same ones that play a role in individual differences in recovery or rate of deterioration. If they are, research on already ill persons could be viewed as especially attractive because it allows for the efficient use of a prospective design, though obviously the "personality factors" that are considered must be viewed in the context of the high stress level under which cancer patients must be assumed to be functioning.

Most of the studies described here used heterogeneous samples of patients with advanced cancers. The heterogeneity can be particularly problematic, as various cancers have differing prognoses. A variable distinguishing good from poor outcome patients might do so simply by distinguishing patients with cancer of one site from patients with cancer of another. This is highlighted by the results of one relevant study (Davies, Quinlan, McKegney, & Kimball, 1973), in which, although an "apathetic-given-up" attitude was associated with early death, it also was associated with degree and site of illness (cf. Derogatis, Abeloff, & McBeth, 1976). Fortunately, in most of the studies described, there was some attempt to compensate for differences in expected longevity associated with site. For a particularly systematic such attempt, see Worden, Johnston, and Harrison (1974).

The classic study in the area is that reported by Blumberg, West, and Ellis (1954). Based largely on MMPI findings, they concluded that persons whose cancer progressed rapidly were anxious, denying, passive, obliging individuals who lacked stress-reducing outlets, even of a neurotic, psychotic, or acting-out sort. However, Krasnoff (1959) and Stavraky (1968) failed to confirm Blumberg et al.'s MMPI findings.

Stavraky (1968) did report projective test data suggesting that those having a favorable outcome had a "high proportion of individuals who had strong hostile drives without loss of emotional control [p. 259]." Somewhat similarly, Weisman and Worden (1975) found that their long survivors were somewhat more resentful and demanding, though not inappropriately so. More generally, they concluded that the short-survival subjects had experienced disruption of emotional ties in childhood and a history of poor, even destructive social relationships as adults. They had poorer relationships with caregivers and were less likely to seek support or to harbor some hope.

This last element, maintaining some hope, also emerged in a study by Achterberg, Lawlis, Simonton, and Matthews-Simonton (1977), who reported that the perception of one's body as unable to fight disease was predictive of poor outcome. Achterberg et al. also reported that their poor outcome group evidenced more denial and a more external locus of control. Paloucek and Graham (1960) also reported that, among cervical cancer patients, poor response to treatment was associated with a hopeless attitude, though this was confounded with the extent to which the woman fitted the classical epidemiological pattern for cervical cancer (bleak childhood, early sexual experience, unsatisfactory marriage).

Derogatis, Abeloff, and Melisaratos (1979) studied women with metastatic breast cancer. When initially evaluated, those who later emerged as long survivors yielded *higher* means on self-report indices of hostility, psychoticism, depression, and guilt than did those with less favorable outcome. They were also rated as *less* well adjusted to their illness and to treatment by their physicians. The groups did not differ on relevant medical variables at the time of psychological evaluation. The difference with respect to hostility is perhaps most noteworthy because it appeared to reflect primarily an unusual lack of hostility among the short-term survivors.

Greer, Morris, and Pettingale (1979) also studied breast cancer patients, in this case nonmetastatic cases. Although numerous variables were not predictive of clinical state at 5-year follow-up—including measures of depression, anger, social adjustment, and usual reactions to stress—there was a relation involving emotional response to cancer assessed 3 months postmastectomy as the predictor; those whose responses were categorized as "denial" (rejection of diagnosis), or "fighting spirit" (optimism and active involvement in recovery) fared better than those who showed a stoic or hopelessness/helplessness reaction.

In summary, absence of hostility has emerged in diverse studies as a correlate of rapid deterioration. Moreover, it relates rather clearly to Kissen's (1969) speculations regarding precursors of lung cancer and to findings regarding correlates of breast cancer (e.g., Greer & Morris, 1975). The predictive studies are much less clear regarding the role of what might generally be viewed as demoralization, with some (Rogentine et al.; Derogatis et al.) seeming to suggest that it is associated with *good* prognosis and others (Achterberg et al.; Greer et al.; Paloucek & Graham, Weisman & Worden) seeming to suggest that, instead, more optimistic patients survive longer. Findings on denial are likewise conflicting. There are a number of possible explanations for the discrepancies, but further research is clearly needed.

A Comprehensive Model

The foregoing focuses on individual differences in coping among cancer patients. Another, perhaps complementary, approach involves a description of the modal, stereotypic person afflicted with cancer. Wortman and Dunkel-Schetter (1979; see also Dunkel-Schetter & Wortman, 1982) have presented such a model, one that focuses on the cancer patient who is in pain and/or is living in dread of deterioration or death. What follows is a summary of this model.

Wortman and Dunkel-Schetter drew the following conclusions from the existing literature, and these served as something of a foundation for their thinking: Some studies suggest that depression is the predominant reaction to having cancer, others that denial is. Claims that there are "stages" (temporally sequenced) in the reaction process are controversial at best. What is clear is that prominent among the difficulties that arise from having cancer are interpersonal problems, and that persons having more satisfactory interpersonal relations cope more adequately with the illness.

The verdict of cancer fosters a state of fear and worry—about the physical effects of the cancer itself, about the quality of care, about the impact upon family—and confronts the patient with a stream of decisions (e.g., choice of physician) that are of great import and for which he or she is unprepared. Patients may feel overwhelmed by their fears, and may in turn fear that their sense of being able to cope is itself abnormal. Although being able to discuss these feelings openly—particularly with loved ones or with others who have or have had cancer—would be most helpful, patients often feel inhibited from doing so. They instead perceive that they should cope heroically and that admitting their true feelings might alienate caregivers and upset loved ones.

Although there is reason to doubt that it is in fact in the best interest of the patient to do so, other persons often feel obliged to be cheerful in the patient's presence. Their true feelings too, of course, are often very uncheerful. They may deal with the discrepancy by avoiding the patient, by communicating superficially and stifling the patient's more open communication, or by giving mixed messages. Others, even loved ones and professionals, may resent the problems caused by the illness and may distance themselves from the patient's plight by blaming the patient for it. This resentment and derogation, when present, may coexist with feelings of sympathy and concern. The result may be ambivalent, confusing communications that are especially difficult for the patient to deal with. Despite others' attempts to hide it, the patient may discern their frustration and rejection, and this may result in a sense of loneliness and greatly diminished worth.

Confronted with this, the patient may try to break through the cloud of cheeriness by emphasizing the negative aspects of the situation or may join in it and emphasize the positive in communications with others. Both approaches are faulty, the former because it may increase others' discomfort and avoidance, the latter because the patient knows that any support that ensues has been elicited on false pretenses.

By way of intervention, Wortman and Dunkel-Schetter (1979) suggest that patients be informed that: "the rejection they receive from others is often independent of their own behavior, and [that] family members . . . be taught that their feelings of anger and guilt toward the patient are normal [p. 244]," perhaps in a family therapy setting. Peer support groups for cancer patients might provide a context for open affective communication and for the exchange of relevant factual information and provide the patient with realization of the normativeness of his or her feelings of being overwhelmed. Professionals' attention to providing direct information regarding common physical and emotional reactions may also be of value in short-circuiting aspects of the distress cycle.

INTERVENTIONS

Turning our attention completely to interventions, the various psychosocial treatment strategies described in the recent literature can be classified in terms of the goals to which they are directed. Three broad treatment goals can be discerned: (1) improving psychosocial functioning; (2) increasing longevity; and (3) minimizing physical discomfort. These goals are often, but not always mutually compatible. For a discussion which overlaps with the following, see Feinstein (1983).

Improving Psychosocial Functioning

Included here are approaches designed to minimize psychological turmoil and social disruption during the illness, to maximize a return to normal functioning if there is recovery, and to help in the maintenance of a sense of dignity and peace in the event of deterioration and death.

Many of the interventions described in the recent literature (Holland & Rowland, 1981; Panagis, 1979) seem not to bear recounting here, as their procedures and goals are not specific to cancer. For instance, a list of interventions for depression in cancer would probably mirror a list of interventions for depression in general. When the patient has cancer, these interventions are ideally carried out in ways that are colored by a sensitivity to concerns common to patients with the particular disease (e.g., sexual concerns in breast cancer; cf. Witkin, 1979) and to an awareness of the limits that medical prognosis places on psychotherapeutic goals. The fact that what appears useful involves existing, rather than novel techniques is paralleled by observations regarding the physical medicine/rehabilitation needs of cancer patients; specifically, Lehmann, DeLisa, Warren, deLateur, Bryant, and Nicholson (1978) noted that many such problems can be dealt with by techniques widely used with noncancer (e.g., stroke) patients but are not dealt with in cancer patients because of the absence of an appropriate referral. Similarly, there are data suggesting that surgeons make psychiatric referrals in only a minority of mastectomy cases in which emotional problems are severe enough to warrant it (Maguire, Tait, Brooke, Thomas, & Sellwood, 1980).

A recurring theme in this literature, relevant to aspects of Wortman and Dunkel-Schetter's (1979) model, has to do with the issue of the patient's *denial* of the reality of the illness and prognosis. There is little consensus or empirical data regarding what the preferred professional stance should be. For instance, Meyerowitz (1980) noted a remarkably high level of sympathy for patient denial in the breast cancer literature, and O'Malley, Koocher, Foster, and Slavin (1979) concluded that denial was a component of readjustment in cancer-surviving children.

On the other hand, two recent studies (Greenwald & Nevitt, 1982; Novack, Plumer, Smith, Ochitill, Morrow, & Bennett, 1979) have documented an increased and predominant tendency of physicians to convey the accurate diagnosis to cancer patients. Related to this trend is the rapid growth of cancer-patient groups, which have an antidenial feature inherent in them by the fact that members will inevitably be confronted with the deterioration and death of other group members (cf. Holland & Rowland, 1981). Indeed, Spiegel, Bloom, and Yalom (1981) have listed as an advantage of support groups for patients with metastases the fact that they bring the members face to face with death, resulting in a process that Spiegel et al. refer to as death desensitization. There is empirical evidence (Gibbs & Achterberg-Lawlis, 1978) in support of the contention that such a process does occur.

As is often the case with newer treatment applications, enthusiasm for psychosocial interventions with cancer patients now exceeds what can be justified on the basis of controlled research. But relevant studies have recently been reported, of which the following two are perhaps the most important.

Gordon et al. (1980) reported a study in which a large number of melanoma, lung, and breast cancer inpatients received either repeated psychosocial assessments (controls), or these assessments plus a series of brief contacts with a counselor during and following hospitalization, according to a flexible protocol. Gordon et al. concluded that the intervention was effective in that counseled patients showed a greater decline of negative affect, a more realistic outlook, and a more active life-style. However, it is not clear that this study should be viewed as strongly supportive of the effectiveness of the interventions, as the statistical inference criteria used were liberal, and on many variables control and intervention groups did not differ.

Somewhat more encouraging results have been presented by Spiegel et al. (1981), who evaluated support groups of women with metastatic carcinoma of the breast, in comparison with similarly ill controls. Groups were led by an expatient (breast cancer in remission) and a professional. It appears that much of the focus was on dealing with death, and the benefits of such groups might or might not be as evident with patients with better prognosis.

Taken together, these and other recent studies (e.g., Maguire et al., 1980) serve primarily to lend credence to clinically based claims of the value of such interventions. They do not provide a basis for conclusions regarding the characteristics of effective interventions, or what patients those interventions are effective with. Although one would like to be able to assume that patients manifesting the most problems are most likely to benefit from intervention, the study by Gordon et al. (1980) casts doubt on it. Specifically, in their study, only persons who manifested relatively *few* psychosocial problems on initial evaluation showed any benefit of intervention.

Increasing Longevity

Literature reviewed in an earlier section suggests a relation among cancer patients between aspects of personal coping and likelihood of early deterioration and death. This raises the possibility that interventions to influence coping might influence longevity. That literature does not make it entirely clear what specific interventions might be warranted. For instance, although it is possible that convincing some cancer patients that they are unable to cope with their illness would extend their lives (cf. Derogatis et al., 1979; Rogentine et al., 1979), most therapists would be reluctant to design a treatment in which this was the central thrust.

Rather, what interventions have been pursued are tied to the findings of poor prognosis among persons with a sense of defeat and hopelessness. These interventions may also be viewed as in the tradition of faith healing, viz, anecdotes in which even metastatic cancer was "cured" upon the patient's arriving at the belief that God had cured him. That such cures do occur seems clear, as does the fact that, in most cases, religious faith does not prevent death.

Turning to recent secular approaches, the reports of Meares(1979) and Simonton, Matthews-Simonton, and Sparks (1980) are prominent examples. Meares has reported having used intensive meditation, fostering a focus on inner experience, in a series of 17 terminal patients, many of whom survived considerably beyond oncologist's expectations. Simonton et al.'s program is more multifaceted, involving individual and group therapy, relaxation exercises, and physical exercise; a major focus is upon guided fantasy relating to one's disease-fighting capacity. Follow-up data are presented on a large sample (e.g., 128 who eventually expired), and it is noted that the average survival times of patients who had undergone this regime were relatively high—usually in excess of twice the longevity predicted from published averages.

Although these results, particularly Simonton et al.'s, are provocative, it would be premature to attribute a beneficial effect to any specific aspect of the intervention. In particular, patients were self-selected (and atypical of cancer patients in a number of respects), and the role of nonspecific, placebo effects was in no way controlled for. Moreover, concern must be raised about the fact that Simonton et al.'s approach places considerable responsibility for one's health upon the patient, incurring risk of a sense of failure and guilt when the disease does progress (cf. Holland & Rowland, 1981). (For that matter, even suggesting to a cancer patient—perhaps on the basis of research such as reviewed earlier in this chapter—that one's personality may have anything to do with the disease may itself be a source of distress, as Sontag (1978) and Surawicz, Brightwell, Weitzel, and Othmer (1976) have noted.)

Reducing Physical Discomfort

Here there are two treatment targets: pain as an aspect of the advanced disease, and nausea (also retching, emesis) as a side effect of chemotherapy. Psychological treatments for the pain include hypnosis and biofeedback. Noyes' (1981) review of the relevant research (only clinical trials) suggests that although these techniques may be helpful for some persons, it is unclear if they are cost-effective in comparison with alternatives (primarily pharmacological).

The role of psychological interventions may be more central in the case of nausea, both because medically oriented antinausea efforts are often somewhat unsuccessful with cancer patients and because the nausea may have an important psychological component. Although there is presumably an unlearned core to the nausea and related symptoms, there are evidently two respects in which learning may exaggerate the problem: (1) retching and emesis may be maintained by secondary gain (operant conditioning); and (2) nausea may be elicited by neutral stimuli associated in the past with chemotherapy (classical conditioning; cf. Neese, Carli, Curtis, & Kleinman, 1980).

The evidence of a learning component in the retching, etc. comes from reports of the effectiveness of behavioral treatment. Specifically, there are case reports (Brunnquell & Hall, 1982; Redd, 1980) in which excessive levels of these behaviors were dealt with by limiting staff repsonses to them. For instance, in the Redd study, the intervention specified that nurses deal very perfunctorily when the patient retched and much more sociably when the patient did not. In all cases, symptom frequency reduced markedly.

With respect to learned or "anticipatory" nausea, the recent work of Burish and Lyles (1981) and of Redd, Andresen and Minagawa (1982) may prove particularly important. Both employed interventions involving relaxation training; Redd et al. also employed hypnotic induction maintained during chemotherapy administration. Both reports documented reduction in nausea and/or emesis. Burish and Lyles also assessed emotional distress surrounding chemotherapy and found improvement on relevant variables. As might be expected from the greater therapist involvement in hypnosis, the benefits of relaxation training only (Burish & Lyles) were shown to generalize beyond the treatment session whereas the benefits of hypnosis (Redd et al.) were not. On the other hand, Redd et al.'s subjects were especially afflicted with anticipatory emesis (as opposed to nausea alone) and it may be that hypnosis is necessary to control this. The authors of both papers suggested that the active elements of their interventions are muscle relaxation and distraction from chemotherapy-related stimuli, but the studies were not designed in such a way as to ascertain the source of their effectiveness. For a more extensive discussion see Redd & Andrykowski (1982).

COMMENT

The literature reviewed in this chapter constitutes a small proportion of the vast number of relevant papers. An attempt has been made to give a balanced portrayal of the state of the field by largely ignoring severely faulted research findings and by deemphasizing theoretical statements based on such findings. The picture that has emerged is somewhat less supportive of the importance of psychological factors than is seen in some other recent surveys of the field (Bahnson, 1980, 1981; Peterson, Popkin, & Hall, 1981). Their more positive tone derives from an inclusion of supportive but faulted research findings, their deemphasis of discouraging findings, and their treatment of diverse findings on diverse cancer sites as providing endorsement of each other. Assuming that the present survey gives a more accurate picture, how can that picture be summarized?

With respect to psychosocial risk factors, the picture is extremely mixed. Though a refreshing tide of prospective studies has appeared in recent years, the findings from most of them are largely negative, and what positive findings there are do not cohere with one another. Most of these have reported only mixed-site cancer results, leaving very open the possibility that very different results would emerge if prospective studies were carried out on more homogeneous samples. When one turns to a site-by-site focus, one in turn must rely predominantly on nonprospective findings. It would seem reasonable to take seriously such findings only when they have arisen in more than one study. Employing this criterion, the following conclusions appear warranted: (1) breast cancer patients include an elevated incidence of persons who rarely express anger (and perhaps of explosive persons too) and of persons who view themselves as self-sacrificing; it is not clear to what extent such results are a reflection of atypical characteristics of control groups used; (2) severity or reoccurrence of melanoma is associated with a view of oneself as being able to cope with the stress of illness; (3) lung cancer persons tend to have had childhoods marked by parental absence and not to admit to personal distress. These conclusions may appear rather paltry in comparison with the enormous literature on which they are derived, but they do suggest that persons who have been advocating a role of psychological factors in cancer may not be entirely misguided. These findings also appear to be the ones that deserve the expense of evaluation in prospective studies. Other findings of cross-sectional studies deserve to be replicated cross-sectionally before the prospective step is taken.

Noteworthy for its absence among replicated findings is evidence for a role of stress in cancer onset. It would appear premature to dismiss this variable, for several reasons: (1) its demonstrated importance in animal studies and in the study of immune system parameters in humans; (2) its appearance as a variable in isolated instances in human cancer; and (3) the fact that possible stress-personality interactions have not been investigated.

Though it has not been detailed in this chapter, one problem with many of the studies lies in their failure to take full account of medical risk factors with which psychological variables may be confounded. Generally, only the most obvious and powerful ones (e.g., smoking in lung cancer) have been considered. Of special interest is the foremost among risk factors: age. In particular, there is logical and empirical (cf. Abse et al., 1974; Becker, 1979; Lehrer, 1981; Morris et al., 1981) reason to suspect that psychological factors may play a greater role in the etiology of cancer among younger persons than among persons who are at risk by virtue of their advanced age. If this is the case, important effects could be obscured by a lack of a sufficient number of young subjects, analyzed separately.

Although there is no reason to believe that site differences are less important with respect to psychological predictors of medical prognosis among cancer patients than with respect to risk factors of becoming ill in the first place, the predominance of mixed-site samples in prognosis studies has not prevented some coherence from emerging. The conclusion that persons who manifest some hostility have a better prognosis than those who do not appears to be as safe as any in the entire field. As previously noted, both persons who feel unable to cope and persons who are hopeful about prognosis have appeared in long-surviving groups, though the two seem somewhat contradictory. Clearly, additional research is needed to resolve this inconsistency, to examine possible site differences, and to ascertain what role, if any, external stress during illness may play in outcome.

The clinical and empirical literature on typical reactions to cancer, and on the subsequent impact on personal and interpersonal functioning, is rich enough that one does not sense a crying need for further research attention. In contrast, there is clearly room for new psychological applications in dealing with the emotional and physical distress of cancer. On the basis of what research there is, advocacy of more widespread use of psychosocial intervention with cancer patients seems justified, although it remains to be shown what patients are benefited by what interventions and why. The use of relaxation and hypnosis in chemotherapy-related nausea is promising enough to deserve extensive clinical attention. The issue of psychological intervention as a way of prolonging life is much more controversial; neither enthusiasm nor ridicule appears warranted at present, and controlled research is needed.

REFERENCES

Abse, D. W., Wilkins, M. M., van de Castle, R. L., Buxton, W. D., Demars, J., Brown, R. S., & Kirschner, L. G. Personality and behavioral characteristics of lung cancer patients. *Journal of Psychosomatic Research,* 1974, *18,* 101–113.

Achterberg, J., Lawlis, G. F., Simonton, O.C., & Matthews-Simonton, S. Psychological factors and blood chemistries as disease outcome predictors for cancer patients. *Multivariate Experimental Clinical Research,* 1977, *3,* 107–122.

Bagley, C. Control of the emotions, remote stress, and the emergence of breast cancer. *Indian Journal of Clinical Psychology,* 1979, *6,* 213–220.

Bahnson, C. B. Stress and cancer: The state of the art, Part 1. *Psychosomatics,* 1980, *21,* 975–981.

Bahnson, C. B. Stress and cancer: The state of the art, Part 2. *Psychosomatics,* 1981, *22,* 207–220.

Becker, H. Psychodynamic aspects of breast cancer: Differences in younger and older patients. *Psychotherapy and Psychosomatics,* 1979, *32,* 287–296.

Blumberg, E. M., West, P. M., & Ellis, F. W. A possible relationship between psychological factors and human cancer. *Psychosomatic Medicine,* 1954, *16,* 277–286.

Brunnquell, D., & Hall, M. D. Issues in the psychological care of pediatric oncology patients. *American Journal of Orthopsychiatry,* 1982, *52,* 32–44.

Burish, T. G., & Lyles, J. N. Effectiveness of relaxation training in reducing adverse reactions to cancer chemotherapy. *Journal of Behavioral Medicine*, 1981, *4*, 65 – 78.

Chesser, E. S., & Anderson, J. L. Treatment of breast cancer: Doctor/patient communication and psychosocial implications. *Proceedings of the Royal Society of Medicine*, 1975, *68*, 793 – 795.

Coppen, A., & Metcalfe, M. Cancer and extraversion. *British Medical Journal*, 1963, *2*, 18 – 19.

Craig, T. J., & Abeloff, M. D. Psychiatric symptomatology among hospitalized cancer patients. *American Journal of Psychiatry*, 1974, *131*, 1323 – 1327.

Dattore, P. J., Shontz, F. C., & Coyne, L. Premorbid personality differentiation of cancer and noncancer groups: A test of the hypothesis of cancer proneness. *Journal of Consulting and Clinical Psychology*, 1980, *48*, 388 – 394.

Davies, R. K., Quinlan, D. M., McKegney, F. P., & Kimball, C. P. Organic factors and psychological adjustment in advanced cancer patients. *Psychosomatic Medicine*, 1973, *35*, 464 – 471.

Deeley, T. J. Cancer of the cervix uteri: An epidemiological survey. *Clinical Radiology*, 1976, *27*, 43 – 51.

Derogatis, L. R., Abeloff, M. D., & McBeth, C. D. Cancer patients and their physicians in the perception of psychological symptoms. *Psychosomatics*, 1976, *17*, 197 – 201.

Derogatis, L. R., Abeloff, M. D., & Melisaratos, N. Psychological coping mechanisms and survival time in metastatic breast cancer. *Journal of the American Medical Association*, 1979, *242*, 1504 – 1508.

Dunkel-Schetter, C., & Wortman, C. B. The interpersonal dynamics of cancer: Problems in social relationships and their impact on the patient. In H. S. Friedman & M. R. DiMatteo (Eds.), *Interpersonal issues in health care*. New York: Academic Press, 1982.

Duszynski, K. R., Shaffer, J. W., & Thomas, C. B. Neoplasm and traumatic events in childhood. *Archives of General Psychiatry*, 1981, *38*, 327 – 331.

Engelman, S. R. *The symbolic relationship of breast cancer patients to their cancer, cure, physician, and themselves*. Paper presented at the American Psychological Association meeting, August 1981.

Ernster, V. L., Sacks, S. T., Selvin, S., & Petrakis, N. L. Cancer incidence by marital status: U.S. third national cancer survey. *Journal of the National Cancer Institute*, 1979, *63*, 567 – 585.

Evans, N. J. R., Baldwin, J. A., & Gath, D. The incidence of cancer among in-patients with affective disorders. *British Journal of Psychiatry*, 1974, *124*, 518 – 525.

Eysenck, H. J. *The causes and effects of smoking*. Beverly Hills, Calif.: Sage, 1980.

Feinstein, A. D. Psychological interventions in the treatment of cancer. *Clinical Psychology Review*, 1983, *3*, 1 – 14.

Fox, B. H. Premorbid psychological factors as related to cancer incidence. *Journal of Behavioral Medicine*, 1978, *1*, 45 – 133.

Fox, B. H. Psychosocial factors and the immune system in human cancer. In R. Ader (Ed.), *Psychoneuroimmunology*. New York: Academic Press, 1981.

Fox, B. H. A psychological measure as a predictor in cancer. In J. Cohen, J. W. Cullen, & L. R. Martin (Eds.), *Psychosocial aspects of cancer*. New York: Raven Press, 1982. (a)

Fox, B. H. Personal communication, July 1982. (b)

Fox, B. H. Psychogenic etiology and prognosis of cancer—Current status of theory. A. Christ, & K. Flomenhaft (Eds.), *Childhood cancer: Impact on the family*. New York: Plenum, in press.

Fox, B. H., & Howell, M. A. Cancer risks among psychiatric patients: A hypothesis. *International Journal of Epidemiology*, 1974, *3*, 207 – 208.

Fras, I., Litin, E. M., & Pearson, J. S. Comparison of psychiatric symptoms in carcinoma of the pancreas with those in some other intra-abdominal neoplasms. *American Journal of Psychiatry*, 1967, *123*, 1553 – 1561.

Freidenbergs, I., Gordon, W., Hibbard, M., Levine, L., Wolf, C., & Diller, L. Psychosocial aspects of living with cancer: A review of the literature. *International Journal of Psychiatry in Medicine*, 1982, *11*, 303 – 329.

Gibbs, H. W., & Achterberg-Lawlis, J. Spiritual values and death anxiety: Implications for counseling with terminal cancer patients. *Journal of Counseling Psychology*, 1978, *25*, 563 – 569.

Goode, D. J., Corbett, W. T., Schey, H. M., Suh, S. H., Woodie, B., Morris, D. L., & Morrisey, L. Breast cancer in hospitalized psychiatric patients. *American Journal of Psychiatry*, 1981, *138*, 804 – 806.

Gordon, W. A., Freidenbergs, I., Diller, L., Hibbard, M., Wolf, C., Levine, L, Lipkins, R., Ezrachi, O., & Lucido, D. Efficacy of psychosocial intervention with cancer patients. *Journal of Consulting and Clinical Psychology*, 1980, *48*, 743 – 759.

Gorzynski, J. G., Holland, J., Katz, J. L., Weiner, H., Zumoff, B., Fukushima, D., & Levin, J. Stability of ego defenses and endocrine responses in women prior to breast biopsy and ten years later. *Psychosomatic Medicine*, 1980, *42*, 323 – 328.

Graham, S., Snell, L. M., Graham, J. B., & Ford, L. Social trauma in the epidemiology of cancer of the cervix. *Journal of Chronic Diseases*, 1971, *24*, 711 – 725.

Greenberg, R. P., & Dattore, P. J. The relationship between dependency and the development of cancer. *Psychosomatic Medicine*, 1981, *43*, 35 – 43.

Greenwald, H. P., & Nevitt, M. C. Physician's attitudes toward communication with cancer patients. *Social Science and Medicine*, 1982, *16*, 591 – 594.

Greer, S., & Morris, T., Psychological attributes of women who develop breast cancer: A controlled study. *Journal of Psychosomatic Research*, 1975, *19*, 147 – 153.

Greer, S., & Morris, T., & Pettingale, K. W. Psychological response to breast cancer: Effect on outcome. *Lancet*, 1979, *2*, 785 – 787.

Grissom, J. J., Weiner, B. J., & Weiner, E. A. Psychological correlates of cancer. *Journal of Consulting and Clinical Psychology*, 1975, *43*, 113.

Grossarth-Maticek, R. Psychosocial predictors of cancer and internal diseases. *Psychotherapy and Psychosomatics*, 1980, *33*, 122 – 128.

Hagnell, O. The premorbid personality of persons who develop cancer in a total population investigated in 1947 and 1957. *Annals of the New York Academy of Sciences*, 1966, *125*, 846 – 855.

Hinton, J. The influence of previous personality on reactions to having terminal cancer. *Omega*, 1975, *6*, 95 – 111.

Holland, J. C., & Rowland, J. H. Psychiatric, psychosocial, and behavioral interventions in the treatment of cancer: An historical overview. In S. M. Weiss, J. A. Herd, & B. H. Fox (Eds.), *Perspectives on behavioral medicine*. New York: Academic, 1981.

Horne, R. L., & Picard, R. S. Psychosocial risk factors for lung cancer. *Psychosomatic Medicine*, 1979, *41*, 503 – 514.

Huggan, R. R. A critique and possible reinterpretation of the observed low neuroticism scores of male patients with lung cancer. *British Journal of Social and Clinical Psychology*, 1968, *7*, 122 – 128.

Jacobs, S., & Ostfeld, A. An epidemiological review of the mortality of bereavement. *Psychosomatic Medicine*, 1977, *39*, 344 – 357.

Jacobs, T. J., & Charles, E. Life events and the occurrence of cancer in children. *Psychosomatic Medicine*, 1980, *42*, 11 – 24.

Jacobsson, L., & Ottosson, J.-O. Initial mental disorders in carcinoma of pancreas and stomach. *Acta Psychiatrica Scandinavica*, 1971, Suppl. 221, 120 – 127.

Jansen, M. A. *Personality variables associated with fibrocystic disease and breast cancer*. Paper presented at the American Psychological Association meeting, August 1981.

Joseph, J. G., & Syme, S. L. Social connection and the etiology of cancer: An epidemiological review and discussion. In J. Cohen, J. W. Cullen, & L. R. Martin (Eds.), *Psychosocial aspects of cancer*. New York: Raven Press, 1982.

Katz, J. L., Ackman, P., Rothwax, Y., Sachar, E., Weiner, H., Hellman, L., & Gallagher, T. F. Psychoendocrine aspects of cancer of the breast. *Psychosomatic Medicine*, 1970, *32*, 1 – 18.

Keast, D. Immune surveillance and cancer. In K. Bammer, & B. H. Newberry (Eds.), *Stress and cancer*. Toronto: C. J. Hogrefe, 1981.

Keehn, R. J. Goldberg, I.D., & Beebe, G. W. Twenty-four year mortality follow-up of army veterans with disability separations for psychoneurosis in 1944. *Psychosomatic Medicine*, 1974, *36*, 27 – 46.

Kellerman, J. A note on psychosomatic factors in the etiology of neoplasms. *Journal of Consulting and Clinical Psychology,* 1978, *46,* 1522 – 1523.

Kerr, T. A., Schapira, K., & Roth, M. The relationship between premature death and affective disorders. *British Journal of Psychiatry,* 1969, *115,* 1277 – 1282.

Kissen, D. M. Psychosocial factors, personality and lung cancer in men aged 55-64. *British Journal of Medical Psychology,* 1967, *40,* 29 – 43.

Kissen, D. M. The present status of psychosomatic cancer research. *Geriatrics,* 1969, *24,* 129 – 137.

Kobasa, S. C., Maddi, S. R., & Kahn, S. Hardiness and health: A prospective study. *Journal of Personality and Social Psychology,* 1982, *42,* 168 – 177.

Kosch, S. G. *Life style variables associated with fibrocystic disease and breast cancer.* Paper presented at the American Psychological Association meeting, August 1981.

Krasnoff, A. Psychological variables and human cancer: A cross-validation study. *Psychosomatic Medicine,* 1959, *21,* 291 – 295.

Lehmann, J. F., DeLisa, J. A., Warren, C. G., deLateur, B. J., Bryant, P. L. S., & Nicholson, C. G. Cancer rehabilitation: Assessment of need, development, and evaluation of a model of care. *Archives of Physical Medicine and Rehabilitation,* 1978, *59,* 410 – 419.

Lehrer. S. Life change and gastric cancer. *Psychosomatic Medicine,* 1980, *42,* 499 – 502.

Lehrer, S. Life change and lung cancer. *Journal of Human Stress.* 1981, *7,* 7 – 11.

LeShan, L. An emotional life-history pattern associated with neoplastic disease. *Annals of the New York Academy of Sciences,* 1969, *164,* 546 – 557.

LeShan, L., & Reznikoff, M. A psychological factor apparently associated with neoplastic disease. *Journal of Abnormal and Social Psychology,* 1960, *60,* 439 – 440.

Lloyd, G. G. Psychological stress and coping mechanisms in patients with cancer. In B. A. Stoll (Ed.), *Mind and cancer prognosis.* Chichester: Wiley, 1979.

Locke, S. E. Stress, adaptation, and immunity: Studies in humans. *General Hospital Psychiatry,* 1982, *4,* 49 – 58.

Locke, S. E., Jemmott, J. B., Kraus, L., Hurst, M. W., Heisel, J. S., McClelland, D. C., & Williams, R. M. *Stressful life change and human immunity.* Paper presented at the American Psychological Association meeting, August 1981.

Maguire, P., Tait, A., Brooke, M., Thomas, C., & Sellwood, R. Effect of counselling on the psychiatric morbidity associated with mastectomy. *British Medical Journal,* 1980, *281,* 1454 – 1456.

Mastrovito, R. C., Deguire, K. S., Clarkin, J., Thaler, T., Lewis, J. L., & Cooper, E. Personality characteristics of women with gynecological cancer. *Cancer Detection and Prevention,* 1979, *2,* 281 – 287.

McCoy, J. W. Psychological variables and onset of cancer. *Dissertation Abstracts International,* 1978, *38,* 4471B.

Meares, A. Meditation: A psychological approach to cancer treatment. *Practitioner,* 1979, *222,* 119 – 122.

Meyerowitz, B. E. Psychosocial correlates of breast cancer and its treatment. *Psychological Bulletin,* 1980, *87,* 108 – 131.

Morris, T., Greer, S., Pettingale, K. W., & Watson, M. Patterns of expressions of anger and their psychological correlates in women with breast cancer. *Journal of Psychosomatic Research,* 1981, *25,* 111 – 117.

Morrison, F. R. Psychosocial factors in the etiology of cancer. *Dissertation Abstracts International,* 1981, *42,* 155 – 156B.

Moss, A. R. Specific risk versus general susceptibility: Social and psychological risk factors for heart disease and cancer mortality in a nine-year prospective study. *Dissertation Abstracts International,* 1980, *40,* 3677B.

Muslin, H. L., Gyarfas, K., & Pieper, W. J. Separation experience and cancer of the breast. *Annals of the New York Academy of Sciences,* 1966, *125,* 802 – 806.

Nesse, R. M., Carli, T., Curtis, G. C., & Kleinman, P. D. Pretreatment nausea in cancer chemotherapy: A conditioned response? *Psychosomatic Medicine*, 1980, *42*, 33 – 36.

Nieburgs, H. E., Weiss, J., Navarrete, M., Strax, P., Teirstein, A., Grillione, G., & Siedlecki, B. The role of stress in human and experimental oncogenesis. *Cancer Detection and Prevention*, 1979, *2*, 307 – 336.

Niemi, T., & Jaaskelainen, J. Cancer morbidity in depressive persons. *Journal of Psychosomatic Research*, 1978, *22*, 117 – 120.

Novack, D. H., Plumer, R., Smith, R. L., Ochitill, H., Morrow, G. R., & Bennett, J. M. Changes in physicians' attitudes toward telling the cancer patient. *Journal of the American Medical Association*, 1979,*241*, 897 – 900.

Noyes, R. Treatment of cancer pain. *Psychosomatic Medicine*, 1981, *43*, 57 – 70.

O'Malley, J. E., Koocher, G., Foster, D., & Slavin, L. Psychiatric sequelae of surviving childhood cancer. *American Journal of Orthopsychiatry*, 1979, *49*, 608 – 616.

Paloucek, F. P., & Graham, J. B. Precipitating factors in cancer of the cervix. *Surgical Forum*, 1960, *10*, 740 – 742.

Panagis, D. M. Supportive therapy: Goals and methods. In B. A. Stoll (Ed.), *Mind and cancer prognosis*. Chichester: Wiley, 1979.

Parkes, C. M., Benjamin, B., & Fitzgerald, R. G. Broken heart: A statistical study of increased mortality among widowers. *British Medical Journal, 1969, 1*, 740 – 743.

Peters, L. J., & Mason, K. A. Influences of stress on experimental cancer. In B. A. Stoll (Ed.), *Mind and cancer prognosis*. Chichester: Wiley, 1979.

Peterson, L. G., Popkin, M. K., & Hall, R. C. W. Psychiatric aspects of cancer. *Psychosomatics*, 1981, *22*, 774 – 789.

Pettingale, K. W., Greer, S., & Tee, D. E. H. Serum IgA and emotional expression in breast cancer patients. *Journal of Psychosomatic Research*, 1977, *21*, 395 – 399.

Pettingale, K. W., Merrett, T. G., & Tee, D. E. H. Prognostic value of serum levels of immunoglobulins (IgG, IgA, IgM and IgE) in breast cancer: A preliminary study. *British Journal of Cancer*, 1977, *36*, 550 – 557.

Rabkin, J. G., & Struening, E. L. Life events, stress, and illness. *Science*, 1976, *194*, 1013 – 1020.

Rassidakis, N. C., Kelepouris, M., Goulis, K., & Karaiossefidis, K. On the incidence of malignancy among schizophrenic patients. *Agressologie*, 1973, *14*, 269 – 273.

Redd, W. H. Stimulus control and extinction of psychosomatic symptoms in cancer patients in protective isolation. *Journal of Consulting and Clinical Psychology*, 1980, *48*, 448 – 455.

Redd, W. H., Andresen, G. V., & Minagawa, R. Y. Hypnotic control of anticipatory emesis in patients receiving cancer chemotherapy. *Journal of Consulting and Clinical Psychology*, 1982, *50*, 14 – 19.

Redd, H., & Andrykowski, M. A. Behavioral intervention in cancer treatment: Controlling aversion reactions to chemotherapy. *Journal of Consulting and Clinical Psychology*, 1982, *50*, 1018 – 1029.

Reznikoff, M. Psychological factors in breast cancer. *Pschosomatic Medicine*, 1955, *17*, 96 – 108.

Riley, V. Biobehavioral factors in animal work on turmorigenesis. In S. M. Weiss, J. A. Herd, & B. H. Fox (Eds.), *Perspectives on behavioral medicine*. New York: Academic, 1981.

Rogentine, G. N., van Kammen, D. P., Fox, B. H., Docherty, J. P., Rosenblatt, J. E., Boyd, S. C., & Bunney, W. E. Psychological factors in the prognosis of malignant melanoma: A prospective study. *Psychosomatic Medicine*, 1979, *41*, 647 – 655.

Rogers, M. P., Dubey, D., & Reich, P. The influence of the psyche and the brain on immunity and disease susceptibility: A critical review. *Psychosomatic Medicine*, 1979, *41*, 147 – 164.

Ross, R. D., Stockdale, F., & Jacobs, C. Cancer Patient Behavior Scale: Scores of cancer patients and healthy adults. *Proceedings of the American Society of Clinical Oncology*, 1978, *19*, 348.

Salmon, P. A. The significance of psychic symptoms in the early diagnosis of carcinoma of the pancreas. *Canadian Medical Association Journal*, 1967, *97*, 767 – 772.

Schmale, A. H., & Iker, H. P. The affect of hopelessness and the development of cancer. *Psychosomatic Medicine*, 1966, *28*, 714 – 721. (a)

Schmale, A. H., & Iker, H. The psychological setting of uterine cervical cancer. *Annals of the New York Academy of Sciences*, 1966, *125*, 807 – 813. (b)

Schmale, A. H., & Iker, H. Hopelessness as a predictor of cervical cancer. *Social Science and Medicine*, 1971, *5*, 95 – 100.

Schonfield, J. Psychological and life-experience differences between Israeli women with benign and cancerous breast lesions. *Journal of Psychosomatic Research*, 1975, *19*, 229 – 234.

Schyve, P. M., Smithline, F., & Meltzer, H. Y. Neuroleptic-induced prolactin level elevation and breast cancer. *Archives of General Psychiatry*, 1978, *35*, 1291 – 1301.

Shekelle, R. B., Raynor, W. J., Ostfeld, A. M., Garron, D. C., Bieliauskas, L. A., Liu, S. C., Maliza, C., & Paul, O. Psychological depression and 17-year risk of death from cancer. *Psychosomatic Medicine*, 1981, *43*, 117 – 125.

Simonton, O. C., Matthews-Simonton, S., & Sparks, T. F. Psychological intervention in the treatment of cancer. *Psychosomatics*, 1980, *21*, 226 – 233.

Sklar, L. S., & Anisman, H. Contributions of stress and coping to cancer development and growth. In K. Bammer & B. H. Newberry (Eds.), *Stress and cancer*. Toronto: C.J. Hogrefe, 1981. (a)

Sklar, L. S., & Anisman, H. Stress and cancer. *Psychological Bulletin*, 1981, *89*, 369 – 406.(b)

Snell, L., & Graham, S. Social trauma as related to cancer of the breast. *British Journal of Cancer*, 1971, *25*, 721 – 734.

Sobel, H. J., & Worden, J. W. The MMPI as a predictor of psychosocial adaptation in cancer. *Journal of Consulting and Clinical Psychology*, 1979, *47*, 716 – 724.

Sontag, S. *Illness as metaphor*. New York: Farrar, Straus and Giroux, 1978.

Spence, D. P., Scarborough, H. S., & Ginsberg, E. H. Lexical correlates of cervical cancer. *Social Science and Medicine*, 1978, *12*, 141 – 145.

Spiegel, D., Bloom, J. R., & Yalom, I. Group support for patients with metastatic cancer. *Archives of General Psychiatry*, 1981, *38*, 527 – 533.

Stavraky, K. M. Psychological factors in the outcome of human cancer. *Journal of Psychosomatic Research*, 1968, *12*, 251 – 259.

Surawicz, F. G., Brightwell, D. R., Weitzel, W. D., & Othmer, E. Cancer, emotions, and mental illness: The present state of understanding. *American Journal of Psychiatry*, 1976, *133*, 1306 – 1309.

Temoshok, L. *Stress and "type C" versus epidemiological risk factors in melanoma*. Paper presented at the American Psychological Association meeting, August 1981.

Thomas, C. B., & McCabe, O. L. Precursors of premature disease and death: Habits of nervous tension. *Johns Hopkins Medical Journal*, 1980, *147*, 137 – 145.

Thomas, C. B., Ross, D. C., Brown, B. S., & Duszynski, K. R. A prospective study of the Rorschachs of suicides: The predictive potential of pathological content. *Johns Hopkins Medical Journal*, 1973, *132*, 334 – 360.

Thomas, C. B., Duszynski, K. R., & Shaffer, J. W. Family attitudes reported in youth as potential predictors of cancer. *Psychosomatic Medicine*, 1979, *41*, 287 – 302.

Tsuang, M. T., Woolson, R. F., & Fleming, J. A. Premature deaths in schizophrenia and affective disorders. *Archives of General Psychiatry*, 1980, *37*, 979 – 983.

Voth, H. M. Cancer and personality. *Perceptual and Motor Skills*, 1976, *42*, 1131 – 1137.

Watson, C. G., & Schuld, D. Psychosomatic factors in the etiology of neoplasms. *Journal of Consulting and Clinical Psychology*, 1977, *45*, 455 – 461.

Watson, C. G., & Schuld, D. Psychosomatic etiological factors in neoplasms: A response to Kellerman. *Journal of Consulting and Clinical Psychology*, 1978, *46*, 1524 – 1525.

Weisman, A. D., & Worden, J. W. Psychosocial analysis of cancer deaths. *Omega*, 1975, *6*, 61 – 75.

Wheeler, J. I., & Caldwell, B. M. Psychological evaluation of women with cancer of the breast and cancer of the cervix. *Psychosomatic Medicine*, 1955, *17*, 256 – 268.

Whitlock, F. A., & Siskind, M. Depression and cancer: A follow-up study. *Psychological Medicine*, 1979, *9*, 747 – 752.

Wirsching, M., Stierlin, H., Hoffmann, F., Weber, G., & Wirsching, B. Psychological identification of breast cancer patients before biopsy. *Journal of Psychosomatic Research,* 1982, *26,* 1 – 10.

Witkin, M. H. Psychological concerns in sexual rehabilitation and mastectomy. *Sexuality and Disability,* 1979, *2,* 54 – 59.

Worden, J. W., Johnston, L. C., & Harrison, R.H. Survival quotient as a method for investigating psychosocial aspects of cancer survival. *Psychological Reports,* 1974, *35,* 719 – 726.

Worden, J. W. & Sobel, H. J. Ego strength and psychosocial adaptation to cancer. *Psychosomatic Medicine,* 1978, *40,* 585 – 592.

Wortman, C. B., & Dunkel-Schetter, C. Interpersonal relationships and cancer: A theoretical analysis. *Journal of Social Issues,* 1979, *35,* 120 – 155.

20   Behavioral Approaches to Pain

Ray Winters
University of Miami

INTRODUCTION

As a sensory experience, pain is unusual. It has both a perceptual and an emotional/motivational component. Both are adaptive functions; the perceptual component localizes the source of the pain and the emotional/motivational component energizes and directs behaviors that potentially minimize tissue damage. People who are congenitally insensitive to pain suffer from an abnormally large number of injuries. Sternbach (1968) describes a girl, congenitally insensitive to pain, who had chewed the tip of her tongue to a pulp by the time she was 2 years old. The same girl, at the age of 3, suffered third-degree burns from kneeling on a hot radiator while she watched children playing outside. Other people have been known to die from ruptured appendices because they did not feel the pain (Sternbach, 1968).

Transmission of Pain Information to the Brain

It is generally believed that free nerve endings are the receptors for pain and the nerve impulses resulting from noxious stimuli are transmitted to the central nervous system (CNS) by small unmyelinated axons or small thinly myelinated fibers. The prevailing view is that tissue damage causes the release of chemical substances, probably *prostaglandins*, that activate free nerve endings. Pain information from the body is transmitted to the thalamus along a number of neuronal pathways. For the most part these pathways are distinct from the pathways conveying other types of somatic information to the brain. Unlike other sensory modalities, projections to the cerebral cortex do not appear to be necessary for the perception of pain. The integrity of regions in the thalamus, however, are.

565

Lesion studies conducted on terminal cancer patients provide evidence that several regions within the thalamus are involved in pain. The *ventral posterior medial* (VPM) and *ventral posterior lateral nuclei* (VPL) appear to mediate cutaneous pain (pinprick) as well as touch and temperature. The *parafascicular* and *intralaminar* nuclei are essential to the perception of deep, chronic pain. Lesions of the *anterior thalamic* and *dorsomedial nuclei* remove the motivational/ emotional component of pain without affecting the perception of deep or cutaneous pain. Neurons of the dorsomedial nucleus project to the prefrontal area of the frontal lobes. One of the symptoms of damage or removal of the prefrontal area is an emotional indifference to pain. Thus, it would appear that the intralaminar VPM, VPL, and parafascicular nuclei of the thalamus are necessary for the perception of pain and that the anterior nucleus and the dorsomedial nuclei are essential to the motivational/emotional component of pain. The latter two nuclei are a part of the limbic system, a neuronal system believed to be involved in emotions (Chapter 4).

Melzack and Wall (1965) have proposed a physiological model to account for the transmission of pain from the spinal cord to the brain. They contend that cells of the *substantia gelatinosa*, a dense nuclear area in the spinal cord, act as a "gating" mechanism to control the flow of nerve impulses to the brain regions subserving pain (Fig. 20.1). The output of *T-cells* (pain transmission cells) receives excitatory input from *L (large) fibers* and *S (small) fibers* from somatic receptors. The large fibers are activated primarily by non-noxious peripheral stimuli (i.e., touch and pressure); collaterals of these axons carry somatic sensory information to the brain. The small fibers convey, for the most part, information about noxious stimuli. The T-cell compares the amount of activity from the S and L fibers. When the amount of activity in the large fibers is high relative to the amount of activity in the S fibers, the spinal gate is closed (as a result of inhibition) and no pain information is transmitted to the brain. The gate is open when the amount of neural activity in the S fibers is high relative to the amount of L fiber activity and a pain message reaches the brain. Another important feature of the model is that the activity of T-cells can be modulated by descending fibers from the brain.

There is some evidence that supports the Melzack and Wall model. Because of the structural characteristics of the receptors that activate the two types of fibers, the L fibers, relative to the S fibers, adapt rather rapidly to a sustained stimulus. After an initial burst of action potentials, there is a substantial reduction in the firing rate of these axons. Intermittent stimulation, however, increases the activity of L fibers and thus would tend to close the gate.

The use of intermittent stimulation for the relief of pain makes sense from common experience. If one's arm hurts the individual rubs it rather than apply continuous pressure. Similarly, the itch (a mild form of pain) from a mosquito bite is relieved by scratching it, not pressing on it. In general, intermittent stimulation allays mild forms of pain. For example, individuals suffering from phantom limb pain find relief by lightly tapping the stump of the removed limb. Whirlpool baths,

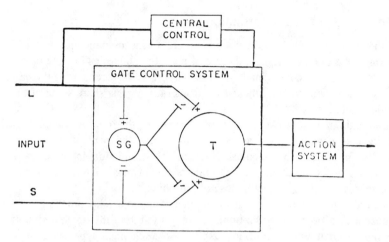

FIG. 20.1.   Schematic diagram of Melzack and Wall (1965) Gate Control model
for pain.
SG: substantia gelatinosa cells
T: transmission cells to the brain
S: small axons
L: large axons

a form of intermittent stimulation, are also effective for mild forms of muscle pain. The *transcutaneous stimulator,* an electrical device used for the relief of pain, delivers intermittent electrical stimulation to the injured region.

The Melzack and Wall model has not been thoroughly tested by controlled experimentation but the studies that have been conducted give only partial support to it. Wall and Sweet (1967) demonstrated that chronic pain could be reduced in patients by stimulating large fibers. Also, patients with a disease that preferentially destroys large fibers gained considerable relief by electrical stimulation of the remaining large fibers (Nathan & Wall, 1974).

There are a number of findings, reviewed by Nathan (1976), that are clearly inconsistent with the Melzack and Wall model. For example there is a great deal of pain in thallium neuropathy yet there is a large decrease in the number of small diameter fibers and very little change in large diameter fibers. Similarly, in polyneuropathy, which is usually painless, there is a disproportionate destruction of large fibers, relative to small fibers.

In general, the results of neurophysiological studies have led to a number of questions regarding the details of the gate control model, particularly in regards to gating mechanism in the spinal cord (Nathan, & Rudge, 1974; Nathan, 1976). Nevertheless, this model has contributed substantially to the understanding of pain mechanisms. The importance of the temporal patterning of stimuli in pain perception has been well established by the model and, perhaps more importantly, it directed attention to the important role of descending fibers from the brain.

CNS Modulation of Pain Information

Two of the most effective treatments for severe forms of pain are electrical stimulation of the brain (ESB) and the use of narcotic analgesics like the opiate derivatives (morphine, codeine) and synthetic narcotics. Research during the past 12 years provides evidence that these two forms of analgesia share some of the same brain mechanisms.

Electrical stimulation of two areas of the brainstem, the *periaqueductal gray* and the *nucleus raphe magnus* are known to reduce the perception of pain substantially. In rats, a few seconds of electrical stimulation in these areas produces an analgesic effect that lasts several hours (Mayer & Liebeskind, 1974), and the effect is as potent as a large dose of morphine.

The analgesia produced by ESB stimulation appears to result from the activation of descending fibers from the brain, thereby inhibiting the transmission of pain messages from the spinal cord. Fig. 20.2 shows a schematic representation of the descending pathway that is believed to mediate the effects of ESB-induced analgesia. Neurons in the periaqueductal gray excite cells in the nucleus raphe magnus. These cells synapse upon an inhibitory interneuron that blocks pain information reaching the spinal cord from afferent neurons. The neurotransmitter between the raphe neuron and inhibitory interneuron is thought to be *serotonin;* an *endorphin* is thought to be the transmitter between the inhibitory interneuron and the afferent sensory neurons.

Evidence for this descending pain pathway comes from several sources. First, when the descending fibers of the nucleus raphe magnus are destroyed the ESB induced analgesia disappears (Basbaum, Marley, & O'Keefe, 1976). Moreover, electrical stimulation in brain regions that produce analgesia cause total inhibition of spinal cord neurons that transmit pain information. This inhibitory effect is selective in that other somatic sensory modalities are unaffected. Excitatory drugs also increase the activity in the periaqueductal gray and produce analgesia (Behbehani & Fields, 1979). Moreover, electrical stimulation of the periaqueductal gray and the administration of excitatory drugs also increase the electrical activity of cells in the nucleus raphe magnus (Behbehani & Fields, 1979). Endorphin receptors have been found in the dorsal gray matter of the spinal cord (Atweh & Kuhar, 1977). Also, analgesia can be produced by direct injection of enkephalin and morphine (endorphin agonists) into the dorsal gray matter (Duggan, 1979). The analgesic effects of these drugs is eliminated by injections of *naloxone* (Yaksh, 1979), an endorphin antagonist.

There are a number of similarities between ESB-induced and morphine-induced analgesia. For example, the drug naloxone, which partially blocks the analgesic effect of ESB (Akil, Mayer, & Liebeskind, 1976), also renders morphine ineffective as a pain reliever. Naloxone is a drug used clinically to counteract the effect of morphine and heroin overdose. Neural activity in the periaqueductal gray increases when animals are given an injection of morphine (Criswell & Rogers, 1978; Urca & Nahin, 1978). Depletion of serotonin with parachlorophenylalanine

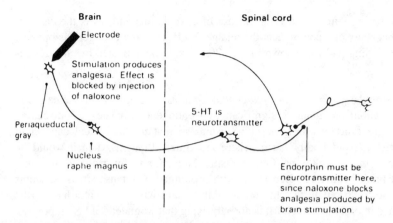

FIG. 20.2. Central control of ascending pain information. Stimulation of peri-aqueductal gray leads to inhibition of pain transmission from the spinal cord to the brain.

or lesions in the raphe nuclei blocks both ESB analgesia and the effects of morphine (Lee & Fennessy, 1970). Descending serotonergic fibers must be intact for both types of pain relief to be effective.

The user of morphine quickly develops *tolerance* to the drug so that increasingly larger doses must be taken. The same holds true for ESB-induced analgesia. In fact *cross-tolerance* between the two types of analgesia has been demonstrated (Mayer & Hayes, 1975). That is, if an individual has become tolerant to morphine he or she will also be tolerant to ESB analgesia, and vice versa. In addition, the two forms of analgesia are additive. Pain relief can be produced by simultaneous administration of low doses of morphine combined with low levels of ESB, which if administered independently would not be strong enough to induce analgesia.

Endogenous Opiates. Findings from several laboratories account for the similarities between ESB- and opiate-induced analgesia. A study by Pert, Snowman, and Snyder (1974) provides strong evidence that many neurons in the brain have, within their cell membranes, opiate receptors. Similarly, Hughes, Smith, Kosterlitz, Fothergill, Morgan, and Morris (1975) identified opiatelike substances in pig brains. They referred to them as *enkephalins*. The enkephalins are similar to morphine but considerably more potent. Terenius and Wahlstrom (1975) found in the cerebral spinal fluid of patients with *trigeminal neuralgia*, a disease that causes facial pain, a substance that has an affinity for opiate receptors. The results of these three studies, and similar experiments, suggest that the brain might produce its own opiates that are secreted during prolonged pain. Morphine would, according to this view, mimic the action of endogenous opiates. Endorphins are another type of endogenous opiate.

The enkaphalins are known to occupy receptor sites in a number of areas of the brain including some regions of the limbic system and along the pain pathways.

Pain-producing stimuli cause the release of enkephalins and, as is the case for morphine, naloxone counteracts the analgesic effect of the endogenous opiates. The descending pathway shown in Fig. 20.2 would be activated by endogenous opiates.

Functional Significance of Endogenous Opiates.   At this point one can only speculate about the adaptive significance of endogenous opiates. As discussed earlier, pain functions as a warning system so that the individual can act to minimize or avoid bodily harm. There are times, though, when it would be adaptive to inactivate the pain mechanisms. Pain, might, for example, interfere with adaptive behaviors when faced with prolonged or intense stress. It seems reasonable to speculate that the brain inhibits pain when behaviors have to be performed in order to survive. It is not surprising that wounded soldiers report not feeling pain until they have reached safety. In this regard it is interesting to note that electrical stimulation of the periaqueductal gray also produces aggressive and defensive behaviors. Also consistent with this hypothesis is the finding that circulatory levels of the endogenous opiate *beta endorphin,* increase during pain. Beta endorphin also is found in the pituitary gland. Adrenocorticotrophic hormone (ACTH), a hormone released by the pituitary into the circulation during times of stress, and beta endorphins have a common chemical precursor.

Also, it is interesting to note that endorphins are released during situations in which an organism is unable to actively cope with a stressor. Normally an animal can tolerate more electrical shock if it is warned by a signal (a flash of light for example) than if the shock is not signaled. This effect is eliminated, however, by naloxone injections (Fanselow, 1979). In a sense, then an animal is experiencing less pain during an unavoidable stressor, if it receives a warning. This mechanism may be important when an individual is experiencing a stressor, but knows about it in advance. An obvious example would be the pain experienced during childbirth. Although childbirth is a painful experience, the release of endogenous opiates may serve to mitigate the pain. Thus one's ability to cope with unavoidable pain may, in part, be mediated by the release of endogenous opiates in the brain.

Other Functions of Endogenous Opiates.   Endorphins may also be neurotransmitters involved in thermoregulation. Local injections of endorphin into the hypothalamus produce changes in body temperature (Martin & Bacino, 1978), and naloxone administration alters the ability of the brain to regulate body temperature (Holaday, Wei, Loh, & Li, 1978). In addition, endorphins may be involved in the brain's reward mechanisms. This is not surprising in view of the fact that opiates such as heroin, morphine, and codeine have euphoric effects upon many of their users. Rats will perform a task so as to receive injections of enkephalins (Belluzzi & Stein, 1977). Furthermore, many of the brain regions that have been shown to be effective in self-stimulation studies (Chapter 4) also contain endorphins. Belluzzi and Stein (1977) found that rats would not self-stimulate in the periaqueductal gray when given injections of naloxone. As discussed in Chapter 4, dopamine is believed to be the transmitter involved in reward, but endogenous opiates also appear to be involved.

Neurophysiological and Neurochemical Basis of Pharmacological Treatment of Pain

There are a number of methods for the treatment of pain including surgical intervention, ESB, behavioral methods such as EMG, biofeedback, relaxation therapy, cognitive restructuring, and the administration of pharmacological agents. Recent advances in our understanding of receptor mechanisms, of how pain information is gated in the CNS, and the role of endogenous opiates in the perceptual and emotional components of pain, has provided a basis for the understanding of many of the methods, particularly the manner in which pharmacological agents relieve pain. Some of these ideas are discussed in this section.

Aspirin. Oral administration of salicylates, like aspirin, is the most common treatment for pain. The FDA estimates that Americans ingest about 19 billion per year. Aspirin is most effective for the relief of low intensity pain from tension headaches, muscle pain, and joint ache; it is often quite effective for rheumatoid arthritis, an inflammatory disease involving the body joints. Aspirin relieves pain by inhibiting the synthesis of *prostaglandins*. Prostaglandins are substances produced by most tissues in the body; they are synthesized from an essential fatty acid, arachidonic acid, but are not stored by body cells. They are known to be involved in the mechanism of blood coagulation, edema, fever, inflammation, and pain. Prostaglandins are secreted when there is tissue damage or inflammation. If the pathological state is not too severe aspirin can be effective in the reduction of the pain mediated by prostaglandins.

For most people the occasional use of aspirin has no adverse effects but chronic ingestion of the drugs has several disadvantages. It may cause nausea for some individuals because it irritates the lining of the stomach. Also it has a stimulating effect on the vomiting reflex mediated by neurons in the brain. It also may cause a loss of blood from the gastrointestinal tract and it prolongs bleeding time. Taking aspirin with alcohol or anticoagulates is ill-advised because of the risks associated with increased bleeding. Many of these risks can be averted by using coated aspirins that are absorbed in the small intestine rather than the stomach.

Aspirin Substitutes. The safest and most effective aspirin substitute is acetaminophen (Tylenol, Valadul, Tempra, & Datril). This drug has the analgesic and antipyretic (fever-reducing) effect of aspirin but is not very effective as an anti-inflammatory agent. This drug does not cause increased bleeding or loss of blood in the gastrointestinal tract; it has less potential for causing nausea and vomiting.

The major risk of this drug is that prolonged use or high doses may cause liver damage.

Narcotic Analgesics.   Salicylates and acetaminophen are quite effective for the reduction of mild or moderate pain, but more potent prescription drugs are required for severe forms of pain. The narcotic analgesics are either direct derivatives of the opium poppy (codeine and morphine) or synthetic drugs that have a similar effect on the central nervous system (e.g. methadone, heroin, Percodan, Demerol).

The narcotic analgesics probably affect both the perceptual and emotional/ motivation components of pain by stimulating opiate receptors in the brain and spinal cord. As mentioned earlier, endorphins appear to be a neurotransmitter that can block transmission of nerve impulses in the spinal cord that convey pain information to the brain. Also, there are opiate receptors in a number of areas within the limbic system.

The major disadvantage of the use of narcotic oralgesics is their addictive properties. A drug is defined as being addictive if it produces *tolerance* and *physical dependency.* Tolerance refers to a progressive decrease in sensitivity to a drug. Thus the user requires a higher dose of the drug to obtain the same effect. Physical dependency is revealed when administration of the drug is discontinued. If the drug is addicting withdrawal symptoms will occur. Among these symptoms are; depression, psychomotor agitation, convulsions, hallucinations, and sleep disturbances. Because of their addictive properties, one goal of most chronic pain treatment programs is the termination of the use of narcotic analgesics.

Local Anesthetics.   These drugs (e.g. procaine, novocaine, xylocaine) are usually applied topically or injected subcutaneously at the site of the body region producing the pain. Local anesthetics prevent increases in membrane permeability to sodium ions that are necessary for the propagation of nerve impulses. Also, they lower the resting membrane permeability to sodium and potassium ions, thereby preventing the generation of nerve impulses.

General Anesthetics.   Injection of general anesthetics, usually barbiturates (e.g., nembutal or pentothal), eliminates pain by decreasing synaptic transmission throughout the CNS. It is generally believed that the reduction in activity within the brainstem reticular formation underlies the loss of consciousness and the analgesic properties of these drugs.

Hypnosis, Acupuncture, and Placebos.   A number of studies have demonstrated the effectiveness of acupuncture (Gaw, Chang, & Shaw, 1975; Mann, Bowsher, Mumford, Lipton, & Miles, 1973). Because acupuncture uses intermittent stimulation, either turning needles or intermittent electrical current, its analgesic effects are consistent with the Gate Control Model of pain. The Gate

Control Model, however, does not account for the fact that the analgesic effects last for several hours after the stimulation is terminated. Because the analgesic effects of acupuncture can be eliminated by naloxone (Mayer, Price, Rafii, & Barber, 1976), the release of endogeneous opiates appears to be involved in the mechanism. Hypnotically induced analgesia has not been found to be blocked to be affected by naloxone injection (Mayer et al, 1976) but placebos have been (Levine, Gordon, & Fields, 1979).

TREATMENT OF CHRONIC PAIN

Chronic pain, as defined by Black (1975) is a syndrome characterized by intractable pain for more than 6 months and complaints about the pain that are not commensurate with existing physical symptoms. In some cases there are no measurable physical dysfunctions or tissue damage. The management of the chronic pain syndrome is particularly difficult and has become a major problem for the health-care community because of the disproportionate time, resources, and health dollars required for its treatment.

Chronic pain treatment programs have several goals, most of which are substantially different from those used to treat pain in the terminally ill. Whereas surgical intervention, ESB analgesia, and the use of narcotic analgesics may be justified for a patient with terminal cancer, chronic pain treatment programs seek to avoid these measures. In fact, one of the major goals of most of these programs is to decrease or eliminate medication intake, particulary addicting drugs like the narcotic analgesics and sedative hypnotic drugs. Because psychological factors play a major role in this syndrome, the purpose of these programs, in addition to withdrawal from addicting drugs, is to provide the patient with coping strategies that enable him or her to: (1) decrease the utilization of health-care facilities; (2) increase motor behaviors; (3) increase work activity; (4) elevate his or her mood, as depression is usually one of the major symptoms. In regard to these goals, the use of sedative-hypnotic drugs is contraindicated because they are CNS depressants and would tend to decrease motor activity, exacerbate depression, and increase the need for the utilization of health-care resources. Similarly, narcotic analgesics, in addition to relieving pain, provide positive reinforcement because of their euphoric effects and the social reinforcement provided by those who dispense the medication. Also, narcotic analgesics and sedative hypnotic drugs probably contribute to the disability of the patient (Fordyce, 1977; Taylor, Zlutnick, Corley, & Flora, 1980).

Social reinforcement provided by significant others, because of the reported pain, may be one of the most difficult problems that these programs face. Social support from loved ones is important for the recovery of the patient but also serves to reinforce the behaviors that the program is trying to modify. Consultation with the family of the patient, therefore, becomes extremely important to the success of the program.

Outcome Results of Treatment Programs

Inpatient Programs. One of the first outcome studies of a program utiilizing an eclectic treatment package for chronic pain was conducted by Sternbach (1974). The program employed behavior modification techniques, treatment contracts, and group therapy. Patients in the programs showed only slight changes in self-report scores of pain but relatively large increments in motor activity, as assessed by walking time, number of laps around a gym, and overall activity. These data were not analyzed statistically. A questionaire sent to patients 6 months after the program showed only small changes in motor activity relative to pretreatment scores but a statistically significant reduction in unit dosage of medication (Cairns, Thomas, Mooney, & Pace, 1976).

Cairns, Thomas, Mooney, and Pace (1976) used behavior modification techniques to treat patients with lower back pain. Follow-up data revealed that 70% of the patients reported significantly less pain or increased motor activity. Seventy-four percent had not utilized health-care facilities after the program and 58% reported that they required less analgesic medication. A number of the patients were given vocational training and 74% of them were either working or in a work preparation program.

In an eclectic program conducted by Gottlieb, Strite, Koller, Madorsky, Hockersmith, Kleeman, and Wagner (1977), vocational counseling, physical reconditioning, individual therapy, family therapy, group therapy, and biofeedback training were given to treat back pain patients. Sixty-eight percent of the group finished the program. A random sample of the program graduates was studied and was found to show a significant improvement in physical functioning and improvement on clinical assessment scales; the clinical assessment scale measured changes in assertiveness and comprehension of the program goals. Also, some of the patients chose to participate in a vocational restoration program. Of the 50 (of 59) patients who completed the program, 40 were evaluated one month after its completion; of these patients 95% had maintained a successful level of vocational rehabilitation. Twenty-three of the 50 were contacted 6 months after the program and of those, 92% were either involved in vocational training or successfully employed.

Swanson, Floreen, and Swenson (1976) used physical therapy, behavior modification techniques, biofeedback, and counseling with the patients and members of the patient's family in a treatment program for 50 patients with pain in the extremities, back, and neck. Twenty-one of the patients were using narcotic analgesics at the beginning of the program but none were using them when they were discharged. Also, at admission, 15 patients were ambulatory, 17 were partially ambulatory, and 2 were not ambulatory at all. After being discharged, 31 patients were completely ambulatory, 13 partially ambulatory, and zero patients were not ambulatory. In a follow-up study examining 26 of the original 50 patients, 5 of them reported a decrement in the intensity and duration of pain, 10 reported that pain remained unchanged, and 6 reported that pain was more intense, or lasted longer, or both; 6 patients did not respond. Eighty percent of the patients in the follow-up study said that they had not sought additional medical treatment. Also 15 patients were using less medication or the same amount of medication, and 6 patients were using more medication; 5 did not respond.

The goal of a treatment program conducted by Fordyce (1977) was to increase exercise, social, and work activities while decreasing medication intake, verbal complaints of pain, and a decrease in activities that had been used to avoid pain. After completion of the program patients showed significant increases in activity and exercise tolerance. Also, narcotic usage decreased from 1.0 morphine unit equivalent to 0.1 units for 13 patients, and 1.0 to 0.2 for 26 patients. For those patients using sedative hypnotic drugs, there was a decrement from 1.5 units to 0.9 units after completion of the program.

Summary.   Behavioral and eclectic chronic pain treatment programs appear to produce some improvements in patients but because of lack of control groups, differences in subject populations, measures of improvement, and follow-up procedures, it is difficult to make meaningful comparisons between various programs. Moreover, outcome measures may vary according to the type of pain that the patient is experiencing. As a case in point, self-report data of patients with low back pain seldom change significantly after treatment, despite the fact that other measures show significant gains. In contrast, headache and abdominal pain patients frequently report complete or near complete cessation of pain (Zlutnick, Corley, & Owens, 1980).

Outpatient Studies.   Many outpatient studies are conducted in laboratories, under controlled conditions, thereby permitting the assessment of individual components of chronic pain treatment programs.

Cognitive Therapy.   Several studies have examined cognitive techniques of pain control. Horan and Dellinger (1974) compared emotive imagery with distraction, and a control in allaying pain due to cold-pressor stimulation. During emotive imagery the subject imagines a particular event (usually pleasant) to distract his or her attention from the pain. Horan and Dellinger report that the emotive imagery group was more tolerant of pain than the other two groups. Other studies that examined the effectiveness of this technique typically have not been able to replicate their findings (e.g., Greene & Reyher, 1972). One study that did support their findings compared the various components of the Lamaze natural childbirth techniques (Stone, Demchick-Stone, & Horan, 1977). These investigators used immersion time in cold water, pain threshold, and self-report as outcome measures and found that the emotive imagery was more effective than focal-point visualization or no treatment.

Relaxation Therapy.   Relaxation therapy appears to be effective in mitigating a number of types of pain. Bobey and Davidson (1970) report that relaxation therapy appears to increase tolerance to radiant heat and pressure pain. Subjects in their experiment were exposed to one of four conditions: cognitive rehearsal, increased anxiety, relaxation therapy, or a control condition. The relaxation group showed significantly higher tolerance scores than the other groups.

McAmmond, Davidson, and Kovitz (1971) found relaxation to be superior to hypnosis and control procedures in stress reactions to analgesic injections and pressure algometer pain. Lehrer (1972) assessed the effectiveness of relaxation therapy upon habituation and reduced skin response to electric shock. The relaxation therapy group was found to be superior to an increased tension group but not to controls. Similarly, a study by Blanchard and Ahles (1979) provides evidence that relaxation therapy and similar techniques lead to a significant reduction in the intensity and frequency of migraine headaches.

Advanced Preparation.   Several studies provide evidence that advanced preparation serves to mitigate pain. Patients in a study conducted by Egbert, Battit, Welch, and Partlett (1964) were provided detailed information about the type and intensity of pain that they might experience postoperatively and that relaxation might help reduce this pain. They also were told that they should expect to be moved around the recovery room after the operation. In comparison to controls, the advanced preparation group requested fewer narcotics following surgery and were sent home on the average of 2 to 7 days earlier.

To prepare patients to undergo a gastrointestinal endoscope examination, Johnson and Rice (1974) described typical sensations patients reported during the procedure and suggested ways that they might cope with the pain. As a result of this procedure patients were found to experience less discomfort than controls.

The results of the studies by Egbert et al, (1964), and Johnson and Rice (1974) are interesting in view of the results of animal studies discussed earlier that demonstrate that endogenous opiates are secreted during a signaled-shock experimental paradigm. Perhaps, advanced preparation serves as a signal that causes the release of endogenous opiates. Also, advanced preparation may have a placebo effect because of the similarity of the patient/doctor social interaction during advanced preparation and when a placebo is given by a doctor to a patient. It will be recalled that placebos also cause the release of endogenous opiates.

Summary.   The studies cited in this section provide evidence that several of the techniques used for chronic patients can be demonstrated to be effective in reducing pain induced in a laboratory setting or during surgical procedures. Because the subjects in these experiments were not chronic pain patients, further experimentation must be conducted to demonstrate the effectiveness of these techniques with this type of clinical population.

TREATMENT AND MANAGEMENT OF BURN PAIN

Burns rank as the third leading cause of traumatic death to adults in the United States. Over two million people are believed to survive serious burns each year. The treatment of burn pain and the psychological effects of the trauma and disfigurement associated with major (third-degree) burns are a topic of major concern to behavioral medicine.

There are three major stages of treatment of burn patients: (1) the resuscitation phase; (2) the acute phase; and, (3) the rehabilitative phase. The medical treatment and psychological reactions during these phases have been described in detail elsewhere (Achterberg-Lawlis & Kenner, 1982; Miezala, 1978); a summary of these reports is given here.

Resuscitation Phase

Medical treatment during the initial stage, which lasts about 72 hours, seeks to maintain general physical health, particularly pulmonary functioning and the maintenance of fluid and electrolytic balances. Also the control of infection is of central concern because the skin is the first line of defense against microrganisms; also necrotic tissue provides an excellent medium for the proliferation of microrganisms. The major concern of the patient, who is often quite alert and rational during this phase, is his or her personal survival.

Acute Phase

The acute phase is the time interval from 72 hours after the burn until grafting occurs. The control and prevention of infection becomes the major concern during this period. Active exercise is usually encouraged to minimize edema and the prevention of the adherence of tendons to surrounding tissues. Also, the patient has a difficult time regulating metabolic functioning so the maintenance of nutritional needs is a major problem during the second stage of recovery. Usually a high protein diet is initiated as soon as possible during the wound-healing stage.

During the acute phase two rather serious psychological periods emerge. The *withdrawal period* is characterized by a decrement in general awareness in which the patient is rather calm and often denies or represses thoughts and feelings regarding what has happened to him or her. This period may elicit adaptive or maladaptive processes (Seligman, 1974). The symptoms of *conservation withdrawal*, an adaptive coping mechanism and *depression withdrawal*, a maladaptive process, are very similar. In the latter case, however, there is a high risk of death following depression and hopelessness. There patients apparently do not have the resources to survive, so psychological interventions are mandatory. In the case of conservation withdrawal, psychological intercession is contraindicated because the withdrawal represents an attempt on the part of the patient to survive.

During the *reactive period* the patient marshals the defense mechanisms that have enabled him or her to deal with stressors experienced prior to the trauma. Thus a wide variety of behaviors may be shown, depending on the coping mechanisms unique to each patient (Miezala, 1978; Steiner & Clark, 1977). It would not be wise to attempt to modify these defensive behaviors because they are probably essential to the recovery of the patient.

Rehabilitative Phase

This phase is defined as the period following the completion of healing. Preservation of new skin tissue, the prevention of infection, and the attainment of optimal behavioral function are the major concerns during this period.

The rehabilitative stage is the period when the patient is required to cope with a long-term adjustment problem that may require significant changes in life-style. It is during this period that the patient requires the greatest amount of emotional support and may require professional help.

About 30% of the patients studied by Andreasen and Norris (1972) had significant adjustment problems related to work or interpersonal relationships during this phase. Similarly Cobb and Lindemann (1943) reported that about 50% of the burn patients they studied had serious psychiatric problems during the rehabilitative phase. Similar figures have been reported by other investigators (Hamburg, Artz, Reiss, Amspacher, & Chambers, 1953; Noyes, Andreason, & Hartford, 1971).

HEADACHE PAIN

There are three major types of headaches in which psychological factors appear to precipitate the pain: migraine, muscle contraction headaches (MCH), and a combination of these two types called the mixed headache. Chronic forms of these headaches are estimated to affect between 10 and 30% of the population of the United States. The National Ambulatory Medical Care Survey indicated that headache symptoms account for about 12 million visits to the doctor's office each year.

In general, headaches are more common among women than among men (Friedman, 1979; Philips, 1977a; Selby & Lance, 1960; Turner & Stone, 1979; Waters, 1971). Lance (1978) reports that 75% of patients with tension headaches were women. The incidence of migraine headache has been reported to be between 23% and 29% in women and 15% to 20% in men (Waters & O'Conner, 1975). A rather extensive survey conducted in Finland (Nikaforow & Hokkanen, 1978) found a significantly higher incidence of headaches among individuals in urban areas and a sharp decline in incidence in adults over 65. Headache is less common among children under 11 years of age (Bille, 1962; Sillanpaa, 1976; Vahlquist, 1955).

Muscle Contraction Headache

In a study that examined 496 headache patients, Philips (1977a) reports that 80% of his sample suffered from MCH. Muscle contraction headache pain is usually bilaterally localized in the frontal, occipital, or suboccipital regions of the head. The most common precipitating factor for MCH appears to be emotional stress (Friedman, 1979; Friedman, Von Storch, & Merritt, 1954; Nikiforow & Hokkanen, 1978). However, the finding that MCH headache may occur in the absence of heightened skeletal muscle activity (Philips, 1978) suggests that social reinforcement (attention) may serve to maintain the symptom.

The exact physiological mechanisms that underlie MCH are still unknown but muscle tension appears to be involved (Dalessio, 1972; Friedman, 1979). Clearly it is not muscle tension per se that underlies the symptoms. Electromyogram levels do not correlate with pain intensity, frequency, or medication use (Philips, 1978). Furthermore, Bakal and Kaganov (1977) found no differences in frontal EMG reactivity in MCH headache patients and control subjects to 80 db auditory stimuli. Philips (1977b) contends that sustained elevations of EMG, rather than absolute levels of EMG, are most relevant to tension headaches. Sustained contractions, according to Friedman (1979), lead to relative ischemia in the muscles that are involved. The ischemia would be expected to cause a release of pain-inducing chemical substances in the muscles. A study by Tunis and Wolff (1954) provides evidence that vasoconstriction of scalp vessels occurs in tension headache subjects. If the capillaries do not dilate, then muscles may become ischemic, or perhaps sustained contraction of the arterioles may be painful. In any case, it is not necessary to postulate that it is the sustained muscle contraction itself that causes the pain. The fact that ergotamine, a vasoconstrictor, can exacerbate MCH pain and the vasodilator alcohol can allay MCH pain (Brazil & Friedman, 1957; Ostfeld, Reis, & Wolff, 1957) attests to the importance of vascular mechanisms in MCH. The fact that aspirin is usually an effective analgesic for MCH suggests that prostaglandins are important in the mechanism.

The typical treatment for MCH is mild analgesics like aspirin or acetaminophen. In cases where the pain is more intense or sustained, sedative – hypnotic drugs or tricyclic antidepressants may be prescribed. Combination drugs are given sometimes for more severe headaches. Of these, Fiorinal is the most widely used one. It contains a short-acting barbiturate, caffeine, aspirin, and phenacetin.

In regard to the effectiveness of various chemical agents, it is interesting to note that placebos are particularly effective for MCH patients. Friedman and Merritt (1957) assessed the effectiveness of various therapeutic agents in the treatment of

MCH and found that 55% of MCH patients reported pain relief following the use of a placebo. This compares to 71% for the most effective drug used—a combination of a mild analgesic, caffeine, and a sedative – hypnotic drug.

A wide variety of behavioral and cognitive techniques have been used to treat MCH. The major assumptions underlying these methods, which are often used in combination (Beaty & Haynes, 1979), is that repeated increases in arousal due to perceived threat lead to a heightened activation of the sympathetic division of the automatic nervous system and sustained muscle tension. Cognitive approaches to MCH reduction, therefore, attempt to modify the appraisal of situations that may elicit putative sympathetic arousal and skeletal muscle contraction. Relaxation training, EMG biofeedback, operant techniques, and systematic desensitization treat the symptoms rather than the causes of the disorder.

Outcome studies of frontal EMG feedback and relaxation therapy experimentation (Budzynski, Stoyva, Adler, & Mullaney, 1973; Chesney & Shelton, 1976; Cox, Freundlich, & Meyer, 1975; Haynes, Griffin, Mooney, & Parise, 1975; Holroyd, Andrasik, & Noble, 1980; Kondo & Canter, 1977; Philips, 1977c) report significant, but equivalent reduction in MCH relative to control procedures. Control procedures in these studies include: false feedback, placebo medication, no treatment, psychotherapy, or symptom-monitoring controls.

Relaxation therapy and biofeedback techniques are the most frequently used nonpharmacological methods to treat MCH. Cognitive restructuring has been shown in one outcome study (Holroyd, Andrasik, & Westbrook, 1977) to be effective in the treatment of MCH but it is apparent that more outcome studies assessing the relative effectiveness of nonbehavioral techniques is required in order to provide more definitive data regarding the clinical utility of these approaches.

Migraine Headaches

It is generally believed (Feuerstein & Gainer, 1982) that migraine headaches result from a two-stage cerebral vascular pathophysiological mechanism in which vasodilation is preceded by vasoconstriction. The precise role of intracranial and extracranial arteries in migraines is not known but arteriolar narrowing is thought to lead to brain ischemia, thereby generating the aura associated with the syndrome. An accumulation of carbon dioxide is thought to trigger arteriolar dilation. Cutaneous vascular ischemia also is thought to occur. The actual headache pain results from the vasodilation component of the response (Edmeads, 1979).

Etiology of Migraines.   Although there is a veritable plethora of studies on the subject, the etiologic factors involved in migraine headache remain elusive. The evidence for a genetic component is, at best, only suggestive (Refsum, 1968; Ziegler, 1978). Even though 25% of migraine patients attribute the onset of the symptoms to diet (Selby & Lance, 1960) there is very little evidence to support this belief (Moffett, Swash, & Scott, 1972; Medina & Diamond, 1978; Shaw, Johnson, & Keogh, 1978).

Psychosocial stress appears to be a major precipitating factor for migraine headaches. Selby and Lance (1960) report that 67% of 388 migraine patients they examined indicated that stress factors triggered the onset of their headaches. Similarly, Henryk-Gutt and Reese (1973) found that 54% of the headache attacks of patients they examined were believed to be precipitated by emotional factors. It is interesting to note that in this study migraine sufferers did not report a higher incidence of stressful events than nonheadache controls.

Hormonal variations may also be a factor that contributes to migraine headaches. Female migraine sufferers often experience symptom relief during pregnancy, particularly if the headaches were previously associated with the menstrual cycle (Lance & Anthony, 1966). Oral contraceptives appear to exacerbate the symptoms (Carroll, 1971; Dalton, 1976; Whitty, Hockaday, & Whitty, 1966).

Adverse weather conditions have been associated with migraine headache, but a controlled study by Wilkinson and Woodrow (1979) failed to reveal any relationship between weather conditions and the disorder. This finding is inconsistent with the results of an earlier study conducted by Sulman, Levy, Lewy, Pfeifer, Superstine, and Tal (1974) which reported that 20 to 30% of their subjects experienced migraine headaches when exposed to sudden, hot, dry winds. The discrepancy between the results of these studies may be due to differences in subject populations or the fact that the weather changes were more gradual in the Wilkinson and Woodrow (1979) study (Feuerstein & Gainer, 1982). The finding that relative humidity and physiological reactivity covary (Waters, Koresko, Rossie, & Hackley, 1979) also suggests a possible role of meteorological factors in migraines. The results of the Waters et al. study and the Wilkinson and Woodrow (1979) study suggest that weather variables may be important, but further investigations are required to confirm the importance of this factor.

The neurochemical changes that occur during sleep may hold a key to the understanding of the etiology of migraine headaches. Plasma norepinephrine levels rise 3 hours prior to the onset of migraines that occur during REM sleep (Hsu, Crisp, Kalucy, Koval, Chen, Carruthers, & Zilkha, 1977). Also, plasma serotonin levels fall at the onset of REM sleep (Dexter & Riley, 1975; Hsu et al, 1977), thus suggesting that changes in norepinephrine and serotonin levels during sleep may be responsible for the vasomotor pattern associated with migraines. Several of the drugs used to treat migraine headache (e.g. tricyclic antidepressant, and sedative – hypnotic agents) depress REM sleep; tricyclic antidepressants are known to elevate serotonin levels.

Selby and Lance (1960) find that about one of every four migraine sufferers attributes the onset of their headaches to the ingestion of a particular type of food (e.g., chocolate or cheese). Controlled experiments that have examined this variable, in general, have not found the ingestion of specific dietary agents and migraine headaches to covary (Medina & Diamond, 1978; Moffett et al., 1972;

Sandler, Youdin, & Hanington, 1974; Shaw, Johnson, & Keogh, 1978). Perhaps, as suggested by Jessup (1978), the association between a particular food and the onset of a migraine headache occurs as a result of classical conditioning.

Biochemical Mechanisms

It appears that serotonin is released from blood platelets at the onset of migraine headache; also, there is an increase in excretion of serotonin's major metabolite, 5-hydroxyindoleacetic acid, during migraine attacks (Curran, Hinterberger, & Lance, 1965; Sicuteri, Testi, & Anselmi, 1961). Furthermore there is an increase in plasma serotonin levels during the preheadache period and a reduction in these levels during the attack (Anthony, Hinterberger, & Lance, 1967; Hilton & Cumings, 1972). Fanchamps (1974) contends that blood platelets release serotonin at the beginning of a migraine attack and this ultimately leads to a reduction in the threshold for pain in the arterial walls. He also argues that there is a reduction in tonus of the extracranial vessels, thereby causing a massive vasodilation in vascular walls that have become more sensitive to pain.

   Treatment of Migraine Headaches.   Medication is the most common treatment of migraine headaches. Behavioral techniques have been employed and these are discussed in Chapter 17. Pharmacological agents can be used as prophylactic measures or to treat the symptoms of the pain during the attack. Methysergide is the most widely used drug to prevent the onset of migraine. It is a serotonin antagonist but its mechanism of action is not fully understood. It may prevent the release of serotonin from blood platelets or perhaps it blocks the action of serotonin at vascular receptor sites. Another prophylactic agent used for migraine headache sufferers is propranolol. This drug is a beta-adrenergic receptor blocker and thus may prevent the onset of migraines by preventing vasoconstriction (Diamond & Medina, 1976; Wideroe & Vigander, 1974). Monoamine oxidase inhibitors, which prevent serotonin enzymatic deactivation breakdown, are also effective prophylactic agents. Vasoconstrictors like ergotamine typically are used to treat the pain of migraine headache once it has been begun.

CONCLUSIONS

Pain is a problem that has a long history in the field of medicine and psychology. The magnitude and complexity of this disorder is enormous and presents a challenge of considerable magnitude to the emerging field of behavioral medicine. The results of controlled experiments and clinical data have led to the synthesis of new pharmacological agents and the application of behavioral and cognitive techniques that serve to advance our understanding of its mechanisms and its treatment.

REFERENCES

Achterberg-Lawlis, J. & Kenner, C. In C. M. Doleys, R. L. Meridith, & A. R. Ceminiro (Eds.), *Burn patients in behavioral medicine: Assessment and treatment strategies.* Plenum Press, 1982.

Akil, H., Mayer, D., & Liebeskind, J. C. Antagonism of stimulation-produced analgesia by Naloxone, a narcotic antagonist. *Science,* 1976, *191,* 961 – 962.

Andreasen, N. J. C., & Norris, A. S. Long-term adjustment and adaptation mechanisms in severly burned adults. *The Journal of Nervous and Mental Diseases,* 1972, *154*(5), 352 – 362.

Anthony, M., Hinterberger, H., & Lance, J. W. Plasma serotonin in migraine and stress. *Archives of Neurology,* 1967, *16,* 544 – 552.

Atweh, S. F. & Kuhar, M. J. Autoradiographic localization of opiate receptors in rat brain. I. Spinal cord and lower medulla. *Brain Research,* 1977, *124,* 53 – 67.

Bakal, D. A., & Kaganov, J. A. Muscle contraction and migraine headache: a psychophysiological comparison. *Headache,* 1977, *17,* 208 – 215.

Basbaum, A. I., Marley, N., & O'Keefe, J. Effects of spinal cord lesions on the analgesic properties of electrical stimulation. In J. J. Bonica & D. Albe-Fessard (Eds.), *Recent advances in pain research and therapy: Proceedings of the first World Congress on Pain.* New York: Raven Press, 1976.

Beaty, E. T., & Haynes, S. N. Behavioral intervention with muscle-contraction headache: A review. *Psychosomatic Medicine,* 1979, *41,* 165 – 180.

Behbehani, M. M. & Fields, H. L. Evidence that an excitatory connection between the periaqueductal gray and nucleus raphe magnus mediates stimulation-produced analgesia. *Brain Research,* 1979, *170,* 85 – 93.

Belluzzi, J. D., & Stein, L. Enkephalin may mediate euphoria and drive-reduction reward. *Nature,* 1977, *266,* 556 – 558.

Bille, B. Migraine in school children. *Acta Paediatrica,* 1962, *51* (Suppl. 136), 1 – 151.

Black, R. G. The chronic pain syndrome. *Surgical Clinics of North America,* 1975, *55,* 4.

Blanchard, D., & Ahles, T. A. Behavioral treatment of psycho-physiological disorders. *Behavior Modification,* 1979, *3,* 518 – 549.

Bobey, J. J. & Davidson, P. O. Psychological factors affecting pain tolerance. *Journal of Psychosomatic Research,* 1970, *14,* 371 – 376.

Brazil, P., & Friedman, A. P. Further observations in craniovascular studies. *Neurology,* 1957, *7,* 52 – 55.

Budzynski, T., Stoyva, J., Adler, C., & Mullaney, D. EMG biofeedback and tension headache: A controlled outcome study. *Psychosomatic Medicine,* 1973, *35,* 484 – 496.

Cairns, D., Thomas, L., Mooney, V., & Pace, J. B. A comprehensive treatment approach to chronic low back pain. *Pain,* 1976, *2,* 301 – 308.

Carroll, J. D. Migraine: General management. *British Medical Journal,* 1971, *2,* 756 – 757.

Chesney, M. A., & Shelton, J. L. A comparison of muscle relaxation and electromyogram biofeedback treatment for muscle-contraction headache. *Journal of Behavior Therapy and Experimental Psychiatry,* 1976, *7,* 221 – 225.

Cobb, S., & Lindemann, E. Coconut Grove burns: Neuropsychiatric observations. *Annals of Surgery,* 1943, *117,* 814 – 824.

Cox, D., Freundlich, A., & Meyer, R. Differential effectiveness of electromyograph feedback, verbal relaxation instructions, and medication placebo with tension headaches. *Journal of Consulting and Clinical Psychology,* 1975, *43,* 892 – 898.

Criswell, H. E., & Rogers, F. G. Narcotic analgesia: Changes in neural activity recorded from periaqueductal gray matter of rat brain. *Society for Neuroscience Abstracts,* 1978, *4,* 458.

Curran, D. A., Hinterberger, H., & Lance, J. W. Total plasma serotonin, 5-hydroxy-induꞁeacetic acid and p-hydroxy-m-methoxymandelic acid excretion in normal and migrainous subjects. *Brain,* 1965, *88,* 997 – 1010.

Dalessio, D. J. *Wolff's headache and other head pain.* New York: Oxford University Press, 1972.

Dalton, K. Migraine and oral contraceptives. *Headache,* 1976, *16,* 247 – 251.

Dexter, J., & Riley, T. Studies in nocturnal migraine. *Headache,* 1975, *15,* 51 – 62.

Diamond, S., & Medina, J. L. Double blind study of propranolol for migraine prophylaxis. *Headache,* 1976, *16,* 24 – 27.

Duggan, A. W. Morphine, enkephalins and the spinal cord. In J. J. Bonica, J. C. Liebeskind, & D. Albe-Fessard (Eds.), *Advances in pain research and therapy* (Vol. 3). New York: Raven Press, 1979.

Edmeads, J. Vascular headache and the cranial circulation: Another look. *Headache,* 1979, *19,* 127 – 132.

Egbert, L. D., Battit, G. E., Welch, C. E., & Partlett, M. D. Reduction of postoperative pain by encouragement and instruction of patients. *New England Journal of Medicine,* 1964, *270,* 825 – 827.

Fanchamps, A. The role of humoral mediators in migraine headache. *Canadian Journal of Neurological Sciences,* 1974, *1,* 189 – 195.

Fanselow, M. S. Naloxone attenuates rat's preference for signaled avoidance. *Physiological Psychology,* 1979, *7,* 70 – 74.

Feuerstein, M., & Gainer, J. *Chronic headache: Etiology and management in behavioral medicine: Assessment and treatment strategies.* In D. M. Doleys, R. L. Meredith, & A. R. Ceminiro (Eds.), *Behavioral medicine, assessment and treatment strategies.* Plenum Press, 1982.

Fordyce, W. E. *Behavioral methods for chronic pain and illness.* St. Louis: C. V. Mosby, 1977.

Friedman, A. P. Characteristics of tension headache: A profile of 1420 cases. *Psychosomatics,* 1979, *20,* 451 – 458.

Friedman, A. P., & Merritt, H. H. Treatment of headache. *Journal of the American Medical Association,* 1957, *163,* 1111 – 1117.

Friedman, A. P., Von Storch, T. C., & Merrit, H. H. Migraine and tension headache: A clinical study of 2000 cases. *Neurology,* 1954, *4,* 773 – 778.

Gaw, A. C., Chang, L. W., and Shaw, I. C. Efficacy of acupuncture on osteoarthritic pain. *New England Journal of Medicine,* 1975, *293,* 375 – 378.

Gottlieb, H., Strite, L. C. Koller, R., Madorsky, A., Hockersmith, V., Kleeman, M., & Wagner, J. Comprehensive rehabilitation of patients having chronic low back pain. *Archives of Physical Medicine and Rehabilitation,* 1977, *58,* 101 – 108.

Greene, R. J., & Reyher, J. Pain tolerance in hypnotic analgesic and imagination states. *Journal of Abnormal Psychology,* 1972, *79,* 29 – 38.

Hamburg, D. A., Artz, C. P., Reiss, E., Amspacher, W. H., & Chambers, R. E. Clinical importance of emotional problems in the care of patients with burns. *New England Journal of Medicine,* 1953, *248,* 355 – 359.

Haynes, S., Griffin, P., Mooney, D., & Parise, M. Electromyographic biofeedback and relaxation instructions in the treatment of muscle-contraction headaches. *Behavior Therapy,* 1975, *6,* 672 – 678.

Henryk-Gutt, R., & Reese, W. L. Psychological aspects of migraine. *Journal of Psychosomatic Research,* 1973, *17,* 141 – 153.

Hilton, B. P., & Cumings, J. N. 5-Hydroxytryptamine levels and platelet aggregation responses in subjects with acute migraine headache. *Journal of Neurology, Neurosurgery and Psychiatry.* 1972, *35,* 505 – 509.

Holaday, J. W., Wei, E., Loh, H. H., & Li, C. H. Endorphins may function in heat adaptation. *Proceedings of the National Academy of Sciences,* (USA), 1978, *75,* 2923 – 2927.

Holroyd, K. A., Andrasik, F., & Noble, J. A comparison of EMG biofeedback and a credible pseudotherapy in treating tension headache. *Journal of Behavioral Medicine,* 1980, *3,* 29 – 39.

Holroyd, K. A., Andrasik, F., & Westbrook, T. Cognitive control of tension headache. *Cognitive Therapy and Research,* 1977, *1,* 121 – 133.

Horan, J. J., & Dellinger, J. K. "In vivo" emotive imagery: A preliminary test. *Perceptual and Motor Skills,* 1974, *39,* 359 – 362.

Hsu, L. K. G., Crisp, A. H., Kalucy, R. S., Koval, J., Chen, C. N., Carruthers, M., & Zilkha, K. Early morning migraine: Nocturnal plasma levels of catecholamines, tryptophan, glucose and free fatty acids, and sleep encephalographs. *Lancet*, 1977, *1*, 447−450.

Hughes, J., Smith, T. W., Kosterlitz, H. W., Fothergill, L. A., Morgan, B. A., & Morris, H. R. Identification of two related pentapeptides from the brain with potent opiate agonist activity. *Nature*, 1975, *258*, 577−579.

Jessup, B. A. The role of diet in migraine: Conditioned taste aversion. *Headache*, 1978, *18*, 229.

Johnson, J. E., & Rice, V. H. Sensory and distress components of pain: Implications for the study of clinical pain. *Nursing Research*, 1974, *23*, 203−209.

Kondo, C., & Canter, A. True and false electromyographic feedback: Effect on tension headache. *Journal of Abnormal Psychology*, 1977, *86*, 93−95.

Lance, J. W. *Mechanism and management of headache* (3rd ed.). London: Butterworth, 1978.

Lance, J. W., & Anthony, M. Some clinical aspects of migraine: A prospective survey of 500 patients. *Archives of Neurology*, 1966, *15*, 356−361.

Lee, J. R., & Fennessy, M. R. The relationship between morphine analgesia and the levels of biogenic amines in the mouse brain. *European Journal of Pharmacology*, 1970, *12*, 65−70.

Lehrer, P. M. Physiological effects of relaxation in a double-blind analog of desensitization. *Behavior Therapy*, 1972, *3*, 193−208.

Levine, J. D., Gordon, N. C., & Fields, H. L. The role of endorphins in placebo analgesia. In J. J. Bonica, J. C. Liebeskind, & D. Albe-Fessard (Eds.), *Advances in pain research and therapy* (Vol. 3). New York: Raven Press, 1979.

Mann, F., Bowsher, D., Mumford, J., Lipton, S., & Miles, J. Treatment of intractable pain by acupuncture. *Lancet*, 1973, *2*, 57−60.

Martin, G. E., & Bacino, C. B. Action of intrahypothalamically-injected beta-endorphin on the body temperature of the rat. *Abstracts, Society of Neuroscience*, 1978, *4*, 411.

Mayer, D. J., & Hayes, R. L. Stimulation-produced analgesia: Development of tolerance and cross-tolerance to morphine. *Science*, 1975, *188*, 941−943.

Mayer, D. J., & Liebeskind, J. C. Pain reduction by focal electrical stimulation of the brain: An anatomical and behavioral analysis. *Brain Research*, 1974, *68*, 73−93.

Mayer, D. J., Price, D. D., Rafii, A., & Barber, J. Acupuncture hypalgesia: Evidence for activation of a central control system as a mechanism of action. In J. J. Bonica & D. Albe-Fessard (Eds.) *Advances in pain research and therapy* (Vol. 1). New York: Raven Press, 1976, 751−754.

McAmmond, D. M., Davidson, P. O., & Kovitz, D. M. A comparison of the effects of hypnosis and relaxation training on stress reactions in a dental situation. *American Journal of Clinical Hypnosis*, 1971, *13*, 233−242.

Medina, J. L., & Diamond, S. The role of diet in migraine. *Headache*, 1978, *18*, 31−34.

Melzack, R., & Wall, P. D. Pain mechanisms: A new theory. *Science*, 1965, *150*, 971−979.

Miezala, P. Post burn psychological adaptation: An overview. *Critical Care Quarterly*, 1978, *1*(3), 93−110.

Moffett, A., Swash, M., & Scott, D. F. Effect of tyramine in migraine: A double-blind study. *Journal of Neurology, Neurosurgery and Psychiatry*, 1972, *35*, 496−499.

Moffett, A., Swash, M., & Scott, D. F. Effect of chocolate in migraine: A double-blind study. *Journal of Neurology, Neurosurgery and Psychiatry*, 1974, *37*, 445−448.

Nathan, P. W. The gate control theory of pain: A critical review. *Brain*, 1976, *99*, 123.

Nathan, P. W., & Rudge, P. Testing the gate-control theory of pain in man. *Journal of Neurology, Neurosurgery and Psychiatry*, 1974, *37*, 1366−1372.

Nathan, P. W., & Wall, P. D. Treatment of post-herpetic neuralgia by prolonged electrical stimulation. *British Medical Journal*, 1974, *3*, 645−647.

Nikaforow, R., & Hokkanen, E. An epidemiological study of headache in an urban and rural population in Northern Finland. *Headache*, 1978, *18*, 137−145.

Noyes, R., Jr., Andreasen, N. J. C., & Hartford, C. E. The psychological reaction to severe burns. *Psychosomatics*, 1971, *12*(6), 416−422.

Ostfeld, A. M., Reis, D. J., & Wolff, H. G. Studies on headache: Bulbar conjunctival ischemia and muscle contraction headache. *Archives of Neurology and Psychiatry,* 1957, *77,* 113 – 119.

Pert, C. B., Snowman, A. M., & Snyder, S. H. Localization of opiate receptor binding in presynaptic membranes of rat brain. *Brain Research,* 1974, *70,* 184 – 188.

Philips, C. Headache in general practice. *Headache,* 1977, *16,* 322 – 329. (a)

Philips, C. A psychological analysis of tension headaches. In S. Rachman (Ed.), *Advances in medical psychology.* Oxford: Pergamon, 1977. (b)

Philips, C. Tension headache: Theoretical problems. *Behavioral Research and Therapy,* 1978, *16,* 249 – 261.

Philips, C. The modification of tension headache pain using EMG biofeedback. In *Behavior research and therapy.* Oxford: Pergamon, 1977. (c)

Refsum, S. Genetic aspects of migraine. In P. J. Vinken & G. W. Bruyn (Eds.), *Handbook of clinical neurology* (Vol. 5). Amsterdam: North Holland, 1968.

Sandler, J. D., Youdim, M. B. H., & Hanington, E. A phenylethylamine oxidasing defect in migraine. *Nature,* 1974, *250,* 335–337.

Selby, G., & Lance, J. W. Observations on 500 cases of migraine and allied vascular headache. *Journal of Neurology, Neurosurgery and Psychiatry,* 1960, *23,* 23 – 32.

Seligman, R. A psychiatric classification system for burned children. *American Journal of Psychiatry,* 1974, *13*(1), 41 – 46.

Shaw, S. W. J., Johnson, R. H., & Keogh, H. J. Oral tyramine in dietary migraine sufferers. In R. Greene (Ed.), *Current concepts in migraine research.* New York: Raven Press, 1978.

Sicuteri, F., Testi, A., & Anselmi, B. Biochemical investigations in headache: Increase in hydroxyindoleacetic acid excretion during migraine attacks. *International Archives of Allergy and Applied Immunology,* 1961, *19,* 55 – 58.

Sillanpaa, M. Prevalence of migraine and other headaches in Finnish children starting school. *Headache,* 1976, *15,* 288 – 290.

Steiner, H., & Clark, W. R. Psychiatric complications of burned adults: A classification. *Journal of Trauma,* 1977, *17*(2), 134 – 143.

Sternbach, R. A. *Pain: A psychophysiological analysis.* New York: Academic Press, 1968.

Sternbach, R. A. *Pain patients: Traits and treatment.* New York: Academic Press, 1974.

Stone, C. I., Demchick-Stone, S. A., & Horan, J. J. Coping with pain: A comparative analysis of Lamaze and cognitive – behavioral procedures. *Journal of Psychosomatic Research,* 1977, *21,* 451 – 456.

Sulman, F. G., Levy, D., Lewy, A., Pfeifer, Y., Superstine, E., & Tal, E. Air-ionometry of hot, dry desert winds (sharav) and treatment with air ions of weather-sensitive subjects. *Journal of International Biometeorology,* 1974, *18,* 313 – 318.

Swanson, D. W., Floreen, A. C., & Swenson, W. M. Program for managing chronic pain. II. Short-term results. *Mayo Clinic Proceedings,* 1976, *51,* 409 – 411.

Taylor, C. B., Zlutnick, S., Corley, M. J., & Flora, J. The effects of detoxification, relaxation and brief supportive therapy on chronic pain. *Pain,* 1980, *8,* 319 – 329.

Terenius, L., & Wahlstrom, A. Morphine-like ligand for opiate receptors in human CSF. *Life Sciences,* 1975, *16,* 1759 – 1764.

Tunis, M. M., & Wolff, H. G. Studies on headache: Cranial artery vasoconstriction and muscle contraction headache. *Archives of Neurology and Psychiatry,* 1954, *71,* 425 – 434.

Turner, D. B., & Stone, A. J. Headache and its treatment: A random survey. *Headache,* 1979, *19,* 74 – 77.

Urca, G., & Nahin, R. L. Morphine-induced multiple unit changes in analgesic and rewarding brain sites. *Pain Abstracts,* 1978, *1,* 261.

Vahlquist, B. Migraine in children. *International Archives of Allergy,* 1955, *7,* 348 – 355.

Wall, P. D., & Sweet, W. H. Temporary abolition of pain in man. *Science,* 1967, *155,* 108 – 109.

Waters, W. E. Epidemiological aspects of migraine. In J. N. Cumings (Ed.), *Background to migraine.* London: Heinemann, 1971.

Waters, W. E., & O'Connor, P. J. Prevalence of migraine. *Journal of Neurology, Neurosurgery and Psychiatry,* 1975, *38,* 613 – 616.

Waters, W. E., Koresko, R. L., Rossie, G. V., & Hackley, S. A. Short-, medium-, and long-term relationships among meteorological and electrodermal variables. *Psychophysiology,* 1979, *16,* 445 – 451.

Whitty, C. W. M., Hockaday, J. M., & Whitty, M. M. The effect of oral contraceptives on migraine. *Lancet,* 1966, *1,* 856 – 859.

Wideroe, T., & Vigander, T. Propranolol in the treatment of migraine. *British Medical Journal,* 1974, *29,* 699 – 701.

Wilkinson, M., & Woodrow, J. Migraine and weather. *Headache,* 1979, *19,* 375 – 378.

Yaksh, T. L. Central nervous system sites mediating opiate analgesia. In J. J. Bonica, J. C. Liebeskind, & D. Albe-Fessard (Eds.), *Advances in pain research and therapy* (Vol. 3). New York: Raven Press, 1979.

Ziegler, D. K. The epidemiology and genetics of migraine. *Research and Clinical Studies in Headache,* 1978, *5,* 21 – 33.

Zlutnick, S., Corley, M. J., & Owens, M. *The assessment and management of chronic pain.* Workshop presented at the annual meeting of the Association for the Advancement of Behavior Therapy, San Francisco, December 1980.

21 Spinal Cord Injury and Neuromuscular Reeducation

Susan S. Hendrick
University of Miami

INTRODUCTION

History

Although history records tremendous advances made by medical science, the treatment of spinal cord injuries showed little progress from ancient Egypt to the mid-20th century. A medical papyrus written 5000 years ago by an Egyptian physician described a spinal cord lesion and advised that it was "an ailment not to be treated [Guttman, 1976, p. 1]." Hippocrates in 400 B.C. advocated high fluid intake and traction for spinal cord injuries. Galen used surgical techniques on the spinal cord and observed that transverse incisions in the cord disrupted function whereas longitudinal incisions did not, at least not in the same way. In the intervening centuries, various surgical and medical techniques were used on cord injuries, particularly mechanical devices for extension and subsequent reduction of the injured spine (Guttman, 1976), though basically, medical intervention remained largely the same. Of those men receiving serious spinal cord injuries during World War I, 80% died within 2 weeks after injury. Those who survived could anticipate major health complications and a shortened life-span. Because the prognosis for the spinal cord injured was so poor, little was attempted in terms of rehabilitation. A defeatist attitude prevailed.

It was primarily during World War II that this attitude began to change. Because many spinal cord injuries were anticipated in England due to both military casualties and civilian victims of air raids in World War II, 12 spinal cord units were created to offer specialized, comprehensive care to the spinal cord injured. These centers were understaffed and without adequate facilities. A major breakthrough was achieved in 1944 with the opening of Stoke Mandeville National

Spinal Injuries Centre. In this place maximum comprehensive physical, and psychosocial rehabilitation of paraplegics and quadriplegics was the central goal (Guttman, 1976). Though increased rehabilitation services to cord injured persons have since been developed in many countries, including the United States, Stoke Mandeville continues as a model facility.

Epidemiological Data

Spinal cord injuries may be caused by both accident and disease. Motor vehicle accidents account for a disproportionately large share of cord injuries, but injuries are also caused by falls, sports-related injuries (including diving accidents), industrial accidents, and combat injuries (Herrmann & Stancil, 1977). Most spinal cord victims are males. This may reflect males' greater risk-taking behavior, more frequent participation in action sports, and dominance in combat situations. The proportion of females increases when one looks at only motor vehicle accidents as a cause (Smart & Sanders, 1976). No one at any age is safe from the possibility of spinal cord injury, but there is a particularly high frequency of spinal cord injuries in people in their 20s and 30s.

Anatomy and Physiology of the Spine

The *spinal column* is composed of 33 bony vertebrae connected by ligamentous tissue and given flexibility primarily by the cartilaginous intervertebral discs. The upper 24 vertebrae are moveable or "true" vertebrae and consist of seven cervical, twelve thoracic, and five lumbar vertebrae. The lower nine vertebrae are fixed or "false" vertebrae and five are fused to form the sacrum while four form the coccyx (Herrmann & Stancil, 1977). Each vertebra is composed of an anterior portion, vertebral body, and posterior portion. The vertebral arch consists of a pair of pedicles, a pair of laminae, and seven processes: four articular, two transverse, and one spinous. The individual vertebrae differ in size and shape depending on location and function. The intervertebral discs also vary in thickness, though they serve as the chief vertebral connection throughout the spinal column. These discs are basically avascular and in some portions of the spine are particularly vulnerable to physical stress such as twisting or lifting (Guttman, 1976). See Fig. 21.1.

The major ligamentous processes are the anterior longitudinal ligament, the posterior longitudinal ligament, and the ligamenta flava, which connects the laminae of adjacent vertebrae. Both the superficial and deep muscles of the trunk are attached to the vertebrae column either directly or through fascie.

The *spinal cord* is a continuation of the medulla oblongata, a part of the brainstem, and extends through the foramen magnum at the base of the brain ending at the second lumbar vertebra, below which it becomes neural filaments termed the "cauda equina" (Gardner, 1961). The cord is typically 45 cm long in males and 42 cm in females and is divided into cervical, thoracic, and lumbar

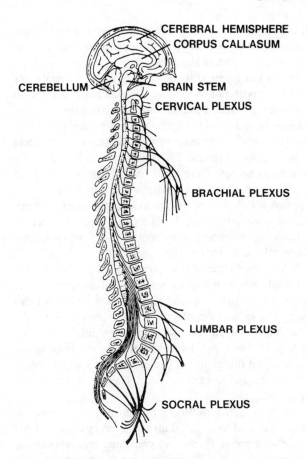

FIG. 21.1 Drawing of the brain and spinal cord (Gardner, 1961).

regions, corresponding to the spinal vertebrae. The cord is protected by three layers of meninges: the dura mater, the arachnoidea, and the pia. Cerebrospinal fluid fills the space between the cord itself and the dura mater. The structure of the cord follows closely that of the brain, as both together form the central nervous system. There are midline grooves on the anterior and posterior portions of the spinal cord. The "anterior median fissure" is occupied by the anterior spinal artery, and "ventral roots" leave from the anterolateral area of the cord. Posteriorly, one finds the posterior median sulcus, posterior spinal arteries, and dorsal roots that enter the posterolateral region.

The interior spinal cord contains grey matter surrounded by white, and in cross-section resembles a butterfly or an "H." In the crossbar of the "H" is the central spinal canal, containing cerebrospinal fluid. The anterior horns of the gray matter are connected to the dorsal roots. The anatomical arrangement of the white matter consists of three bundles or columns of nerves called funiculi: anterior, lateral, and posterior. These funiculi conduct a great variety of afferent nerve impulses and connect the dorsal and ventral spinal root fibers with both the spinal cord and the brain. Spinal roots and nerves are shown in Fig. 21.2.

The dorsal and ventral roots just mentioned comprise 31 pairs of spinal roots that are divided into anterior and posterior roots. They connect horizontally with the spinal cord in the cervical region but take a downward turn so that the bundle of roots in the spinal canal below the ending of the spinal cord resembles the tail of a horse (thus the name "cauda equina"). The anterior roots contain efferent fibers whereas the posterior contain afferent fibers. The spinal cord is larger in the cervical and lumbosacral regions because these areas contain heavier bundles of spinal roots; the spinal roots compose part of the peripheral nervous system.

The spinal cord is supplied with blood by the anterior spinal artery, anterior radicular artery, and posterior spinal arteries, and is fairly well supplied except in the mid-thoracic region. The cord's venous system connects to the venous system of the lungs, and the abdominal and pelvic cavities.

The primary purpose of the spinal column is to provide a secure and flexible protection for the spinal cord, which transmits sensory and motor impulses between the brain and the trunk and extremities and also serves as the major locus of reflex activity in the body. The spinal roots described earlier are attached to the cord at fixed intervals. Each dorsal root joins the corresponding ventral root within the same cord segment to form a spinal nerve. Every spinal nerve leaves the spinal canal and divides into ventral and dorsal rami. The ventral rami supply nerve impulses to the limbs and the sides and front of the body. The dorsal rami supply the muscles and skin of the back.

Particular spinal nerve branches, plus sympathetic trunks (long nerve trunks on each side of the vertebrae that extend from the skull to the coccyx) and related ganglia, supply the viscera with motor fibers and constitute the sympathetic portion of the autonomic nervous system. The parasympathetic portion is composed of branches of certain cranial nerves plus branches of the second and third sacral nerves that connect to the pelvis.

The gray matter of the central spinal cord has essentially the same structure and function throughout but is modified locally because of the size and number of neurons it contains. The white matter contains funiculi, described earlier, and spinospinal or propriospinal fibers, which both originate and terminate within the spinal cord itself. These "local" fibers link various parts of the spinal cord and allow coordinated activity (essentially reflex arcs) to occur within the cord itself and thus account for the significant amount of reflex motor activity that can return to parts of the body below a complete spinal cord lesion.

Spinal Cord Injuries

All injuries to the spinal cord do not involve permanent damage and loss of function, as a "spinal concussion" may occur when a missile strikes the vertebral

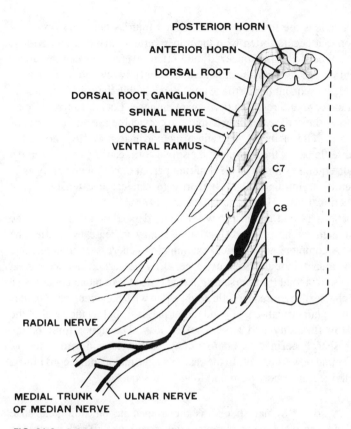

POSTERIOR HORN

ANTERIOR HORN

DORSAL ROOT

DORSAL ROOT GANGLION

SPINAL NERVE

DORSAL RAMUS

VENTRAL RAMUS

C6

C7

C8

T1

RADIAL NERVE

MEDIAL TRUNK   ULNAR NERVE
OF MEDIAN NERVE

FIG. 21.2   Spinal roots and nerves (Gardner, 1961).

column and does not injure the cord itself but nevertheless creates local trauma (e.g., hemorrhage, edema) resulting in temporary paralysis (Adams, 1970). It is not the extensiveness of this paralysis that is of prime importance, but rather its reversibility.

Most spinal injuries are considerably more serious, however, and result in at least some irreversible damage. Spinal cord injuries can be classified as "fracture-dislocations," "pure fractures," and "pure dislocations" and occur at a ratio of 3:1:1 (Adams, 1970). These injuries occur because of force applied to the spinal column from some distance, force that causes vertical compression of the spinal column and immediate flexion, or possibly abrupt extension of the neck. The strength, direction, and point of impact of the force will affect the type and severity of the spinal injury; different impacts precipitate different injuries (Adams, 1970).

Over half of all spinal fractures are compression injuries, usually due to falls in which the spine is hyperflexed or jackknifed. Most of these injuries occur at the junction between the relatively fixed thoracic spine and the movable lumbar spine (Herrmann & Stancil, 1977).

Fracture dislocations are the most serious spinal injuries because of the vertebral dislocation that occurs, often with the upper vertebra displaced anteriorly, and with the spinal cord caught, squeezed, and often severed between the upper and lower vertebrae. The cord may be either partially or fully severed, but even if it is merely bruised, subsequent hemorrhage and edema within the spinal canal may put pressure on the cord and result in permanent damage. Localized trauma may progress up or down the cord, extending damage to cervical segments not immediately adjacent to the site of injury. Extradural hemorrhage may flow down the spinal canal and settle below the bottom of the spinal cord, causing pressure and a subsequent cauda equina symptom with resulting partial or complete paralysis in the lower extremities. Intramedullary hemorrhage can cause extensive nerve damage and functional loss (Herrmann & Stancil, 1977).

The extent of sensory and motor loss will usually depend on the extent of the initial injury, though we have noted that damage may increase even after the original trauma. A complete neurological examination is necessary to determine the full range of injury, though this must necessarily be carried out with great caution. In the case of a total transverse lesion (the type of lesion that concerns us throughout this chapter), there can be little doubt about what has occurred. There is complete, usually symmetrical sensory and motor paralysis below the level of the lesion, marked by flaccidity and tendon reflex loss. The upper limit of the paralysis may be sharply defined by a border of hyperesthesia, and there is loss of voluntary bladder and bowel control. In the case of such a major spinal cord injury, effects can be divided into short-term and long-term sequelae.

Short-Term Effects.   "Spinal shock" is the immediate physiological state occurring after spinal cord trauma and involves the cessation of all reflex action of spinal segments and affected areas below the level of the lesion. Plantar reflexes are absent, no thermoregulation exists, and bony areas of the body become particularly prone to ulceration. This period of shock may last from 2 weeks to 3 months or longer. During this time, the spinal cord patient must be assisted in bladder and bowel function, rotated to avoid decubitus ulcers, progressively raised on a tilt table to reduce hypotensive crises, aided in respiratory function, and carefully monitored for complications such as autonomic hyperflexia, hypertension, hypothermia, and bradycardia.

Long-Term Effects.   The full extent of spinal cord injury is often not known for some time, as concussions and partial lesions may heal, with full or nearly full functional recovery ensuing. Variability in type and extent of injuries as well as remediable problems such as cord edema make long-term prediction difficult for a physician treating a spinal cord patient, at least for the first 6 months after injury.

For the complete transverse cord lesions we are concerned with, Gardner (1961) describes the general progression after spinal cord injury as typically "spinal shock" to "minimal reflex activity" to "flexor spasms" to "alternating flexor and extensor spasms." Muscles are intact, and the isolated portion of the cord regains automatic functions, with reflex arcs influenced by local stimuli such as touch or temperature. All sensation below the lesion remains absent, however. Note that the difference between vertebral column level of injury and functional cord level may be up to two spinal segments. With the return of certain reflex processes will come relief of some of the functional loss experienced during spinal shock, though much function is irrevocably lost.

TREATMENT OF SPINAL CORD INJURY

Early Management

Medical care of the spinal cord injured continues to improve, though controversy exists over exactly what constitutes good medical care (e.g., Guttman, 1976; Miller, 1977). Most authorities agree that patients with acute spinal cord injuries can best be managed at comprehensive regional centers especially designed to offer multimodal treatment. At Stoke Mandeville, 90% of the patients are brought in within 24 hours after injury (Miller, 1977). Both care and speed of transport are essential, and physicians typically administer corticosteroids or other medications to reduce edema of the injured cord. Though surgical laminectomy has traditionally been used to stabilize a fractured spine and thus prevent further cord damage, Guttman (1976) holds that it is difficult to tell in the early postinjury period whether or not the fracture is unstable. Because he has found that few fractures remain unstable for an extended period of time, he believes laminectomy is seldom warranted, may cause more damage than it prevents, and can be better replaced by graduated reduction of the fracture. His reduction method consists of horizontal placement on rubber packs with turning of the patient every 2 hours. Various types of motorized beds or frames such as the Stryker frame are also used for turning spinal cord patients. Of course laminectomy is still widely employed (Herrmann & Stancil, 1977).

Guttman lists the following criteria as possible reasons why surgery would be useful at a later time: (1)persistent or recurrent instability of spine; (2)restitution of neural function; (3)treatment of spasticity and contractures; and (4)treatment of pain [1976, p. 175]."

After initial treatment such as immediate first aid, antibiotics (for open wounds), transport to a spinal center, and decisions about surgical intervention, various medical treatments are essential to the spinal cord patient's survival.

Urinary Treatment

Urinary tract infection is a primary danger following cord injury. Though Guttman (1976) believes that catheterization does not need to be started for several hours after spinal cord injury, Graham (1977) recommends intervention immediately after injury with either intermittent catheterization or insertion of an indwelling catheter. The eventual treatment goal is for the patient to be catheter-free (with sterile urine), and Graham describes a bladder training program that involves clamping the catheter for progressively longer periods of time and then draining the bladder, to encourage reflex voiding. Intermittent catheterization is also used and appears to leave less residual infection in patients when they eventually become catheter-free. If the bladder does not achieve reflex voiding, male patients usually have surgery of the vesicle neck and sphincter that will allow urine to be voided after very limited muscular contraction of the bladder. After such surgery, most male patients will require an external urinary appliance (e.g., "Texas special," "gizmo"), commonly a condom with a hole in the end that is connected to a rubber tube attached to a leg bag that holds the urine and is periodically emptied. Female patients cannot use an external appliance, and most wear indwelling catheters. Interestingly, upper level cord injuries allow for return of reflex action to the bladder, whereas lower injuries may interrupt the reflex arc of the bladder's detrusor muscle and thus result in a flaccid bladder. The goal of the rehabilitation team is to get each cord patient as close to natural function as possible and to have him or her assume bladder care. This is often possible for all but the high-level quadriplegics. Antibiotics are administered when necessary to correct infection. Suprapubic cystotomies are much less often used now as surgical intervention either immediately following or sometime after a spinal cord injury.

Bowel Treatment

The spinal cord patient will have to be aided in bowel function throughout the spinal shock period by use of enemas, suppositories, and manual evacuation, though after that period many patients can assume responsibility for their own bowel care. The patient should follow a consistent schedule daily or every other day and, with the aid of proper positioning, gentle massage of the abdomen, digital stimulation of the anal area, and judicious use of mild laxative or stool softeners can achieve satisfactory bowel function. Diet is important to both bowel and bladder function, and the patient is encouraged to drink an adequate amount of liquid as well as consume a diet high in protein and in fibre content.

A possible complication in spinal cord injuries that is directly related to bladder and bowel function is "autonomic hyperflexia." Symptoms of this disorder may include vague abdominal discomfort, flushing and sweating of the skin above the lesion, nasal congestion, and pounding headache. Objective medical findings include hypertension, both systolic and diastolic, and associated bradycardia. The customary causes of this disorder, which is really a type of hypertensive crisis, is distension of the bladder or bowel due to failure to properly evacuate, or systemic infection (Gruber, 1978). Typical treatment will consist of removing the precipitating cause after elevating the patient's head. Occasionally, an alpha adrenergic blocker will be administered.

Exercise and Movement

A typical patient problem is hypotension when in an upright position. This results from pooling of blood in the gut and lower extremities when the patient is raised and the inadequate body response in terms of sympathetic vasoconstriction and increased cardiac output to continue cerebral blood flow (Belson, 1978). Although this condition tends to stabilize over time, early therapeutic use of a tilt table and consistent periods of time spent in vertical positions are good preventive measures.

Physical therapy is an integral part of recovery for the spinal cord patient, and Ofir and Hofkosh (1977) list three stages during which the spinal cord patient requires treatment: acute stage, intermediate stage, and final stage. In the acute stage after injury, a paraplegic can be given range of motion (ROM) exercises of the lower extremities, primarily to prevent contractures, and a quadriplegic may receive passive range of motion exercises and assistance in proper positioning.

During the intermediate stage, paraplegics may receive range of motion exercises for both lower and upper extremities as well as active exercises for the upper body. A progressive exercise program may be set up that involves progressive resistance exercises, hydrotherapy, tilt table, and additional mat activities. The spinal cord injured patient needs to develop the intact musculature to its maximum. Although in the intermediate stage, the quadriplegic may be restricted to an electric bed or Stryker frame, a definite exercise program can be instituted. Full range of motion of major joints (i.e., scapula and elbow) must be maintained along with range of motion of the lower extremities. Active, active – assistive, and isometric exercises are started for the intact musculature, and great attention is given to achieving more adequate respiratory function, because respiratory effectiveness is seriously compromised for the high-level quadriplegic. The physical therapist can also offer help with skin care, give hydrotherapy, and institute progressive time on the tilt table.

During the final or stable stage in a paraplegic's recovery, the patient may have a comprehensive program of activities, including activities of daily living, sports activities, and continued exercise. The nonambulatory (chairbound) paraplegic must be maintained in full range of motion exercises as well as upper body strengthening exercise. Upper body exercises are primarily for the purpose of effecting independent transfers to and from a wheelchair. The quadriplegic in the final stage can increase greatly his or her exercise activities. Strengthening, stretching, and balancing activities are instituted and are followed by the teaching of dressing and transfer techniques. The patient's natural spasticity may sometimes actually aid in dressing and transfer because of the limb rigidity (Ofir & Hofkosh, 1977). Medication can sometimes control spasticity; however, according to Herrmann and Stancil, 1977: "it has been said that spasms give a sense of 'wholeness' to the patient which is lost in anesthetic flaccidity [1977, p. 17]." The exercise and activity programs instituted by the physical therapist and other members of the rehabilitation team must be continued by the patient and his or her family on a posthospitalization basis if the maximum possible degree of functioning is to be maintained.

Independence Training

In addition to physical therapy, the cornerstone of recovery is independence training, including teaching of activities for daily living (ADL), ambulation training, and the use of prosthetic devices. During concentrated rehabilitation, a patient is given various functional motor tests to determine capabilities and is then entered into an intensive ADL program during which he or she gains as much independence as possible in eating, dressing, grooming, bladder and bowel care, health care, mobility, and any other activities necessary for work, recreation, or daily living. This program requires professional help from a physical therapist, occupational therapist, and orthotist. Although the paraplegic retains many former skills and can be fairly easily taught additional compensatory ones, the quadriplegic can find even small tasks monumental and may work long hours to learn to lift a cup and drink from it. During this painstaking, often frustrating learning period, a patient's high motivation is paramount. In addition to self-care skills, spinal cord patients may also learn various homemaking skills, usually in a living – learning model area especially designed for teaching the injured.

Ambulation is a primary concern for spinal cord patients and may be considered a possibility for patients with lesions below T − 1 or occasionally for quadriplegics with higher lesions. A patient will begin to learn to walk with braces, between parallel bars. Training ends when the patient can put on and take off braces, make transfers, manage stairs, learn how to fall and how to get up, and to ambulate outside.

Orthotic devices are necessary in spinal cord rehabilitation, particularly for the quadriplegic. Devices include splints such as the balanced forearm orthosis and externally powered splints, headsticks for typing, adapted personal care objects (i.e., razors, toothbrush), dressing hooks, mouthsticks, overhead slings, hand and wrist cuffs, eating devices, tiltboards and standing devices, and automobiles and vans. Tremendous technical skill has gone into developing a wide array of self-help devices for the spinal cord injured.

Sexual Implications

Because we discuss sexual implications and alternatives thoroughly later in the chapter, we just briefly note here the immediate sexual results of traumatic spinal cord injury. Before injury, typical male sexual response includes erection, ejaculation and emission, orgasm, and involution. After injury, and after spinal shock has subsided, reflex erections are possible for over 90% of individuals (Geiger, 1979).

Ejaculation occurs in some cases, and fertility may be retained. Though the full sensation of orgasm does not occur, there may be some muscular relaxation and a cessation of chronic muscle spasms for a period after ejaculation. This sequence exists for cervical and thoracic lesions, but with lumbar lesions, the reflex arc for reflex erection and ejaculation is interrupted. In this situation, Geiger (1979) has reported some incidence of psychologically induced or "psychic" erections, even when reflex erections are not possible.

For women, typical sexual response includes excitement, plateau, orgasm, and resolution. After cervical and thoracic injuries, there may be general physiological excitement above the lesion and specific sensual stimulation of erogenous areas above the lesion such as the mouth, ears, nose, eyes, breasts, and armpits, which contribute to sexual satisfaction. With lumbar injuries, reflex lubrication may be cut off, but psychic components may be present. Information on female orgasm and resolution is quite limited. Spinal cord injury typically does not affect female fertility, and successful pregnancy is possible.

Long-Term Complications

Careful and constant attention to health factors is always required of the spinal cord injured patient. Bowel and skin care are important, and a patient must learn to reposition himself or herself frequently to avoid decubiti.

Renal complications account for half the deaths of the spinal cord injured, so urinary care remains a constant concern. Frequent evaluations of urinary function are recommended, as is immediate attention to any infection. Autonomic hyperflexia is a danger. Consistent exercise, passive movement, and repositioning are necessary to prevent both deep venous thrombosis and contractures.

A continuing complication of spinal cord injury is "osteoporosis" and spontaneous bone fractures. A typical result of spinal cord injury is atrophy of the soft tissues, particularly the muscles and skeletal tissues. Most frequently affected are the pelvis and the femur. Therapy consists of frequent turning in the early stages and movement in later stages, high protein diet, and padded splints. Because no pain will be experienced below the lesion, the only clues to an injury may be swelling and warmth on the skin around the affected area.

Respiratory infections are particularly dangerous long-term complications for quadriplegics, as the quadriplegic has lost the use of the intercostal and abdominal muscles and is dependent on diaphragmatic breathing (Gruber, 1978). In Gruber's words: "He has compromised pulmonary reserve; his vital capacity has been decreased; his maximum breathing capacity has been decreased; his cough reflex is ineffectual; and his ability to clear his airways is impaired [p. 23]." Therefore, any indication of respiratory infection or difficulties must be treated vigorously. Patterns of health care established by the patient and significant others during hospitalization must be continued throughout the patient's lifetime.

PSYCHOSOCIAL ASPECTS OF SPINAL CORD INJURY

Adjustment to Injury

Only a person with a spinal cord injury can understand the variety of emotions that such an injury can create. Nevertheless, professionals who work with the spinal cord injured must attempt as fully as possible to understand both the shock and the readjustment that follow injury.

Eisenberg and Gilbert (1978) present a "stage" theory of emotional reaction to spinal cord injury. The first stage, "shock," can be described as a somewhat impersonal emergency reaction characterized by detachment. The individual is not yet fully aware of what has occurred. The second stage, "impact," is manifested by disorganization, helplessness and despair. Feelings of grief and loss are extreme, and the individual may keep reliving the traumatic experience that resulted in the injury. The third stage is "retreat," characterized by denial of the implications of the injury and a desire to ward off a final diagnosis of disability. The fourth and final stage is "adaptation," which is the longest and most complicated stage. A patient's realistic acceptance of physical deficit is necessary for comprehensive rehabilitation, and a patient who accepts the injury and begins rehabilitation may expect that gaining mastery over his or her environment will proceed smoothly. However, rehabilitation is replete with frustrations, roadblocks, and negative learning. Recovery is often a case of "two steps forward, one step back." The nature of the adjustment process is cyclic, so several cycles of depression, retreat, and adaptation may be necessary to complete adjustment. The early reaction of grieving or mourning is discussed by several authors (Cull & Hardy, 1977; Wright, 1960), and the feeling of loss (similar to the loss of a loved one through death) is central to the mourning process. Following the time of mourning may be a period when many psychological defenses are used to deal with disability. They include denial and withdrawal (noted earlier), regression, repression, reaction formation, fantasy, rationalization, and projection. These may be followed by identification and compensation, which are healthier defenses (Cull & Hardy, 1977).

What affects a person's progress toward acceptance of disability and full participation in rehabilitation? Stewart and Rossier (1978) have discussed several factors. The first factor is the person's place in the life cycle; injury may mean different things to an adolescent in the midst of identity formation and to a middle-aged adult who is contemplating retirement. According to Stewart and Rossier, "The question 'why me?' draws attention to the feeling of guilt often associated with paralysis [p. 76]." The meaning to the individual of the paralyzed body parts is quite important, for when bowel and bladder functions are disrupted, almost primitive feelings of doubt and shame can arise in a patient. Sexual function loss may vary in importance, but for some it represents a tremendous loss. Paralysis of the lower extremities and resulting wheelchair confinement require considerable adjustment. Discussing the phenomenon of "eye contact," Stewart and Rossier point out that "people in wheelchairs must continually look upwards at their peers [p. 77]" and may often feel that they face the world in a "one-down" situation. The paralysis of upper extremities can necessitate a degree of dependency not experienced by an individual since infancy. Although the cord injured person also experiences the normal developmental life crises of the able-bodied, such crises may be magnified.

Katz, Gordon, Iversen, and Myers (1978) compared postinjury depression to preinjury depression and found that a pretrauma history of positive coping skills and healthy family background was related to significantly less depression both pre- and post-injury. Lawson (1978) found a high level of depression surrounding important postinjury events such as hospital admission and discharge, and noted that: "an extended period of depression or grief . . . appears to be counterproductive to posthospital adjustment [p. 578]." Fogel and Rosillo (1971) discovered that rehabilitation progress was positively related to: (1) realistic evaluation of life problems (including disability and rehabilitation) and making rational decisions about them; (2) successful coping with stress; (3) infrequent use of rationalization as a defense mechanism; and (4) assumption of a dominant rather than a submissive role in interpersonal interactions. Obviously, many of the factors contributing to successful psychological adjustment and rehabilitation after spinal cord injury are those that also contribute to healthy behavior among the able-bodied population.

Stewart and Rossier (1978) discuss several classifications of character types and how each can best be treated during the hospital stay. The "dependent overdemanding patient" needs extra reassurances that he or she will not be abandoned by the staff. The "orderly, controlled patient" can be helped to achieve some feeling of personal control by detailed explanations of physical condition and treatment. The "long-suffering and self-sacrificing patient" needs to retain some measure of acknowledged pain and suffering in order to be able to also accept whatever functional recovery is present. The "paranoid patient" requires careful and detailed explanations of all procedures and treatment. The "patient with feelings of superiority" can often profit from reassurance that he or she is still an esteemed human being. Finally, the "unloved and aloof" patient may require times of privacy and aloneness to balance out the volume of human contact encountered during rehabilitation. The character types just listed are general ones, and themes from various types may be found in any one patient. Additional research has proposed other behavior styles after disability (Cull & Hardy, 1977).

An interesting phenomenon that may occur after spinal cord injury is "body image distortion." Conomy (1973) studied 18 traumatically injured spinal cord patients and 10 patients with congenital spinal problems. He found that all the traumatic and none of the congenital patients had some disruption of the body schema. Such disruptions included: (1) disordered perception of the body in space (proprioceptive body image), usually manifesting the feeling that the legs are floating up off the bed with flexion at the hips and extension at ankles or knees (while in fact the legs are supine); (2) disordered perception of posture and movement (disorder of kinetic body image), usually resulting in an impression of muscular work (such as bicycling) and muscle fatigue; and (3) disorders of perception of somatic bulk, size, and continuity (somatic body image), accompanied by the feeling of swollen feet or legs and no perception of diminution of trunk size or limb length (pp. 843 – 847). Such distortions of body image can seem almost like hallucinations and can badly frighten a patient who does not expect the situation to occur. Explanations for these fleeting distortions include alternate routes for postural and kinetic information going from the brain to the lower extremities and the possibility that some afferent neurons exist at the injury site (p. 850). Although body image distortion has frequently been compared to the "phantom limb" phenomenon occurring after limb amputation, the phenomena are in fact quite different, because after spinal cord injury, the limbs are still intact. Although *intra*personal factors such as preinjury personality style, self-esteem, and coping abilities are significant in a spinal cord patient's reaction to disability, of equal importance are the *inter*personal factors involving the patient's family.

The Family

The injured patient's family experiences an initial "crisis reaction" to the injury that parallels the patient's experience of "shock" (Eisenberg & Gilbert, 1978). The family is numb, unable to plan ahead, and extremely dependent on health care personnel for information and support during this period. Because family members may be initially concerned about whether the patient will live, their distress is increased when they are unable to see the patient or can visit only for limited periods of time. Harris, Patel, Greer, and Naughton (1973) suggest that facilities be set up in a hospital so that close relatives of the injured person can spend the night and be available to the patient. This could mitigate some of the fear and isolation experienced by both patient and family. In addition, family members can offer emotional support and sensory stimulation to the patient who is experiencing sensory deprivation in a strictly physical sense.

Not all family members can offer support, however, for they have their own crises to handle. A typical family response is "guilt," often brought on by parents' feelings that they should have prevented the injury in some way (Stewart & Rossier, 1978). Another reason for guilt is the many things that were "done or not done" by the family members before the patient's injury. Shame, overcompensation, or extreme reliance upon religion are other frequent family defenses (Eisenberg & Gilbert, 1978). Denial is used by a family in much the same way it is used by the patient; the losses seem too great to bear, so denial is the only acceptable alternative. Basic education about the short- and long-term implications of the disability may reduce family anxiety. Didactic and therapeutic groups are useful for concrete, logistical planning as well as for ventilation of feelings (Miller, Wolfe, & Spiegel, 1975). Harris et al. (1973) believe it is useful to have families of spinal cord injured persons meet each other to provide emotional support as well as offer practical ideas for care.

The single individual other than the patient who is most affected by the injury is usually the patient's spouse. Role changes occur immediately, as, at least for a time, the injured person can no longer assume his or her roles in the family. Thus roles of income attainment, household maintenance, child rearing, and the like must be assumed by the spouse or other family members. In addition, responsibilities for giving physical care to the patient may fall on an already overworked spouse. Peterson (1979) found that role flexibility was required in many marriages where one of the spouses was disabled, and that *congruence* of role expectations and subsequent role performance was related to marital satisfaction. The author also found a definite relationship between one spouse's physical handicap and the presence of marital stress. Sexual problems can provide a major source of stress to a couple in which one spouse has a spinal cord injury.

Guttman (1976) briefly discusses the marital aftermath of spinal cord injury. He cites a 1964 survey of 1505 spinal cord injured patients who had been treated at Stoke Mandeville Centre; 65% of these patients were married either before or after hospital admission. The total divorce rate in this group was 7.3% (p. 501). In fact, the divorce rate was lower for the couples who were married before the spinal cord injury than for those married after injury. Although injury creates understandable stresses, it does not appear to lead to a particularly high divorce rate or to exclude the couple from substantial marital satisfaction. It is undoubtedly beneficial for both patients and spouses faced with spinal cord injury to have some ongoing counseling during the rehabilitation process (Eisenberg & Gilbert, 1978).

Counseling Approaches

The Rehabilitation Unit.   Comprehensive rehabilitation consists of physical, vocational, recreational, individual, and marital therapy; each with its own set of treatment goals, but all coordinated in their efforts to effectively treat the spinal cord injured patient.

Physical therapy has as its goal the restoration of the best possible physical functioning, including ambulation when possible. A variety of exercises and devices are needed to facilitate this, including mat and resistance exercises, hydrotherapy, and bracing (for ambulation). Transfer training (i.e., from bed to wheelchair) is also taught. Occupational therapy includes training with orthotic devices, work preparation, and self-care (both personal and home care).

Vocational counseling typically begins about 6 months after hospital discharge and initially involves detailed medical, social, and psychological evaluation, and work tolerance tests. Patient and counselor cooperate in career selection, which may involve retraining via college or technical school. Governmental economic aid is available to most cord injured patients, and there are estimates that 63% of paraplegics and 48% of quadriplegics are reemployed after injury (Smart & Sanders, 1976). Problems intrinsic to the patients themselves combine with extrinsic factors such as institutional barriers and governmental disability allowances to reinforce sick role behavior and thence unemployment for many cord injured patients. Kemp and Vash (1971) found that postinjury productivity of spinal cord patients was positively related to: (1) having more goals; (2) paying less attention to physical loss; (3) being creative; and (4) having interpersonal support.

Recreational therapy acknowledges that a handicap need not limit the individual's participation in sports and other recreational activities. Wheelchair sports were introduced over 30 years ago as "remedial exercise" for cord patients, and today wheelchair sports include archery, swimming, polo, basketball, bowling, track and field, fencing, billiards, and lawn bowls. It is estimated that over 10,000 men and women are now actively engaged in wheelchair sports, and the International Stoke Mandeville Games (informally called the wheelchair olympics) have grown to include over 70 nations. Effort has been made to keep wheelchair sports as close to the original sports as possible, and Labanowich (1978) notes that when the sports are radically altered so as to become easier for disabled participants, the sports lose their excitement and potential for learning.

Individual counseling focuses on facilitating the patient's emotional adjustment, though counseling needs vary from patient to patient, and some patients require no psychological intervention (Grzesiak, 1979). The severity of a patient's reaction to injury does not necessarily correspond to the injury's severity, so less seriously injured patients may actually experience greater psychological decompensation. Maximum patient self-sufficiency is a goal of all rehabilitation team members, and Vineberg and Willems (1971) found that patients in advanced stages of rehabilitation had higher activity levels than early stage patients. Most of the patient's hospital contacts occur with paraprofessional rather than professional medical personnel.

Sexuality After Spinal Cord Injury

Sexual Function.   As noted earlier in the chapter, sexual function varies after spinal cord injury according to the type of lesion: cervical, thoracic, or lumbar. It is also affected by completeness or incompleteness of the lesion, as more residual function remains when a lesion is incomplete. In his study of 150 spinal cord patients, Comarr (1970) found that male patients with complete upper motor neuron lesions had a 96.4% incidence of reflex erections but only a 1.3% incidence of ejaculation and orgasm. Patients with lower lesions had a 24.2% erection rate and a 15% rate of ejaculation and orgasm. Patients with incomplete lesions also had higher rates of erection, ejaculation, and orgasm than did lower lesion level patients. Comarr also found that over one-third of his patients did not even attempt sexual activity. In reviewing the literature on sexual function, Griffith, Tomko, and Timms (1973), in an analysis of nine previous surveys, found that erection occurred in 54% to 87% of the subjects, with erection rates varying from 7% of men with complete lower motor neuron lesions to 99% with incomplete upper lesions. Ejaculation occurred at a much lower rate, with as few as 1% of men with complete upper lesions reporting ejaculation whereas up to 70% of those with incomplete lower lesions did so. Griffith et al. consider male procreation to be difficult, though Guttman (1976) cites frequent incidences of spinal cord injured males fathering children subsequent to injury. The literature on psychogenic erections of males with lower lesions is variable, though such erections definitely do occur (Geiger, 1979).

Less information is available on female sexual response, both because fewer females receive spinal cord injuries and also because female sexuality is thought to be less disrupted by traumatic spinal cord injury (Bregman & Hadley, 1976). Women have sexual responses similar to men, as reflex lubrication is possible with upper level lesions whereas a more psychogenic sexual response is possible with a lower lesion.

Two basic differences between female and male sexual response however, are that: (1) impaired female response is much less obvious than impaired male response; and (2) female fertility is usually unimpaired by spinal cord injury (Geiger, 1979). Research on female sexuality is increasing, however. Griffith and Trieschman (1975) found that although sexuality may actually increase for women following injury, women may also be more affected than men by the discrepancy between their appearance and cultural standards of beauty and wholeness. Bregman and Hadley (1976) noted that women reported the first sexual experience after injury to be the most uncomfortable one, and after that, comfort increased as long as there was completely open communication between sexual partners. Although bladder and bowel function and apparatus had to be considered in relation to sexual encounters (true also for males), such considerations did not necessarily impede sexual satisfaction.

Other researchers (Fitting, Salisbury, Davies, & Mayclin, 1978) explored self-concept and sexuality in spinal cord injured women and found that the majority enjoyed sex before and after injury. In terms of self-concept, 33% of the women reported feeling less attractive after injury, 17% felt more attractive, and 50% reported no change. Many of the women saw themselves as more assertive, independent, honest, and empathic after their injury. Sexuality in relation to self-concept has been studied for both men and women, and Teal and Athelstan (1975) note that psychosocial factors relating to sexual adjustment include self-concept and self-worth, identity and social role, and body image.

Although sex was at one time virtually ignored in the rehabilitation of the spinal cord injured, we now recognize that although sexual function may be impaired by injury, it is not necessarily lost, and in fact libido is virtually unaffected (Singh & Magner, 1975).

Sex Counseling. Sexuality counseling for the spinal cord injured has developed primarily within the last decade. For some patients, regaining sexual performance is the highest priority during rehabilitation. General answers must necessarily be given to questions arising soon after injury because sexual function may not have stabilized. Sex counseling may be part of more generalized counseling on other issues or may be presented as a specialized program.

The University of Minnesota has developed sex counseling within a workshop structure, serving spinal cord injured persons and their partners as well as many able-bodied persons, usually professionals who work in some capacity with disabled persons (Cole, Chilgren, & Rosenberg, 1973; Held, Cole, Held, Anderson, & Chilgren, 1975). The workshops include explicit sexual material to demythologize sex and desensitize participants, content lectures, and several small group discussion sessions. Spinal cord injured adults and their spouses frequently work with professional staff members in designing and implementing the workshops. Additional sexuality counseling programs are discussed in a comprehensive review by Chipouras (1979).

Politics of the Handicapped

Handicapped persons have become a vocal political minority in the United States within the past few years. Passage of the Rehabilitation Act of 1973 and the Developmental Disabilities Act initiated various vocational rehabilitation programs, research, training, special projects, and grants-in-aid to many states. Amendments to these acts have expanded services in the areas of housing, transportation, and barrier-free access to public places. Such services are expensive. Smart and Sanders (1976) estimate that the total (lifetime) expected societal costs for the spinal cord injuries occurring in *motor vehicle accidents alone* in the United States during 1974 may exceed $559 million dollars. This figure includes direct costs (e.g., hospitalization, medical supplies, attendant care, vocational rehabilitation) as well as indirect costs (e.g., losses attributable to the unrealized productivity of the individuals involved). Spinal cord injury is a low incidence disease, but one that results in catastrophic personal and financial costs.

NEUROMUSCULAR REEDUCATION

Introduction

The range of neurological, neurospinal, and neuromuscular disorders is very wide and cannot be comprehensively addressed in a single volume, much less a single chapter. Thus we have chosen to deal in depth with only spinal cord injury, presenting it comprehensively in terms of etiology, treatment, and psychosocial concomitants. Although etiology differs in nearly every instance of neurological and neuromuscular disorder (e.g., stroke occurs differently from cerebral palsy, which is in turn different from epilepsy), similar treatment/rehabilitation techniques are used for many of these disorders. One such technique is biofeedback.

Biofeedback, described by Pomerleau (1979) as one of "the two major intervention techniques in behavioral medicine [p. 656]" selectively applies operant conditioning methods to control visceral, somatomotor, and central nervous system action. "Biofeedback methodology (then) consists of providing feedback of a physiological response in an instrumental learning paradigm for the purpose of learning control of that response [Brucker, 1979, p. 2]." Biofeedback has become an increasingly important tool of psychologists in the past decade and is directly applicable to neuromuscular and neurological disorders in the learning of skeletal (voluntary) and visceral (autonomic) responses.

Skeletal Muscle Reeducation

Pioneer work by Basmajian and others in the use of electromyography (EMG) to teach subjects to control firing of single motor neuron units opened the way for the use of EMG in rehabilitation.

The opportunity for rehabilitation/reeducation of muscles exists with many neuromuscular disorders, notably cerebrovascular accident (stroke), poliomyelitis, cerebral palsy, torticollis, nerve injury, and of course spinal cord injury. Biofeedback is a useful diagnostic tool that can reveal whether a cord injured patient has some residual motor function, thus signaling a partial rather than a complete lesion. In the case of stroke, control of limb musculature is largely, but not completely, contralateral; approximately 75 − 80% of the corticospinal fibers cross to the opposite side of the spinal cord, whereas 20 − 25% descend ipsilaterally. Consequently, after many cases of stroke, considerable functional potential remains, which can be augmented by neuromuscular training. When paresis (weakening) rather than paralysis is present, biofeedback can help determine the motor units most amenable to reeducation.

As early as 1960, Marinacci and Horande used EMG feedback to generate partial recovery of motor unit function in a hemiparalytic stroke patient, and in 1964, Andrews elicited strong muscle action in 17 of 20 hemiplegic patients using EMG feedback. However, the somewhat anecdotal nature of the material may be the reason that follow-ups to these studies were not immediate. Brudny and his colleagues reviewed treatment of 114 patients, many of whom were the victims of cerebrovascular accidents (Brudny, Korein, Grynbaum, Friedmann, Weinstein, Sachs-Frankel, & Belandres, 1976). They found that EMG feedback was therapeutically useful for most subjects, and in the case of the hemiparetic group, 20 of the 39 treated patients retained significant long-term gains. Basmajian has used biofeedback in the treatment of paralytic foot drop after stroke, and in one study (Basmajian, Kukulka, Narayan, & Takebe, 1975), found that a group of patients treated with a combination of therapeutic exercise and biofeedback had 100% greater gains in range of movement (ROM) and dorsiflexion than did a similar group treated only with exercise. However, although functional improvement in the exercise/biofeedback group was noted, there was no significant change in nerve conduction velocity or spasticity (Takebe, Kukulka, Narayan, & Basmajian, 1976). Swann, VanWieringen, and Fokkema (1976) demonstrated little superiority of EMG biofeedback over conventional physical therapy, but methodological difficulties limit generalization of their results. Methodological and statistical difficulties mar most of the studies using EMG biofeedback in the treatment of stroke patients, however, results are sufficiently impressive for biofeedback to be included in many comprehensive programs of neuromuscular reeducation (Brudny, Korein, Grynbaum, Belandres, & Gianutsos, 1979; Epstein, Malone, & Cunningham, 1978).

The use of EMG feedback in treating poliomyelitis is less definitive but predates biofeedback's use with stroke patients. Marinacci (1955) worked with more than 20 polio patients for periods of up to 2 years, providing EMG feedback to teach the patients to retrain motor units by means of gentle voluntary movement and passive exercising of limbs by a physical therapist. Although Marinacci reported increases in muscle strength and volume for some patients, reports were essentially anecdotal, and no controlled studies on the application of EMG biofeedback to polio patients have thus far been reported (Keefe & Surwit, 1978).

The use of EMG feedback in treating cerebral palsy patients has been minimal, though Brudny and colleagues (Brudny, Korein, Levidow, Grynbaum, Lieberman, & Friedmann, 1974) successfully treated one subject with cerebral palsy as part of a larger study, and Wolpert and Wooldridge (1975) successfully applied EMG feedback to normalize head position in a cerebral palsied adolescent. Cataldo, Bird, and Cunningham (1978) successfully induced improvement in muscle control in three cerebral palsy patients, using various forms of EMG feedback. Additional work with cerebral palsy includes a combination of visual feedback and motor activity to teach a functional motor response (Sachs, Martin, & Fitch, 1972), a head control device (with visual or auditory feedback) to teach control and stabilization of the head (Harris, Spelman, & Hymer, 1974; Wooldridge & Russell, 1976), and a portable electronic switch device placed in a subject's shoe to give auditory feedback of foot dragging (Spearing & Poppen, 1974).

One neuromuscular disorder that has proved quite responsive to EMG biofeedback is torticollis, a disorder that may be static or spastic and that involves overdevelopment of the sternocleidomastoid and upper trapezius muscles on one side of the head relative to an underdevelopment of the same muscles on the opposite side of the head, causing a patient's head to turn to one side. Feedback is used to help a patient strengthen the underdeveloped sternocleidomastoid muscle and relax the relatively overdeveloped one. Cleeland (1973) applied both EMG feedback and aversive cutaneous shock (to the fingertips) to nine victims of torticollis and one of retrocollis. Subjects lowered the feedback signal and reduced the shock by moving their head into a normal midline position, that position being attained after a shaping process. Follow-up taken at about 19 months posttraining showed a stable therapeutic improvement for six of ten patients. Brudny, Grynbaum, and Korein (1974) administered visual and auditory feedback to nine torticollis patients unimproved after traditional therapy. After training, three patients could maintain indefinite head control for very short periods. In a similar study (Brudny et al., 1976), 20 of the 48 treated patients showed significant improvement. Although various authors (Brucker, 1979; Keefe & Surwit, 1978) believe EMG biofeedback to be promising in torticollis treatment, all agree that control procedures and other methodological improvements must be instituted.

EMG feedback has also proved useful in treating various nerve injuries. Jacobs and Felton (1969) first applied EMG feedback to 10 patients with diagnosed injury of the nerve leading to the upper trapezius muscle and compared these 10 to a group of normal subjects. Both groups demonstrated lower EMG activity when given biofeedback, and after extended feedback training, muscle injured patients could lower their activity to that exhibited by normals. Booker, Rubow, and Coleman (1969) used EMG biofeedback with a female patient suffering from a facial injury, whose face was asymmetrical at rest. As a consequence of surgery, partial reinnervation of the facial muscles was accomplished using neural pathways that originally innervated the trapezius and sternomastoid muscles. The patient was then taught, using EMG feedback, to perform facial movements involving nerves that had previously innervated muscles used in shoulder movement. Although other researchers have used EMG feedback with a few patients (Brudny et al., 1976; Marinacci & Horande, 1960) only the Jacobs and Felton (1969) study had a control procedure. Thus one must be careful about generalizing the efficacy of EMG feedback in the treatment of peripheral nerve injuries.

Brudny et al. (1974) included two spinal cord patients, with lesions at C − 5 and C − 6 levels respectively, with 36 neuromuscular disordered patients treated by audio and visual biofeedback. Although traditional physical therapy had effected little improvement in the cord patients, substantial improvement was noted after feedback training, and therapeutic gains were retained at 2-year follow-up.

Although EMG biofeedback shows some promise as a therapeutic tool in rehabilitation after stroke, poliomyelitis, cerebral palsy, torticollis, nerve injury, spinal cord injury and other neuromuscular disorders, improved methodology is clearly required before therapeutic results can be given the full attention they deserve.

Autonomic System Interventions

EMG feedback has been applied to the autonomic nervous system in the treatment of postural hypotension (Brucker, 1979). A spinal cord patient with a 3-year-old lesion at T − 3 was fitted with long leg braces but was unable to stand or walk because of severe postural hypotension. Through the use of EMG biofeedback, the patient learned both to voluntarily increase his blood pressure and to perceive changes in his pressure. Various measures taken during the training procedure indicated that "the subject had learned to directly control an autonomic response without skeletal muscle mediation [p. 33]." In another instance, Brucker (1979) used auditory biofeedback to train 10 spinal cord patients with lesions ranging from C − 3 to T − eleven to raise their blood pressure. After initial training, nine of the ten subjects learned to make reliable voluntary increases in blood pressure with the feedback present. Towards the end of training, they were able to do the same with the feedback absent. Two patients were given additional training for postural hypotension, and both patients learned to successfully control their pressure to the point where they could maintain a normal sitting position for several hours.

Conditioning the Neurogenic Bladder

Several spinal cord injured patients with spastic neurogenic bladders have been treated by Ince, Brucker, and Alba (1977, 1978a, 1978b) with classical conditioning techniques. In three separate studies, utilizing electrical stimulation of the abdomen as the unconditioned stimulus and electrical stimulation of the inner thigh as the conditioned stimulus, a reliable response of voiding was finally obtained using the conditioned stimulus alone. Although subjects initially pushed themselves up off their wheelchair seats to void, they subsequently learned to apply the CS themselves and void while seated. Additional testing revealed that after voiding in this manner, residual amounts of urine remaining in the bladder were within safe limits. In discussing the practical implications of this type of reflex conditioning, Ince points out that there is a decreased total amount of urine output when subjects are fully seated and that spontaneous voidings ("leaks") occur between administrations of the CS. Thus the conditioning technique requires further refinements.

Summary

In the last three decades, comprehensive treatment and rehabilitation have been developed for spinal cord injured patients. Most spinal cord injuries are caused by motor vehicle accidents, falls, sports and industrial accidents, and combat injuries.

Most severe spinal cord injuries are fracture-dislocations that result in displacement of the vertebrae and partial or total severation of the spinal cord. Initial damage may increase after the original trauma due to edema and hemorrhage. "Spinal shock" frequently occurs after injury and in humans may last up to several months. Effects of the injury include paralysis and loss of sensation below the injury and disruption of bladder, bowel, and sexual function. Additional complications include postural hypotension, autonomic hyperflexia, decubiti, respiratory infections, and contractures. Treatment and rehabilitation consist of physical therapy, occupational therapy, vocational counseling, and psychological intervention.

Psychological adjustment to spinal cord injury usually occurs in several stages and is affected by the patient's preinjury personality style and methods of coping as well as the time and circumstances of the injury. The patient's family reacts strongly to the injury and may profit from supportive counseling as they relate to the patient and assume new responsibilities. Although injury puts great stress on marriages, the divorce rate for the spinal cord injured is no higher than that for the general population.

Most spinal cord patients are reemployable after suitable rehabilitation and training, and getting patients working again is one way to offset the tremendous direct and indirect costs of spinal cord injuries. Sexual function is variable for the cord injured. Overall, more males retain some ability to achieve erection than can experience ejaculation and orgasm. Female sexuality and fertility are somewhat less impaired. Sexual counseling is an important component of rehabilitation for patients and their partners.

Neuromuscular disorders require some of the same rehabilitation techniques as does spinal cord injury. EMG biofeedback has been used with some success in the rehabilitation of stroke, poliomyelitis, cerebral palsy, torticollis, nerve injury, and some aspects of spinal cord injury. Classical conditioning techniques have been used to evoke reflex conditioning in the neurogenic bladder. Although methodology needs to be improved and practical results of biofeedback need to be clarified, it is clearly a new frontier of rehabilitation.

REFERENCES

Adams, R. D. Diseases of the spinal cord. In M. M. Wintrobe, G. W. Thorn, R. D. Adams, I. L. Bennett, Jr., E. Braunwald, K. J. Isselbacher, & R. G. Petersdorf (Eds.), *Harrison's principles of internal medicine* (6th ed.). New York: McGraw-Hill, 1970.

Andrews, J. M. Neuromuscular re-education of the hemiplegic with the aid of the electromyograph. *Archives of Physical Medicine and Rehabilitation,* 1964, *45,* 530 – 532.

Basmajian, J. V., Kukulka, C. G., Narayan, M. G., & Takebe, K. Biofeedback treatment of foot-drop after stroke compared with standard rehabilitation technique: Effects on voluntary control and strength. *Archives of Physical Medicine and Rehabilitation,* 1975, *56,* 231 – 236.

Belson, P. Autonomic nervous system dysfunction in recent spinal cord injured patients: A physical therapist's perspective. In M. G. Eisenberg & J. A. Falconer (Eds.), *Treatment of the spinal cord injured.* Springfield, Ill.: Charles C. Thomas, 1978.

Booker, H. E., Rubow, R. T., & Coleman, P. J. Simplified feedback in neuromuscular retraining: An automated approach using electromyographic signals. *Archives of Physical Medicine and Rehabilitation,* 1969, *50,* 621 – 629.

Bregman, S., & Hadley, R. G. Sexual adjustment and feminine attractiveness among spinal cord injured women. *Archives of Physical Medicine and Rehabilitation,* 1976, *57,* 448 – 450.

Brucker, B. S. Biofeedback and rehabilitation. In L. P. Ince (Ed.), *Behavioral psychology in rehabilitation medicine: Clinical applications.* Baltimore: Williams & Wilkins, 1979.

Brudny, J., Grynbaum, B., & Korein, J. Spasmodic torticollis: Treatment by feedback display of the EMG. *Archives of Physical Medicine and Rehabilitation,* 1974, *55,* 403 – 408.

Brudny, J., Korein, J., Grynbaum, B. B., Belandres, P. V., & Gianutsos, J. G. Helping hemiparetics to help themselves: Sensory feedback therapy. *Journal of the American Medical Association,* 1979, *241,* 814 – 818.

Brudny, J., Korein, J., Grynbaum, B. B., Friedmann, L. W., Weinstein, S., Sachs-Frankel, G., & Belandres, P. V. EMG feedback therapy: Review of treatment of 114 patients. *Archives of Physical Medicine and Rehabilitation*, 1976, *57*, 55 – 61.

Brudny, J., Korein, J., Levidow, L., Grynbaun, B. B., Lieberman, A., & Friedmann, L. W. Sensory feedback therapy as a modality of treatment in central nervous system disorders of voluntary movement. *Neurology*, 1974, *24*, 925 – 932.

Cataldo, M. F., Bird, B. L., & Cunningham, C. E. Experimental analysis of EMG feedback in treating cerebral palsy. *Journal of Behavioral Medicine*, 1978, *1*, 311 – 322.

Chipouras, S. Ten sexuality programs for spinal cord injured persons. *Sexuality and Disability*, 1979, *2*, 301 – 321.

Cleeland, C. S. Behavioral techniques in modification of spasmodic torticollis. *Neurology*, 1973, *23*, 1241 – 1247.

Cole, T. M., Chilgren, M. D., & Rosenberg, P. A new programme of sex education and counselling for spinal cord injured adults and health care professionals. *Paraplegia*, 1973, *11*(2), 111 – 124.

Comarr, A. E. Sexual function among patients with spinal cord injury. *Urology International*, 1970, *25*(2), 134 – 168.

Conomy, J. P. Disorders of body image after spinal cord injury. *Neurology*, 1973, *23*, 842 – 850.

Cull, J. G., & Hardy, R. E. Psychotherapeutic concerns in aiding the spinal cord-injured individual. In J. G. Cull & R. E. Hardy (Eds.), *Physical medicine and rehabilitation approaches in spinal cord injury*. Springfield, Ill.: Charles C. Thomas, 1977.

Eisenberg, M. G., & Gilbert, B. M. Individual and family reaction to spinal cord injury: Some guidelines for treatment. In M. G. Eisenberg & J. A. Falconer (Eds.), *Treatment of the spinal cord injured*. Springfield, Ill.: Charles C. Thomas, 1978.

Epstein, L. H., Malone, D. R., & Cunningham, J. Feedback influenced EMG changes in stroke patients. *Behavioral Modification*, 1978, *2*, 387 – 402.

Fitting, M. D., Salisbury, S., Davies, N. H., & Mayclin, D. K. Self-concept and sexuality of spinal cord injured women. *Archives of Sexual Behavior*, 1978, *7*, 143 – 156.

Fogel, M. L., & Rosillo, R. H. Correlation of psychologic variables and progress in physical rehabilitation: III. Ego functions and defensive and adaptive mechanisms. *Archives of Physical Medicine and Rehabilitation*, 1971, *52*, 15 – 21.

Gardner, E. *Fundamentals of neurology* (3rd ed.). Philadelphia: W. B. Saunders, 1961.

Geiger, R. C. Neurophysiology of sexual response in spinal cord injury. *Sexuality and Disability*, 1979, *2*, 257 – 266.

Graham, S. D. The urological care of the cord-injured. In J. G. Cull & R. E. Hardy (Eds.), *Physical medicine and rehabilitation approaches in spinal cord injury*. Springfield, Ill.: Charles C. Thomas, 1977.

Griffith, E. R., Tomko, M. A., & Timms, J. A. Sexual function in spinal cord-injured patients: A review. *Archives of Physical Medicine and Rehabilitation*, 1973, *54*, 539 – 543.

Griffith, E. R., & Trieschman, R. B. Sexual functioning in women with spinal cord injury. *Archives of Physical Medicine and Rehabilitation*, 1975, *56*, 18 – 21.

Gruber, A. An internist's perspective on the problem: An overview of some significant medical problems. In M. G. Eisenberg & J. A. Falconer (Eds.), *Treatment of the spinal cord injured*. Springfield, Ill.: Charles C. Thomas, 1978.

Grzesiak, R. C. Psychological services in rehabilitation medicine: Clinical aspects of rehabilitation psychology. *Professional Psychology*, 1979, *10*, 511 – 520.

Guttman, L. *Spinal cord injuries: Comprehensive management and research* (2nd ed.). London: Blackwell Scientific Publications, 1976.

Harris, P., Patel, S. S., Greer, W., & Naughton, J. A. Psychological and social reactions to acute spinal paralysis. *Paraplegia*, 1973, *11*(2), 132 – 136.

Harris, F. A., Spelman, F. A., & Hymer, J. W. Electronic sensory aids as treatment for cerebral palsied children. *Physical Therapy*, 1974, *54*, 354 – 365.

Held, J. P., Cole, T. M., Held, C. A., Anderson, C., & Chilgren, R. A. Sexual attitude reassessment workshops: Effect on spinal cord injured adults, their partners and rehabilitation professionals. *Archives of Physical Medicine and Rehabilitation,* 1975, *56,* 14 – 18.

Herrmann, R. W., & Stancil, M. L. Types of spinal cord injuries and their effects. In J. G. Cull & R. E. Hardy (Eds.), *Physical medicine and rehabilitation approaches in spinal cord injury.* Springfield, Ill.: Charles C. Thomas, 1977.

Ince, L. P., Brucker, B. S., & Alba, A. Conditioning bladder responses in patients with spinal cord lesions. *Archives of Physical Medicine and Rehabilitation,* 1977, *58,* 59 – 65.

Ince, L. P., Brucker, B. S., & Alba, A. Conditioned responding of the neurogenic bladder. *Psychosomatic Medicine,* 1978, *40*(1), 14 – 24. (a)

Ince, L. P., Brucker, B. S., & Alba, A. Reflex conditioning in a spinal man. *Journal of Comparative and Physiological Psychology,* 1978, *92,* 796 – 802. (b)

Jacobs, A., & Felton, G. S. Visual feedback of myoelectric output to facilitate muscle relaxation in normal persons and patients with neck injuries. *Archives of Physical Medicine and Rehabilitation,* 1969, *50,* 34 – 39.

Katz, V., Gordon, R., Iversen, D., & Myers, S. J. Past history and degree of depression of paraplegic individuals. *Paraplegia,* 1978, *16*(1), 8 – 14.

Keefe, F. J., & Surwit, R. S. Electromyographic biofeedback: Behavioral treatment of neuromuscular disorders. *Journal of Behavioral Medicine,* 1978, *1*(1), 13 – 24.

Kemp, B. J., & Vash, C. L. Productivity after injury in a sample of spinal cord injured persons: A pilot study. *Journal of Chronic Disease,* 1971, *24,* 259 – 275.

Labanowich, S. Wheelchair sports: Their meaning for the physically disabled. In M. G. Eisenberg & J. A. Falconer (Eds.), *Treatment of the spinal cord injured.* Springfield, Ill.: Charles C. Thomas, 1978.

Lawson, N. C. Significant events in the rehabilitation process: The spinal cord patient's point of view. *Archives of Physical Medicine and Rehabilitation,* 1978, *59,* 573 – 579.

Marinacci, A. A. *Clinical electromyography.* Los Angeles: San Lucas Press, 1955.

Marinacci, A. A., & Horande, M. Electromyogram in neuromuscular reeducation. *Bulletin of the Los Angeles Neurological Society,* 1960, *25,* 57 – 71.

Miller, D. K., Wolfe, M., & Spiegel, M. H. Therapeutic groups for patients with spinal cord injuries. *Archives of Physical Medicine and Rehabilitation,* 1975, *56,* 130 – 135.

Miller, J. M. The role of regional cord injury centers in the rehabilitation of the spinal cord-injured. In J. G. Cull & R. E. Hardy (Eds.), *Physical medicine and rehabilitation approaches in spinal cord injury.* Springfield, Ill.: Charles C. Thomas, 1977.

Ofir, R., & Hofkosh, J. M. The role of the physical therapist in treatment of the spinal cord-injured patient. In J. G. Cull & R. E. Hardy (Eds.), *Physical medicine and rehabilitation approaches in spinal cord injury.* Springfield, Ill.: Charles C. Thomas, 1977.

Peterson, Y. The impact of physical disability on marital adjustment: A literature review. *The Family Coordinator,* 1979, *28,* 47 – 51.

Pomerleau, O. F. Behavioral medicine: The contribution of the experimental analysis of behavior to medical care. *American Psychologist,* 1979, *34,* 654 – 663.

Sachs, D. A., Martin, J. E., & Fitch, J. L. The effect of visual feedback on a digital exercise in a functionally deaf cerebral palsied child. *Journal of Behavior Therapy and Experimental Psychiatry,* 1972, *3,* 217 – 222.

Singh, S. P., & Magner, T. Sex and self: The spinal cord-injured. *Rehabilitation Literature,* 1975, *36,* 2 – 10.

Smart, C. N., & Sanders, C. R. *The costs of motor vehicle related spinal cord injuries.* Washington, D.C.: Insurance Institute for Highway Safety, 1976.

Spearing, D. L., & Poppen, R. The use of feedback in the reduction of foot dragging in a cerebral palsied client. *Journal of Nervous and Mental Disease,* 1974, *15,* 148 – 151.

Stewart, T. D., & Rossier, A. B. Psychological considerations in the adjustment to spinal cord injury. *Rehabilitation Literature,* 1978, *39*(3), 75 – 80.

Swaan, D., VanWieringen, P. C. W., & Fokkema, S. E. Auditory electromyographic feedback therapy to inhibit undesired motor activity. *Archives of Physical Medicine and Rehabilitation*, 1976, *57*, 9 – 11.

Takebe, K., Kukulka, C. G., Narayan, M. G., & Basmajian, J. V. Biofeedback treatment of foot drop after stroke compared with standard rehabilitation technique. Part 2. Effects on nerve conduction velocity and spasticity. *Archives of Physical Medicine and Rehabilitation*, 1976, *57*, 9 – 11.

Teal, J. C., & Athelstan, G. T. Sexuality and spinal cord injury: Some psychosocial considerations. *Archives of Physical Medicine and Rehabilitation*, 1975, *56*, 264 – 268.

Vineberg, S. E., & Willems, E. P. Observation and analysis of patient behavior in the rehabilitation hospital. *Archives of Physical Medicine and Rehabilitation*, 1971, *52*, 8 – 14.

Wolpert, R., & Wooldridge, C. P. The use of electromyography as biofeedback therapy in the management of cerebral palsy: A review and case study. *Physiotherapy Canada*, 1975, *27*, 5 – 9.

Wooldridge, C. P., & Russell, G. Head position training with the cerebral palsied child: An application of biofeedback techniques. *Archives of Physical Medicine and Rehabilitation*, 1976, *57*, 407 – 414.

Wright, B. A. *Physical disability—a psychological approach*. New York: Harper & Row, 1960.

Author Index

Numbers in *italics* denote pages with bibliographic information.

Subject Index